Concise Textbook of
Pathology

Concise Textbook of
Pathology

Editor

Ganga S Pilli MD, PhD

Professor
Department of Pathology
JN Medical College
KLE Academy of Higher Education and Research
(A Deemed to be University)
Belagavi, Karnataka, India

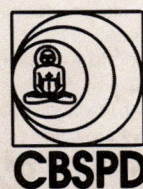

CBSPD

CBS Publishers & Distributors Pvt Ltd

New Delhi • Bengaluru • Chennai • Kochi • Kolkata • Lucknow • Mumbai
Hyderabad • Jharkhand • Nagpur • Patna • Pune • Uttarakhand

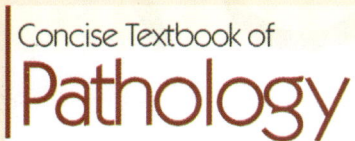

Concise Textbook of
Pathology

ISBN: 978-93-89688-57-3

First Edition: 2021
Reprint: 2023, **2024**

Published by **Satish Kumar Jain** and produced by **Varun Jain** for

CBS Publishers & Distributors Pvt Ltd

4819/XI Prahlad Street, 24 Ansari Road, Daryaganj, New Delhi 110 002, India.
Ph: 011-23289259, 23266838   Website: www.cbspd.com
                                                             e-mail: delhi@cbspd.com

Corporate Office: 204 FIE, Industrial Area, Patparganj, Delhi 110 092
Ph: 011-4934 4934   Fax: 011-4934 4935   e-mail: publishing@cbspd.com; publicity@cbspd.com

Branches

• **Bengaluru:** Seema House 2975, 17th Cross, KR Road, Banasankari 2nd Stage, Bengaluru 560 070, Karnataka, India
  Ph: +91-80-26771678/79   Fax: +91-80-26771680   e-mail: bangalore@cbspd.com
• **Chennai:** 7, Subbaraya Street, Shenoy Nagar, Chennai 600 030, Tamil Nadu, India
  Ph: +91-44-26680620, 26681266   Fax: +91-44-42032115   e-mail: chennai@cbspd.com
• **Kochi:** 42/1325, 1326, Power House Road, Opp KSEB, Power House, Ernakulum Kochi 682 018, Kerala, India
  Ph: +91-484-4059061-65,67   Fax: +91-484-4059065   e-mail: kochi@cbspd.com
• **Kolkata:** 147, Hind Ceramics Compound, 1st Floor, Nilgunj Road, Belghoria, Kolkata-700056, West Bengal, India
  Ph: +033-25633055, 033-25633056   e-mail: kolkata@cbspd.com
• **Lucknow:** Basement, Khushnuma Complex, 7 Meerabai Marg (Behind Jawahar Bhawan), Lucknow-226001, UP, India
  Ph: +0522-4000032   e-mail: tiwari.lucknow@cbspd.com
• **Mumbai:** PWD Shed, Gala no 25/26, Ramchandra Bhatt Marg, Next to JJ Hospital Gate no. 2, Opp. Union Bank of India, Noorbaug, Mumbai-400009, Maharashtra, India
  Ph: 022-66661880/89   e-mail: mumbai@cbspd.com

Representatives

• **Hyderabad**	0-9885175004	• **Jharkhand**	0-9811541605	• **Nagpur**	0-8692091830
• **Patna**	0-9334159340	• **Pune**	0-9664372571	• **Uttarakhand**	0-9716462459

Printed at Goyal Offset Works Pvt. Ltd, Sonipat, Haryana, India

to
My parents,
My family members,
and
My dear students
for their
constant encouragement

Foreword

Knowledge of pathology is very important for successful medical practitioner. It is rightly said that to be a good clinician, the knowledge of basic subjects is very essential. Those who are good in understanding the pathophysiology of a disease can treat the patient better with confidence. Subject of pathology which is learnt in II MBBS curriculum forms the basis for understanding the disease process. For any physician, to give the appropriate care for his patients, an appropriate diagnosis has to be made. Sound knowledge of the basic subjects and investigations form an important component in the whole process, may be in subjects of pathology, microbiology or biochemistry.

There are many voluminous books in the subject of pathology which are difficult for the undergraduate students to go through them and assimilate the knowledge. The present book is dealt in a simple and lucid style with easily understandable diagrams and flow charts.

The book is divided into four main sections namely, Haematology, General Pathology, Systemic Pathology I and Systemic Pathology II covering different important chapters with emphasis on theory as well as some practical skills and covers the MCI identified competencies. The book is also useful for the MBBS phase II students in preparation of examination in pathology as well as other phase students in competitive examinations in medicine. There are many original and schematic diagrams of gross and microscopic pictures and line diagrams.

The author Dr Ganga S. Pilli has already got the experience of writing textbook for medical subjects and her books are in demand by the medical and paramedical students, so much that the editions of these books are being brought out. She has a rich experience in the field of pathology for having worked as Lecturer, Assistant Professor, Associate Professor and Professor of Pathology for a period of almost 35 years in a reputed department of our college. She was heading of the department during the years 2012 to 2014. The knowledge of pathology gained through this book will be of a real benefit to the undergraduate students of medical, dental, allied health science courses including medical laboratory technology course, nursing and AYUSH courses. The necessary theory and practical material provided in this book will enrich the knowledge and will improve the skills of the students. I am sure this book will be accepted by all the students and teaching fraternity of pathology.

I congratulate Dr Ganga S. Pilli for the bold venture and hope she will continue to bring out more books for the benefit of the students and wish her all the success in her future endeavors.

Prof. VD Patil

Ex-Registrar, KLE Academy of Higher Education and Research
(KLE University)
and
Former Principal, JN Medical College, Belagavi

Preface

Pathology is a medical speciality concerned with the study of diseases which leads to the structural and functional changes in the human body. Pathology is basis for all the practicing physicians and surgeons. Knowledge of pathology plays a very important role in the field of medicine for accurate diagnosis and patient care. The subject of pathology which is learnt in MBBS course forms the basis for this. There are many voluminous books dealing extensively with various aspects of pathology written by foreign and Indian authors. Subject of pathology has grown to a great extent especially in molecular and cytogenetic areas, the identification of these abnormalities has led to personalized treatment in many of the diseases. There is a need for concise textbook with updated information, to meet the academic requirements of all undergraduate students studying pathology.

The idea of bringing out this book was evolved while teaching pathology to the undergraduate and postgraduate students over a period of 35 years. The *Practical Pathology and Quick Review,* which has seen second edition, has made my job easier. This book has been written in an easy language and in a simple and lucid style with the help of illustrations for the benefit of wise as well as ordinary students studying pathology in various fields of medicine (medical, dental, laboratory technology, other allied health sciences, nursing and AYUSH courses).

The salient features of the book are:

1. The book is divided into four main sections namely, Haematology, General Pathology, Systemic Pathology I and Systemic Pathology II.

2. In each section, different important chapters are covered.

3. The book emphasizes on theory as well as some practical skills.

4. The book covers the recent MCI competencies.

5. The book is also useful for the students in preparation of examination to answer long answers, short assays and short answers and to face viva-voce in pathology.

5. After main four sections, at the end has "Similes in Pathology", "Know your Scientists", and "Pearls to Know".

6. MCQs covering various topics which will help the students in preparation for MBBS II pathology as well as competitive examinations in medicine are also included at the end of each chapter.

7. The book is designed with illustrations of gross and microscopic pictures with original as well as schematic diagrams and line diagrams.

The book has seen its first edition through CBS Publishers who have made the book to reach the students studying Pathology nationwide.

The legacy of authoring a book is to follow the footprints of my father (Prof. SS Nanjannavar) who is a retired professor from Karnatak University, Dharwad and a noted author of many books in the field of geography. He is the main source of inspiration for me to continue this noble task of writing a book in order to serve the cause of student community in particular and medical education in general. It is hoped that this book would be of great help to the students and serve as a ready reference book to those who are studying pathology.

I will be failing in my duty if I do not express my sincere gratitude to Dr Prabhakar Kore, Chancellor and Dr Vivek Saoji, Vice-chancellor of KLE University, Belgaum for providing me all the facilities. I extend my grateful thanks to Dr VD Patil, Ex-registrar, KAHER (Deemed to be University), Belgaum for writing a foreword to this book and constantly encouraging for this difficult task of authoring books. I also thank our present registrar of KAHER, Dr VA Kotiwale. I sincerely thank my Principal, Dr Niranjana Mahantshetti and my colleagues at the department.

I offer my special thanks to Dr (Mrs) AV Dhaded, former Professor of Pathology, JN Medical College, Belagavi and to Dr Bhagyashri Hungund, Professor of Pathology, JN Medical College, Belgaum for giving valuable suggestions. I am grateful to all my co-authors who have reduced my work pressure. I thank Prof. Uday V Kokatnur, who inspite of his busy schedule, stood next to me for drawing nice diagrams. I also thank Mahantesh Nanjannavar for editing the pictures. I am thankful to my postgraduate students for their timely help.

I am grateful to my husband Dr Sharanabasava C Pilli, for his constant encouragement and support. Similarly, I appreciate the patience and co-operation of my children—Vijay and Veena and daughter-in-law and son-in-law during the preparation of this book.

Constructive suggestions from the teachers and students of pathology are most welcome for the improvement of this book in the subsequent editions.

Ganga S Pilli

Acknowledgements

1. I acknowledge the help rendered by all the co-authors in preparation of the manuscript.

2. I am thankful to CBS Publishers and Distributors. I would like to put on record the sincere efforts of Mr YN Arjuna (Senior Vice-President Publishing, Editorial and Publicity) and his team comprising of Ms Ritu Chawla (GM Production), Mr Tarun Rajput, Mr Surendra Jha and Ms Baljeet Kaur, for bringing out book in the present form.

Ganga S Pilli

List of Contributors

Chhatre A
Consultant Pathologist
Chhatre Diagnostics
Belagavi, Karnataka, India

Hawal M
Former Assistant Professor
Department of Pathology
USM Medical College and Consultant Pathologist
Belagavi

Hemanth V
Assistant Professor of Pathology
Shimoga Institute of Medical Sciences
Shimoga, Karnataka, India

Kanetkar SR
Professor and Head
Department of Pathology
Krishna Institute of Medical Sciences
Karad, Maharashtra, India

Kanodia KV
Professor
Department of Pathology, Lab. Medicine, Transfusion Services
and Immunohematology, GR Doshi and KM Mehta Institute of
Kidney Diseases and Research Centre and Dr HL Trivedi Institute
of Transplantation Sciences, Civil Hospital Campus
Asarwa, Ahmedabad, India

Kavita GU
Professor
Department of Pathology
SS Institute of Medical Sciences and Research Centre
Davangere, Karnataka, India

Kini U
Retd. Professor
St. John's Medical College
Bengaluru

Nigam LA
Assistant Professor
Department of Pathology, Lab. Medicine, Transfusion Services
and Immunohematology, GR Doshi and KM Mehta Institute of
Kidney Diseases and Research Centre and Dr HL Trivedi Institute
of Transplantation Sciences, Civil Hospital Campus
Asarwa, Ahmedabad, India

Panduranga C
Associate Professor
Department of Pathology, ESI Medical College and PGIMSR
Rajaji Nagar, Bengaluru, Karnataka

Patel RD
Professor
Department of Pathology, Lab. Medicine, Transfusion Services
and Immunohematology, GR Doshi and KM Mehta Institute of
Kidney Diseases and Research Centre and Dr HL Trivedi Institute
of Transplantation Sciences, Civil Hospital Campus
Asarwa, Ahmedabad, India

Patil PV
Former Professor and HOD
Department of Pathology
JN Medical College
Belagavi, Karnataka, India

Pattanashetti M
Assistant Professor
Kodagu Institute of Medical Sciences
Madikeri

Pilli GS
Professor
Department of Pathology
JN Medical College
KLE Academy of Higher Education and Research
(A Deemed to be University)
Belagavi, Karnataka, India

Pruthvi D
Professor
Department of Pathology
SS Institute of Medical Sciences and Research Centre
Davangere, Karnataka, India

Shashikala P
Professor and HOD
Department of Pathology
SS Institute of Medical Sciences and Research Centre
Davangere, Karnataka, India

Shukla D
Former Assistant Professor
Department of Pathology
Krishna Institute of Medical Sciences
Karad, Maharashtra, India

Sridevi HB
Associate Professor
Department of Pathology
Kasturba Medical College, Mangalore
Manipal Academy of Higher Education
Manipal, Karnataka, India

Suresh PK
Associate Professor
Department of Pathology
Kasturba Medical College, Mangalore
Manipal Academy of Higher Education
Manipal, Karnataka, India

Susmitha MS
Associate Professor
Department of Pathology
Shimoga Institute of Medical Sciences
Shimoga, Karnataka, India

Suthar KS
Associate Professor
Department of Pathology, Lab. Medicine, Transfusion Services and Immunohematology, GR Doshi and KM Mehta Institute of Kidney Diseases and Research Centre and Dr HL Trivedi Institute of Transplantation Sciences, Civil Hospital Campus
Asarwa, Ahmedabad, India

Vanikar AV
Professor and Head
Department of Pathology, Lab. Medicine, Transfusion Services and Immunohematology, GR Doshi and KM Mehta Institute of Kidney Diseases and Research Centre and Dr HL Trivedi Institute of Transplantation Sciences, Civil Hospital Campus
Asarwa, Ahmedabad, India

Wani R
Consultant Obstetrician and Gynaecologist
KLE Dr Prabhakar Kore Hospital and Research Centre
Belagavi, Karnataka, India

Contents

Contents

ADCC	Antibody dependent cell mediated cytotoxicity
ADH	Antidiuretic hormone
AD	Autosomal dominant
ADP	Adenosine diphosphate
AIHA	Autoimmune haemolytic anaemia
AFP	Alpha-fetoproteins
ALIP	Abnormal localisation of immature precursors
ANCAs	Antineutrophil cytoplasmic antibodies
APLA/APS	Antiphospholipid antibody
APTT	Activated partial thromboplastin time
AR	Autosomal recessive
AS	Aortic stenosis
Beta 2M	Beta 2 microglobulin (β2 microglobulin)
BCC	Basal cell carcinoma
BM	Bone marrow
CCF	Congestive cardiac failure
CaCl2	Calcium chloride
CIN	Carcinoma in situ
CFTR	Cystic fibrosis transmembrane conductance regulator
CMMI	Chronic myelomonocytic leukaemia
CMP	Cardiomyopathy
CMV	Cytomegalovirus
CNS	Central nervous system
CRAB	Calcium (elevated), renal failure, anaemia, bone lesions
CT	Computerised tomography
CV	Cardiovascular
DCIS	Duct carcinoma in situ
DIC	Disseminated intravascular coagulation
DVT	Deep vein thrombosis
EBV	Epstein-Barr virus
ECM	Extracellular matrix
ER	Estrogen receptors
FH	Familial hypercholesterolemia
fl	Femtolitres
FSGS	Focal segmental glomerulosclerosis
GCT	Giant cell tumour
GERD	Gastroesophageal reflux disease
GGT	Gamma glutamyl transpeptidase
G6PD	Glucose-6-phosphate dehydrogenase
HA	Haemolytic anaemia
Hb	Haemoglobin
HCC	Hepatocellular carcinoma
HCG	Human chorionic gonadotropin
HCl	Hydrochloric acid
HD	Hodgkin disease
HDL	Heavy density lipoproteins
HDN	Haemolytic disease of newborn
HELLP	Hemolysis, elevated liver enzymes, low platelet count
HLA	Human leucocyte antigen
HNPCC	Hereditary non-polyposis colorectal cancer
HPV	Human papilloma virus
HS	Hereditary spherocytosis
HSIL	High grade squamous intraepithelial lesion
HT	Hypertension
IC	Integrated circuit
IDL	Intermediate density lipoproteins
IL	Interleukin
IM	Infectious mononucleosis
INF	Interferon
IHC	Immunohistochemistry
IHD	Ischaemic heart disease
ITP	Idiopathic thrombocytopenic purpura
KOH	Potassium hydroxide
LCA	Left coronary artery
LDH	Lactate dehydrogenase
LDHD	Lymphocyte depleted Hodgkin disease
L and H	Lymphocytic and histiocytic
LDL	Low density lipoproteins
LN	Lymph node
LSIL	Low grade squamous intraepithelial lesion
MCD	Minimal change disease
MCHC	Mean corpuscular haemoglobin concentration
MCV	Mean corpuscular volume
MDS	Myelodysplastic syndrome
MGN	Mesangial glomerulonephritis
MEN	Multiple endocrine neoplasia
MGG stain	May-Grunwald-Giemsa stain
MI/MR	Mitral incompetence/mitral regurgitation
MA	Macrocytic anaemia
MHA	Microcytic hypochromic anaemia
MM	Multiple myeloma
MPGN	Membranoproliferative glomerulonephritis
NaOH	Sodium hydroxide
NADPH	Nicotinamide adenine dinucleotide phosphate

NAIT	Neonatal autoimmune thrombo-cytopenia
NNA	Normocytic normochromic anaemia
NO	Nitric oxide
NP	Niemann-Pick disease
OD	Optical density
OS	Osteosarcoma
PCV	Packed cell volume
PAS stain	Periodic acid-Schiff stain
PLAP	Placental alkaline phosphatase
POEMS	Polyneuropathy, organomegaly, endo-crinopathy, myeloma protein and skin changes
PNH	Paroxysmal nocturnal hemoglobinuria
PRCA	Pure red cell aplasia
PSGN	Post-streptococcal glomerulonephritis
PT	Prothrombin time
PV-B19	Parvovirus B19
RA	Refractory anaemia
RARS	Refractory anaemia with ring sidero-blasts
RAEB	Refractory anaemia with excess blasts
RBC	Red blood cell
RCA	Right coronary artery
ROS	Reactive oxygen species
RPGN	Rapidly progressive glomerulonephritis
RS cells	Reed-Sternberg cells
SBC	Simple bone cyst
SIADH	Syndrome of inappropriate secretion of ADH
SLE	Systemic lupus erythematosus
TLR	Toll-like receptor
TNF	Tumour necrosis factor
US	Ultrasound
V	Voltage
VLDL	Very low density lipoproteins
vWD disease	von Willebrand disease

Haematology and Blood Banking

Bone Marrow and Haemopoiesis

FORMATION OF BLOOD ELEMENTS FROM GESTATIONAL LIFE TO ADULT LIFE

Cellular differentiation, proliferation and maturation of blood cells take place in the haematopoietic tissue, i.e. in the bone marrow. Mature cells are released into the peripheral blood.

Development of haematopoiesis takes place at different places during gestational period and after birth and it is as below:

1. Yolk sac—begins on 19th day of gestation and lasts up to 3 months.
2. Liver along with spleen, kidney, thymus, and lymph nodes—3rd month to 24 weeks of gestation.
3. Bone marrow—3rd trimester onwards and throughout life.

HAEMATOPOIETIC MARROW ARCHITECTURE (Fig. 1.1)

Nucleated cells of RBC series constitute 25–30% of marrow cells and are produced near the sinusoids. Erythroblastic island is composed of erythoblasts in varying states of maturation. Least mature cells are towards the centre of the island and more mature cells towards the periphery.

Granulocytes are produced in the nests, close to the trebaculae and arterioles. At the metamyelocyte stage, they begin moving towards the sinusoids.

Lymphocytes are produced in lymphoid tissues (nodules) which are randomly dispersed throughout marrow. Lymphoid stem cells may leave the bone marrow and travel to thymus where they mature into T lymphocytes. Some lymphocytes remain in bone marrow where they mature into B lymphocytes.

Megakaryocytes lie adjacent to the endothelium of sinusoidal walls and discharge platelets directly into

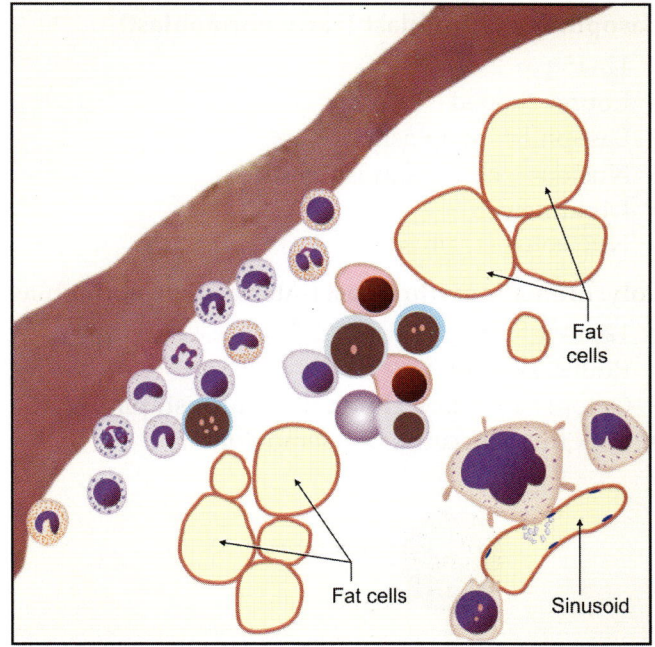

Fig. 1.1: Topography of bone marrow cells of different series (paratrabecular area—myeloid series, near the sinusoids—megakaryocytic series, in between area—erythroid series) (schematic)

lumen of sinuses. Cytoplasmic processes of megakaryocyte penetrate the sinus wall and pinch off to form platelets.

ERYTHROID SERIES

It is an orderly process through which peripheral concentration of RBCs is maintained in a steady state.

Bone marrow maturation of normoblast occurs in orderly and well-defined sequence.

The process involves gradual decrease in cell size, together with condensation and eventual expulsion of nucleus.

As normoblasts mature, there is gradual increase in haemoglobin production. Normoblast generally spends 5–7 days in proliferating and maturing compartment of the marrow.

After maturation in the marrow, the reticulocytes are released into the marrow sinuses and gain access to peripheral blood. It continues to mature in blood for 1 or 2 days.

Description of Erythroid Series Cells (Fig. 1.2)

Erythroblast (Normoblast)

- 14–20 μ, round shaped, nucleus round.
- Nucleus large occupies 4/5th of the cell and cytoplasm is 1/5th of the cell.
- The cytoplasm is basophilic.
- The nucleus has nucleoli (1–2).
- Dividing cell.

Basophilic erythroblast (early normoblast)

- 12–15 μ
- Round shaped
- Basophilic cytoplasm
- Nucleus—chromatin is dense
- Dividing cell
- Nucleolus (1) present.

Polychromatic erythroblast (intermediate normoblast)

- 12–14 μ
- Round shaped
- Cytoplasm is polychromatic (purplish pink)
- Pink tint is because of haemoglobin.

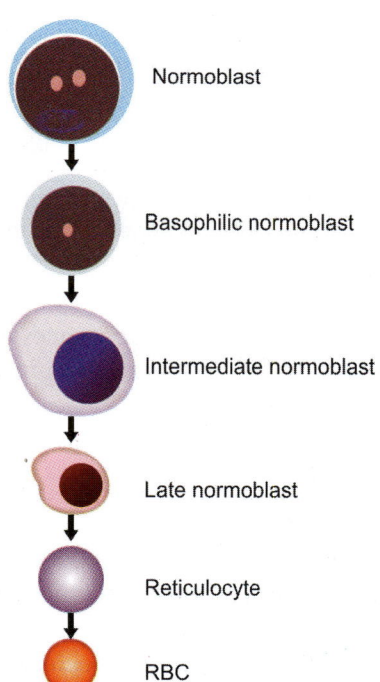

Fig. 1.2: Erythroid series cells (schematic)

- Nucleus—chromatin clumped.
- No division, cell develops by maturation.

Orthochromatic erythroblast (late normoblast)

- 12–14 μ
- Round shaped
- Cytoplasm—more pinkish because of increased content of Hb
- Nucleus small and pyknotic with blue black colour
- The cell matures into reticulocyte.

Reticulocyte

- 8 μ
- Slightly larger than normal RBCs
- Biconcave discoid shaped
- Cytoplasm—polychromatic, contains RNA material which can be stained with supravital stains.
- Matures to RBCs in 1–2 days.

Red Blood Cell

- 7.2 μ
- Biconcave, discoid shaped
- Central 1/3rd is pale, peripheral 2/3rd pinkish.

MYELOID SERIES (Fig. 1.3)

Myeloblast

- 15–20 μ, round shaped
- Nucleus—round, occupies 4/5th of the cell and cytoplasm is 1/5th of the cell.
- Nuclear chromatin less coarser than that of lymphoblast
- The cytoplasm is basophilic.
- The nucleus has 4–5 nucleoli.
- Dividing cell
- Sometimes Aner rod is found in the cytoplasm. It is purplish pink in colour.

Promyelocyte

- Nucleus—round
- Nuclear chromatin coarse
- Cytoplasm has primary granules which are dusty and purplish pink
- Nucleoli are few, 1–2 in number.
- Other features are similar to myeloblast.
- Dividing cell.

Myelocyte

- Nucleus is round.
- Nuclear chromatin still coarser, no nucleoli.
- Cytoplasm less basophilic and abundant.

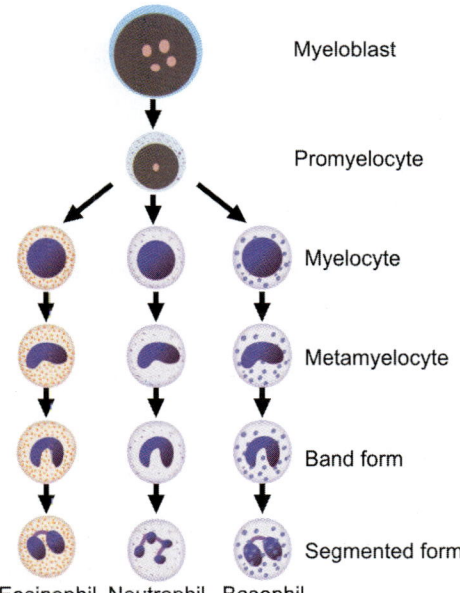

Fig. 1.3: Myeloid series cells (schematic)

- Specific granules also appear in the cytoplasm. Depending upon these granules, the cells are called neutrophilic myelocyte, basophilic myelocyte and eosinophilic myelocyte.

Metamyelocyte

- Nucleus is kidney shaped.
- Cytoplasm is similar to earlier cell.

Band Form (Stab Form)

- Nucleus more bent and attains U shaped. The degree of indentation is greater than 50% of the nuclear diameter.
- Cytoplasm is similar to earlier cell.
- These band forms mature to segmented forms.

Neutrophil (Polymorphonuclear Leucocyte, Segmented Neutrophilic Granulocyte)

- 12–14 µ
- Nucleus lobulated, has 2–5 lobes.
- Cytoplasm has primary and secondary granules which are dusty and purplish pink coloured.
- A sex chromatin (drumstick) may be present in some of the neutrophils attached to one of the lobes.

Eosinophil

- 14–16 µ
- Nucleus has two lobes (spectacular shaped), cytoplasm has coarse granules which stain reddish or orange coloured.
- The granules do not overlap the nucleus.

Basophil

- 14–16 µ
- Nucleus has two lobes.
- Cytoplasm has large round to oval deeply staining basophilic granules.

Note: Eosinophil and basophil are slightly larger than neutrophil.

LYMPHOID SERIES (Fig. 1.4)

Lymphoblast

- Nucleoli are 1–2.
- Other features are similar to myeloblast.

Prolymphocyte

- Nucleoli are 0–1.
- This cell divides and produces a large lymphocyte which matures to small lymphocyte.

Large Lymphocyte

- 12–16 µ
- Nucleus round or indented
- Cytoplasm abundant, sky-blue or pale-blue coloured, a few azurophilic granules may be present.

Small Lymphocyte

- 6–10 µ
- Nucleus round or indented
- Cytoplasm scanty and pale-blue coloured

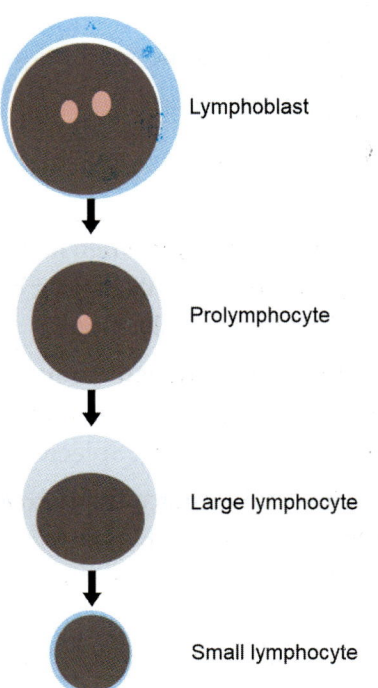

Fig. 1.4: Lymphoid series cells (schematic)

MONOCYTE SERIES (Fig. 1.5)

Monoblast

- Nucleus round or indented or convoluted
- Other features are similar to myeloblast.

Promonocyte

- Nucleus indented, can have clefts or convolutions.
- Cytoplasm has azurophilic purplish pink granules.
- Other features are similar to promyelocyte.

Monocyte

- 14–20 µ
- Nucleus lobulated, indented, kidney shaped or has convolutions.
- Nucleus has fine chromatin.
- Cytoplasm grey blue, ground glass and abundant, fine azurophilic purplish pink
- Granules may be present sometimes, cytoplasm has vacuoles.

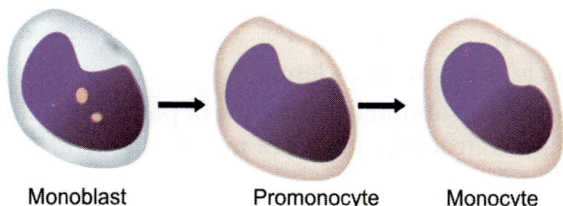

Fig.1.5: Monocyte series cells (schematic)

MEGAKARYOCYTIC SERIES (Fig. 1.6)

Megakaryoblast

- Nucleus and cytoplasmic features are similar to myeloblast.

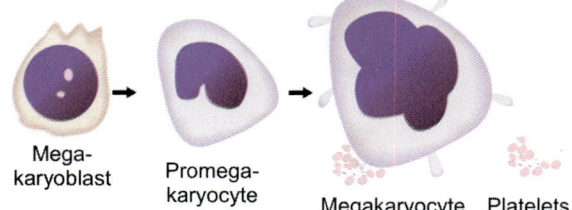

Fig. 1.6: Megakaryocytic series cells (schematic)

Promegakaryocyte

- Nucleus is bigger than megakaryoblast.
- Nucleus is lobulated because of endoreduplication of nucleus.
- Cytoplasm basophilic, stains light blue and has azurophilic purplish pink granules.

Megakaryocyte

- Largest cell in the bone marrow
- 30–90 µ
- Nucleus lobulated (4–16 lobes)
- Chromatin clumped
- Cytoplasm has azurophilic granules.
- Platelets are formed by the protrusion of the pseudopodia of the megakaryocyte cytoplasm into the bone marrow sinusoids.

Platelets

- 1–4 µ
- Approximately 1/3rd of an RBC size
- No nucleus
- Cytoplasm is light blue, has azurophilic purplish pink granules.

SELF-ASSESSMENT EXERCISE

1. **What happens to red cells when haem is removed?**
   A. Cannot bind oxygen B. Cannot bind iron
   C. Both   D. None

2. **Erythropoietin is produced from:**
   A. Heart   B. Bone marrow
   C. Kidney   D. Spleen

3. **Haemopoiesis takes place in all *except*:**
   A. Bone marrow   B. Spleen
   C. Liver   D. Kidney

4. **Time taken for normoblast to reticulocyte is:**
   A. 5 to 7 days
   B. 10 days
   C. 4 weeks
   D. 15 days

5. **Time taken for reticulocyte to develop into RBC is:**
   A. 4 days   B. Half a day
   C. 1 to 2 days   D. One week

Answers

1. A   **2.** C   **3.** D   **4.** A   **5.** C

Red Blood Cell Disorders

RED BLOOD CELLS

Red blood cells are biconcave discs of 7.2 μ in diameter, containing haemoglobin. The cell lacks nucleus and bound by highly deformable and elastic cell membrane. The cell membrane is attached to cytoskeletal proteins. The normal lifespan is 120 days.

STRUCTURE OF RED CELL MEMBRANE

The red cell membrane is composed of lipid bilayer which is traversed by several transmembrane proteins.

The cell membrane and underlying cytoskeleton together is called stroma. The cytoskeleton is made up of spectrin (alpha and beta chains), ankyrin, actin, band 4.1, band 4.2 and transmembrane proteins (band 3 and glycophorin). Band 4.1 binds to spectrin and also to glycophorin. Ankyrin links to spectrin. Band 3 with the help of 4.2 protein is linked to ankyrin and thus to spectrin. These proteins give the red cell, a deformable state while passing through the capillaries. Deficiency in any of these proteins can cause membrane abnormalities (Fig. 2.1).

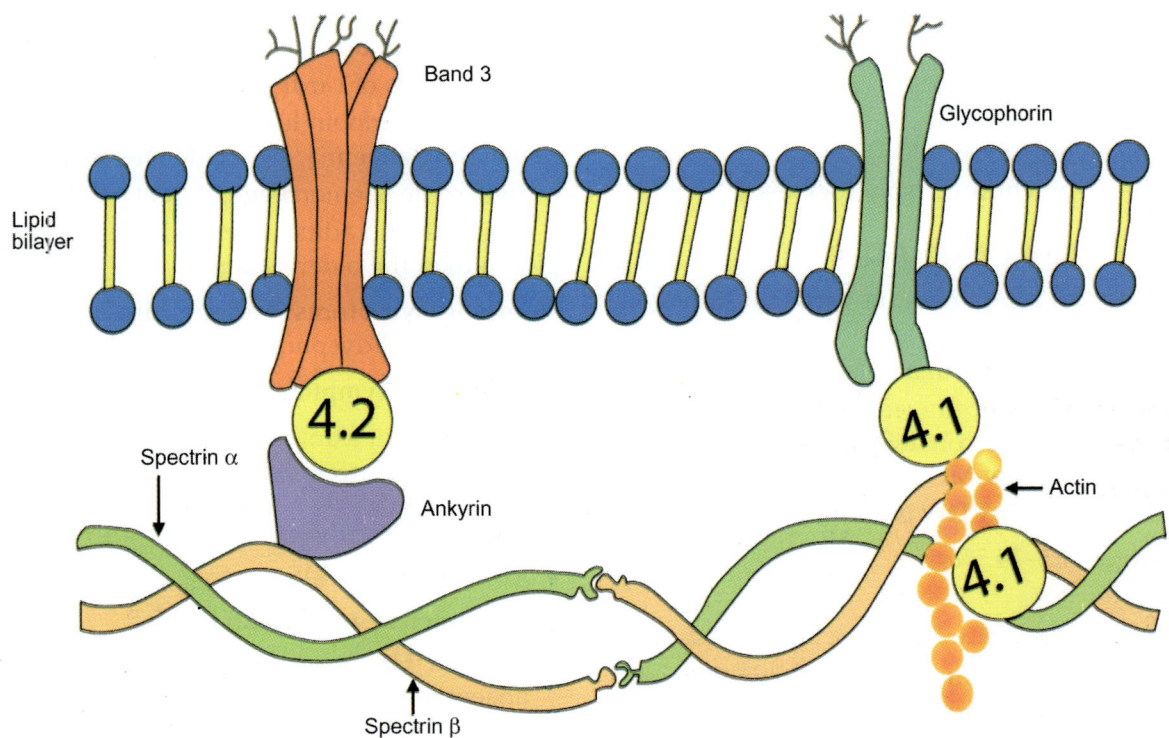

Fig. 2.1: Structure of red cell membrane

RED CELL INDICES

Mean Corpuscular Volume (MCV)

MCV indicates volume of red cells. It is expressed in femtolitres (fl)

$$MCV = \frac{Haematocrit \times 10}{RBC\ count\ in\ millions}$$

Normal range: 80–98 fl: Normocytes
- <80 fl: Microcytes
- >100 fl: Macrocytes

Mean Corpuscular Haemoglobin (MCH)

MCH indicates amount of Hb per red cell. It is expressed in pg (picograms)

$$MCH = \frac{Hb\,(g/dl) \times 10}{RBC\ count\ in\ millions}$$

Normal range: 26–34 pg

Less than 26 pg: Decreased MCH—seen in microcytic hypochromic anaemia.

More than 34 pg: Increased MCH—seen in macrocytic anaemia.

Mean Corpuscular Haemoglobin Concentration (MCHC)

MCHC denotes average concentration of haemoglobin in the red cells.

$$MCHC = \frac{Hb\,(g/dl) \times 10}{Haematocrit\,(\%)}$$

MCHC is expressed in g/dl.

Normal range is 31–37g/dl
- <31 g/dl—hypochromic
- >37 g/dl—hyperchromic (spherocytosis)

Red Cell Distribution Width (RDW)

RDW provides an assessment on variation in red cell volume.
- In early iron deficiency anaemia, RDW is increased with normal MCV.
- In established case of iron deficiency anaemia, RDW is increased with low MCV.
- In thalassaemia trait, RDW is normal with low MCV.

Normal range: 11.5–14.5%

ANAEMIAS

Anaemia is defined as reduced haemoglobin (Hb) level or oxygen carryng capacity or reduced red cell counts below the lower extreme of the normal range for that age and sex of the patient.

In a case of anaemia, the following questions need to be answered.
  I. Is the patient anaemic?
 II. What type of anaemia on symptoms and investigations?
III. What is the cause?

It is considered as anaemia, if Hb values as below.
1. Adult male: Hb less than 13 g/dl
2. Adult female: Hb less than 12 g/dl
3. Children up to 6 years: Hb less than 11 g/dl
4. 7 to 14 years: Below 12 gm/dl

History in Anaemia
- Family history of anaemia, splenomegaly, jaundice and splenectomy
- Exercise intolerance
- Pallor and jaundice
- Bleeding tendency
- Malnutrition, malabsorption and alcoholism
- Multiple pregnancies and menorrhagia
- Hypothyroidism

Clinical Manifestations of Anaemia

The symptoms and signs of anaemia may be due to:
  i. Anaemia itself
 ii. The disorder which is causing anaemia

The level of haemoglobin, when symptoms start, depends upon:
  i. The rate of development of anaemia, and
 ii. The status of cardiovascular system of the patient.

The haemoglobin level may be higher with rapidly developing anaemia, e.g. acute haemorrhage.

In chronic haemorrhage, it may be at lower level.

Children and adults tolerate lower levels of haemoglobin than the older patients.

Common symptoms: Fatigue, tiredness, palpitation and exertional dyspnoea

Less common symptoms: Fainting, giddiness and angina

Signs: Pallor of skin, conjunctiva and nail beds
High cardiac output states

Findings on Examination of an Anaemia Patient
- **Skin changes:** Pallor
- **Conjunctiva and sclera:** Pallor
- **Retina:** Haemorrhages (especially in cases of anaemia with thrombocytopenia)
- **Mouth:** Pale tongue and lips
- Splenomegaly

- Hepatomegaly
- **Abdominal mass (epigastric mass, iliac mass, etc.):** Carcinoma stomach, carcinoma colon, etc.
- **Lymphadenopathy (superficial):** Chronic lymphocytic leukaemia, lymphoma, or secondaries
- Bony tenderness.

Evidences to Diagnose Anaemia

- Symptoms of anaemia
- Signs of anaemia
- Investigation findings

Type of Anaemia

Examination of peripheral smear is important to know the type of anaemia along with indices. The important indices are:

- Mean corpuscular volume (MCV)
- Mean corpuscular haemoglobin (MCH)
- Mean corpuscular haemoglobin concentration (MCHC)
- Red cell distribution width (RDW)

Classification of Anaemia (Tables 2.1 and 2.2)

Table 2.1	Pathophysiological classification
I. Blood loss: Acute and chronic	
II. Impaired red cell production	
a. Inadequate supply of nutrients	
Iron deficiency	
Vitamin B_{12} deficiency	
Folic acid deficiency	
Protein calorie malnutrition	
b. Depression of erythropoietic activity	
c. Anaemia associated with chronic disorders	
Infections	
Connective tissue disorders	
Inflammatory disorders	
Disseminated malignancy	
d. Anaemia in renal failure	
e. Aplastic anaemia	
f. Replacement of bone marrow	
Leukaemia	
Lymphoma	
Myeloproliferative neoplasms (MPNs)	
Multiple myeloma (MM)	
Myelodysplastic syndrome (MDS)	
III. Excessive red cell destruction (haemolytic anaemias)	
Intrinsic defects of red cells	
Extrinsic defects of red cells	

Table 2.2	Morphological classification
Normocytic normochromic anaemia: MCV, MCH and MCHC within normal range	
Microcytic hypochromic anaemia: MCV—low, MCH and MCHC—decreased, RDW—increased, MCV—less than 70 fl	
Macrocytic anaemia: MCV—more than 100 fl, MCH—increased, MCHC—normal	
Dimorphic anaemia: Two population of cells with hypochromia	

DDs for Normocytic Normochromic Anaemia

1. Acute blood loss
2. Haemolytic anaemia
3. Chronic renal failure (erythropoietin deficiency)
4. Anaemia of chronic disorders: Infections
5. Microangiopathic haemolytic anaemia (HA)
6. Autoimmune HA
7. Transfusion reactions
8. Burns

DDs for Microcytic Anaemia (Mnemonics—TICS)

1. **T**halassaemia
2. **I**ron deficiency anaemia
3. Anaemia of **C**hronic diseases
4. **S**ideroblastic anaemia

DDs for Macrocytic Anaemia—Megaloblastic Marrow

1. Vitamin B_{12} deficiency
2. Folic acid deficiency
3. MDS

DDs for Macrocytic Anaemia—Non-Megaloblastic Marrow

1. **A**lcohol
2. Chronic liver disease (cirrhosis)
3. Congenital bone marrow (BM) failure (Schwamann-Diamond syndrome—BM dysregulation, sketetal abnormalities and exocrine pancreatic insufficiency)
4. **T**hyroid: Hypothyroidism
5. **R**eticulocytosis

IRON DEFICIENCY ANAEMIA

Iron deficiency anaemia occurs due to reduced intake, decreased intestinal absorption, increased utilization or chronic blood loss (Tables 2.3 and 2.4). As a result, there is reduction in concentration of Hb in circulating red blood cells below normal for that particular age and sex.

Sources of Iron

- The main source of iron is diet. Though diet contains around 10 to 20 mg of iron, only 1 mg is absorbed.
- High iron content is present in red meat, legumes and green leafy vegetables.

Many factors influence iron absorption.

1. Gastric acid, ascorbic acid, acidic foods (citrus) convert ferric to ferrous iron and enhance iron absorption. Amino acids also enhance absorption of inorganic iron.
2. Tannates (tea), carbonates, calcium, phosphates, oxalates, and phytates reduce iron absorption.
3. Hepcidin, a hormone produced by liver, regulates iron absorption. If body iron stores are less, hepcidin secretion reduced and ferroportin, hephaestin and DMT1 (divalent metal iron transporter) are over expressed and ferric iron absorption increases.

Iron Absorption

- Ferric iron (Fe^{3+}) is reduced to ferrous iron (Fe^{2+}) by ferric reductase enzyme (duodenal cytochrome b) of duodenum.
- Ferrous iron is absorbed in proximal part of intestine mainly from first part of duodenum.
- Two steps are required: Mucosal uptake of ferrous iron and transfer of it from enterocytes to lamina propria to enter circulation.
- In mucosa, iron in ferrous form is transported mainly by DMT1 and to small percentage by mobiferrin-integrin-paraferrin channels.
- Ferrous iron from enterocytes to lamina propria require ferroportin and hephaestin to be converted to ferric iron which can enter circulation.
- Once released into circulation, ferric iron is transported in combination with transferrin and reaches tissues.
- The iron released from senescent RBCs is recycled.

Table 2.3	Etiological factors for iron deficiency anaemia in different stages of life

Causes: Major etiological factors for iron deficiency anaemia in different stages of life:

Females in reproductive life
- Pregnancy—number and frequency
- Miscarriages
- Lactation
- Pathological blood loss—causes are mentioned below
- Deficient diet/inadequate iron intake

Adult males and post-menopausal females
- Pathological blood loss—causes are mentioned below

Infants and children
- Deficient diet/inadequate iron intake
- Diminished iron stores at birth

Table 2.4	Causes of iron deficieny anaemia: According to etiology

Inadequate iron intake: This is the major cause of iron deficiency anaemia in infants and children. In adults, it may occur due to:
- Poor economic status
- Iron content may be lower with vegetarian diet
- Dietary fads or dislikes

Pathological blood loss
- Menorrhagia
- GI bleeding
  - Peptic ulcer
  - Carcinoma stomach
  - Carcinoma colon
  - **Chronic aspirin ingestion/ NSAID use**
  - Oesophagitis
  - Oesophageal varices
  - Haemorrhoids
  - **Hookworm infestation**
  - Hiatus hernia
  - Angiodysplasia
  - Diverticulosis
  - Meckel's diverticula
  - Colitis or inflammatory bowel disease
- Bleeding disorder
- Pulmonary lesions with bleeding
- Haemoglobinuria and haemosiderinuria (chronic intravascular haemolysis)
- Haemodialysis
- Haematuria (chronic)
- Frequent blood donation each time 200–250 mg iron/unit—blood is lost

The causes for decreased absorption of iron are:
- Gastric surgery
- Achlorhydria
- Sprue/coeliac disease
- Pica (non-nutritive substances like clay, chalk, sand, etc.)

Etiological factors of iron deficiency anaemia are shown in Tables 2.3 and 2.4.

Clinical Features

Clinical features most commonly occur with long-standing iron deficiency states.

Following are the clinical features:
- Pallor, fatigue, weakness, dyspnoea
- Anxiety, irritability, angina, sleepiness, palpitation
- Changes in the tongue like atrophy of papillae resulting in **pale bald tongue.**

- Changes in the nails—longitudinal ridging, flattening and **koilonychia** (spoon-shaped nails) or nails that are weak or brittle.
- Poor appetite
- Unusual obsessive food craving, known as pica
- **Plummer-Vinson syndrome** (Paterson-Brown-Kelly syndrome): Dysphagia due to formation of oesophageal webs, iron deficiency anaemia, glossitis and cheilitis. Spleen may be enlarged, most commonly seen in postmenopausal females.
- **Tayanc-Prasad syndrome** (growth retardation, hypogonadism, hepatosplenomegaly, zinc and iron deficiency, geophagia).

Approach to a patient with iron deficiency anaemia, investigations and grading of iron stores in bone marrow are shown in Tables 2.5, 2.6 and 2.7; Figs 2.2 and 2.3.

Table 2.5	Approach to a patient with iron deficiency anaemia

History

Females in reproductive period: Menorrhagia, pregnancies—number and frequency, miscarriages, iron deficient diet, GI blood loss, hematuria, epistaxis, haemoptysis, GI surgery, aspirin ingestion

Males and post-menopausal females: Iron deficient diet, haematemesis, melaena or per rectal bleeding (GI blood loss due to haemorrhoids, oesophageal varices, bleeding due to GI malignancies), haematuria, epistaxis, haemoptysis, GI surgery, aspirin ingestion

Infants and children: Dietary history regarding supplemental feeding, prematurity, multiple births, iron deficiency in mother, GI disturbances, blood loss of any cause

Physical and systemic examination

Examination of any mass, rectal examination, pelvic examination in females, telangiectasias of face and mouth

Relevant investigations commonly required
- Examination of faeces for occult blood and hookworm
- Urine microscopy for haematuria
- GI endoscopy or barium swallow study: Peptic ulcer, hiatus hernia
- Ca stomach, oesophageal varices, Meckel's diverticulum
- Barium swallow studies of oesophageal varices in a cirrhotic patient show multiple serpiginous filling defects of lower one-third of the oesophagus.

Colonoscopy: Carcinoma colon, caecum, ulcerative colitis, diverticula, angiodysplasia

Sigmoidoscopy: Carcinoma rectum, ulcerative colitis

Relevant investigations occasionally required
- Chest X-ray and bronchoscopy (haemoptysis)
- Cystoscopy (haematuria)
- Liver function tests (cirrhosis)

Table 2.6	Blood picture, bone marrow and biochemical findings in iron deficiency anaemia

1. **Complete blood count**
   - Low haemoglobin
   - Low haematocrit
   - Reduced RBC count

2. **RBC indices**
   - Low MCV
   - Low MCH
   - Low or normal MCHC
   - Increased RDW

3. **Peripheral smear**

   RBCs: RBCs show anisocytosis and poikilocytosis

   Majority of the RBCs are microcytic hypochromic, ring/pessary type cells, pencil-shaped cells, target cells, polychromatic cells are present

   WBCs: Count and distribution normal

   Platelets: Count and morphology normal

4. **Bone marrow examination**
   - Depleted iron stores (Perls' stain)
   - Erythroid series—erythroid hyperplasia, micronormoblastic reaction
   - Granulopoiesis—normal
   - Megakaryopoiesis—normal

5. **Iron studies**
   - Serum Iron: ↓
   - Serum ferritin ↓ in general, values less than 10 µg/L are indicative of iron deficiency
   - TIBC: ↑, TIBC is 1/3rd saturated under normal conditions
   - Plasma transferrin ↑
   - Transferrin saturation: ↓ (normal 6–33%), <5% definitely indicates iron deficiency
   - Transferrin receptor: ↑ free erythrocyte protoporphyrin

6. **Stool examination: Hookworm infestation**

   Normal values:
   - **Serum iron:** Male—27–138 µg/dL, female—33–102 µg/dL
   - **Serum ferritin:** Male—29–248 µg/L, female—10–150 µg/dL
   - **TIBC:** Male—174–351 µg/dL, female—194–372 µg/dL
   - **Plasma transferrin:** Male—194–348 µg/dL, female—181–416 µg/dL
   - **Free erythrocyte protoporphyrin:** 17–27 µg/dL
   - **Transferrin saturation:** 6–33%

Differential diagnosis for microcytic anaemias
- Iron deficiency anaemia
- Thalassaemia, HbC, HbE, etc.
- Sideroblastic anaemia
- Lead poisoning
- Anaemia of chronic diseases (sometimes)

Table 2.7	Grading of iron stores in bone marrow aspiration
0	No iron granules seen
1+	Small granules in reticulum cells (seen only with oil immersion)
2+	Few small granules in reticulum cells (seen only with low power)
3+	Numerous small granules in all cells
4+	Large granules in small clumps
5+	Dense large clumps of granules
6+	Large deposits obscuring marrow picture

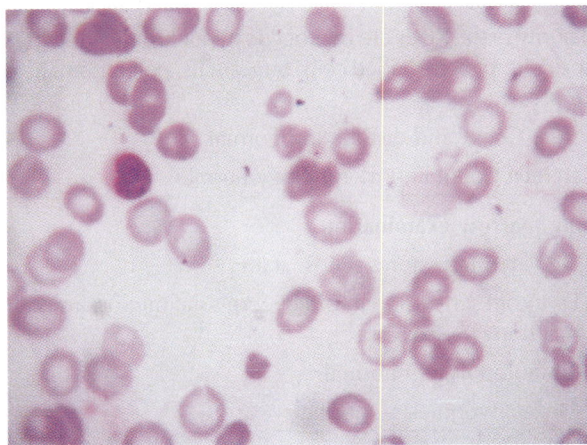

Fig 2.2: Peripheral smear to show microcytic RBCs

MEGALOBLASTIC ANAEMIA

Megaloblastic anaemias are macrocytic anaemias characterised by distinctive cytological and functional abnormalities in peripheral blood and bonemarrow cells due to impaired DNA synthesis, resulting in erythroid precursors that are enlarged and show failure of nuclear maturation (megaloblasts).

Etiology

Megaloblastic anaemias result from conditions in which nucleic acid synthesis is abnormal as:
• **Vitamin B_{12} deficiency**
• **Folic acid deficiency**

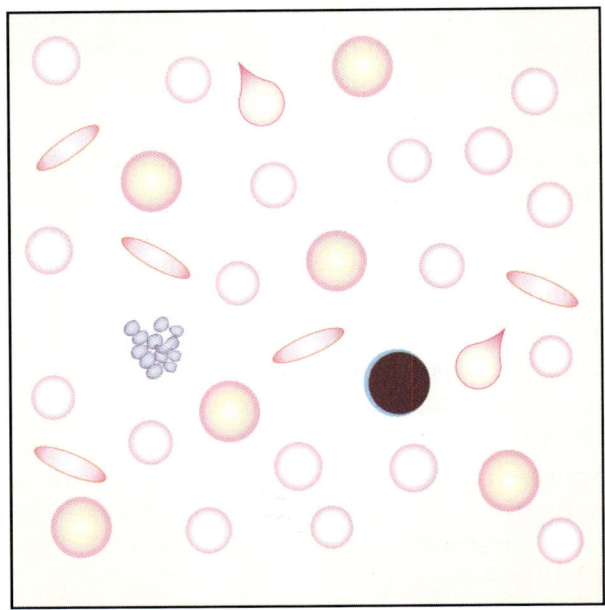

Fig: 2.3: Microcytic hypochromic anaemia (schematic)

Vitamin B_{12} is mainly obtained from foods of animal origin; **kidney, heart and liver are richest sources.** Lesser amounts are present in **muscle meat, fish, eggs, cheese, and milk. Vegetarian diet has no vitamin B_{12}.** The vitamin B_{12} is in the form of adenosylcobalamin and hydroxocobalamin and these are bound to proteins in the food.

Folate is present in diet, largely attached to methyl group and is in an inactive form. It is distributed in plant and animal tissues. The richest sources are liver, kidney, yeast and green leafy vegetables. Spinach and cabbage have good source of folates. Milk has low folate content.

Information about vitamin B_{12} and folic acid is given in Table 2.8.

Absorption of Vitamin B_{12}

When food passes through the stomach, vitamin B_{12} is released from the dietary proteins by the action of acid and proteolytic enzymes.

Vitamin B_{12} first combines with **R protein (haptocorrin)** released from the saliva. As this **vitamin**

Table 2.8	Information about vitamin B_{12} and folic acid	
	Vitamin B_{12}	**Folic acid**
Availability in diet	Vegetarian: Poor Non-vegetarian–meat: Rich	Vegetarian: Rich Non-vegetarian–meat: Moderate
Effect on cooking	10–30% loss	60–90% loss
Daily requirement in adults	2–4 µg	200 µg
Daily intake in adults	5–30 µg	100–500 µg
Absorption site	Ileum	Duodenum and jejunum
Body stores	2–5 mg	5–20 mg

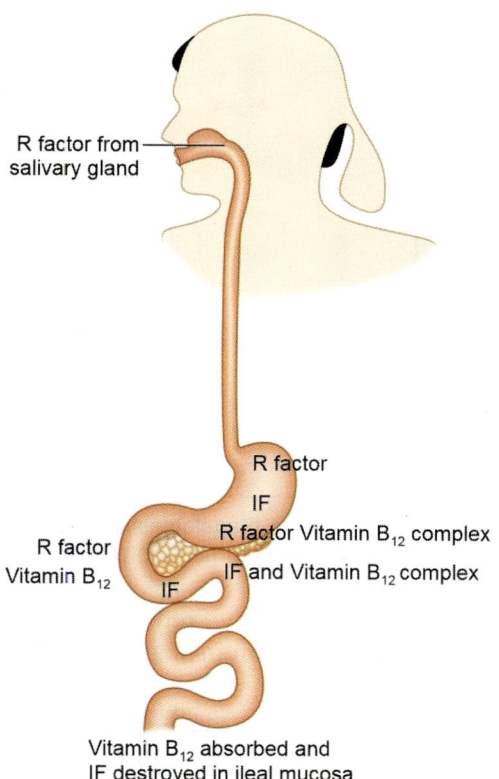

Fig. 2.4: Vitamin B$_{12}$ absorption (schematic)

B$_{12}$ and R complex proceeds to small intestine, the **R protein is degraded by pancreatic enzymes and vitamin B$_{12}$ is released.** The **vitamin B$_{12}$ rapidly combines with the intrinsic factor (IF) secreted by parietal cells** of fundus and body of stomach. **Vitamin B$_{12}$ and IF complex pass in the ileum which is site of absorption.** The vitamin B$_{12}$ and IF complex bind to the receptors (cubilin/amnionless) on the surface of the brush border cells and vitamin B$_{12}$ and IF complex are taken up. IF gets destroyed. Vitamin B$_{12}$ in the circulation will be bound to transport protein called transcobalamin II. Transcobalamin I acts as storage protein (Fig. 2.4).

Absorption of Folate

Folate is absorbed from the duodenum and upper jejunum and to a lesser extent from lower jejunum and ileum. The polyglutamate folates are cleaved to monoglutamate folate and undergo further reduction and methylation and circulate in the blood as methyl-tetrahydrofolate.

Folate is stored in the liver in polyglutamate form. It is required for:

- Methylation of homocysteine to methionine
- Synthesis of thymidine monophosphate from deoxy-uridylate monophosphate in DNA synthesis.

Role of Vitamin B$_{12}$ and Folic Acid

Role of vitamin B$_{12}$ and folic acid is shown in Fig. 2.5.

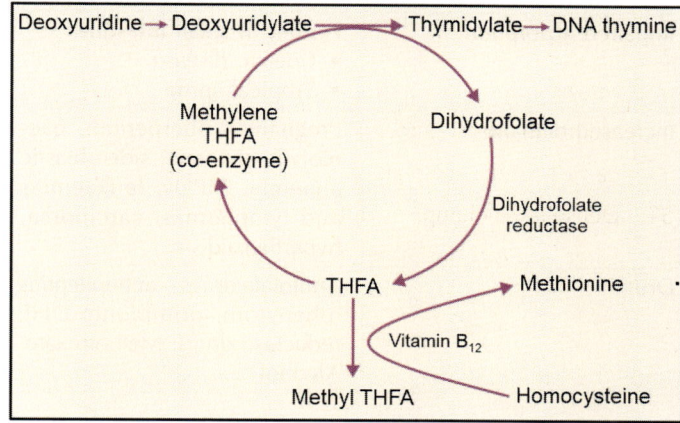

Fig. 2.5: Role of vitamin B$_{12}$ and folate in DNA synthesis

Notes

1. In deficiency of vitamin B$_{12}$ and folic acid, homocysteine levels are increased.

2. Vitamin B$_{12}$ is also required for conversion of methyl-malonyl-CoA to succinyl-CoA. In deficiency of vitamin B$_{12}$, methylmalonyl-CoA accumulates and some of it is hydrolysed to methylmalonic acid which is detected in serum and urine.

3. THFA is required for synthesis of glutamic acid. In absence of folic acid, formiminoglutamic acid (FIGLU) is elevated and excreted in urine.

4. In vitamin B$_{12}$ deficiency, **methyl THFA gets accumulated and this is known as folate trap.**

Causes of megaloblastic anaemia are shown in Tables 2.9 and 2.10.

Table 2.9	Causes of megaloblastic anaemia due to vitamin B$_{12}$ deficiency
Mechanism	**Disorder**
Decreased intake	**Nutritional deficiency**
Impaired absorption	**Gastric causes** • Pernicious anaemia • Gastrectomy—total or partial **Intestinal causes** • Coeliac disease • Tropical sprue • Fish tapeworm infestation • Bacterial overgrowth (blind loop syndrome) • Surgical resection of ileum

Table 2.10	Causes of megaloblastic anaemia due to folate deficiency
Mechanism	**Disorder**
Decreased intake	Nutritional deficiency
Impaired absorption	**Lesions of small intestine** • Coeliac disease • Tropical sprue
Increased demand	Pregnancy, puerperium, hae-molytic anaemia, sideroblastic anaemia, MPDs, leukaemias and lymphomas, carcinoma, hyperthyroidism
Drugs	Antifolate drugs—antiepileptics (phenytoin, primidone) DHF reductase drugs: Methotrexate Alcohol

Clinical Features

These patients present with general features of anaemia.

Following are the other features:

- Glossitis
- Peripheral neuropathy and subacute combined degeneration of spinal cord in vitamin B_{12} deficiency anaemia
- Dementia
- Folate deficiency may also cause diarrhoea and glossitis.

Pathology

Red Cell Changes

- Hb is moderately to markedly reduced, in the range of 5–10 g/dl, may go down as below as 2–3 g/dl.
- PCV is reduced.
- MCV >100 fl
- MCH increased
- MCHC normal
- Reticulocyte count is normal or slightly increased (2–3%).
- Erythropoiesis changes from normoblastic to megaloblastic.

Megaloblasts differ from normoblasts and show nuclear–cytoplasmic asynchrony.

- They are larger (increased cytoplasm).
- Show delayed nuclear maturation
- But normal cytoplasmic haemoglobinization
- Sieve-like nuclear chromatin

Peripheral Smear (Fig. 2.6)

RBCs: There is moderate to marked anisocytosis and poikilocytosis.

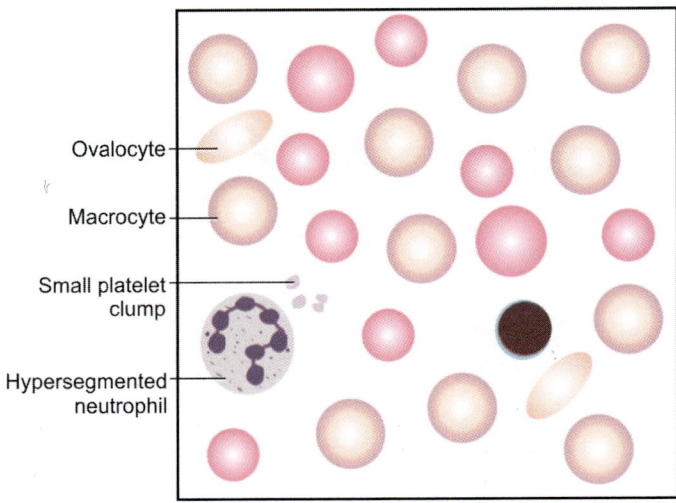

Fig. 2.6: Peripheral smear in megaloblastic anaemia showing macrocytes and hypersegmented neutrophil

There is macrocytosis (large red cells with elevated MCV) and marked variation in size (anisocytosis) and shape (poikilocytosis)

- Oval forms (macro-ovalocytes) are prominent, and
- Evidence of dyserythropoiesis: Basophilic stippling Cabot rings, Howell-Jolly bodies

Megaloblastic anaemias are, therefore, **macrocytic anaemias,** if morphologic classification is used.

A few nucleated RBCs with megaloblastic change may be seen.

Changes in white blood cells: Neutrophils show hypersegmented nuclei, with many cells showing more than 5 nuclear lobes.

Platelets: Normal or reduced.

Pancytopaenia is seen in 10–20% cases of megaloblastic anaemias.

Bone Marrow Changes (Figs 2.7 and 2.8)

Megaloblastic Marrow

- These are large cells compared to normal nucleated erythroid precursors.
- The nucleus has open sieve-like chromatin.
- There is evidence of dyserythropoiesis.
- Nuclear maturation lags behind the cytoplasmic maturation.
- Late normoblasts have open chromatin.
- Giant metamyelocytes are present.
- Mitosis increased.
- Marrow is hypercellular.
- M: E ratio increased (1:1 or 2 : 1).
- Megakaryocytes may be normal or reduced. They may large and hyperlobated.
- In pure megaloblastic anaemia, iron stores may be increased.

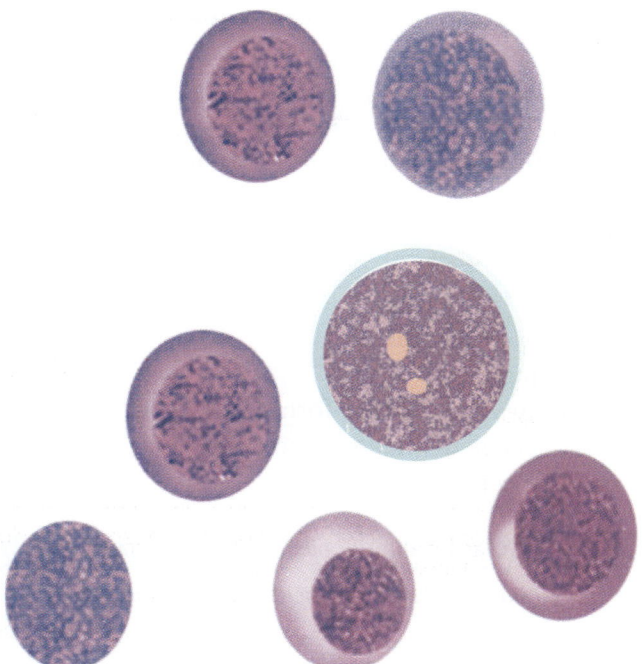

Fig. 2.7: Bone marrow in megaloblastic anaemia: Megaloblasts and other erythroid series cells with nuclei showing open chromatin (schematic)

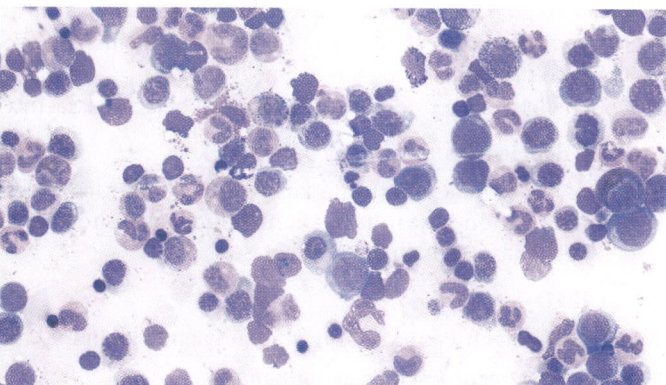

Fig. 2.8: Bone marrow in megaloblastic anaemia: Marrow aspirate showing megaloblasts and other erythroid series cells with nuclei showing open chromatin

Delayed maturation leads to accumulation of erythrocyte precursor cells. The bone marrow is *hypercellular and contains large numbers of megaloblasts*; as a result of **intramedullary haemolysis or ineffective erythropoiesis,** many megaloblasts undergo destruction in the bone marrow before maturation and this:

* Aggravates anaemia with
* Mild elevation of serum bilirubin and lactate dehydrogenase (LDH isoenzymes 1 and 2).

Megakaryocytic series are also affected.

Due to affection of all the series and ineffective erythropoiesis, there may be **pancytopenia, leukopenia or thrombocytopenia** in these patients.

Megaloblastic anaemia should be suspected upon finding in the peripheral blood the following features:

* Macrocytic anaemia with
* Hypersegmented neutrophils.

Biochemical and Other Investigations

1. **Serum vitamin B$_{12}$ levels** decreased in vitamin B$_{12}$ deficiency anaemia.
2. **Serum** and urinary excretion of **methylmalonic acid** level is increased in vitamin B$_{12}$ deficiency.
3. Homocysteine levels are elevated in vitamin B$_{12}$ and folic acid deficiency.
4. **Schilling test in vitamin B$_{12}$ deficiency:**

   * **1st step:** Radioactive (RA) vitamin B$_{12}$ (^{58}Co-B$_{12}$) is given orally. Immediately 1,000 µg of non-RA vitamin B$_{12}$ is given by IM to saturate vitamin B$_{12}$ binding proteins. Urine is collected for 24 hours. In normal health, more than 10% of RA vitamin B$_{12}$ is excreted in urine.
   * **2nd step:** If 1st step is abnormal, the test is repeated with IF.
   Interpretation: If the test turns normal with IF, the diagnosis of pernicious anaemia is made or IF deficiency may be because of gastrectomy. If still abnormal, it is because of ileal pathology or blind loop syndrome.

5. **Deoxyuridine suppression test:** Pre-incubation of normal bone marrow cells with deoxyuridine will suppress the subsequent utilization of radiolabelled thymidine into DNA. In vitamin B$_{12}$ or folic acid deficiency, this suppression is low. By adding vitamin B$_{12}$ or folic acid, one can know which deficiency exists.
6. **Homocysteine levels:** Increased in both vitamin B$_{12}$ and folic acid deficiencies.
7. **Serum bilirubin:** Increased in both vitamin B$_{12}$ and folic acid deficiencies.
8. **Serum LDH levels:** Increased in both vitamin B$_{12}$ and folic acid deficiencies.
9. **Serum ferritin levels:** Increased in both vitamin B$_{12}$ and folic acid deficiencies.
10. **Antibodies to intrinsic factor and parietal cells:** In pernicious anaemia.
11. **Serum folate levels:** Decreased in folate deficiency anaemia.
12. **Red cell folate levels:** Decreased in folate deficiency anaemia.
13. **Formiminoglutamic acid (FIGLU) test:** This an intermediate product in conversion of histidine to glutamate which is excreted in urine in folate deficiency.

Normal Values

1. Serum cobalamin levels—200–900 ng/l, <100 ng/l in megaloblastic anaemia due to vitamin B_{12} deficiency.
2. Serum methylmalonic acid >0.4 µmol/l.
3. Serum folate levels up to 5.0 µg/l, <3 µg/l in megaloblastic anaemia due to folate deficiency.
4. Homocysteine levels: Males—14–15 µmol/l; females—12–14 µmol/l.
5. Red cell folate levels >160 µg/l.

Microbiological Assay in Vitamin B_{12} Deficiency Anaemia

Two micro-organisms *Euglena gracilis* and *Lactobacillus leichmani* are vitamin B_{12} dependent organisms and vitamin B_{12} in the serum is determined by comparing the growth of the organisms.

Microbiological Assay in Folic Acid Deficiency Anaemia

The folate activity can be assessed by methyl tetrahydrofolate. This compound is microbiologically active for *Lactobacillus casei* which is used for assay.

Stool Examination for Parasite

In vitamin B_{12} deficiency: Stool examination for proglottids of fish tapeworm *D. latum*. (Rare in India)

Diagnosis of megaloblastic anaemia

1. Oval macrocytes in peripheral smear
2. Hypersegmented neutrophils
3. Megaloblastic hypercellular marrow
4. Response to vitamin B_{12}/folate therapy

Other causes of macrocytic anaemia

1. Alcoholism
2. Hepatic causes
3. Hypothyroidism
4. Increased reticulocyte count—haemolysis
5. Drugs

HAEMOLYTIC ANAEMIAS

Definition

Haemolytic anaemia (HA) results from premature destruction of erythrocytes. The normal red cell lifespan is 120 days. In haemolytic anaemia, the lifespan of RBCs is shortened by varying degrees and in many cases they survive for only a few days.

Patient may not always be anaemic because of bone marrow compensation.

Anaemia in haemolytic anaemia develops due to:

- Reduced lifespan
- Aplastic crisis
- Haemolytic crisis

Classification of haemolytic anaemia is given in Table 2.11.

Clinical Features

- Pallor
- Intermittent jaundice
- Splenomegaly
- Gallstones—in chronic forms
- Crisis—aplastic, haemolytic
- Ankle ulcers

Table 2.11	Classification of haemolytic anaemia (HA)

HA due to intrinsic (intracorpuscular) abnormalities

CONGENITAL

Membrane abnormalities

- Membrane skeleton proteins: Spherocytosis, elliptocytosis
- Membrane lipids: Abetalipoproteinaemia

Disorders of haemoglobin synthesis

- Deficient globin synthesis: Thalassaemia syndromes
- Structurally abnormal globin synthesis (haemoglobinopathies): Sickle cell anaemia, unstable haemoglobins
- Double heterozygous disorders: Sickle cell beta thalassaemia

Enzyme deficiencies

- Glycolytic enzymes: Pyruvate kinase, hexokinase, enzymes of hexose monophosphate shunt: glucose-6-phosphate dehydrogenase, glutathione synthetase

ACQUIRED

Membrane defect: Paroxysmal nocturnal haemoglobinuria

HA due to extracorpuscular abnormalities

ACQUIRED

Immune mechanisms

- Antibody mediated: Warm antibodies/cold antibodies
- Transfusion reactions: Incompatible blood transfusion
- Erythroblastosis fetalis (haemolytic disease of the newborn)
- Autoantibodies: Idiopathic (primary), drug-associated, systemic lupus erythematosus

Non-immune mechanisms

Mechanical trauma to red cells

- Microangiopathic haemolytic anaemias: Thrombotic thrombocytopenic purpura, disseminated intravascular coagulation
- Prosthetic heart valves
- March haemoglobinuria

Miscellaneous causes

- Infections: Malaria
- Burns
- Lead poisoning

While investigating a case of haemolytic anaemia, following questions need to be answered.

1. Is the anaemia of haemolytic nature?
2. If haemolytic anaemia is present, what is the site of destruction?

   Intravascular or extravascular?
3. What is the etiology?

The haemolytic nature is determined by:

1. Increased destruction of red cells with haemoglobin breakdown
2. Bone marrow regeneration

Site of destruction is determined by:

- In intravascular destruction, there is release of free haemoglobin due to destruction of RBCs in the circulation.
- In extravascular haemolysis, there will be removal of senescent RBCs from reticuloendothelial cells. Haemoglobin is released and catabolised within the macrophages. Indirect bilirubin may be increased but free haemoglobin is not detected in the plasma.

Mechanism of Haemoglobin Breakdown
(Figs 2.9 and 2.10)

1. Haemoglobin present in RBCs is broken down in reticuloendothelial (RE) cells as globin and haem. Globin enters protein pool. Porphyrin ring of haem is cleaved by haemoxidase to biliverdin and CO. Biliverdin is reduced to bilirubin by biliverdin reductase.

   Iron released combines with iron binding proteins and is carried to bone marrow for re-utilisation or to be stored in body iron stores.

Bilirubin in plasma forms firm complex with albumin and reaches liver. In liver, bilirubin combines with glucuronic acid to form bilirubin glucuronide (conjugated bilirubin) and excreted in bile ducts. Conjugated bilirubin is water soluble, passes into intestine and reduced by intestinal bacterial flora to urobilinogen. **About 10–20% of the urobilinogen enters the portal vein and excreted back into bowel (enterohepatic circulation). Some amount of urobilinogen enters the systemic circulation and excreted in kidneys.** Rest is excreted in stools.

2. **In haemolytic anaemia, excess haemoglobin released (a) first combines with haptoglobin. (b)** If binding capacity of haptoglobin exhausted, the remaining, **haemoglobin is converted to methaemoglobin** which is broken down to **ferrihaem and globin.** (c) Ferrihaem binds to haemopexin and thus prevents glomerular filtration. Ferrihaem–haemopexin complex is removed by liver.

   If binding capacity of haemopexin exceeds, ferrihaem binds to albumin in 1:1 molar ratio and forms methaemalbumin. Some of the free haemoglobin may be present in plasma as haemoglobinaemia and also produce haemoglobinuria and haemosiderinuria.

   Thus, in HA, there can be reduced levels of haptoglobin and haemopexin, increased levels of methaemoglobin with haemoglobinaemia, methaemalbuminaemia, haemoglobinuria and haemosiderinuria (Fig. 2.11).

The etiology is established by:

- Clinical features, and
- Special investigations.

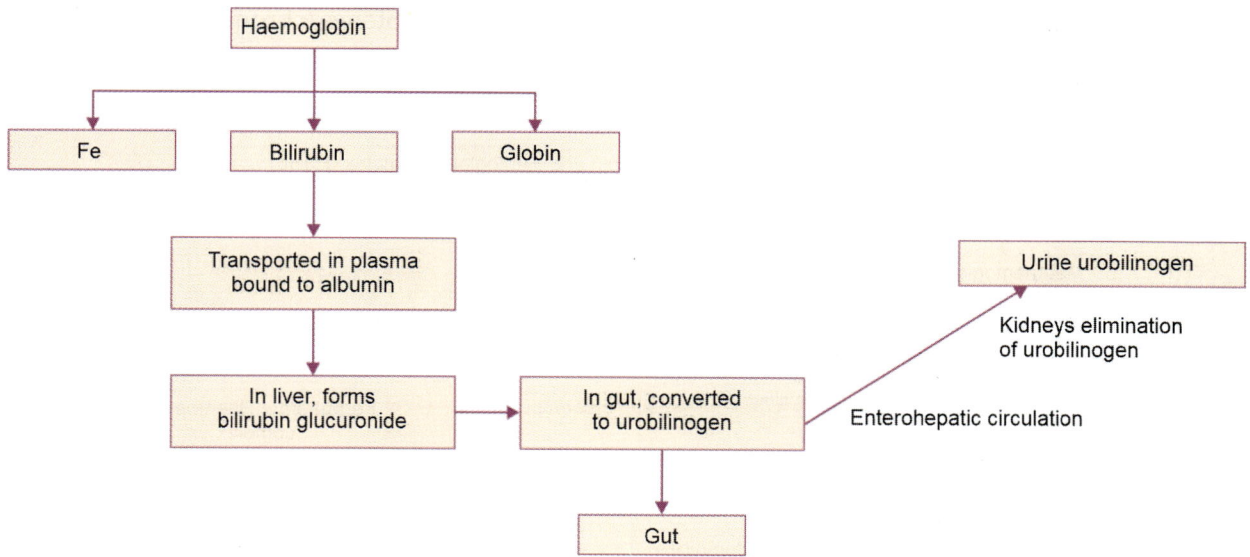

Fig. 2.9: Flowchart showing haemoglobin breakdown

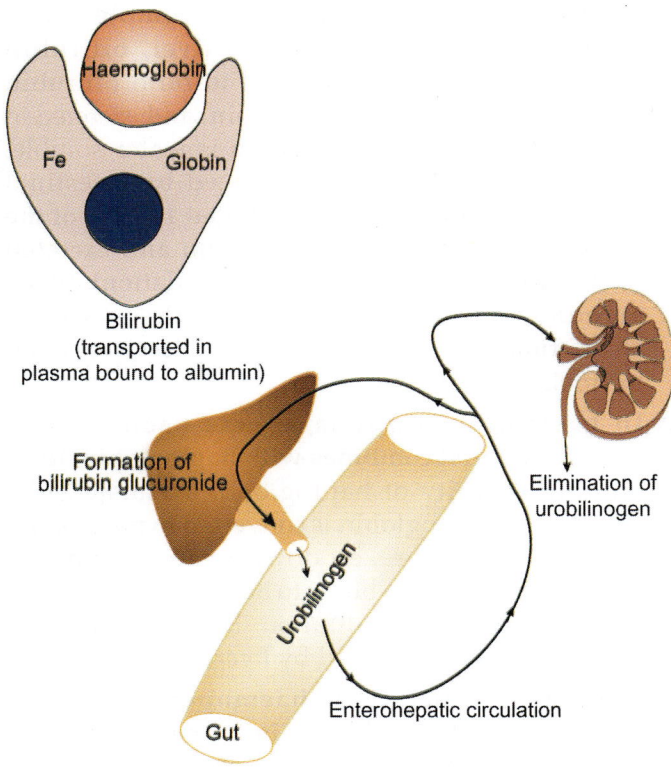

Fig. 2.10: Haemoglobin breakdown (schematic)

General Aspects

Age: **Neonatal period history of hyperbilirubinaemia:**
- Isoimmunisation
- Congenital haemolytic anaemia (hereditory spherocytosis, G6PD deficiency)
- Congenital infection

3–6 months period history of hyperbilirubinaemia:
- Congenital disorder of haemoglobin synthesis
- Defects in haemoglobin (Hb) structure

Gender: X-linked disorders—G6PD deficiency, PK deficiency

Race:
- Haemoglobin S and C—Blacks
- β-thalassaemias—Whites
- β-thalassaemias—Black races

Ethnicity: Thalassaemias—mediterranean origin. G6PD deficiency—Jews, Greeks, Filipinos.

Infection: Infection-induced HA (usually non-immune—malaria, babesiosis, *C. perfringens*).

Inheritance: Family history of anaemia, jaundice, gall-stones, splenomegaly.

General Physical Examination

Observe for the following:
- **Skin:** Jaundice, petechiae, purpura.
- Cavernous haemangioma, history of complications during pregnancy (HELLP syndrome—haemolysis-elevated liver enzymes and low platelet count), microangiopathic HA.
- **Ulcers on lower limbs:** S and C haemoglobin-opathies, thalassaemias, sickle cell anaemia.
- **Facies and bones:** Frontal bossing, prominence of malar and maxillary bones, thinning of cortical bone, spontaneous fractures, hand-foot syndrome.
- Extramedullary haematopoiesis
- **Eyes:**
  – *Tortuosity of conjunctival and retinal vessels:* HbS and HbC.
  – *Microaneurysm of retinal vessels:* S and C haemo-globinopathies.
  – *Cataracts:* G6PD deficiency, galactosaemia with HA in newborns.
  – *Vitreous haemorrhage:* S haemoglobinopathy.
- **Spleen and liver:** Enlargement seen in most HAs.
- **Gallbladder:** Stones (chronic haemolysis, congenital haemolytic anaemias).

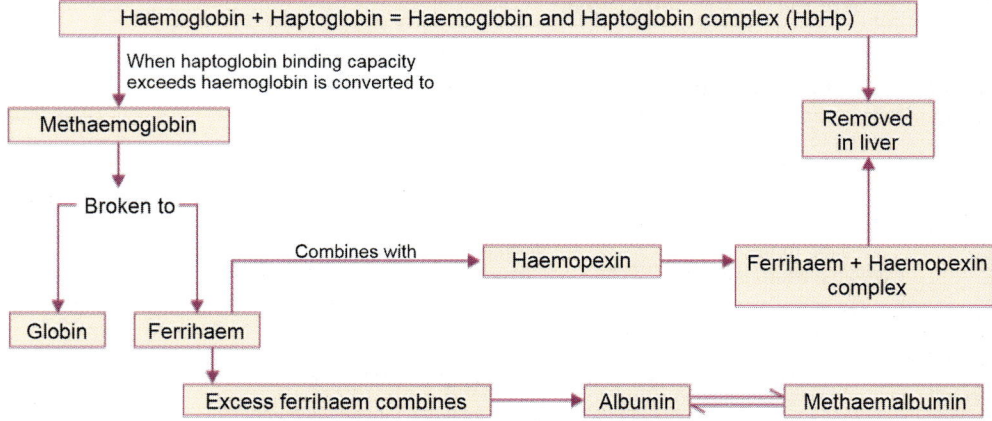

Fig. 2.11: Flowchart showing blood changes in HA

Laboratory Evidence of Haemolysis in Haemolytic Anaemia (Table 2.12, Fig. 2.12)

Table 2.12	Laboratory evidences for haemolysis

Evidence for increased red cell destruction

- Jaundice and hyperbilirubinaemia
- Reduced plasma haptoglobin (<250 mg/l in HA, normal range: 0.3 to 2.0 g/l)
- Reduced haemopexin (normal range 0.5 to 1.0 g/l)
- Increased plasma LDH (up to 800 IU/l) (N = 207 IU/l)
- Evidences of intravascular haemolysis
  Haemoglobinaemia (100–200 mg/dl in HA, normal <0.6 mg/dl)
  Haemoglobinuria
  Methaemoglobinaemia/methaemalbuminaemia
  Increased urine and faecal urobilinogen
  Decreased glycosylated haemoglobin
- Evidences of extravascular haemolysis
  Positive Coomb's test
  Splenomegaly

Evidence for compensatory erythroid hyperplasia

Peripheral smear

- Reduced haemoglobin
- Elevated reticulocyte count—marked polychromasia
- Nucleated RBCs

Bone marrow

- Erythroid hyperplasia
- Reduced M/E ratio

Radiological changes

- Deforming changes in the skull and long bones—frontal bossing

Evidences of red cell damage

- Spherocytosis—HS, immune HA
- Increased red cell fragility
- Fragmented RBCs
- Schistocytes—mechanical damage
- Heinz bodies, bite/blister cells
- Compensated erythroid hyperplasia
- Compensated haemolytic state: A state of haemolysis in which the resulting increased erythrocyte production is able to keep up with accelerated RBC destruction, thus preventing development of anaemia.
- Reticulocytosis
- Macrocytosis/polychromasia
- nRBCs in peripheral blood
- Leucocytosis
- Normoblastic erythroid hyperplasia—bone marrow

Reduced red cell lifespan

Measurement of red cell survival no longer routinely done—Cr 51(N t½ = 25–35 days)

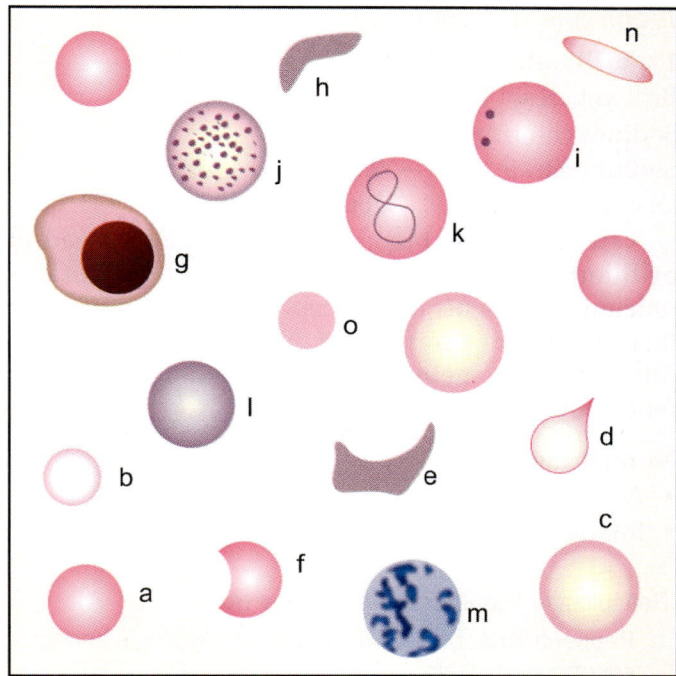

Fig. 2.12: Various red blood cells (poikilocytes): (a) Normal RBC (b) Microcyte; (c) Macrocyte; (d) Tear drop cell; (e) Schistocyte; (f) Bite cell; (g) Nucleated RBC; (h) Sickle cell; (i) Howell-Jolly body; (j) Basophilic stippling; (k) Cabot ring; (l) Poly-chromatophilic cell; (m) Reticulocyte; (n) Pencil-shaped cell; (o) Spherocyte

Some of the important investigations are given below.

1. Reticulocyte Count

This count is one of the important investigations in diagnosis of haemolytic anaemia. It must be remembered that the reticulocytes are juvenile red cells. They contain remains of ribosomes and ribonucleic acids which are present in large amounts in nucleated precursors. Ribosomes and RNA material react with certain dyes: Such as brilliant cresyl blue and new methylene blue to form a blue precipitate of granules or filaments. This reaction takes place in supravital stains. In Romanowsky stained smears, the reticulo-cytes take up diffusely basophilic tint. Most immature reticulocytes have the largest amount of granules and filaments, whereas less immature cells have least granules and filaments.

The number of reticulocytes reflects the erythro-poietic activity. After the cells have been released from the bone marrow, within one day they mature into RBCs. In some cases, increased erythopoietin stimuli result in premature release of reticulocytes with longer time of maturation in circulation. In such cases, reticulocyte maturation time and corrected reticulocyte count are to be deduced by using plasma iron turn over data.

Technique of Reticulocyte Count

1% brilliant cresyl blue

Brilliant cresyl blue	– 1.0 g
Sodium chloride	– 0.7 g
Sodium citrate	– 0.6 g
Distilled water	– 100 ml

New methylene blue can also be used instead of brilliant cresyl blue. New methylene blue stains reticulum filaments more deeply and more uniformly than the brilliant cresyl blue. New methylene blue is different from methylene blue; the latter is a poor reticulocyte stain.

Normal range:

- Adults and children—0.2 to 2.0%
- Infants—2 to 6%

Notes

Reticulocyte should be differentiated from:

1. Pappenheimer bodies which are usually single and less commonly multiple.
2. HbH undergoes denaturation with brilliant cresyl blue or even with new methylene blue.
3. Heinz bodies are stained lighter than reticulocytes with new methylene blue stain.

Reticulocytes also can be counted employing fluorescent microscopy. In that case, one volume of acridine orange to one volume of blood is mixed for 2 minutes, and then make smears and observe under fluorescent microscopy.

Procedure for Demonstration of Reticulocytes

2–3 drops of new methylene blue and equal drops of blood are added to 75 × 10 mm glass or plastic tube. After mixing well keep at 37°C in an incubator for 15–20 minutes. Mix well again before preparing smears; smears should be well spread and the cells should be well stained. Interpret under oil immersion.

Counting of Reticulocytes (Fig. 2.13)

Adjustable diaphragms, paper or cardboard diaphragms could be used for counting the reticulocytes. In paper or cardboard diaphragms, circle/square is cut and inserted in the eyepiece. RBCs counted with this diaphragm should be roughly 50. Such 20 fields are observed, so that roughly 1000 RBCs are inspected. In all these 20 fields, the reticulocytes ('n' cells) are counted.

Calculation

In 1000 RBCs = 'n' reticulocytes

For 100 RBCs = 100 × n /1000

The result is expressed in percentage.

Example: In 20 fields (1000 RBCs), 20 reticulocytes are counted.

Hence, reticulocytes count is: (100 × 20)/1000 = 2%.

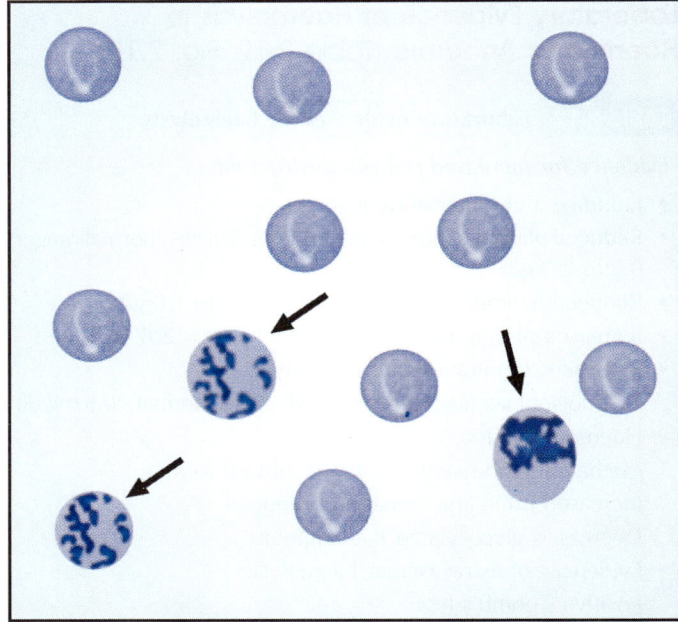

Fig. 2.13: Reticulocytes (arrows)

Corrected Reticulocyte Count

Counting of circulating reticulocytes is the simplest and very reliable sign of accelerated erythrocyte production.

The percentage of reticulocytes can increase either because there are more reticulocytes in the circulation or because there are fewer mature cells. In anaemias, however, some prefer to correct the reticulocyte count by multiplying the percentage of reticulocytes by patient's haematocrit and then dividing the result by normal haematocrit.

Corrected reticulocyte count = Reticulocyte percentage × Patient's haematocrit/0.45

However, corrected counts are not the perfect indices of production, as the percentage of reticulocytes could be altered by premature release from the marrow (shift). A reticulocyte production index (RPI) has been proposed to correct this shift.

RPI = Corrected reticulocyte count / 2 (maturation time correction)

2. Sickling Phenomenon

This test detects the presence of Hb-S; because of the decreased solubility of the abnormal haemoglobin at low oxygen tension (Fig. 2.14).

Methods: The two methods followed are:

i. Mix equal volume of blood and freshly prepared 2% sodium metabisulphite (0.2 g in 10 ml distilled water) on a slide. Place a cover slip. Seal the coverslip edges with vaseline or paraffin wax. Inspect for the resulting sickling under low power.

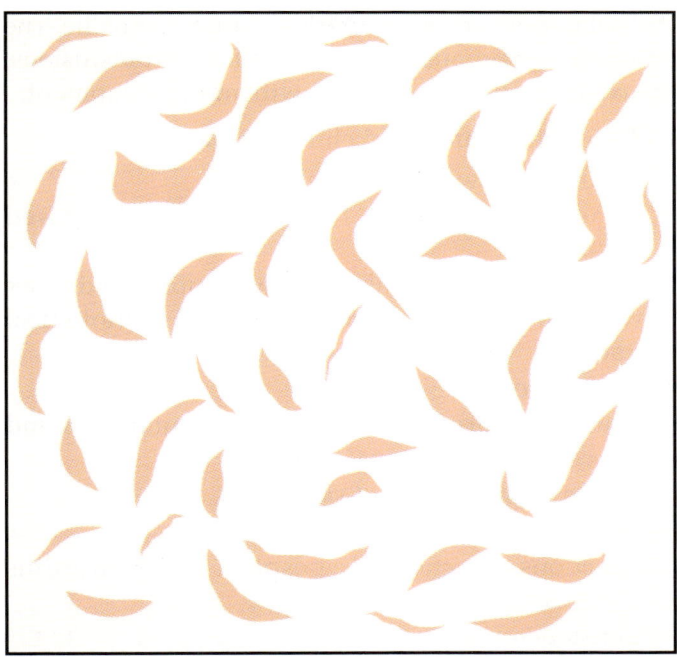

Fig. 2.14: Sickling (schematic)

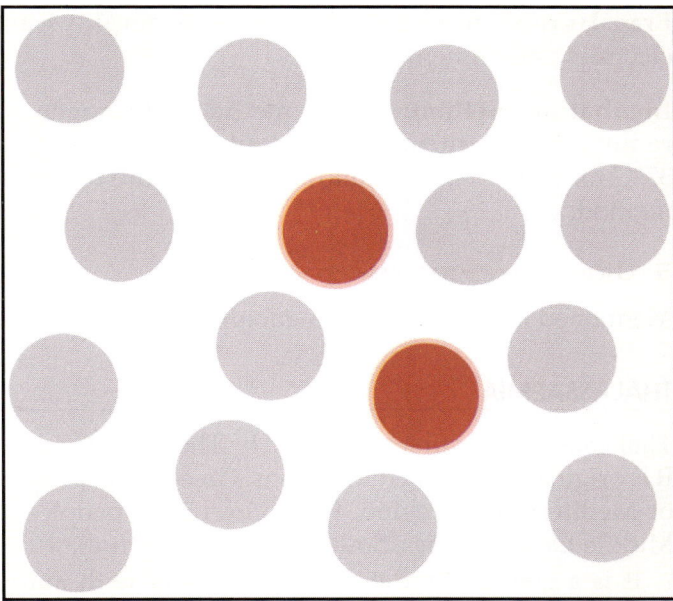

Fig. 2.15: Cells with foetal Hb and normal cells as ghost cells (schematic)

ii. Two volumes of 0.114 M-sodium dithionite ($Na_2S_2O_4$) are mixed with three volumes of 0.114 M-disodium hydrogen phosphate (Na_2HPO_4) to give a final pH of 6.8. Sodium dithionite solution freshly prepared should be added to disodium hydrogen phosphate just before use. About 50 μl of the reagent is mixed with 10 μl of blood, then seal the sides of the coverslip and observed for sickling.

Sickling is visible immediately in HbS disease and within about 60 minutes in HbS trait. If this test is positive, then haemoglobin electrophoresis should be undertaken.

3. Foetal Haemoglobin

i. Alkali haematin method

ii. Acid elution method: Kleihaur, Braun and Betke in 1957 introduced this method. This method detects HbF containing cells; and their detection in maternal circulation has provided valuable information on the pathogenesis of haemolytic disease of the newborn. It must be noted that the HbF containing cells resist acid elution better than the normal cells. They appear as darkly staining cells amongst pale staining ghost cells. Occasional cells (reticulocytes) stain to an intermediate degree and are less easy to evaluate (Fig. 2.15).

4. Osmotic Fragility (OF)

The rate of haemolysis is determined by the structure of the red cells. If the red cells are placed in 0.85% salt solution, the water neither enters nor leaves the cells. At lower concentrations of salt, the water enters the cells, eventually swells, ruptures and haemolyse the cells. When the rate of haemolysis is increased; the fragility of red cells is said to be increased. Similarly, when the rate of haemolysis is decreased, the fragility of the red cells is said to be decreased (Table 2.13).

Methods

Following are the different methods to test for osmotic fragility.

Sanford method: Blood is added to graded series of 12 hypotonic salt solutions; the extent of haemolysis is noted after a period of 2 hours.

Dacie method: Add heparinised blood to graded series of 12 hypotonic salt solutions buffered to pH of 7.4 and allow them to stand for 30 minutes. Centrifuge, read the degree of haemolysis spectrophotometrically and plot the percentage of haemolysis against the percentage of salt concentrate.

Table 2.13	Causes of increased and decreased OF
OF increased	**OF decreased**
Spherocytosis	Iron deficiency anaemia
Aquired autoimmune haemolytic anaemia	Thalassaemia major
Erythroblastosis foetalis	Sickle cell anaemia
Burns	Obstructive jaundice
Chemical poisons	Polycythemia vera
	Haemoglobin 'C' disease

Fragiligraph method: This method employs an electronic instrument.

Incubation method: In this method, fibrinogen is removed; then incubate the defibrinated blood at 37°C for 24 hours, then follow the procedure of Dacie method.

5. Other Investigations

Mentioned later in specific haemolytic anaemia topics.

THALASSAEMIA

Thalassaemia was first recognised by Thomas B. Cooley. It is originally described in Italians, Greeks, and people of Mediterranean region. It also occurs in people of Middle East countries, South East Asia and India.

It is a genetically determined disorder with auto-somal dominant inheritance. There will be reduction in the rate of synthesis of normal haemoglobin polypeptide chains. Thus, there is less amount of adult haemoglobin (HbA).

Classification

Normally, alpha and beta chains are produced under separate genetic control and in normal state the synthesis is balanced. There are two main groups of thalassaemia—one affecting synthesis of alpha chains (α thalassaemia) and the other affecting beta chains (β thalassaemia).

Pathogenesis

In β thalassaemia, there is less amount of Hb-A. There is production of gamma and delta chains, thus there is increased production of Hb-F and Hb-A2. Due to lack of β chains, the alpha chains accumulate, aggregate and interfere in erythroid cell maturation and function, resulting in premature destruction of RBCs.

In α thalassaemia, the levels of HbA, Hb-F and HbA2 are reduced. The beta and gamma chains accumulate and form Hb H (β_4) and Hb Barts (gamma 4). α thalassaemia and β thalassaemia are inherited co-dominantly and have homozygous and heterozygous states.

Clinical Features

Beta thalassaemia occurs in main two forms—β thalassaemia major and β thalassaemia minor. β thalassaemia major, also called Cooley's anaemia, is usually a severe illness characterised by total suppression of beta chains. β thalassaemia minor or trait is mild form. The third form, if the severity falls in between the two, it is thalassaemia intermedia. These do not require transfusions or may require sporadically.

Thalassaemia major manifests by first year of life. The anaemia is insidious. With regular blood transfusions, the child can have normal growth and development.

Inadequately transfused child can have:

- Retarded growth and development
- Anaemia—weakness, lethargy, fever, decreased appetite
- Changes in the skeletal system with mongoloid facies with thinning of cortical bone and pathological fractures
- Osteoporosis
- Extramedullary haemopoiesis can form masses and can compress the spinal cord.
- Brown pigmentation of skin
- Hepatosplenomegaly
- Infections (functional hyposplenism), pericarditis due to streptococcal infection
- Gallstones
- Bleeding tendencies
- Secondary leukopenia and thrombocytopenia
- Cardiac failure
- Recent years, numerous reports of thrombotic complications—possibly procoagulant phospholipids are exposed on RBCs and platelets and haemostatic system is activated. Also endothelial injury and iron overload are possible pathological mechanisms.

The consequences of repeated transfusions like iron accumulation in liver, heart, pancreas, etc., haemo-chromatosis with organ dysfunction can develop and death is usually by 2–3 decades. Pancreatic haemo-siderosis can lead to diabetes mellitus and cirrhosis develops with deposition of iron in liver. Cardiac haemosiderosis leads to arrhythmias, heart block and chronic congestive heart failure.

Bone Changes

- Hyperplastic marrow
- Frontal bossing and maxillary hypertrophy
- Hair-on-end appearance of skull on X-ray

Laboratory Findings (Fig. 2.16)

- Microcytic hypochromic anaemia (Hb of 3–9 g/dl), anaemia is severe
- Anisopoikilocytosis
- Nucleated RBCs
- Polychromasia (reticulocytes increased)
- Schistocytes, dacrocytes, ovalocytes, target cells
- Basophilic stippling
- Decreased MCV, MCH, MCHC, PCV
- HbF and HbA2: Increased in beta thalassaemia
- Decreased osmotic fragility.

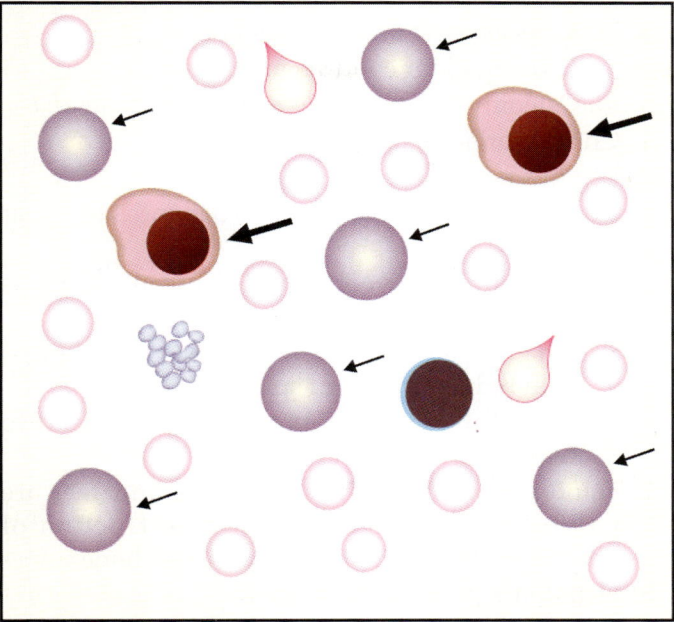

Fig. 2.16: Peripheral smear in thalassaemia major (thick arrow—nucleated RBCs, thin arrow—polychromatophilic cells)

- Increased serum uric acid
- Normal free RBC protoporphyrin
- Necked eye single test tube red cell osmotic fragility (NESTROF) test **positive in thalassaemia minor**
- Serum hepcidin: Reduced

Bone Marrow

- Normoblastic erythroid hyperplasia
- Increased macrophages
- Inclusion bodies in normoblast—methyl violet
- Prussian blue stain—abundance of iron

Lab findings—Hb electrophoresis: The following procedures can be done.
- Citrate agar electrophoresis at alkaline or acid pH
- Capillary electrophoresis
- Automated high performance liquid chromatography
- Isoelectric focusing
- Globin chain electrophoresis

HEREDITARY SPHEROCYTOSIS

Hereditary spherocytosis (HS) has autosomal dominant inheritance. Primarily, the red cells have membrane skeletal disorder of vertical protein interaction. There is defective or absent spectrin molecules, protein 4.2, ankyrin and band 3 protein. Most common amongst these are deficiency of spectrin and ankyrin.

Mechanism

In hereditary spherocytosis, the common defect is spectrin deficiency and spectrin lacks the ability to attach to protein 4.1. Functionally, it is associated with increased permeability to sodium, which passively enters and actively sent out of the cells. This requires ATP. Hypoxia, glucose deprivation and reduced deformity of the cells are the main problems in these cells than the normal ones. These RBCs are delayed in the splenic sinusoids for longer time, with loss of cell membrane with sphering and more rigidity.

Laboratory Findings

1. Moderate/mild/no anaemia
2. Reticulocytosis (5–20%)
3. Nucleated RBCs
4. The peripheral blood smear shows characteristic **microspherocytes**, which appear small, dark, round with no central pallor and decreased diameter
5. Polychromasia
6. Normal/decreased MCV
7. Increased MCHC—hyperhaemoglobin
8. Hyperbilirubinaemia
9. Negative antiglobulin test
10. Increased osmotic fragility (OF)
11. Mild cases with incubation, OF is increased. Blood incubated for 24 hrs at 37°C. Normal RBCs also show increased fragility on incubation—due to swelling. HS cells lose membranes more readily than normal RBCs when incubated. This test has increased sensitivity and is the most reliable diagnostic test for HS.
12. Autohaemolysis
13. Cryohaemolysis

Other tests:

1. Glycerol lysis test
2. Flow cytometry analysis of red cell labelling with eosin-5′-maleimide: Lower intensity of red cells in HS cells than red cells in other HA. This has high specificity and sensitivity.

Autohaemolysis test: This is a screening test for HA with membrane and enzyme defects.

It measures spontaneous haemolysis of blood which is incubated at 37°C for 48 hrs. Blood is incubated at 37°C for 24–48 hrs. After 24 hrs, thoroughly mix the contents by gently swirling. After 48 hrs, estimate PCV, Hb and estimate spontaneous lysis by colourimetry or spectrometry at 540 nm. Normal—0.2 to 2% lysis is seen at 48 hrs. With added glucose—0 to 0.9% lysis is seen at 48 hrs.

Cryohaemolysis: This is specific for hereditary spherocytosis. The cryohaemolysis is dependent on molecular defects of RBC membrane. HS cells are particularly sensitive to cooling at 0°C in hypertonic saline. Normal—3 to 15% lysis, HS—>20% lysis.

Glycerol lysis test: This is the time taken for 50% haemolysis of a blood sample in a buffered hypotonic saline glycerol mixture. Glycerol retards the osmotic swelling of red cells. EDTA blood (20 µl) is diluted in a solution of 9.3 mmol of sodium phosphate and buffered glycerol solution (pH 6.90). Fall in absorbance at 625 nm is measured. Rate of haemolysis is measured.

Optical density to fall to half of initial value (AGLT) is >30 min for normal RBCs and for HS cells <5 min.

SICKLE CELL ANAEMIA

Sickle cell anaemias are hereditary disorders in which red cells contain HbS. Haemoglobin-S differs from HbA in substitution of valine for glutamic acid in 6th position from the N-terminal end of beta chains. Homozygous state manifests early in life than the trait.

Geographical Distribution and Prevalence

HbS is prevalent in Africa, Mediterranean countries, and India. Black population of USA and Latin America has this gene. In India, it is found in Orissa, Andra Pradesh and Madhya Pradesh.

HbS begins to sickle at oxygen tension 50–60 mmHg. HbS cells are sensitive to pH. The decrease in pH from 7.4 to 7.2 results in:

1. Failure of sodium and potassium pump. Sodium enters and potassium leaves the cells.
2. There is increased calcium ion concentration.
3. RBCs get sickled.
4. Sickled RBCs abnormally adhere to endothelial cells
5. In deoxygenated condition, the viscosity of plasma proteins increases.

Clinical Features

Following are the clinical features:
1. Dactilitis and pain
2. Acute chest syndrome
3. Priapism
4. CNS events
5. Aplastic crisis: Due to parvovirus infection
6. Haemolytic crisis
7. Veno-occlusive crisis
8. Sequestration crisis
9. There is increased susceptibility to infections due to hypofunctioning of spleen.

10. Infections:
    i. *S. pneumoniae* until 5 years of age
    ii. *E. coli* in older children and adults
    iii. Osteomyelitis: *Staphylococcus* and *Salmonella*
11. Chronic organ damage
12. Leg ulcers
13. Common age of presentation is 3 months to 1 year of age.
14. The height and weight are reduced. There is delayed puberty.
15. Spleen gradually enlarges. After 5–6 years, there is gradual reduction size of spleen.
16. Multiple infarcts and fibrosis of spleen lead to decreased size (autospenectomy).
17. Hand and foot syndrome: Hands and feet are painful and swollen. There is destruction of phalanges, metacarpal and metatarsal bones.
18. Hepatomegaly and gallstones
19. Cardiomegaly with systolic murmurs

Laboratory Investigations (Fig. 2.17)

1. Haemoglobin: Low (5–10 g/dl)
2. HbF: Positive
3. TC: Increased (20–$30 \times 10^9/l$)
4. Platelets: Normal or increased
5. Peripheral smear: Usually normocytic normochromic anaemia, with normal MCV and MCHC. With deoxygenated states, sickled cells may be present.
6. Occasional target cells and Howell-Jolly bodies are present.
7. Reticulocytes may range 10–20%.
8. ESR: Low as with sickled cells rouleaux formation does not take place.
9. Serum folate and red cell folate levels are low.
10. Serum haptoglobin and hemopexin: Low.
11. Serum iron and ferritin and transferritin saturation: Increased

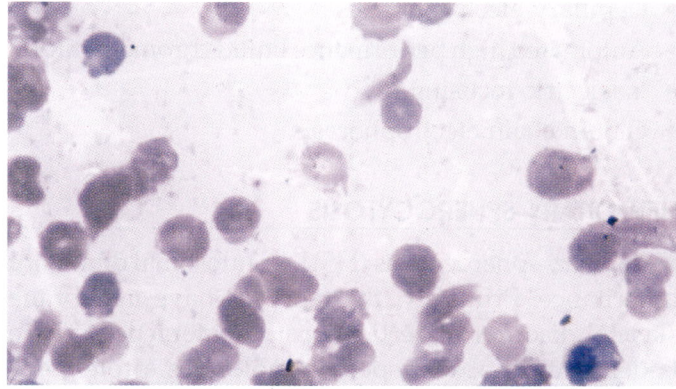

Fig. 2.17: Peripheral smear in sickle cell anaemia. Note sickled RBCs, nucleated RBC and increased polychromatophilic cells

12. Free haemoglobin and methaemalbumin: May be present.
13. Sickle test: Positive
14. Haemoglobin solubility tests: Positive
15. Family studies
16. Hb electrophoresis for HbS and HbA

Sickling test: Refer to investigations in HA.

Solubility test: Sickle cell Hb is insoluble in deoxygenated state in a solution of dithionate in phosphate buffer. Crystals formed refract light and solution to appear turbid. Positive test—HbS. The test does not differentiate between homozygous and heterozygous states.

OTHER HAEMOLYTIC ANAEMIAS

Autoimmune Haemolytic Anaemia, G6PD Deficiency Haemolytic Anaemia and Paroxysmal Nocturnal Haemoglobinuria (PNH)

Autoimmune Haemolytic Anaemia

These are haemolytic anaemias due to development of antibodies directed against antigens on the surface of patients own cells.

These antibodies are usually IgG type and less commonly IgM or IgA and some bind complement.

Autoimmune haemolytic anaemia can be due to following causes:
1. Idiopathic
   a. Warm antibodies: IgG and C3 or Only IgG DCT positive
   b. Cold antibodies: Paroxysmal cold haemoglobunuria (PCH), cold haemagglutination disease (CHAD)
2. Secondary
   Drugs: M-dopa, mefenamic acid, L-dopa, procainamide
   These act by two mechanisms:
   i. Drug adsorption on the RBC surface and antibodies are formed against this.
   ii. Drug combines with proteins and antibodies formed against this complex on the surface, activates complement.
   Red cells coated with IgG and C3 or only with IgG are destroyed by the spleen (extravascular destruction. CHAD is associated with malignant lymphoma, CLL, SLE, Waldenstorm's macroglobulinaemia, infectious mononucleosis, and mycoplasma.

G6PD Deficiency Haemolytic Anaemia

Glucose-6-phosphate dehydrogenase (G6PD) enzyme is required to generate nicotinamide adenine dinucleotide phosphate (NADPH) in pentose phosphate shunt pathway. NADPH is required:

1. To get rid of oxygen free radicals, thus to protect red cells from oxidative stress.
2. To keep sulfhydryl groups of haemoglobin in reduced state.

G6PD deficiency is an X-linked recessive disorder.

These patients can have non-immune haemolytic anaemia when exposed to the following:
1. Fava beans
2. Drugs and chemicals:
   • Oxidant drugs: Dapsone, quinine
   • Antimalarials: Primaquine, chloroquine, mepacrine
   • Antipyretics: Phenacetin, aspirin, probenecid
   • Antibiotics: Sulfonamides, chloramphenicol, cotrimoxazole

Diagnosis: HA due to G6PD is suspected in following situations:
• Prolonged neonatal jaundice causing kernicterus is probably due to G6PD deficiency.
• Haemolysis due to:
   – Infections
   – Drugs
   – Chemicals

Classification (WHO)
• Class I: Less than 10% activity, severe deficiency with chronic HA
• Class II: Less than 10% activity, severe deficiency with intermittent haemolysis
• Class III: 10–60% activity, mild deficiency, haemolysis with stressors only
• Class IV: Non-deficient, no sequelae
• Class V: Increased enzyme activity, no sequelae

Investigations
• Hb: Low
• Reticulocyte count: Increased
• PS: Haemolytic anaemia with presence of bite cells
• Heinz body stained with supravital stains: Crystal violet, new methylene blue, bromocresol green
• Lactate dehydrogenase: Increased
• Haptoglobin: Reduced
• Direct antiglobulin test: Negative
• Brilliant cresyl blue reduction test
• Methaemoglobin reduction test (MRT): Positive with deficiency of G6PD
• Ascorbate cyanide test (ACT)
• Cytochemical test on PS

- Beutler fluorescent spot test: Identifies NADPH produced by G6PD under UV light. In G6PD, it should be absent.
- Quantitative G6PD enzyme assay
- Detection of gene mutation

Brilliant cresyl blue reduction test: Patient's blood hemolysate + G6PD + NADP + brilliant cresyl blue, incubate. If G6PD present, NADP → NADPH which turns blue colour of brilliant cresyl blue → Colourless. Time taken is inversely proportional to the amont of G6PD present. The test is done along with controls (normal blood). It is a specific test for G6PD deficiency.

Methylene blue reduction test: Sodium nitrite converts Hb to Hi (meth HB). Adding methylene blue should stimulate pentose phosphate pathway to produce G6PD and reduce methaemoglobin. But in G6PD methaemoglobin persists. Control blood—red colour, blood with G6PD—brown colour.

Ascorbate cyanide test: G6PD deficient cells develop inclusion bodies, while normal cells do not. G6PD-deficient cells cannot reduce hydrogen peroxide.

Procedure: Patient's blood + Sodium ascorbate + Sodium cyanide + glucose, incubate.

Sodium ascorbate + Hb → H_2O_2. Sodium cyanide inhibits RBC catalase (inhibitor of H_2O_2 formation). Using glucose, RBC converts H_2O_2 → H_2O by action of G6PD.

In cells deficient with G6PD, methaemoglobin forms which is brown colour. It is a most sensitive screening test for detecting heterozygotes of G6PD deficiency. It is not a specific test as it is positive in PNH, defects of HMP shunt and PK deficiency.

Paroxysmal Nocturnal Haemoglobinuria (PNH)

It is uncommon disorder characterised by chronic haemolytic anaemia with intermittent haemoglobinuria.

Pathogenesis: It is an acquired stem cell mutation defect, there is defect is in cell membrane. With a mutated gene for phosphatidylinositol glycan complement A (PIGA), there is deficiency of glycophosphatidylinositol (GPI) on the red cell membrane. GPI serves as anchoring proteins, the important ones which inhibit complement being CD59 and CD55. It is life-threatening and intracorpuscular membrane disorder. It is characterised by destruction of RBCs. In these patients, there is haemolysis of red cells by complement activation which are triggered by acidosis.

CD55 is also called inhibitor of decay accelerating factor (DAF). With the absence of CD55, there is formation of C3 convertase (C4bC2a). CD59 is a membrane inhibitor for reactive lysis (MIRL). It protects the membrane from attack by C5–C9 complex. PNH is usually associated with aplastic anaemia and MDS.

Classification of PNH
- PNH I: Normal expression of anchoring proteins
- PNH II: Partial expression of anchoring proteins
- PNH III: Negative expression of anchoring proteins

Clinical features: Following are the clinical features:
1. PNH commonly appears in third or fourth decade and affects both sexes equally.
2. Onset is insidious, and presents with symptoms of anaemia, most often with haemoglobinuria (cola-coloured urine).
3. Haemolysis occurs typically during sleep, whether sleep is during day or night.
4. PNH has a clinical triad of haemolytic anaemia, bone marrow failure and venous thrombosis.
5. Attacks of haemolysis are precipitated by stress, infection, pregnancy, vaccination, menstruation.

Investigations
- Hb: Low
- Peripheral smear: Normocytic hypochromic anaemia or microcytic hypochromic anaemia or aplastic anaemia
- Bone marrow: Normoblastic hypercellular or aplastic reticulocytosis
- Coomb's test: Negative
- Unconjugated bilirubin: Increased
- Free haemoglobin in blood: Increased
- Methaemoglobin: Increased
- Serum haptoglobin: Low
- Serum LDH: Increased
- Urine: Urobilinogen—increased, haemoglobin—present, iron—present, tubular epithelial cells
- Ham's test: Postive
- Sucrose lysis test: Postive

Other tests
1. Gel card test for CD55 and CD59
2. Monoclonal antibodies to GPI-AP flow cytometry for CD55 and CD59 expression
3. Fluorescent aerolysin (FLAER): Aerolysin is a bacterial toxin that binds to RBCs via PGI anchors and initiates haemolysis. A modified non-haemolytic molecule of aerolysin toxin can detect PNH cells.

Ham's acidified test: The principle of the test is, the cells undergo lysis in acidified serum of the patient's own serum or from another normal person at 37°C. About 10–50% lysis is observed in positive test. The activation of complement occurs though alternate pathway.

Sucrose lysis test: PNH cells lyse when suspended in isotonic solution of sucrose, if serum is present. Take one part of patient's whole blood and nine parts of sucrose solution. Incubate for 30 min at 37°C. Observe the supernatant for haemolysis. Lysis of more than 10% indicates positive test.

PANCYTOPENIA, APLASTIC ANAEMIAS AND BONE MARROW FAILURE SYNDROMES
(Fanconi's Anaemia and Pure Red Cell Aplasia)

Pancytopenia

When anaemia, leukopenia and thrombocytopenia are simultaneously present, it is termed as pancytopenia.

Causes

1. Central defect with bone marrow
2. Peripheral destruction in spleen

Hypocellular marrow

i. Aplastic anaemia
ii. Fanconi anaemia
iii. Cytotoxic drugs
iv. Radiotherapy
v. MDS hypoplastic
vi. Transfusion associated graft versus host disease (TA-GVHD)
vii. Aplastic crisis in haemolytic anaemia

Cellular marrow

i. Bone marrow infiltration: Lymphomas, macroglobulinaemias, multiple myeloma, metastasis
ii. Hypersplenism
iii. Megaloblastic reaction: Vitamin B_{12} and folic acid deficiency
iv. SLE, Sjögren syndrome, sarcoidosis
v. Infections: Tuberculosis, brucellosis, kala-azar
vi. Miscellaneous: Storage diseases (Gaucher, Niemann-Pick disease)

Primary diseases with cellular marrow

i. Subleukaemic acute leukaemia
ii. Hairy cell leukaemia
iii. Myelofibrosis

iv. PNH
v. MDS
vi. Marrow necrosis

The etiology can be determined from clinical features, blood and bone marrow examination and trephine biopsy.

The relevant details required in investigation of pancytopenia are the following:

1. **History:**
   - Age, sex, occupation, diet
   - Exposure to drugs, chemicals or radiation
   - Bone pain, fever, night sweats, malaise, weight loss, pruritus
   - Splenic enlargement

2. **Physical examination:** Lymph node enlargement, splenomegaly, bone tenderness, tumour or deformity of bone, hepatomegaly, gum hypertrophy, portal hypertension, metastasis to bones especially from lung and prostate cancer.

3. **Laboratory investigations:** Peripheral smear: Note for anisocytosis, poikilocytosis, leukoerythroblastic reaction, increased or decreased granules in neutrophils, hypo- or hypersegmentation of neutrophils and rouleaux formation
   - ESR.
   - Haemogram: All cells reduced.

Additional investigations:
- Bone X-ray: Multiple myeloma, metastasis, lymphomas.
- Chest X-ray: Tuberculosis, carcinoma lung, lymphomas
- Serum acid phosphatase and alkaline phosphatase
- Serum electrophoresis: MM and macraglobulinaemia
- DNA antibody: SLE
- Urinary BJ proteins: Multiple myeloma
- Liver biopsy: Tuberculosis, hypersplenism, lymphomas

Important findings in some of the disorders:
- Myelofibrosis has marked poikilocytosis with tear drop cells and LE reaction.
- MDS: Anaemia, pseudo-Pelger-Huet anomaly and giant platelets.
- Megaloblastic anaemia: Anaemia, hypersegmented neutrophils.

Aplastic Anaemia

It is a serious and chronic disease. It is less common. Ehrlich introduced this term in the year 1888. There is reduced production of blood elements at the bone marrow level.

It has pancytopenia with hypocellular bone marrow without infiltration or fibrosis.

It is a life-threatening bone marrow failure. It is associated with high mortality, if not treated.

To diagnose aplastic anaemia, following, at least two, should be present:

1. Hb: <10 g/dl
2. Platelet count: <50,000/dl
3. Leucocyte count: <1500/dl

Classification of Aplastic Anaemia

Inherited: BM failure syndromes (Fanconi's anaemia, dyskeratosis congenita, Shwachman-Diamond syndrome, Pearson syndrome)

Aquired:

1. Idiopathic
2. Secondary
   a. Physical agents: Irradiation
   b. Chemical agents: Benzene, arsenic
   c. Exposure to cytotoxic drugs
   d. Idiosyncratic drugs: Chloramphenicol, NSAIDs, anticonvulsant drugs, antidiabetics, antithyroid drugs, sulphonamides, antimalarials, chemicals like benzene, heavy metals, etc.
   e. Infections: Infectious mononucleosis (IM), Epstein-Barr virus (EBV), parvovirus B19 (PV-B19), hepatitis virus
   f. Paroxysmal nocturnal haemoglobinuria (PNH)
   g. Immune mediated: Systemic lupus erythematosus (SLE), TA-GVHD

Idiopathic causes account for 70–80% of the aplastic anaemia cases.

Common secondary causes include cytotoxic drugs, irradiation, infections and drug idiosyncrasy.

Idiosyncratic drug reactions: These are unpredictable adverse reactions, dose independent, do not occur in all patients, patient specific, when they occur, they are life-threatening.

Clinical Features

The clinical features of anaemia in general be present, most common being weakness fatigability, lassitude and dyspnoea on exertion.

The bleeding manifestations are due to reduced platelets, e.g. petechiae, epistaxis, menorrhagia, bleeding from gums, GI bleeding and cerebral haemorrhage which is most fatal, if occurs.

Infection due to reduced WBCs is the common finding in these patients.

Investigations

- Hb: <7 g/dl
- PS: Normocytic normochromic anaemia (NNA)/ macrocytic anaemia (MA) with leukopenia and thrombocytopenia and relative lymphocytosis.
- Retic count: Reduced/subnormal.
- Bone marrow and trephine biopsy: Hypocellular/ acellular marrow. Fat cells increased. All the cell series are reduced.
- Plasma cells and lymphocytes are prominent.

Management of aplastic anaemia: Identify and eliminate the causative agent, supportive care, immunosuppressive therapy, and stem cell transplantation.

Bone Marrow Failure Syndromes (BMFS)

These can be inherited or acquired.

The inherited BMFS with pancytopenia are: Fanconi's anaemia, dyskeratosis congenita, Shwachman-Diamond syndrome, Pearson's syndrome.

The inherited BMFS with single cell cytopenias are: Pure red cell aplasia (Diamond-Blackfan syndrome), neutropenia (Kostmann syndrome, Shwachman-Diamond syndrome), thrombocytopenia (amegakaryocytic thrombocytopenia with absent radii—TAR).

The acquired BMFS are: Acquired aplastic anaemia, PNH, secondary pure red cell aplasia (PRCA), myelodysplastic syndrome (MDS) primary and secondary, AML—hypoplastic type, myelofibrosis primary and secondary, due to HIV infection, thrombocytopenia, agranulocytosis due to various causes.

Fanconi's Anaemia

This is a rare AR inherited chronic disorder with bone marrow failure. Mean age of occurrence is 8–9 years. These patients have:

   i. Pancytopenia
  ii. Chromosomal breakages
 iii. Increased cancer susceptibility

Clinical Features

1. Patients may have short stature, microcephaly, hypoplastic thumb, skeletal abnormalities, e.g. micrognathia, broad basal bridge, and renal abnormalities.
2. Bleeding manifestations
3. Infections due to neutropenia
4. Malaise
5. Sore throat

6. Ulceration: Mouth and pharynx
7. Fever
8. Chills and sweating

Important investigation findings include:
1. RBCs are normocytic normochromic with neutropenia and thrombocytopenia.
2. Haemoglobin: May be 7–8 g/dl
3. May develop aplastic anaemia or leukaemia

Pure Red Cell Aplasia (PRCA)

Pure red cell aplasia can be:
1. **Congenital:** Diamond-Blackfan syndrome
2. **Aquired:**
   Primary:
   - Autoimmune (SLE, NHL, transient erythroblastopenia of childhood)
   - Pearson syndrome
   - Idiopathic
   Secondary:
   - Thymoma associated
   - Virus induced (EBV, PV-B19, hepatitis)
   - Drug induced
   - Miscellaneous: Bacterial infections, tuberculosis, idiopathic

Congenital Pure Red Cell Aplasia
(Diamond-Blackfan Syndrome)

The congenital pure red cell aplasia which is also called Diamond-Blackfan syndrome is of AD, AR or sporadic inheritance. There is positive family history. There is progressive anaemia may be within first few weeks of birth and well established by one year of age.

Investigations
- Hb and PCV: Low
- Reticulocyte count: Low
- PS: Macrocytosis
- Bone marrow (BM): Paucity of erythroid series
- Other series: Normal

Clinical Features
- Cleft palate or high-arched palate
- Epicanthal folds
- Ear abnormalities
- Flat nasal bridge
- They have pale skin, sleepiness, irritability, rapid heart beat, heart murmur
- Treatment: Steroids, blood transfusions, stem cell transplant.

ANAEMIA OF CHRONIC DISEASES

In anaemias of chronic diseases, anaemia may be mild to moderate. There is failure to transport iron from reticuloendothelial cells to RBCs. Serum ferritin may be normal or increased. Anaemia of chronic disease can be of multifactorial etiology. The following are the causes:
1. Infections/inflammations
2. Malignancies
3. Collagen vascular diseases
4. Uraemia
5. Endocrine diseases
6. Liver diseases

Pathogenesis

Some of the factors which play role in development of anaemia in chronic diseases can be the following:
1. Haemolysis of senescent RBCs which cannot survive due to stress of fever or cytokines
2. Disturbances in iron homeostasis: Impaired flow of iron from RE system to erythroblasts
3. Reduced erythropoietin (EPO) production
4. Blood loss and haemolysis
5. Hepcidine, an acute phase reactant produced by liver may play role in intestinal iron absorption and iron release from macrophages.
6. Anaemia of renal diseases can be due to:
   - Reduced erythropoietin production
   - Short lifespan in haemodialysis
   - Neocytolysis: Haemolysis of young red cells
   - Infections
   - Haemolysins
7. Malignancies:
   - Due to blood loss in carcinomas
   - Reduced erythropoietin response
   - BM infiltration
   - Impaired renal function
   - Nutritional deficiency because of anorexia, vomiting and dyspepsia
   - Myelosuppressive effect of chemotherapy
8. Liver diseases:
   - GI bleeding
   - Oesophageal varices
   - Haemorrhoids
   - Peptic ulcers
   - Nutritional folate deficiency in alcoholism
   - Hypersplenism
   - Haemolytic anaemia due to increase in membrane cholesterol which undergoes splenic sequestration
   - Depression of erythropoiesis

Investigations

- Hb: Low (8–12 g/dl)
- PS: NNA or MHA
- Serum ferritin: Normal/increased
- Serum iron and TIBC: Decreased
- Acute phase reactants: Increased.

SIDEROBLASTIC ANAEMIA (SA)

These are group of disorders, where marrow shows marked dyserythropoiesis and abnormal intra-mitochondrial accumulation of iron in erythropoiesis. Aqiured causes are common than the inherited causes.

Absorption of Iron

Non-haem iron gets absorbed in duodenum into enterocyte by DMT1 (divalent metal iron transporter 1).

DMT1 is increased in iron deficiency anaemia. Dietary iron is Fe^{+++}, duodenal enzyme ferric reductase reduces it to Fe^{++}. This ion is transported across the basolateral membrane to plasma by ferroportin.

Hephastin again converts Fe^{++} to Fe^{+++} state.

Role of Hepcidin in Iron Regulation

Hepcidin is a iron regulator protein, released by liver. Hepcidin is a peptide of 25 amino acids and is excreted by the kidney. Chronic inflammation releases IL-6 which increases hepcidin production by the hepatocytes.

Hepcidin degrades the receptor (ferroportin) and regulates intestinal iron absorption, plasma iron concentration, and tissue iron distribution. Hepcidin binds to ferroportin which is located on the basolateral surface of the enterocytes and plasma membrane of RE cells. When iron stores are high, hepcidin blocks the release of iron from macrophages, hepatocytes and enterocytes and thus inhibits iron absorption. When iron stores are low, hepcidin expression is suppressed, thus increasing the iron absorption.

Classification of Sideroblastic Anaemias

Hereditary/Congenital Sideroblastic Anaemias

- Heritable: X-linked SA
- Associated with erythropoietic protoporphyria
  - Autosomal
  - Congenital

- Associated with genetic disorders
  - X-linked with ataxia
  - Thiamine responsive SA
  - Myopathy, lactic acidosis and SA
  - Mitochondrial cytopathy (Pearson syndrome)

Aquired Sideroblastic Anaemias

- Primary acquired clonal:
  - RA with ringed sideroblasts
  - RA with ringed sideroblasts and thrombocytosis
  - RA with multilineage dysplasia
- Secondary/reversible:
  - Drugs and chemicals
  - Alcoholism
  - Copper deficiency
  - Inflammatory diseases

X-linked Sideroblastic Anaemia

It is an X-linked AR disorder, males are affected, they are anaemic.

The condition is noted in childhood and adulthood.

Defect is due to mutation of erythroid specific gene called delta-ALA gene.

Didmoad syndrome: It has AR inheritance, is a neuronal degenerative disorder. It is associated with SA, neutropenia and thrombocytopenia. Anaemia responds to thiamine.

Investigations

- Anaemia is moderate to marked.
- RBCs are microcytic and hypochromic.
- MCV and MCH are reduced.
- Serum iron is increased.
- There is complete saturation of iron binding capacity.
- There is increased intestinal absorption.
- Hepcidin is reduced.
- Iron glutted mitochondria present in normoblasts.
- Ringed sideroblasts present (criteria for ringed sideroblasts: Iron granules large, granules >5, should be perinuclear location extending around at least 1/3rd of the nucleus).

Treatment

- Pyridoxine
- Folic acid
- Phlebotomy
- Chelation therapy

SELF-ASSESSMENT EXERCISE

1. 3.2% sodium citrate is used in following laboratory studies:
   A. Coagulation studies
   B. Blood counts
   C. Peripheral smear preparation
   D. Reticulocyte count

2. Which is true about heparin?
   A. Forms complex with antithrombin-3
   B. Chelates calcium
   C. Inhibits protein C
   D. Inhibits protein S

3. Defect of red cell membrane is present in:
   A. Thalassaemia
   B. PNH
   C. Spherocytosis
   D. Microangiopathic haemolytic anaemia

4. AIHA is diagnosed by detecting autoantibodies by:
   A. Direct Coomb's
   B. Indirect Coomb's
   C. IF
   D. ELISA

5. Following is encountered with inherited aplastic anaemia:
   A. Eosinophilia
   B. Fanconi's anaemia
   C. PNH
   D. Dimorphic anaemia

6. Storage form of iron is:
   A. Ferritin
   B. Transferrin
   C. Hepcidin
   D. Ferroportin

7. Iron is absorbed in:
   A. Duodenum
   B. Jejunum
   C. Ileum
   D. Ascending colon

8. Iron absorption is facilitated by:
   A. Hepcidin
   B. Ferroportin
   C. Ferritin
   D. Transferrin

9. Vitamin B_{12} absorption requires all *except*:
   A. IF factor
   B. R factor
   C. Enterocytes receptors
   D. Acidic medium

10. Megaloblastic anaemia is seen in:
    A. Ileal resection
    B. Mentrier disease
    C. Resection of colon
    D. Peptic ulcer

11. Schilling test with less than 10% RA-B_{12} excretion is present in:
    A. Ileal resection
    B. Mentrier disease
    C. Resection of colon
    D. Peptic ulcer

12. In pancreatic disease, following deficiency can be present:
    A. Vitamin B_{12}
    B. Iron
    C. FA
    D. Iron and FA

Answers

1. A	2. A	3. C	4. A	5. B	6. A	7. A	8. A
9. D	10. A	11. A	12. A				

Disorders of White Blood Cells

LEUKOCYTOSIS AND LEUKOPENIA—CAUSES

Causes of Neutrophilia (Fig. 3.1)

- Acute infections with cocci
- Tissue injury—infarctions, burns, surgery and necrosis inducing processes
- Haemorrhage
- Neoplasms
- Stress states and hyperactivity conditions like convulsions, tachycardia, labour, severe colic, delirium—tremens
- Inflammatory disorders—collagen disorders, gout and rheumatic fever
- Metabolic disorders—diabetic ketoacidosis
- Corticosteroid administration
- Miscellaneous causes

Lymphocytosis (Fig. 3.2)

Absolute lymphocyte count of about 4×10^9 cells/l is called lymphocytosis.

Relative lymphocytosis: Lymphocyte count is normal but when neutrophil count is reduced, there appears a relative increase in lymphocytes.

Causes of Lymphocytosis

Viral: Pertussis, mumps, measles, influenza and infectious mononucleosis. Atypical lymphocytosis is observed in EB virus infection, CMV infection and infective hepatitis. In atypical lymphocytosis, enlarged pleomorphic lymphocytes are observed. Turk cell is a reactive lymphocyte with basophilic cytoplasm and it resembles plasma cell.

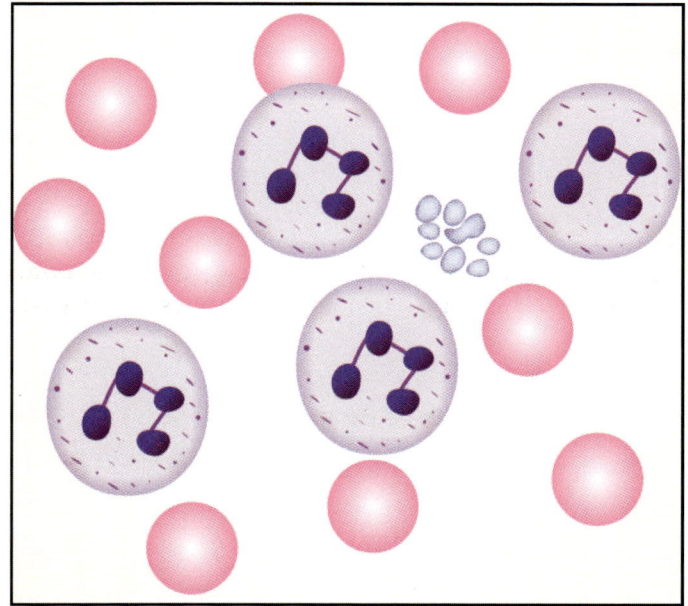

Fig. 3.1: Neutrophilia

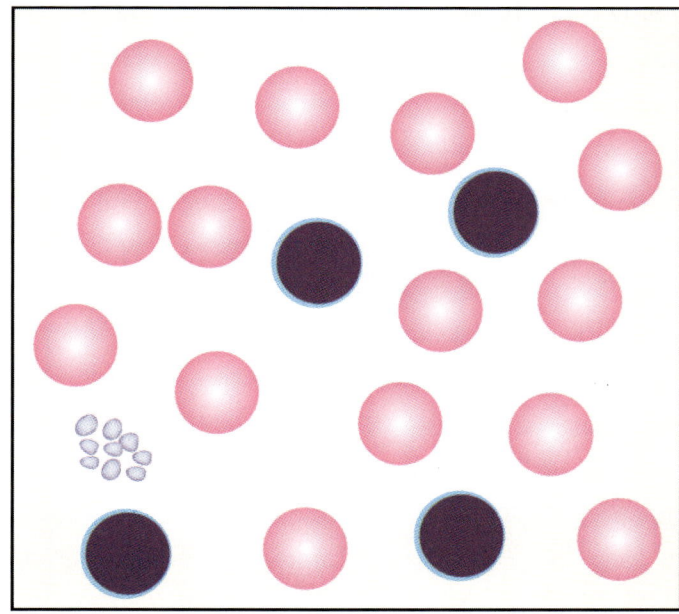

Fig. 3.2: Lymphocytosis

Chronic bacterial infections like tuberculosis, syphilis, typhoid and such other chronic infections.

Eosinophilia (Fig. 3.3)

The eosinophil count in the peripheral blood of normal individuals range between 0.002 and 0.5×10^9 cells/l. In differential count, the eosinophils range between 1 and 6 cells and more than 8 is considered as increase and the absolute count is more than 0.5×10^9 cells/l is called eosinophilia.

Causes of Eosinophilia

- Allergy to extrinsic agents such as vegetables, animal products, parasites, drugs and blood products
- Neoplasms—lymphoproliferative malignancies (Hodgkin's disease), carcinomas
- Certain vasculitis and collagen disorders—polyarteritis nodosa
- Dermatological conditions—pemphigus and dermatitis herpetiformis
- Loeffler's syndrome
- Familial
- Post-splenectomy
- Miscellaneous

Monocytosis

When the absolute monocyte count exceeds the limit of 0.8×10^9 cells/l, then that condition is called monocytosis.

Causes of Monocytosis

- Infections like tuberculosis, malaria, bacterial endo-carditis, typhoid, kala-azar, parasitic and protozoal diseases

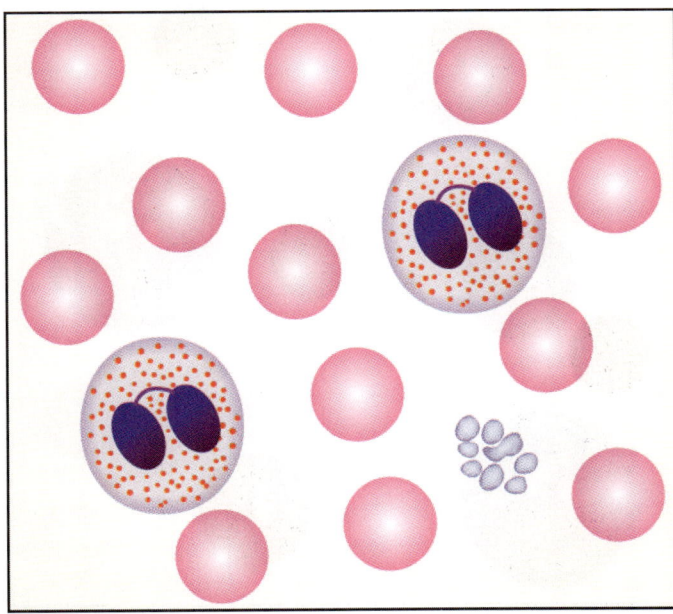

Fig. 3.3: Eosinophilia

- Ulcerative colitis
- Sarcoidosis
- Certain cases of acute myeloid leukaemia
- Chronic myeloid leukaemia
- Myelodysplastic syndrome

Basophilia

Basophils are increased in chronic myeloid leukaemia.

Lymphopenia

Absolute count below the limit of 1.5×10^9 cells/l is called lymphopenia.

Causes of Lymphopenia

- Pancytopenia
- Advanced Hodgkin's disease
- Prodromal phase of viral infections due to depletion of helper T cells, e.g. AIDS
- Corticosteroid therapy

Neutropenia

Causes of Neutropenia

- Conditions that replace normal haemopoietic cells like acute leukaemia, myelofibrosis, lymphoma, multiple myeloma, myelodysplastic syndrome
- Infections—typhoid, viral infections, sepsis
- Megaloblastic anaemia
- Aplastic anaemia
- Iron deficiency anaemia
- Drugs and radiation—marrow depression
- Chronic idiopathic neutropenia
- Hypersplenism
- Cytotoxic therapy
- Cyclic neutropenia

LEUKAEMIAS

Leukaemia is the clonal expansion of a single transformed stem cell resulting in accumulation of immature and non-functional haematopoietic cells in the bone marrow and body organs. Mainly leucocytes are affected.

Etiology and Leukaemogenesis

- Activation of proto-oncogene to oncogene, e.g. t(8;14).
- Formation of chimeric transcription factor t (15;17) RAR/PML transcription repressors block differentiation—AML.
- Formation of fusion protein with enhanced tyrosine kinase activity—t(9;22) BCR/ABL enhanced tyrosine kinase activity.

- Inactivation of tumour suppressor gene pathway-RB1 p53.

Leukaemias are broadly classified as acute or chronic depending upon age of onset, course of disease, clinical presentation. Comparison between acute and chronic leukaemias is given in Table 3.1.

Table 3.1	Comparison of acute and chronic leukaemias	
	Acute	**Chronic**
Age	All ages	Adults and old age
Clinical onset	Sudden	Insidious
Course of disease	Weeks to months	Months to years
Predominant cells	Blasts and few Mature forms	Mature forms
Anaemia	Mild to severe	Mild
Thrombocytopenia	Mild to severe	Mild
WBC count	Variable	Increased

ACUTE LEUKAEMIAS

These are stem cell disorders characterised by malignant neoplastic proliferation of a transformed cell. **Classic triad** of acute leukaemia is **anaemia, infections and bleeding.**

Two major categories are:
1. Acute myeloid leukaemia (AML) or acute non-lymphoid leukaemia
2. Acute lymphoblastic leukaemia (ALL)

Clinical Presentation

Age: Common during 2–10 years of age.

Symptoms: Fatigue, pallor, fever, weight loss, bone pains.

Signs: Hepatosplenomegaly, lymphadenopathy, anaemia, neutropenia, thrombocytopenia.

General Laboratory Findings (Figs 3.4 to 3.6)

Peripheral smear: Leucocyte count usually increased but may be normal or decreased. There can be presence of lymphoblasts or myeloblasts in the peripheral blood. Platelets are usually reduced.

Bone marrow: Hypercellular with lymphoblasts or myeloblasts equal to or >20%.

Other investigations of leukaemias:
1. Hyperuricaemia and increased LDH [due to increased cell turnover]
2. Impairment of renal function [leukaemic infiltration]
3. CNS—frequent site for extramedullary spread, CSF should be analyzed for presence of blasts
4. Cytochemistry
5. Flow cytometry
6. Cytogenetics

Classification of ALL (FAB Classification)

L1: Small, homogenous blasts, scanty cytoplasm, indistinct nucleoli.

L2: Large, heterogenous blasts, indented nuclei, one or more nucleoli, abundant cytoplasm, minimal cytoplasmic vacuolation.

L3: Large, homogenous blasts, abundant basophilic cytoplasm with prominent cytoplasmic vacuolations (Burkitt's lymphoma).

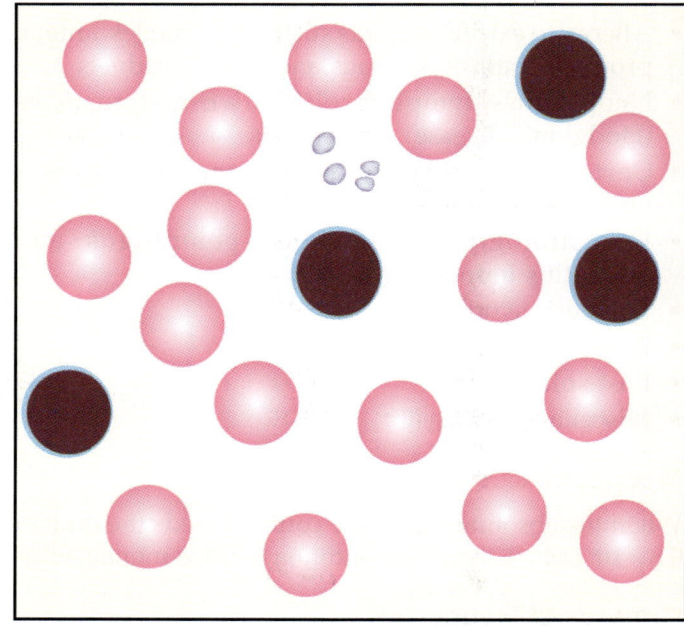

Fig. 3.4: Peripheral smear in acute leukaemia (ALL – L1)

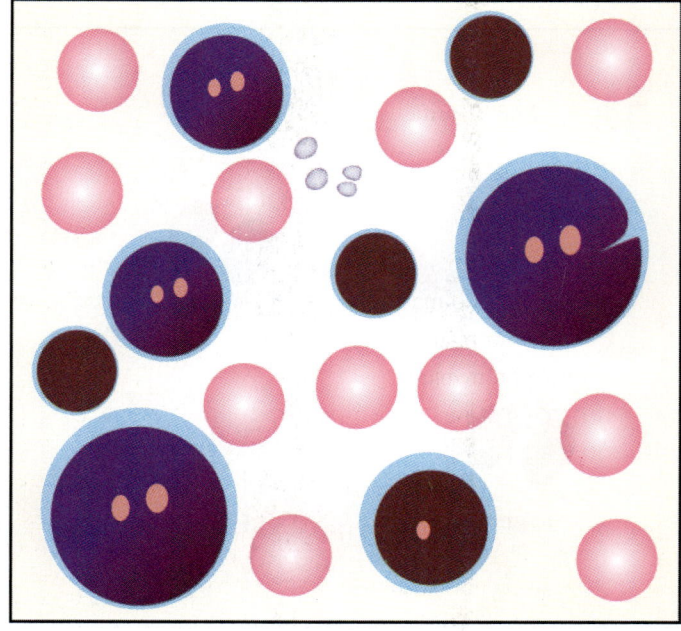

Fig. 3.5: Peripheral smear in acute leukaemia (ALL – L2)

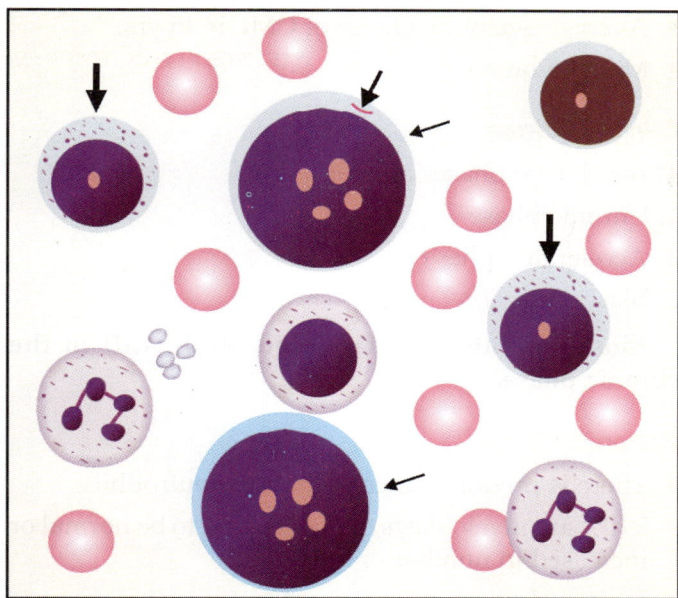

Fig. 3.6: Peripheral smear in acute leukaemia (AML). Note myeloblasts—thin arrow (one myeloblast with Auer rod) and promyelocytes—thick arrow

Acute Myeloid Leukaemia

- The defect primarily affects the common myeloid progenitor cell (CMP).
- Myeloblasts in peripheral blood or bone marrow should be >20%. [WHO, 2001]
- According to the FAB classification, AML is classified as given in Table 3.2.

The 2016 revision to the WHO classification of myeloid neoplasms.[2]

I. AML with recurrent genetic abnormalities:
  - AML with t(8;21) (q22;q22); RUNX1-RUNX1T1
  - AML with inv(16) (p13;q22) or t(16;16) (p13.q22), CBFB/MYH11
  - APML with t(15;17) (q22;12), PML-RARA and variants
  - AML with t(9;11) (p22;q23); MLLT3- MLL
  - AML with t(6;9) (p23;q34); DEK-NUP214
  - AML with inv(3) (q21q26.2); RPN1-EVI1
  - AML (megakaryoblastic) with t(1;22) (p13;q13); RBM15-MKL1
  - AML with BCR-ABL (provisional)
  - AML with mutated NPM1
  - AML with bialleilic mutated CEBPA
  - AML with mutated RUNX1

II. AML with myelodysplasia related changes

III. Therapy related myeloid neoplasms

IV. AML–NOS
  - AML with minimal differentiation
  - AML without maturation
  - AML with maturation
  - Acute myelomonocytic leukaemia
  - Acute monoblastic leukaemia
  - Pure erythroid leukaemia
  - Acute megakaryocytic leukaemia
  - Acute basophilic leukaemia
  - Acute panmyelosis with myelofibrosis

V. Myeloid sarcoma

VI. Myeloid proliferations related to Down syndrome

VII. Blastic plasmacytoid dendritic cell neoplasms

VIII. Acute leukaemia of ambiguous lineage

IX. B lymphoblastic leukaemia/lymphoma

X. T lymphoblastic leukaemia/lymphoma lymphoblastic leukaemia/lymphoma

Table 3.2	FAB classification—acute myeloid leukaemia			
		Morphology	Myeloperoxidase (MPO)	Sudan Black B (SBB)
Mo	Acute myeloblastic leukaemia (AML): Minimally differentiate	>30% blasts; no granules	–ve	–ve
M1	AML with no maturation	>30% blasts, few granules +/- Auer rods	+ve	+ve
M2	AML with maturation	>30% blasts, granules common, + Auer rods	+ve	+ve
M3	Acute promyelocytic leukaemia	>30% blasts, prominent granules, ++ Auer rods	++	++
M4	Acute myelomonoblastic leukaemia	>30% blasts, >20% monocytes, + Auer rods	+	+
M4eos	Acute myelomonocytic leukaemia with eosinophilia	>30% blasts, >20% monocytes, >5% abnormal eosinophils, + Auer rods	+	+
M5 a/b	Acute monoblastic leukaemia With or without maturation	>30% blasts, >80% monoblasts with or without maturation	+/–	+/–
M6	Acute erythroleukaemia	>30% myeloblasts, >50% erythroblasts, + Auer rods	+(myeloblasts)	+(myeloblasts)
M7	Acute megakaryocytic leukaemia	>30% megakaryoblasts, cytoplastic budding +	–	–

Laboratory Findings in AML

Peripheral blood

- **WBCs:** TC—elevated, may exceed 1 lakh/cmm.

  50% of the cases may have normal or decreased counts at the time of presentation

  DC—presence of myeloblasts [WHO >20%]

  Myeloblast in AML—typically 20 µm in diameter. Nucleus composed of dispersed chromatin and variably has 3–4 prominent nucleoli. Cytoplasm may show Auer rod.
- **RBCs:** Decreased in number.
- **Platelets:** Reduced, hypogranular and occasional giant platelets may be present.

Buffy coat smear: Undertaken, if strong suspicion of AML but no blasts in the peripheral smear.

Bone marrow examination: It is typically—hypercellular with predominance of blasts (≥20). The myeloblasts are common. Monoblasts, erythroblasts and megakaryoblasts may be encountered.

Cytochemistry in AML and ALL

Myeloperoxidase stain

- Primary and secondary granules of granulocytic series are positive. Auer rods in myeloblast, other subsequent precursor granulocytes are positive.
- Lymphoblast: Negative

Sudan black B

- Myeloid series cells
- Myeloblasts: Positive
- Lymphoblasts: Negative

Non-specific esterase (with alpha naphthyl acetate as base): Stains monoblasts, promonocytes and monocytes.

Periodic acid-Schiff

- Magenta color
- Lymphoblasts: Block positivity
- Erythroblasts

CHRONIC MYELOID LEUKAEMIA (CML)

It is a **clonal stem cell** disorder characterized by the acquisition of an oncogenic BCR/ABL fusion protein [usually the result of a reciprocal translocation (9;22) (q34;q11)] and by proliferation of granulocytic elements at all stages of differentiation.

- t(9;22) is also referred to as the Philadelphia chromosome.

- Average age of incidence of CML is 45 yrs.
- Men > women

Clinical Phase

Three clinical phases are:

1. Chronic phase
2. Accelerated phase
3. Blast crisis.

Most patients are diagnosed while still in the chronic phase.

Chronic Phase

- There is predominance of mature neutrophils.
- <10% are myeloblasts, platelets tend to be normal or increased in number or low.
- Increased percentage of myelocytes.
- Low leucocyte alkaline phosphatase activity (low LAP score).
- There is basophilia, some patients can have eosinophilia.
- Platelet count normal or increased.

Accelerated Phase

- Myeloblasts: 10–19% in PS or BM
- 20% or more basophils in the PS
- Persistent thrombocytopenia, unrelated to therapy
- Persistent splenomegaly, unresponsive to therapy
- Persistent increasing total count, unresponsive to therapy
- Cytogenic evidence of clonal evolution

Blast Phase

1. Blasts ≥20%
2. Extramedullary blast proliferation
3. Large aggregates/clusters of blasts in the bone marrow

Clinical features indicating a more difficult-to-control marrow proliferative state are suggestive of progression. These include:

1. Rapidly rising WBC count that is more refractory to treatment
2. Increasing splenomegaly
3. Fever, bone pain, and weight loss
4. Laboratory features include more immature cells in the peripheral blood or marrow
5. Increasing eosinophils or basophils
6. The appearance of more chromosome anomalies.

Diagnostic Approach to CML (Figs 3.7 to 3.10 and Table 3.3)

1. Peripheral blood smear and marrow biopsy.
2. Ph+ chromosome by karyotypic analysis or the presence of the BCR-ABL translocation by Southern blot or polymerase chain reaction (PCR) assays confirms the diagnosis.

Peripheral Blood

1. There is a predominance of mature neutrophils.
2. Basophils are increased in number.
3. Increased percentage of myelocytes (so-called myelocyte bulge).

4. <10% are myeloblasts
5. Many patients may also demonstrate eosinophilia.
6. Platelets tend to be normal or increased in number.
7. **Low to absent leucocyte alkaline phosphatase activity (low LAP score)**

Differential Diagnosis of CML[3]

1. Chronic myelomonocytic leukaemia (CMML)
2. Juvenile myelomonocytic leukaemia (JMML)
3. Atypical CML
4. MDS/myeloproliferative diseases, unclassifiable

Differences between chronic myeloid leukaemia and leukaemoid reaction are given in Table 3.3.

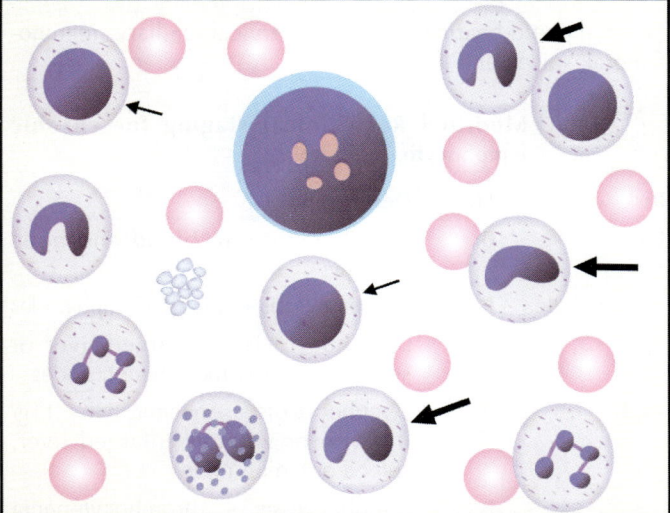

Fig. 3.7: Peripheral smear in CML (thin arrow—myelocytes; thick arrow—metamyelocytes; short arrow—band forms)

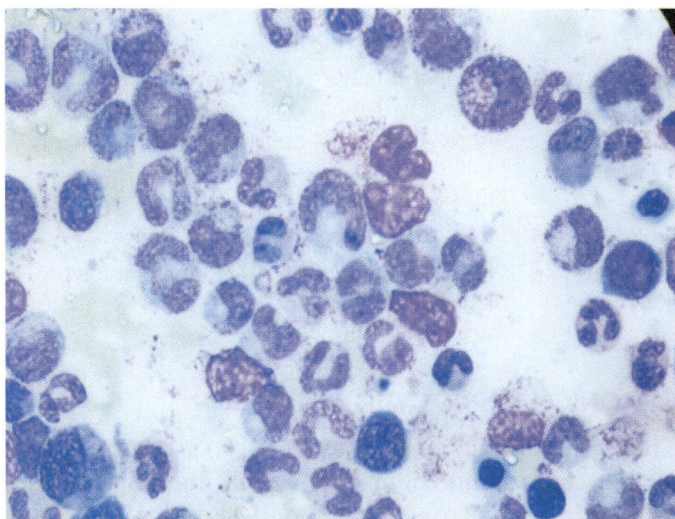

Fig. 3.8: Bone marrow in CML

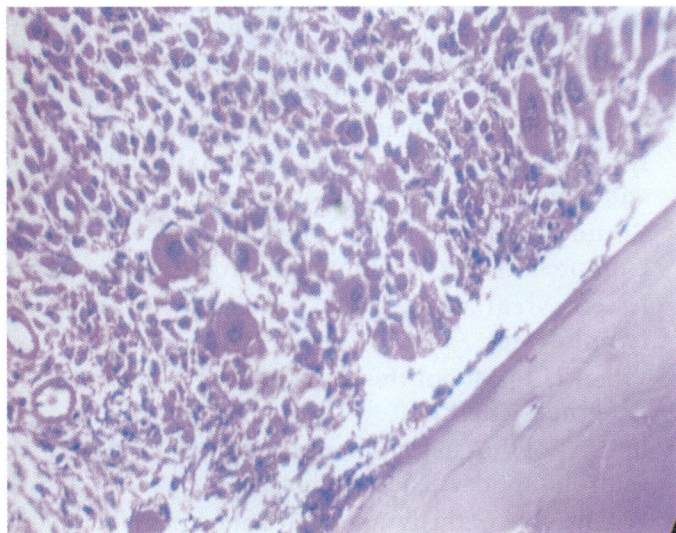

Fig. 3.9: Trephine biopsy in CML (Note plenty of megakaryo-cytes)

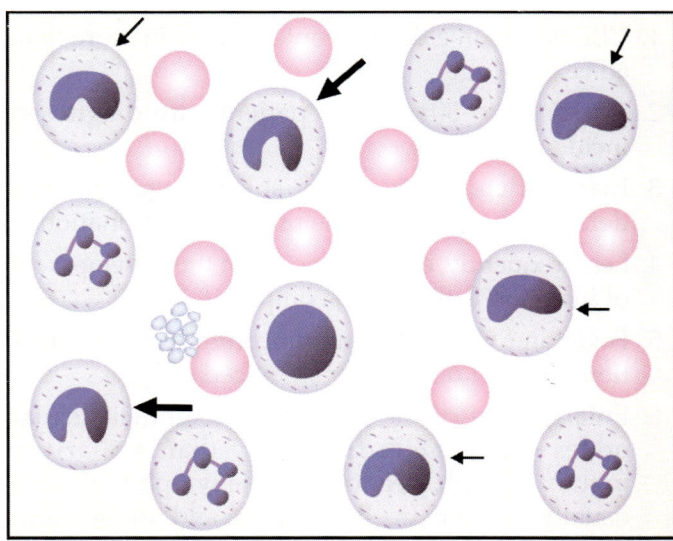

Fig. 3.10: Leukaemoid reaction (Note metamyelocytes—thin arrow; band forms—thick arrow and increased neutrophils) (schematic)

Table 3.3	Differences between chronic myeloid leukaemia and leukaemoid reaction	
Laboratory parameter	**CML**	**Leukaemoid reaction**
Leucocytes	Blasts and promyelocyte in peripheral blood; toxic changes usually absent; eosinophilia and basophilia; neutrophilia with single lobed nuclei and hypogranular forms may be present	Toxic granules; Dohle bodies and vacuoles present; blasts and promyelocytes rare; no absolute basophilia or eosinophilia
Platelets	Often increased with abnormal morphological forms present; occasional micromegakaryocytes	Usually normal
Erythrocytes	Anaemia usually present; variable anisocytosis; poikilocytosis; NRBCs present	Anaemia may be present, but NRBCs not present
LAP/NAP	Low	Increased
Chromosome Karyotype	Ph chromosome or BCR/ABL translocation present	Normal karyotype

CHRONIC LYMPHOCYTIC LEUKAEMIA

Chronic lymphocytic leukaemia (CLL) is characterised by the accumulation of mature-appearing lymphocytes in the blood, marrow, lymph nodes, and spleen. The CLL cells are monoclonal B lymphocytes that express CD19, CD5, and CD23, with weak or no expression of surface immunoglobulin (Ig), CD20, CD79b and FMC7.

Clinical Findings

1. CLL occurs in elderly people usually in more than 60 years of age.
2. About 70 to 80% of the patients are diagnosed incidentally.
3. Lymphadenopathy and/or splenomegaly may be detected during a routine physical examination.
4. Less frequently, enlarged nodes or the development of infection is the initial complaint.
5. Fever and weight loss are uncommon at presentation but may occur with advanced stage.
6. Enlargement of the cervical and supraclavicular nodes occurs more frequently than axillary or inguinal lymphadenopathy. The lymph nodes are usually discrete, freely movable, and non-tender.
7. Usually mild to moderate enlargement of the spleen is present.
8. Enlarged tonsils and mesenteric or retroperitoneal lymphadenopathy is less common.
9. Anaemia and thrombocytopenia occur in later stages.
10. CLL patients may present with autoimmune haemolytic anaemia (AIHA).

Prognosis depends upon the stages. Binet and modified Rai Clinical stagings are given in Tables 3.4 and 3.5.

Table 3.4	Binet Staging System for CLL
Stage	**description**
A	≤2 lymphoid-bearing areas enlarged
B	≥3 lymphoid-bearing areas enlarged
C	Presence of anaemia (Hb <10 g/dl) or thrombocytopenia (platelet count <100,000/L)

Five lymphoid-bearing areas are: Cervical, axillary, inguino-femoral, spleen and liver

Table 3.5		Modified Rai Clinical staging for chronic lymphocytic leukaemia
Risk	**Stage**	**Description**
Low	0	Lymphocytosis in blood and bone marrow
Intermediate	I	Lymphocytosis + enlarged lymph nodes
	II	Lymphocytosis + enlarged liver or spleen with or without lymph nodes
High	III	Lymphocytosis + Anaemia (Hb <11g/dl) with or without enlarged liver, spleen or lymph nodes
	IV	Lymphocytosis + Thrombocytopenia (platelet count <1,00,000/cmm) with or without anaemia or enlarged liver, spleen or lymph nodes

Peripheral Blood and Bone Marrow (Figs 3.11 and 3.12)

- In most patients, there is **increased number of mature lymphocytes** in the peripheral blood and bone marrow. These cells have the morphologic appearance of normal small to medium-sized lymphocytes with **clumped chromatin, inconspicuous nucleoli, and scant cytoplasm**.
- **Smudge cells** (basket cells or shadow cells of Gumprecht) are commonly seen in the blood smear.
- In **classical CLL, >90% of cells are mature lymphocytes**.
- When **11 to 54% of the cells are prolymphocytes, it is termed CLL/PLL.**
- If ≥55% of the cells are prolymphocytes, it is termed as prolymphocytic leukaemia.
- When >15% of the lymphocytes are plasmacytoid or cleaved and <10% are prolymphocytes, it is termed atypical CLL.

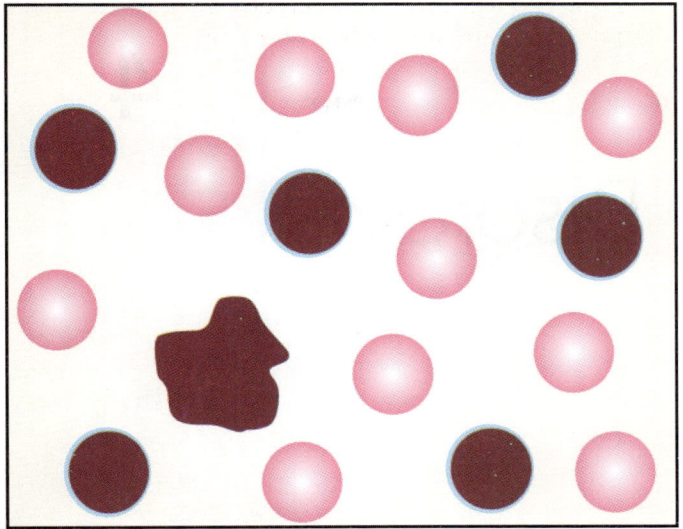

Fig. 3.11: Peripheral smear in CLL. Note increased number of mature lymphocytes and a smudge cell

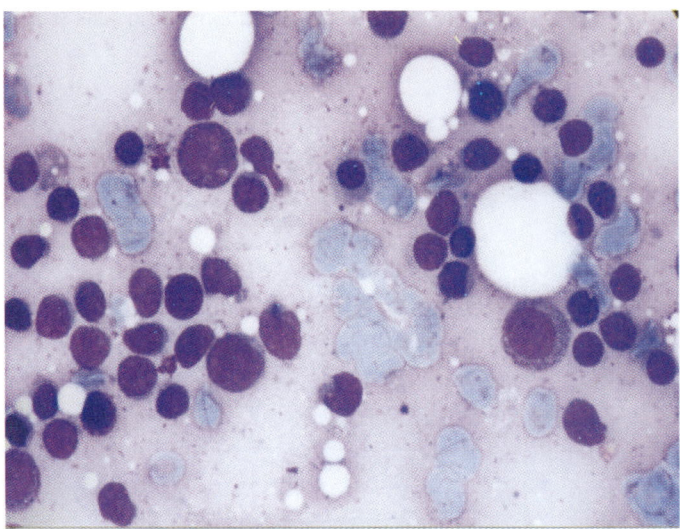

Fig. 3.12: Bone marrow in CLL

SELF-ASSESSMENT EXERCISE

1. **Tartrate resistant acid phosphatase positivity is characteristic of:**
   A. AML M3   B. Hairy cell leukemia
   C. ALL   D. CLL

2. **A patient having bleeding due to DIC and his BM with 20% blasts possibility is:**
   A. AML-M1   B. AML-M3
   C. ALL   D. CML with blast crisis

3. **Mediastinal mass is seen in:**
   A. ALL   B. AML
   C. CLL   D. CML

4. **Regarding T-ALL, all are true *except*:**
   A. Mediastinal mass
   B. Unfavourable prognosis
   C. Recurrence
   D. Acounts 40–50% of ALL cases

5. **Auer rods are present in blast cells of:**
   A. AML
   B. B-ALL
   C. T-ALL
   D. MDS

6. **True for B-ALL is:**
   A. Relatively good prognosis
   B. Never occurs in children
   C. Morphology sufficient for diagnosis
   D. Indolent disease

7. **Good indicator of ALL:**
   A. B lineage marker positivity
   B. T cell lineage marker positivity
   C. Older children
   D. Involvement of CNS

Answers

| 1. B | 2. B | 3. A | 4. D | 5. A | 6. A | 7. A |

Plasma Cell Disorders

MULTIPLE MYELOMA/PLASMA CELL DYSCRASIAS

Plasma cell dyscrasias constitute the following:

Malignant proliferation:

1. Multiple myeloma (MM)
2. Waldenstrom macroglobulinaemia (WM)
3. Plasmacytoma
4. Heavy chain disease

Relatively benign:

1. Monoclonal gammapathy of undetermined significance (MGUS)
2. Smouldering MM
3. Primary systemic amyloidosis
4. POEMS syndrome

Multiple Myeloma

Definition: Multiple myeloma is a malignat disorder characterised by proliferation of a single clone of plasma cells in the bone marrow. There will be lytic lesions of bones, increased monoclonal gammaglobulins and hypercalcaemia.

Pathogenesis: IL-6 plays role in proliferation of plasma cells and lytic lesions of bone.

The different diagnostic criteria and clinical findings are given in Tables 4.1 and 4.2.

Clinical presentation of multiple myeloma is given in Table 4.3.

Laboratory Evaluation

- CBC with peripheral smear (Figs 4.1 to 4.3)
- Chemistry panel (creatinine, calcium, lactic dehydrogenase—LDH, β_2 microglobulin—$\beta_2 M$)
- Immunofixation electrophoresis

Table 4.1	International Myeloma Working Group criteria for diagnosis[4]
M protein in serum or urine	
Clonal bone marrow plasma cells > or equal to 10% or plasmacytoma biopsy proven	
Myeloma-related organ dysfunction—CRAB a. Calcium elevation >11.5 mg% b. Renal insufficiency serum creatinine >1.96 mg% c. Anaemia <10 g/dl d. Bone lesions: Lytic/osteoporosis	
In the absence of end organ damage, clonal plasma cells ≥60%	
In updated International myeloma working group, myeloma is considered when CRAB features are present in a patient with smouldering MM	

Table 4.2	Revised criteria International Myeloma Working Group 2014[5]
In asymptomatic patients following criteria can label the patient as MM	
1. Clonal bone marrow plasma cells greater than or equal to 60%	
2. Free light chain ratio more than 100	
3. MRI showing more than one focal lesion	

Table 4.3	Clinical presentation of multiple myeloma	
Age: Old age (median age 65 years)	Elevated ESR markedly raised often >100 mm/hr
Insidious onset	Hypercalcaemia BJ proteins
Weakness, fatigue	BJ proteins
Pallor	Renal failure
Bone pains	Hyperviscocity: Hypergamma-globulinaemia
Pathological fractures	Amyloidosis
Recurrent infections	Marrow failure
Cord compression	

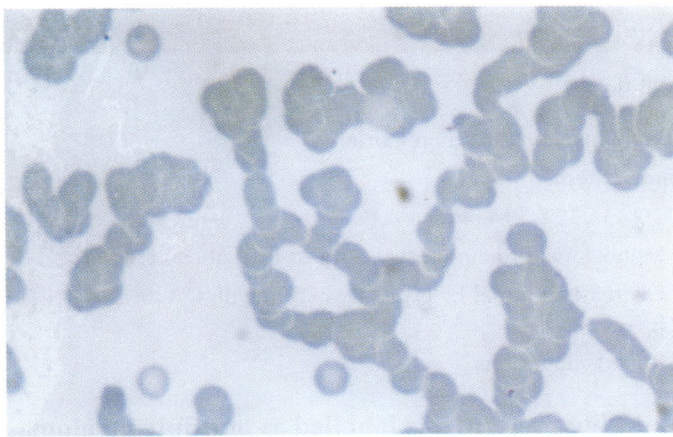

Fig. 4.1: Peripheral smear, note rouleaux formation

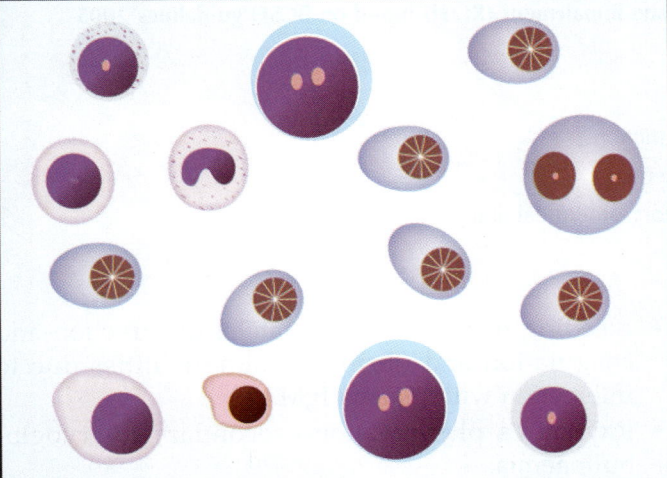

Fig. 4.2: Bone marrow with increased plasma cells in multiple myeloma (schematic)

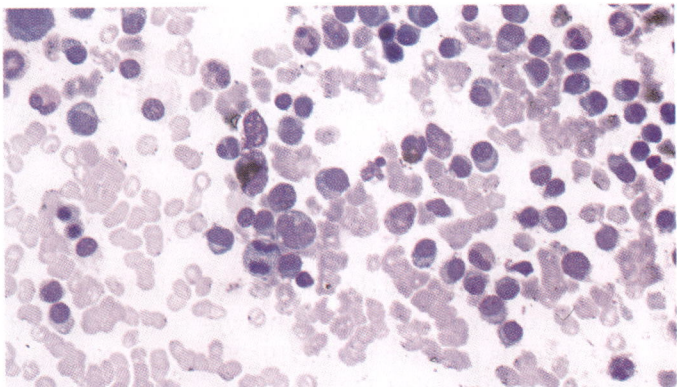

Fig. 4.3: Bone marrow aspirate in multiple myeloma

- Serum free light chain (FLC)
- Urinalysis/24 hr urine for protein
- Bence Jones protein
- Bone marrow examination
- Immunophenotype, cytogenetics

- Skeletal survey/CT/MRI/PET
- Plasma cell labelling index

Staging of Multiple Myeloma

Durie-Salmon staging takes into account haemoglobin, calcium levels, bone lesions on X-ray, M-component (IgG and IgA), Bence Jones proteins and myeloma cell mass.

The International Staging System (ISS) from International Myeloma Working Group of 2005, takes into account beta 2 microglobulin which reflects tumour mass and reduced renal function and reduced serum albumin in multiple myeloma is mainly because of inflammatory cytokines such as IL-6 secreted by myeloma cells. Table 4.4 shows ISS staging for MM.

Table 4.4	ISS staging for MM	
Stage	Criteria	Median survival
I	Serum albumin >3.5 g% Beta 2 microglobulin <3.5 mg/l	62 months
II	Not meeting criteria I and II Serum albumin <3.5 g% Beta 2 microglobulin <3.5 mg/l or Beta 2 microglobulin 3.5 mg/l to 5.5 mg/l Irrespective of serum albumin level	44 months
III	Beta 2 microglobulin. 5.5 mg/l	29 months

R-ISS from International Myeloma Working Group of 2015[6] takes into account ISS criteria, chromosomal abnormalities and serum LDH levels.

The chromosomal abnormalities for CD138 positive plasma cells detected by interphase fluorescent in situ hybridization (iFISH) include del17p, t(4;14)(p16;q32) or t(14;16)(q32;q23). In low risk, none of these is present; while in high risk, at least one of the abnormalities is present (Table 4.5).

LDH is a relevant biomarker and when increased above the normal levels denote aggressiveness and high proliferation or the presence of tumour mass in particular extramedullary and extraosseous disease.

Table 4.5	Risk stratification of multiple myeloma: 2016 update on diagnosis, risk stratification and management[7]
High risk: del17p, t(14:20) or t(14;16)(q32;q23).
Intermediate risk: t(4:14)(p16;q32) and gain 1q21
Standard risk: All others (Trisomies, t(11;14), t(6:14)

The older criteria for diagnosis of MM are given in Table 4.6.

Table 4.6 Diagnostic criteria for multiple myeloma (Salmon Durie)

Major criteria	Minor criteria
1. ≥30% bone marrow plasma cells	1. 10% to 30% BM plasma cells
2. M band in serum: Serum IgG ≥3.5 g/dl or Ig A ≥2 g/dl	2. Monoclonal protein present but less than above criteria
3. Urinary kappa and lambda ≥1 g/24h	3. Decreased normal Ig levels (IgM <50mg/dl, IgA<0.1g/dl, IgG<0.6g/dl)
4. Biopsy proven plasmacytoma	4. Bone Lytic lesions

When one major and one minor or 3 minor including 1 and 2 are present, it is labelled as multiple myeloma.

Criteria for myeloma-related organ or tissue impairment (ROTI) for end organ damage are given in Table 4.7.

Table 4.7 End organ damage: Myeloma-related organ or tissue impairment (ROTI) based on BCSH guidelines 2005

1. Bone lesions—lytic lesions, osteoporosis
2. Anaemia—below 10 g/dl
3. Renal disease—serum creatinine >1.96 mg%, renal tubular dysfunction
4. Susceptibility to infections—neutropenia, (hypogammaglobulinaemia)
5. Hypercalcemia—myeloma cells secrete osteoclast activating factors, serum calcium >11.5 mg%
6. Others: Hyperviscosity, amyloidosis, recurrent bacterial infections

WALDENSTROM'S MACROGLOBULINAEMIA (WM)

The disease is named after Jan Gosta Waldenstrom.

Definition: Waldenstrom's macroglobulinaemia is one of the malignant monoclonal gammopathies which is chronic, indolent and lymphoproliferative disorder. It is characterised by high levels of macroglobulinaemia (IgM), elevated serum viscosity and presence of lymphoplasmacytic infiltrate in the bone marrow and body organs.

Pathogenesis

Monocyte surface receptors are activated—IL-6 triggers increase of IgM.

Criteria for Diagnosis

More than 10% of clonal plasma lymphoid cells in bone marrow, IgM monoclonal band on protein electrophoresis.

Clinical Features

- Elderly patient
- Hyperviscosity syndrome: Visual disturbances/blurred vision, double images, stroke, slurred speech, weakness of one side of the body, headache, hearing problems.
- Neurological symptoms, anti-myelin activity with peripheral neuropathy.
- Hepatosplenomegaly and lymphadenopathy present.

- Bleeding manifestations, platelet dysfunction and coagulation and fibrinogen abnormalities due to interaction with plasma IgM.
- Raynaud's phenomenon—secondary to cryoglobulinaemia.
- Infections
- Increased incidence of lymphoma, MDS and leukaemia.

Investigations

- Haemoglobin reduced
- Normocytic normochromic anaemia with lymphocytosis
- Platelets reduced
- Rouleax formation due to IgM proteins
- ESR increased
- Biochemistry: M band (IgM) on protein electrophoresis
- Bone marrow: Plasma lymphocyte cells increased. Plasma cells positive for CD19, 20 and 22. Negative for CD5, CD10 and CD23.
- X-ray: Diffuse osteopenia

MONOCLONAL GAMMOPATHY OF UNDETERMINED SIGNIFICANCE (MGUS)

MUGS (non-IgM): All three criteria to be met.[5]

1. Serum non-IgM monoclonal proteins <3 g/dl
2. Clonal plasma cells <10%

3. Absence of end organ damage (CRAB criteria) or other features attributable to plasma cell disorder.

MUGS (IgM): All three criteria to be met.[5]
1. Serum IgM monoclonal proteins <3 g/dl
2. Clonal plasma cells <10%
3. Absence of end organ damage (CRAB criteria) or other features attributable to plasma cell disorder.

SMOULDERING MM

Smouldering MM: Both criteria to be met.
1. Serum monoclonal protein (IgG/IgA) more or equal to 3 g/dl or urinary monoclonal protein 500 mg/24 hrs or clonal plasma cells 10–60%.
2. No myeloma defining events or amyloidosis.

SELF-ASSESSMENT EXERCISE

1. Signs and symptoms of multiple myeloma:
   A. Bony pain
   B. Pathological fracture
   C. Anaemia
   D. All of the above

2. Multiple myeloma is diagnosed by:
   A. Symptoms
   B. Peripheral smear
   C. Bone marrow
   D. All of the above

3. Most dangerous in multiple myeloma:
   A. Infections
   B. Fracture bones
   C. Anaemia
   D. Hyperviscocity syndrome

4. Following is not a feature of MUGS:
   A. M proteins less than 3 g/dl
   B. BM plasma cells less than 10%
   C. No evidence of end organ damage
   D. Normal free light chain ratio

5. Smouldering multiple myeloma, all are true except:
   A. Serum monoclonal protein (IgG/IgA) more or equal to 3 g/dl
   B. Urinary monoclonal protein >500 mg/24 hrs
   C. Clonal plasma cells 10–60%
   D. Evidence of end organ damage

6. 10% of haematological malignancies and 1% of all cancer is:
   A. MM
   B. WM
   C. MUGS
   D. SMM

Answers

   1. D   **2.** D   **3.** A   **4.** D   **5.** D   **6.** A

Myeloproliferative/Chronic Myeloproliferative Disorders

Chronic myeloproliferative disorders (CMPDs) are group of disorders characterised by clonal expansion of abnormal haemopoietic stem cells. These can manifest as increased platelets, RBCs or WBCs and sometimes as increased fibrosis in the bone marrow with extramedullary haemopoiesis. The word CMPD used in WHO 2008 classification is replaced by myeloproliferative neoplasms (MPNs) and this category also includes mast cell diseases.[8]

The BCR-ABL negative JAK2 mutation positive disorders are PV, ET, PMF and CML is BCR-ABL positive disorder. Mastocytosis has KIT D816V mutations.

In the 2016 revision of WHO classification of tumours of the haematopoietic and lymphoid tissues, the following changes are made in MPN and MDS (Table 5.1):

1. The primary myelofibrosis is categorized as early (prefibrotic) and fibrotic types.
2. The haemoglobin criterion for PV is lowered to prevent underdiagnosis.
3. Neutrophilic leukaemia (CNL) now includes specific mention of *CSF3R* T618I or other activating *CSF3R* mutation as a major diagnostic criterion. Diagnosis is still permitted in the absence of this mutation, if neutrophilia is present for three months with no identifiable cause or if another clonal finding is identified.
4. The diagnostic criteria for essential thrombocythemia now adds *CALR* and *MPL* mutations to *JAK2* mutation as major findings, a change that also affects primary myelofibrosis.

PRIMARY MYELOFIBROSIS

Primary myelofibrosis has progressive anaemia and splenomegaly. It is a JAK2 V617F mutations positive disorder. These patients are transfusion dependent.

Table 5.1	The 2016 WHO classification MPN and MDS/MPN[9]

1. MPN

- Chronic myeloid leukaemia (CML) BCR-ABL1+
- Chronic neutrophilic leukaemia (CNL)
- Chronic eosinophilic leukaemia, not otherwise specified (CEL-NOS)
- Polycythaemia vera (PV)
- Essential thrombocythemia (ET)
- Primary myelofibrosis (PMF)
  - Pre-fibrotic stage
  - Fibrotic stage
- MPN unclassifiable
- Mastocytosis

2. MDS/MPN

- CMML
- aCML, BCR-ABL1 negative
- JCMML
- MDS/MPN with ringed sideroblasts and thrombocytosis (MDS/MPN-RS-T)
- MDS/MPN unclassifiable

Proposed Revised WHO Criteria for Pre-PMF

Major Criteria

1. Increased megakaryocytes with atypia, without reticulin and collagen—grade I
2. Not meeting WHO criteria of BCR-ABL+ CML, ET, PV, MDS or myeloid neoplasms
3. Demonstration of JAK2 mutations, CALR, or MPL mutation

Minor Criteria

1. Leucoerythroblastosis
2. Leucocytosis $\geq 11 \times 10^9/l$
2. Increased serum lactate dehydrogenase
3. Anaemia not attributed to a co-morbid condition
4. Palpable splenomegaly

Overt PMF: Pre-PMF criteria with increased mega-karyocytes with atypia with reticulin and/or collagen (fibrosis—grade II or III).

All three major criteria and at least one minor criteria should be met to diagnose PMF.

Patients have low grade fever, cachexia, night sweats and portal hypertension.

Investigations

- **Hb:** <10 g/dl
- **PC:** >10 L/decreased
- **TC:** >20000/leukopenia
- **LDH:** Increased
- **PS:** There is leukoerythroblastosis. Tear drop cells are plenty.
- **BM:** Shows dry tap. It has cellular phase and fibrotic phase (Table 5.2).

Table 5.2	Grading of myelofibrosis
MF-0	Scattered linear reticulin with no intersections
MF-1	Loose network with intersections especially in perivascular area
MF-2	Diffuse dense increase in reticulin with extensive intersections, associated with osteosclerosis
MF-3	Diffuse dense increase in reticulin with extensive intersections and thick fibres of collagen, associated with osteosclerosis

POLYCYTHAEMIA VERA

Polycythaemia vera (PV) is a clonal chronic MPD, insidious onset, and is characterised by absolute increase in red cell mass along with leucocytosis, thrombocytosis and splenomegaly. This has an autosomal dominance type of inheritance. Average age of occurrence is 60 years of age.

Clinical Features

Classical features are splenomegaly, erythrocytosis and thrombocytosis. JAK2 V617F mutation is positive.

The 2008 WHO Criteria for PV

Major criteria

1. Hb >18.5 g/dl in males and >16.5 g/dl in females
2. JAK2 V617F or similar mutation JAK2 exon 12 mutation

Minor criteria

1. Trilineage hypercellular bone marrow
2. Subnormal serum erythropoietin level
3. EEC (endogenous erythroid colony) growth *in vitro*

For diagnosis, either both major with one minor or first major with two minor criteria should be present.

WHO Criteria PV 2016

Major criteria

1. Hb >16.5 g/dl in men
   Hb >16 g/dl in women
   PCV >49% in men and >48% in women or increased red cell mass
2. BM hypercellularity with trilineage proliferation (panmyelosis)
3. JAK2 V617F or similar mutation JAK2 exon 12 mutation

Minor criteria

1. Subnormal erythropoietin (EPO) levels

For diagnosis of PV, all three major or the first two major and the minor criteria should be present.

The most frequent cause of mortality in poly-cythaemia vera is venous thrombosis due to increased red cell mass. The whole blood viscocity is increased.

The symptoms are:

1. Headache
2. Weakness
3. Pruritus
4. Dizziness
5. Excessive sweating
6. Visual disturbances
7. Thrombosis

On Physical Exmaination

1. Cyanosis
2. Conjunctival plethora
3. Hepatomegaly
4. Splenomegaly
5. Hypertension

PV may transform into MF and acute leukaemia.

ESSENTIAL THROMBOCYTOSIS (Table 5.3)

Essential thrombocytosis (ET) is a myeloproliferative disorder with sustained proliferation of megakaryocytes with increased number of platelet count more than $450 \times 10^9/l$.

These patients have bone marrow with megakaryocytic hyperplasia, splenomegaly and haemorrhage or thrombotic episodes. JAK2 V617F mutation is positive.

Average age of occurrence is 50 years. This is inherited as an autosomal dominant pattern. The defect is in the thrombopoietin gene.

Table 5.3	The revised 2016 WHO diagnostic criteria for ET

Major

1. Sustained platelet count 4.5 L/cmm
2. Megakaryocytic proliferation with large and mature morphology with hyperlobated nuclei
3. Not meeting WHO criteria of BCR-ABL+ CML, PV, MDS or myeloid neoplasms
4. Demonstration of JAK2 mutations, CALR, or MPL mutation

Minor

1. Presence of clonal marker or absence of evidence for reactive thrombocytosis

Note: For diagnosis, all four major criteria or first 3 major and the minor criterion to be met.

Clinical Features

Thrombotic and hemorrhagic episodes, headache, paraesthesia, visual disturbances and seizures.

Lab Findings

Total count: Increased

Platelet count: Increased

Peripheral smear: Leucoerythroblastic blood picture, tear drop cells plenty, mild eosinophilia and mild basophilia

Uric acid levels: Increased

JAK2 V617F mutation: Positive

Bone marrow: Megathrombocytes, enlargement of megakaryocytes with hyperlobulation of nuclei.

MASTOCYTOSIS

Mast cell disease/mastocytosis has increased accumulation of morphologically and immunophenotypically abnormal mast cells in one or more organs of the body. These have mutations of C-KIT (KITD816V) and FIP1L1-PGGFRA. The mast cells are hypogranular and the nuclei are monocytoid.

The clinical features include skin rash, musculoskeletal symptoms and organomegaly. Spleen is enlarged. These patients have weight loss, hypoalbuminaemia and malabsorption.

Diagnosis and Investigations

- Abnormal mast cells, splenomegaly, cytopenias diagnostic findings.
- **Total count:** Low, neutropenia
- **Hb:** Low <10 g/dl
- **Platelet count:** Less than 100000/dl
- **Hypoalbuminaemia:** Present
- **CD117 and CD25:** Positive
- **Mast cells:** Tryptase positive on IHC
- **Serum tryptase:** More than 20 ng/ml
- Marked osteosclerosis.

SELF-ASSESSMENT EXERCISE

1. **All are true for JAK2 mutation *except*:**
   A. Janus kinase 2 mutated
   B. DNA fragment involved
   C. Philadelphia chromosome positive
   D. Myeloproliferative disease

2. **For polycythaemia vera, all are true *except*:**
   A. Increased blood viscocity
   B. Vascular stasis
   C. Thrombotic tendency
   D. ESR is increased

3. **In secondary polycythaemia, serum erythropoietin is:**

   A. Increased   B. Decreased
   C. None of the above   D. All of the above

4. **For PV patients, following drugs can be used:**
   A. Hydroxyurea   B. Imatinib
   C. None   D. Both

5. **For ET diagnosis, all are true *except*:**
   A. Platelet count should be more than 4.5 L cells/cmm.
   B. Thrombotic events
   C. Uric acid increased
   D. Philadelphia chromosome positive

Answers

1. C   2. D   3. A   4. D   5. D

Myelodysplastic Syndrome (MDS)

The diagnosis of **myelodysplastic syndrome (MDS)** is considered with unexplained persistent cytopenias.

Etiology and Pathogenesis of MDS

MDS is a clonal stem cell disorder. The peripheral cytopenia is thought to be due to apoptosis.

The erythrocytic precursors have decreased response to erythropoietin (EPO). The terminally differentiated cells have functional defects. The mature granulocytes have decreased myeloperoxidase activity. Platelets have impaired aggregation properties.

The various etiological factors are:

- Radiation
- Benzene
- Alkylating agents (secondary MDS)
- PNH aplastic anaemia may transform into MDS

MDS may co-exist with other haematological malignancies like:

1. Multiple myeloma
2. Hairy cell leukaemia
3. Chronic lymphocytic leukaemia
4. Non-Hodgkin's lymphoma

Cytogenetic and Molecular Abnormalities

- 60% of the patients have normal karyotype.
- Most common abnormality is trisomy 8.
- 5q deletion is common in old age.
- Other abnormalities: Monosomy 5 or 7, loss of chromosome 7, deletion of long arm of 5, 7, 11, 13 and 20q deletion is common in patients with refractory anaemia. Therapy related MDS has partial or complete loss of chromosome 5 or 7.

Classification of MDS (Table 6.1)

1. Primary (de novo)
2. Secondary (chemo-/radiotherapy for malignancies)

Table 6.1	Classification of MDS (WHO 2016)
• MDS with single lineage dysplasia
• MDS with ringed sideroblasts (MDS-RS)
• MDS with multilineage dysplasia
• MDS with excess blasts
• MDS with 5q deletion
• MDS unclassifiable

Tables 6.2 and 6.3 are showing the older classifications of MDS by FAB (1982) and WHO (2008).

Table 6.2	FAB (1982) classification of MDS	
Subtypes	**Blood findings**	**BM picture**
Refractory anaemia (RA)	Blasts <1%	Blasts <5%, RS <15%
Refractory anaemia with ring sideroblasts (RARS)	Blasts <1%	Blasts <5%, RS >15%
Refractory anaemia with excess blasts (RAEB)	Blasts > or equal to 5%	Blasts 5–19%
Refractory anaemia with excess blasts (RAEB-1)	Blasts >5%	21–30%
Chronic myelomonocytic leukaemia (CMML)	Blasts <5%, monocytosis (≥1000/dl)	Variable

Table 6.3 WHO (2008) classification of MDS		
Subtype	**PS picture**	**BM picture**
Refractory cytopenias with unilineage dysplasia Refractory anaemia Refractory neutropenia Refractory thrombocytopenia	Unicytopenia or bicytopenia No/rare blasts	Unilineage dysplasia ≥10% of cells in one myeloid lineage with <5% blasts; <15% ring sideroblasts.
Refractory anaemia with ring sideroblasts (RARS)	Anaemia ≥15% ring sideroblasts, <5% blasts	Erythroid hyperplasia with dyserythropoiesis
Refractory cytopenias with multilineage dysplasia (RCMD)	Bi/pancytopenia No/rare blast No Auer rod <1 × 10⁹/l monocytes	Dysplasia in ≥10% of the cells of ≥2 myeloid lines <5% blasts in the marrow >15% ringed sideroblasts
Refractory anaemia with excess blasts (RAEB)-1	<5% blasts Bi/pancytopenia No Auer rods <1 × 10⁹/l monocytes	5–9% blasts, no Auer rod Dysplastic changes in ≥1 haematopoietic cell line
Refractory anaemia with excess blasts (RAEB)-2	5–19% blasts Cytopenias Auer rods <1 × 10⁹/l monocytes	10–19% blasts, Auer rod± Myelodysplasia of ≥1cell line
MDS unclassified	No blasts (≤1%) Cytopenia only	<5% blasts, cytogenetic abnormality + Granulocytic or megakaryocytic dysplasia. (Unequivocal dysplasia in ≥1 myeloid cell line cytogenetic abnormality)
MDS-5q del	<1% blasts Anaemia Platelets ↑/N	<5% blasts ↑/N megakaryocytes with hypolobated nuclei Isolated del 5q No Auer rods
Childhood MDS	<2% blasts Dysplastic changes in >10% of neutrophils	Dysplastic changes in >10% erythroid precursors Dysplastic changes in >10% gran. Precursors Micromegakaryocytes, dysplastic changes in megakaryocytes.

Clinical Syndromes

Patients with MDS present with symptoms of ineffective haemopoiesis. They are:
- Age: Old age, average age 65 years
- Gradual onset of pallor
- Recurrent infections—due to neutropenia
- Bleeding
- Easy bruising
- Fatigue
- Lethargy
- Dyspnoea on exertion
- Splenomegaly which is just palpable in one-fourth of the MDS cases.
- Bleeding manifestations
- History of previous chemo- and radiotherapy gives clue for secondary MDS.

MDS with 5q Deletion
- This is common in old patients.
- For many patients, it may be stable for long time and rarely rapidly progress to acute myeloid leukaemia.
- The bone marrow is hypoplastic, there are mononuclear micromegakaryocytes.

- There is macrocytic anaemia.
- Supportive care is the most appropriate treatment.

Laboratory Investigations in MDS
- Low reticulocyte count,
- Platelets reduced in 25% of the cases
- Pancytopenia in 50% of the cases.
- **Peripheral smear:** Normocytic nomochromic anaemia (NNA)/microcytic hypochromic anaemia (MHA)/ macrocytic anaemia (MA), macroovalocytes, acanthocytes, macrocytic anaemia. Rule out vitamin B₁₂ and folic acid deficiency anaemias.
- Hypogranular neutrophils, pseudo-Pelger-Huet anomaly present.

Bone Marrow Findings
Immature myeloid precursors from paratrabacular area are dipslaced in the centre, i.e. abnormal localisation of immature precursors (ALIP).

Erythroid series: Megaloblastic erythroid precursors. Ringed sideroblasts: Iron staining granules encircling more than one-third of the nucleus.

Dysplasia in All Lineages

Myeloid cells: Neutrophils have reduced cytoplasmic granules, hypolobated/hyposegmented neutrophils (pseudo-Pelger-Huet anomaly), hypersegmentation of neutrophils.

Megakaryocytes: Micromegakaryocytes present. About 50% of the MDS cases have thrombocytopenia.

In 15% of the MDS patients, bone marrow is hypercellular.

The International Prognostic Scoring System (IPSS)

Clinically MDS is classified as low-risk, intermediate-risk and high-risk groups. The classification predicts MDS disease transforming into acute leukaemia.

Table 6.4 shows the new IPSS—revised for MDS.[10]

Table 6.4	The new IPSS—revised for MDS							
Prognostic variable	0	0.5	1	1.5	2	3	4
Marrow blasts%	Less than or equal 2		>2 to < 5%		5 to 10%	>10%	
Karyotype*	Very good		Good		Intermediate	Poor	Very poor
H (g/dl)	More than or equal 10		8–10	<8			
Platelets	More than or equal 1L	50,000-1L	<50,000				
Absolute	More than or equal 0.8	<0.8					
Neutrophil count							

IPSS risk group: Very low: 1.5; Low: >1.5–3; Intermediate: >3–4.5; High: 4.5–6; Very high: >6

*Karyotype: Very good (–y, del 11q); Good (normal, del 5q, del 12p, del 20q); Intermediate (del 7q, +8, +19); Poor (-7, inv3 -7/del 7q); Very poor: >3 abnormalities

SELF-ASSESSMENT EXERCISE

1. **Chromosomal abnormality in MDS are all** *except*:
   A. Monosomy 7
   B. 5q deletion
   C. Deletion 12p
   D. Philadelphia chromosome

2. **In MDS, following are present** *except*:
   A. Infections
   B. Bleeding
   C. Splenomegaly
   D. Normal cell counts

3. **Pelger-Heut anomaly is:**
   A. Neutrophils with less lobes
   B. Eosinophils with no lobulation

C. Basophil with no lobulation
D. All of the above

4. **It is true for MDS patients:**
   A. Supportive therapy
   B. Treatment with immunomodulatory drug
   C. Bone marrow confirmation
   D. All of the above

5. **Following are true for MDS** *except*:
   A. Refractory anaemia
   B. Bleeding
   C. Infections
   D. Iron is given

Answers

1. D   2. D   3. A   4. D   5. D

Bleeding Disorders

Bleeding disorders or haemorrhagic disorders can be because of any of the following:

1. Vascular defects
2. Platelet abnormalities
3. Coagulation disorders

Vascular Defects

These can be aquired or congenital.

Aquired

- Simple easy bruising
- Senile purpura
- Non-thrombocytopenic purpura: Infections, drugs, uraemia, Cushing's disease and adrenocorticosteroid administration
- Scurvy
- Miscellaneous disorders: Orthostatic purpura, mechanical purpura, fat embolism
- Systemic disorders: Collagen disease especially polyarteritis nodosa.

Congenital: Osler-Rendu-Weber disease, Ehlers-Danlos disease.

Platelet Abnormalities

- These can be thrombocytopenia or functional defects
- Causes of thrombocytopenia: Aquired or functional defects

Aquired Causes

Common causes:

1. Idiopathic thrombocytopenic purpura (ITP)—acute or chronic
2. Drugs and chemicals
3. Leukaemias
4. Aplastic anaemias
5. Bone marrow infiltration
6. Hypersplenism
7. Disseminated lupus erythematosus

Less common causes:

1. HIV infection
2. Megaloblastic anaemia
3. Liver disease
4. Alcoholism
5. Massive blood transfusion
6. DIC
7. Food allergy

Functional Defects

1. Membrane receptor defects—Glanzmann's thrombasthenia, Bernard-Soulier syndrome
2. Enzyme defects
3. Granule defects

Coagulation Disorders

1. Haemophilia A, haemophilia B
2. von Willebrand disease
3. Other factor deficiency disorders—Factor I (fibrinogen), Factor II (prothrombin), Factor V, Factor VII, Factor X, Factor XI, Factor XII and Factor XIII.

PLATELET ABNORMALITIES

Thrombocytopenia

Thrombocytopenia is reduction of peripheral blood platelets below the lower normal limit of $150 \times 10^9/l$. The platelet count should be always confirmed by inspection of platelets on peripheral smear. Classifications of thrombocytopenia is given in Table 7.1.

Table 7.1	Classification of thrombocytopenia

Aquired
Common causes

Primary ITP: Acute/chronic
Secondary ITP
- Drugs and chemicals
- Leukaemias
- Aplastic anaemia
- Bone marrow infiltration: Multiple myeloma, lymphoma, myelofibrosis, carcinoma
- Hypersplenism
- SLE
- Infection

Less common causes

Infection including HIV, liver disease, alcohol, blood transfusion, DIC

Rare causes

Thrombotic thrombocytopenic purpura, postpartum thrombo-cytopenia, post-transfusion purpura, haemangiomas

Neonatal and congenital
- Immune: AI, NAIT
- Infections
- Drugs administration to mothers
- Wiskott-Aldrich syndrome
- May-Hegglin anomaly
- Bernard-Soulier syndrome
- Glanzmann thrombasthenia

IDIOPATHIC THROMBOCYTOPENIC PURPURA (Immune Mediated)

Idiopathic thrombocytopenic purpura (ITP) is an acquired disorder with thrombocytopenia due to antibody formation. An international working group has used the term primary for idiopathic, to denote ITP with no identifiable cause. This is classified depending upon duration as:
1. Acute
2. Chronic
   or
1. Newly diagnosed
2. Persistent (3–12 months)
3. Chronic (>12 months)

Clinical Features

The bleeding due to thrombocytopenia is spontaneous. Following are the sites of bleeding.
1. Skin is common site of bleeding.
2. Petechiae are usually common. These are pinhead sized. When fresh, red in colour, with time changes in colour due to absorbing blood. Petichiae occur in crops or group, common on arms, legs, neck, and on upper part of chest.
3. Echymosis may occur. These vary in size, initially purple in colour.

4. Bleeding from nose is less common, in the form of epistaxis as compared to bleeding from skin, gums, hematuria, menorrhagia and metrorrhagia. Melena is less common. Haematemesis and haemoptysis occur less commonly.
5. Bleeding from internal organs less common but serious especially cerebral haemorrhage and spinal cord and meninges.
6. Bleeding from joint is rare.

On Examination

- Subconjuntival and retinal haemorrhage are common. Spleen is enlarged slightly and only in 10% of the cases.
- Lymph nodes and liver are not palpable.
- Jaundice is absent (except for extensive hemorrhage).
- Fever is usually absent.

Primary ITP is more common in children and adults. In children peak age is 2–4 years with equal frequency in boys and girls. Prevalence of ITP increases with age in adults. There is female preponderance

Acute ITP: Childhood ITP has an acute abrupt onset and is commonly a few weeks after viral fever or immunisation and is self limited. It is more common in late winter and spring seasons and resolves within weeks or few months. 20% of acute ITP can go for chronic ITP.

Chronic ITP: Adult ITP has no antecedent viral infection. It is persistent or chronic with no precipitating event.

Differences between acute and chronic ITP are given in Table 7.2.

Pathogenesis

In ITP, the possible mechanisms are:
1. The antibodies develop to platelet glycoprotein complex GPIIb/IIIa and GPIb. The platelets coated with the antibodies are recognised by the Fc receptor of splenic macrophages.
2. Dysregulation of T cells with CD8+ T cell-mediated cytotoxicity and platelet destruction.

The monoclonal antibody specific immobilisation of platelet Ag (MAIPA): Positive (50–65%).

Treatment

Parents of children with ITP need assurance. Short course of intravenous immunoglobulins and anti-D (Rh-positive individuals) can be given. Splenectomy is not indicated. ITP in adults requires prednisolone and intravenous immunoglobulin shows initial response. Immunosuppressant drugs are used in refractory cases.

Table 7.2	Differences between acute and chronic ITP		
Features	Acute		Chronic
Age	Children (2–6 yrs)		Adult
Sex	Equal		F: M = 3:1
Seasonal variation	Spring time		None
Preceding infection	80%		Unusual
Associated AI disorder (SLE)	Uncommon		Common
Onset	Acute		Chronic
Platelet count	<20000/cmm		<40–80000/cmm
Eosinophilia and lymphocytosis	Common		Rare
Duration of illness	2–6 weeks		Months to years

Investigations in ITP are shown in Table 7.3 and Fig. 7.1.

Table 7.3	Laboratory investigations in ITP
Hb	Normal/decreased (proportional to degree of blood loss)
TC	Normal
Platelet count	Decreased (below normal to less than 10×10^9/l)
BT	Prolonged
CT	Normal
ESR	Normal
PS	Normocytic hypochromic and microcytic hypochromic
Auto-antibody to platelets	Present
BM	Erythroid and myeloid series normal. Megakaryocytes increased which are often in clusters. Immature megakaryocytes often with hypogranular and hypolobation present. Cytoplasm is basophilic. Erythroid hyperplasia, if anaemia is severe.

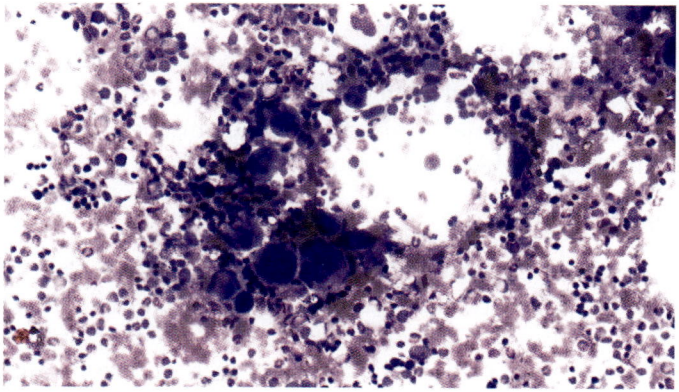

Fig. 7.1: Bone marrow in ITP (Note clustering of immature megakaryocytes)

INHERITED THROMBOCYTOPENIAS

Bernard-Soulier Syndrome (Synonyms: BSS, Gaint Platelet Syndrome, vWF Receptor Deficiency)

It is rare autosomal recessive inherited disorder characterised by large platelets, low platelet count and prolonged bleeding time (Table 7.4).

There is absence or decreased expression of a membrane glycoprotein GPIb–IX–V complex which binds to vWF in adhesion of platelets to subendothelial collagen.

Symptoms: Easy brusing, epistaxis, menorrhagia, GI bleeding.

Table 7.4	Lab investigations in Bernard-Soulier syndrome[11]
Platelet count	Decreased, gaint platelets seen
Hb	Normal/decreased
BT	Increased
Platelet aggregation studies	Do not aggregate in response to ristocetin even after adding normal plasma. Normal function with ADP, epinephrine and collagen

Bernadt MC and Andrews RK. Bernard-Soulier syndrome. Haematologica 2011;96:355–359.

Glanzmann's Thrombasthenia

Glanzmann's thrombasthenia (GT) is rare AR bleeding disorder characterised by lack of platelet aggregation. There is qualitative and quantitative abnormalities GPIIb/IIIa complex ($\alpha IIb\beta 3$) integrins receptor which are required for platelet adhesion. Platelets fail to aggregate in response to all agonist including ADP, thrombin and collagen (Table 7.5).

Clinical Features

The disease begins at birth or shortly thereafter. Mucocutaneous bleeding, epistaxis, bleeding gums, GI bleeding can be seen.

Table 7.5	Laboratory investigations in Glanzmann's thrombasthenia
Platelet aggregation	Absent with ADP, thrombin and collagen, response to ristocetin is normal
Platelet count	Normal
Clot retraction time	Prolonged
PT	Normal
APTT	Normal
BT	Increased
RBC count	Decreased
PS	NNA/MHA (due to bleeding)

Grey Platelet Syndrome (Table 7.6)

Grey platelet syndrome (GPS) is characterised by a reduction in α-granules of platelets. Platelets appear large, pale and grey on Romanowasky stains. It is an AR disorder with reduced or absent α-granules.

α-granules contain many adhesive proteins (vWF). There is defect in mutation of NBEL2 gene which is critical for development of α-granules.

α-granules are essential for normal platelet activity. They secrete fibrinogen and vWF, adhesive proteins which mediate platelet–platelet and platelet–endothelial interaction.

Clinical Features

Following are clinical features in grey platelet syndrome.
1. Mild to moderate bleeding.
2. Moderate thrombocytopenia.
3. Decrease or absent α-granules.
4. Both sexes equally affected. It presents at birth.

Table 7.6	Lab investigations in grey platelet syndrome
Platelet count	Normal/decreased
Platelet α-granules	Absent/reduced

COAGULATION DISORDERS

The main aim of coagulation during vessel injury is:
1. To produce thrombin, to aid activate platelets, and
2. To form fibrin from fibrinogen.
3. Once the punctured/injured vessel is closed, coagulation inactivation takes place.

Both intrinsic and extrinsic pathways lead to formation of prothrombin activator (Xa). Prothrombin in presence of thromboplastin, Ca^{++} and platelets is converted to thrombin. This acts on fibrinogen to form fibrin (Fig. 7.2).

Extrinsic pathway: Tissue trauma releases TF, converts VII to VIIa, Ca^{++} VIIa and TF converts X to Xa. Now Xa along with Va and Ca^{++} is PT activator.

Intrinsic pathway: Damage to blood cells or exposure to collagen, activation of XII to XIIa, in presence of HMK acts on XI to XIa, Ca^{++} to IX to IXa, IXa, Ca^{++} and VIIIa acts on X to Xa.

Plasminogen activator, released by endothelium, converts plasminogen to plasmin, which breaks down fibrin mesh.

The different coagulation factors along with site of their production are listed in Table 7.7.

Table 7.7	Coagulation factors
I : Fibrinogen: Liver
II: Prothrombin: Liver
III: Thromboplastin: Endothelium and platelets
IV: Ca^{++} (from bone and GI absorption)
V: Labile factor
VI: Not named
VII: Stable factor (proconvertin, serum prothrombin convertion accelerator): Liver
VIII: Anti-hemophilic factor: Endothelium
IX: Christmas factor: Liver
X: Stuart F: Liver
XI: Hageman factor
XII: Fibrin stabilising factor
Vitamin K dependant factors: X, IX, VII and II

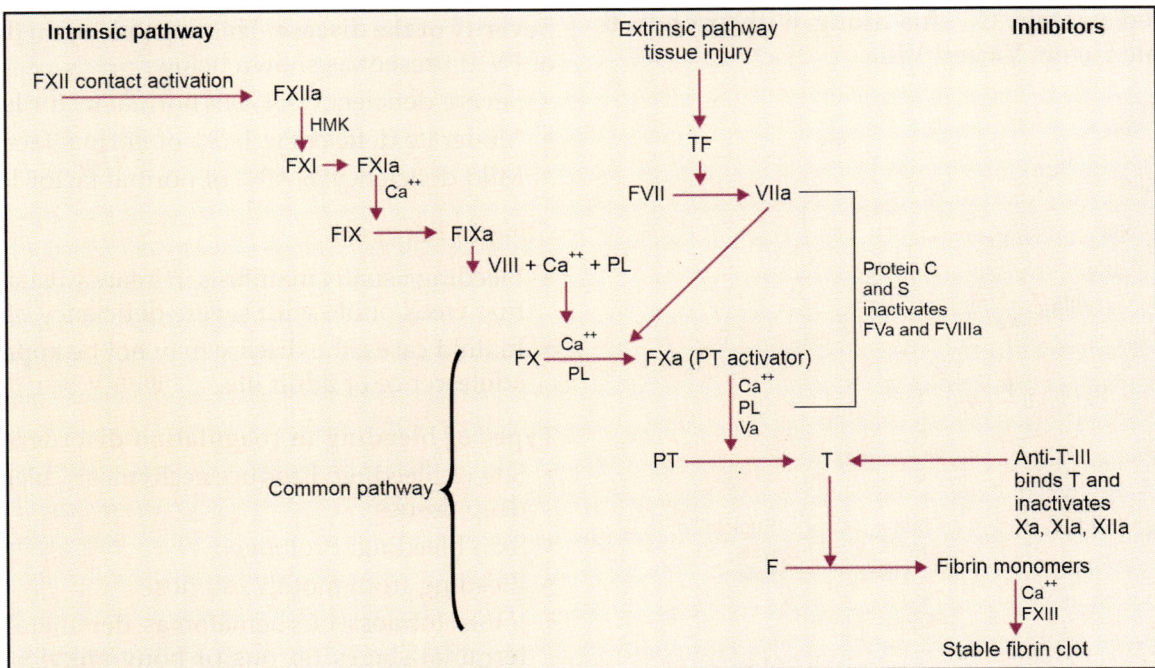

Fig. 7.2: Mechanism of coagulation (Anti-T: Anti-thrombin; T: Thrombin)

Table 7.8 shows classification of congenital coagulation disorders.

Table 7.8	Classification of congenital coagulation disorders
Common	
Haemophilia A (factor VIII deficiency, classical haemophilia)	
Haemophilia B (factor IX deficiency, Christmas disease)	
von Willebrand disease	
Less common	
Fibrinogen deficiency	
PT deficiency	
V deficiency	
VII deficiency	
X deficiency	
XI deficiency	
XII deficiency	
XII deficiency	
Fletcher factor (prekallikrein) deficiency	
Fitzgerald factor (HMWK) deficiency	

Common Tests in Coagulation Disorders

Common tests done in coagulation disorders are shown in Fig. 7.3.

Important Information

1. PT normal and APTT prolonged in factors VIII, IX, prekallikrein, HMWK deficiency and with presence of inhibitors.
2. PT increased in defects of factors V, VII, X and fibrinogen deficiency.
3. Vitamin K dependent coagulation factors are: Factors II, VII, IX and X.
4. vWF from endothelium
5. Factor VIII is always in combination with vWF.
6. Protein C, thrombomodulin, and thrombin form activated protein C. This along with protein S inactivate factors Va and VIIIa.

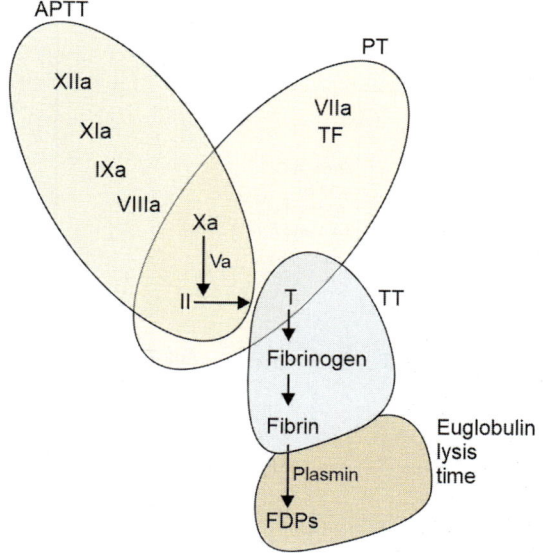

Fig. 7.3: Important tests in coagulation disorders

7. Protein C cannot cleave factor Va Leiden.
8. Heparin-like molecules from endothelium activate antithrombin-III. This binds thrombin and inactivated vitamin K dependent activated factors.
9. PGI2 and NO produced by endothelial cells have antiplatelet effect.

HAEMOPHILIA A AND B

Haemophilia A and B are hereditary congenital disorders of males inherited as X-linked disorders. Females are the carriers and males are the sufferers.

Haemophilia A

The functional unit of FVIII (FVIIIc) deficiency is called haemophilia and FIX deficiency as haemophilia B. The FVIII is always as in combination with vWF. Factor VIII is located on Xq28. Factor VIII is a glycoprotein, synthesized in liver under the control of X-linked gene.

Prevalence: 1:20000 to 1:10000.

Inheritance

- X-linked recessive pattern
- Males are sufferers and females are carriers.
- A male haemophiliac passes his abnormal X gene to all his daughters, who will be carriers, while son will not get X gene from father and they are normal.
- A carrier female may not have any symptoms, as another normal X allele from mother present.
- The carrier female can have four possible outcomes with each pregnancy, i.e. haemophiliac male sufferer, carrier and two other normal children.

Severity of the disease: This depends upon the amount of FVIII present as shown below:
- Severe deficiency: <1% of normal factor levels
- Moderate deficiency: 1–5% of normal factor levels
- Mild deficiency: 6–40% of normal factor levels.

Clinical Features

- Bleeding usually manifests in infancy usually during first week of life with severe deficiency of FVIII.
- In mild cases, the disease may not be apparent until adolescence or adult life.

Types of bleeding in coagulation disorders:
- Site of bleeding: Produce ecchymosis, bleeding into deep tissues
- Skin bleeding: Prolonged
- Bleeding from mouth and nose
- Joints: Intraosseous hematomas, demineralisation, in terminal stages fibrous or bony ankylosis. This is called chronic haemophilic arthropathy.

- CNS bleeding
- Urogenital bleeding
- GIT bleeding

Complications of Bleeding

a. Local pain
b. Anaemia bacause of bleeding
c. Fever
d. Arthritis
e. Sequelae of haematoma
f. Deformities of joints.

Diagnosis

a. Sex
b. Age of onset
c. Type of bleed
d. Heredity
e. Male child with abnormal bleeding
f. History of male relative of maternal side family
g. Bleeding in a male relative with minor procedure, e.g. tooth extraction

Laboratory Investigations

1. Hess test (tourniquet test): Normal
2. BT: N
3. CT: Increased
4. APTT: Increased (N; 30–35 secs), APTT corrected by normal plasma
5. PT: N
6. TT:N
7. Factor VIII assay: Low/reduced
8. DNA studies

Haemophilia B

In haemophilia B, there is deficiency of FIX in the blood. It is less common than Factor VIII deficiency.

Prevalence: 1; 40000.

Inheritance: It is similar to FVIII.

Clinical features: Clinical features are similar to FVIII deficiency, however, occurs in milder form.

Laboratory diagnosis: Same as for factor VIII except for FIX deficiency.

VON WILLEBRAND DISEASE

von Willebrand disease (vWD) is an inherited disorder of autosomal dominance character and occasionally autosomal recessive. It is located on chromosome 1 and affects both sexes.

vWF is produced by endothelial cells.

Functions

1. vWF protects FVIII from protein C inactivation. With vWF, FVIII is 5 times more in concentration.
2. It helps adhesion of platelets to the subendothelial collagen when there is injury to the vessel wall.

Prevalence: 1% of population are affected.

Clinical Features

In majority of the cases, bleeding is mild, with easy bruising and epistaxis. Mucocutaneous haemorrhages are common rather than haemathrosis and deep tissue bleeding. Family history of bleeding is present. Patients may bleed up to 36 hrs with minor procedures.

Investigations

- PC: Normal
- BT: Prolonged
- Hess test (tournoquet test): Positive
- APTT: Slightly prolonged due to reduced FVIIIc activity.
- Platelet aggregation: Absent with restocetin (diagnostic for vWD)
- vWF assay: Reduced
- FVIII activity: Reduced

Treatment: Cryoprecipitate, recombinent vWF and FVIII can be given.

FIBRINOGEN DEFICIENCY

It is a rare disorder. It is AD or AR disorder. It may affect both sexes. Bleeding follows trauma, small lacerations and patients do not bleed excessively. Afibrinogenaemia cases generally bleed postnatally, because of bleeding from the umbilical cord and/or following circumcision. The normal volume of fibrinogen in the blood is from 2 to 4 g/l. Fibrinogen defects can of three tytes: Afibrinogenaemia, hypofibrinogenaemia and dysfibrinogenaemia.

Afibrinogenaemia: This has AR inheritance. In this, there is complete absence of fibrinogen. The fibrinogen level is <0.2 g/l of plasma. This causes serious bleeding.

Hypofibrinogenaemia: This has AR inheritance. In this, fibrinogen is **lower level** than normal, between 0.2 g/l and 0.8 g/l. This is less frequent than afibrinogenaemia. The bleeding may be mild, moderate or severe.

Dysfibrinogenaemia: This has AD or AR inheritance. The fibrinogen level is normal (2 to 4 g/l), but the fibrinogen does not **function properly.**

Prevalence: About 1 person in 1 million population is affected by this condition. The affected person rarely suffer from haemorrhagic problems. They may have thrombosis states.

Treatment: Fibrinogen concentrate, cryoprecipitate and fresh frozen plasma (FFP).

Investigations

- CT: Clot not formed
- PT: No clot
- APTT: No clot
- TT: No clot
- TGT: Normal
- Fibrinogen levels: Absent/reduced/normal levels, functionally abnormal.

SELF-ASSESSMENT EXERCISE

1. **Normal platelet count is found in:**
   A. Von Willebrand diseases
   B. ITP
   C. Dengue fever
   D. Wiskott-Aldrich syndrome

2. **Normal platelet count is found in:**
   A. ITP
   B. Dengue fever
   C. Wiskott-Aldrich syndrome
   D. Henoch-Schonlein purpura

3. **Newborn bleeding with circumcision, possibility is:**
   A. Factor VIII deficiency
   B. Factor XI deficiency
   C. Factor XII deficiency
   D. Factor IX deficiency

4. **History of prolonged bleeding from umbilical stump, now cerebral haemorrhage at the age of 1 year, possibility is:**
   A. Factor XIII deficiency
   B. Factor II deficiiciency
   C. Factor VII deficiency
   D. Factor XI deficiency

5. **Factor V Leiden gene mutation, all are true *except*:**
   A. Activated protein C cannot breakdown activated factor V Leiden
   B. Produces venous thrombosis
   C. PCR screening useful for detection of factor V Leiden
   D. Protein C can easily inactivate activated factor V Leiden

Answers

1. A   2. D   3. A   4. A   5. D

Blood Groups and Transfusion Reactions

BLOOD GROUPS

There are several blood groups. They are ABO, MNSs, P, Rh, Lutheran, Kell, Lewis, Kidd, Duffy, Diego, Yt, Xg, Ii, Dombrock, etc. Amongst these, ABO and Rh systems are important.

ABO Blood Groups

The red cell surface has antigens. The antigenic characters of red cells are inherited. The antigen detection of blood groups is based upon haemag-glutination reactions. This is a serological reaction of red cells with the corresponding antibody, as determined in the laboratory. There are naturally occurring ABO group antibodies of IgM type in the serum of the patients. The serum contains the antibody for that antigen missing on the cell surface. Some information about ABO system is given in Table 8.1.

Table 8.1	Blood groups in general population, antigens and antibodies		
Blood group	General population	Antigens	Antibodies
AB	3–8% (least common)	A and B	Nil
A	20–40%	A	Anti-B
B	20–40%	B	Anti-A
O	40–48% (most common)	Nil	Anti-A, Anti-B

Note: Racial variations in the frequency of these groups are noticeable. 'O' is most common and AB is least common. Percentage of all groups varies.

Purpose of ABO blood grouping:

i. Blood transfusion
ii. Medicolegal purposes, i.e. in cases of disputed paternity.

Procedure

Red cell suspension with 0.9% NaCl is prepared. Take a slide with three concavities or two concavities. Label the concavities as anti-A and anti-B. In a slide with three concavities, the central one is used for control.

One drop of anti-sera A (blue coloured) is put in the concavity labelled as anti-A and one drop of anti-sera B (yellow coloured) in concavity labelled as anti-B. Add one drop of blood diluted with normal saline to all the concavities. The central concavity containing only saline diluted blood acts as control. Take a glass rod; mix well, each time using different ends. Care is taken not to contaminate one another. Observe for agglutination after 5 to 10 minutes (Fig. 8.1).

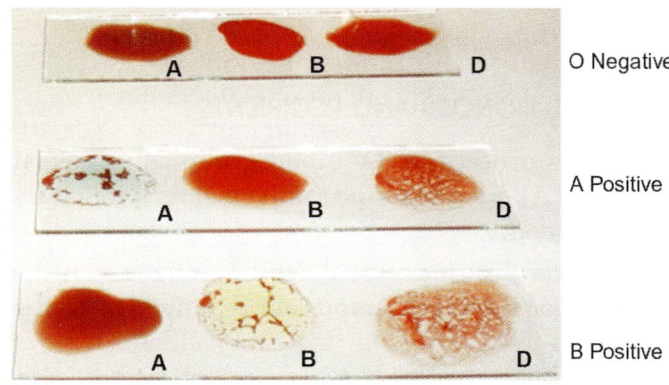

Fig. 8.1: Blood grouping by slide method

Agglutination	Blood group
Present in both anti-A, anti-B concavities	'AB'
Absent in both concavities	'O'
Present in only anti-A concavity	'A'
Present in only anti-B concavity	'B'

Note: When doubtful agglutination is present, the agglutination may be checked under microscope.

The antibodies in ABO system are naturally occurring complete antibodies and they can be easily detected by saline agglutination tests.

Blood Group Antigens

- The antigenic determinants or epitopes are small portions of molecules recognised by antibodies.
- **ABO antigens are carbohydrate in nature.** They are oligosaccharide chains anchored to glycoproteins or glycolipids of the RBC membrane.
- They are **highly immunogenic**.
- A and B antigens **differ in only the terminal sugar**.
- There is terminal sugar **N-acetyl galactosamine in A group**.
- And terminal sugar **galactose in B group**.
- There is no A or B antigen in O blood group. There is **absence of terminal sugars in O phenotype**.

Antibodies

- In ABO system, there are natural antibodies.
- They are present in the serum/plasma.
- They are **IgM type** and have high molecular weight and hence cannot pass through the placenta.
- These antibodies react well at 4°C, room temperature or at 37°C.
- Some times IgG antibodies may be produced in O blood group patients which can cause haemolytic transfusion reactions and haemolytic disease of newborn.

UNIVERSAL DONORS AND RECIPIENTS

The earlier concept of **'O' blood group as universal donor** and **AB blood group as universal recipient** does not hold good.

'O' blood group person have no antigens on the red cells but have anti-A and anti-B antibodies in the serum.

When given to recipient, these antibodies can destroy some of the recepient's red cells.

Hence, 'O' blood, better not to be given to A, B or AB persons. **However, washed 'O' red cells can be given.**

Earlier notion of AB person as a universal recipient, as they have A and B antigen on the red cells does not hold good. A or B blood groups will have antibodies against AB blood group antigens and can destroy some red cells of the AB recipient. Hence A or B blood groups

better not to be transfused to AB blood group patient. However, AB plasma can be given to A, B or O persons as it does not have any antibodies.

Hence, **washed O red cell packs** and **AB plasma** are **universal donors**.

ABO SUBGROUPS

Subgroups of A: A_1 and A_2.

These two phenotypes are best differentiated using lectin that is extracted from the seeds of Dolichos biflorus which reacts only with A_1 cells.

A_1 accounts for 80% of blood group A.

A_2 accounts for 20% of blood group A.

A_2 reacts weakly and misdiagnosed as 'O' blood group.

A_2 gene has two nucleotides different from A_1 gene which results in diminished enzymatic activity and subsequently weakened antigen expression.

If A_2 is misdiagnosed as 'O' blood group, there is no harm; however if A_2 is misdiagnosed as 'O' and if this blood is given to 'O' recipient, the anti-A and anti-B antibodies of the recipient might cause the early distruction of tranfused blood.

A_2 and A_2B individuals can produce anti-A_1 antibodies.

Approximately 4% of A_2 individuals and up to 25% of the A_2B individuals can have anti-A_1 antibodies in their serum.

The number of other subgroups of A has been described. This appears to result from inheritance of rare alleles of ABO locus and include Aint, A_3, A_x, A_m, Aend, Ael, Abuntu and Afinn. Except for Aint and A_3, many of these subgroups are weakly reactive or non-reactive with anti-A antibodies.

Subgroups of B: As described for A blood group, subgroups of B are also reported. Reactions of these red cells with anti-B are weak and variable.

Bombay Blood Group

This phenotype arises when two hh genes are inherited at the Hh locus. Such individuals are unable to convert type II paragloboside to H antigen. Hence, they are unable to make A or B antigens. These individuals produce anti-H, anti-A and anti-B as naturally occurring antibodies. On initial testing, Bombay blood group red cells appear to be of group 'O' but when this blood is transfused to 'O' blood group patients, these patients produce haemolytic reactions.

LABORATORY TESTS DONE ON A UNIT OF BLOOD DONATED

Following are the tests:

1. Haemoglobin estimation
2. Blood grouping and crossmatching
4. Screening for unwanted antibodies
5. Screening for transfusion transmissible infections: Indian Govt (Food and Drug Control Act) recommends following 5 tests to be mandatory.
   - HIV 1 and 2
   - Hepatitis B
   - Hepatitis C
   - Syphilis
   - Malaria

Tests must be performed at each donation regardless of number of earlier donations.

Rh System (Rh Typing)

The Rh system is so named because the original antibody was raised by injecting red cells of rhesus monkeys into rabbits and guinea pigs, also reacted with human cells. The Rh system is a gene complex which gives rise to various combinations of three alternative antigens C or c, D or d and E or e as originally suggested by Fisher. The Rh locus is on chromosome 1. Amongst these antigens, D antigen is the most immunogenic and it is convenient to classify the individual as Rh-D positive or Rh-D negative, depending on the presence of the Rh-D antigen. For Rh-D antigen detection, usually slide agglutination procedure is routinely done; whenever doubt arises tube technique is followed.

Slide agglutination method: One drop of anti-D (IgG Rh antibody) and one drop of blood are mixed well, observe for agglutination after 2 minutes.

Note: False negative result may be observed when room temperature is less and the test may need pre-warming of the slide.

Rh confirmation by tube technique: This is done with controls; wash the cells with saline 3 times (5 drops of blood). Take 1 drop of cell suspension and 1drop of anti-D; incubate at least for 30 minutes. Add antihuman globulin serum. Centrifuge for 1 minute and observe for agglutination.

Weak D Phenotype (D^u Phenotype)

Because of immunogenicity, the D antigen is the most clinically important antigen in the Rh blood group system. The donor and the recipient are tested for the presence or absence of the D antigen. The D positive recipients can receive D positive blood components and they can as well receive D negative blood components. On the other hand, D negative recipients should be transfused with only D negative blood components. Although D typing on the vast majority of blood samples is straight forward, some variants of weak D typing may be encountered. These weak D typings are usually labelled as D negative on an immediate spin reading, but they are D positive when indirect antiglobulin test is conducted. This weak variant is described as D^u phenotype (weak D). Reasons for this variant include a transposition effect, genetically transmissible D^u and D categories.

When a C-producing Rh gene (without D) is in transposition, weakened expression of D antigen may be observed. These cells may fail to react with anti-D sera at immediate spin but they react strongly at antiglobulin phase of testing. This type of D^u is also called high grade D^u.

Some D^u phenotypes arise from inheritance of specific Rh genes. This type D^u is referred to as the low grade D^u. Among the blacks, a variant of R^0 gene may produce lesser amounts of D antigen. Among the whites, such diminished production is more frequently associated with variant R^1 or variant R^2 gene.

Among individuals with alloanti-D in the serum of D positive individuals, D Ag is proposed to be a mosaic, composed of genetically distinct pieces. A majority of D positive individuals have inherited Rh genes that produce all pieces of the mosaic; however, some may inherit most of the pieces but not all the pieces of the antigen. Such individuals are at a risk during pregnancy and transfusion, to produce anti-D to the portion of D antigen, they lack on their red cells. These are grouped as D categories. Some of these are D positive on immediate spin, however, others appear to be D-negative on immediate spin and demonstrate positive D with antiglobulin phase of testing. So most D category individuals are not apparent until they present with alloanti-D in their serum.

Hence, D^u testing for donor cells is necessary to avoid immune response, if transfused to D-negative recipient.

CROSSMATCHING

Purpose

This is done to ensure absence of incompatibility between the blood to be transfused and the blood of recipient.

Major crossmatching is important, in which the serum of the recipient and the cells of the donor are mixed. The purpose of the major crossmatch is that the recipient's serum should not contain isoantibodies to the donor's red cells. Minor crossmatching is meant to detect isoantibodies in the serum of the donor because they are capable of reacting with the recipient's red cells. This test is not mandatory.

Procedure of Major Crossmatch

Prepare 2% red cell suspension of donor cells in saline. Add 2 drops of recipient's serum and 2 drops of red cell suspension, centrifuge at 1500 RPM for one minute and check for agglutination both macroscopically and microscopically. If positive, the test detects IgM antibodies.

If there is no agglutination, then incubate in waterbath at 37°C for 15 minutes. Wash 3 times with saline. Thereafter, follow the procedure of Coomb's test. Check for agglutination; if positive, it denotes IgG antibodies.

Procedure of Minor Crossmatch

Similar procedure as above is followed using red cells of the recipient and the donor's serum.

COOMB'S TEST

Purpose: This test detects incomplete antibodies (IgG).

Requirements: Small glass test tubes (10 × 75 mm), pipettes, normal saline, centrifuging machine, Coomb's serum and the blood to be investigated into.

Coomb's serum (anti-human globulin serum): This is obtained by immunizing rabbits with human serum. Broad-spectrum antisera contain anti-IgG and anti-complement components. Specific antisera against heavy chains of IgG, IgM and IgA can be prepared.

Direct Coomb's Test

Wash the test red cells 3–4 times with minimum of 3 ml of saline per wash and prepare 10–20% of red cell suspension in saline. About 2 drops of red cell suspension and 2 drops of Coomb's serum are mixed. Wait for 5 minutes. Centrifuge for 1 min/1500 RPM. Check for agglutination with naked eye or under microscope.

Test can be conducted with fourfold dilution of Coomb's serum (1:4, 1:16, 1:64, 1:256, 1:1024, and 1:4096).

Coomb's test with broad-spectrum antisera is non-specific. It would agglutinate a wide range of proteins, drugs and corresponding antidrug antibodies.

Indications

- Haemolytic disease of the newborn
- Autoimmune haemolytic anaemia
- Haemolytic transfusion reaction (incompatible blood transfusion).

Indirect Coomb's Test

Prepare red cell suspension of a known antigenicity ('O' cells). In a test tube, place 2 drops of serum to be tested. To this, add 2 drops of 10–20% red cells suspension ('O' blood group cells). Incubate for 30 minutes to 2 hours. If no agglutination, then wash for 3 times. Thereafter follow the steps of direct Coomb's test.

Indications

1. Detection of IgG antibodies to Rh factor (pregnant patients)
2. Detection of autoantibodies in the serum of patients with autoimmune haemolytic anaemia.

Note: These tests should be conducted with controls.

Sources of Errors

1. Red cells need to be washed adequately before adding anti-human globulin serum. Otherwise neutralization of anti-human globulin serum may occur.
2. Adequate incubation period is necessary.

TRANSFUSION REACTIONS

Transfusion reaction is defined as any unfavourable event that occurs during or after a transfusion of blood and its components. **The transfusion reactions can be classified as given in Table 8.2.**

Table 8.2	Transfusion reactions

Acute transfusion reactions—immunological
- Febrile non-haemolytic transfusion reactions (FNHTR)
- Allergic reactions
- Anaphylactic and anaphylactoid reactions
- Acute haemolytic transfusion reactions (AHTRs)
- Transfusion related acute lung injury (TRALI)

Acute transfusion reactions—non-immunological
- Bacterial contamination
- Transfusion-associated circulatory overload (TACO)
- Physical and chemical
- Haemolysis
- Metabolic derangements

Delayed transfusion reactions—immunological
- Delayed haemolytic transfusion reactions
- Transfusion-associated graft-versus-host disease (TA-GVHD)
- Post-transfusion purpura

Delayed transfusion reactions—non-immunological
- Iron overload
- Post-transfusion haemosiderosis
- Transfusion-transmitted diseases

Febrile Non-Haemolytic Transfusion Reaction (FNHTR)

This is a frequent kind of reaction, occurs in 1:200 cases.

Definition: 1°C temperature rise associated with transfusion of blood when there is no medical explanation for fever other than blood transfusion.

Causes: Patient has immunologic sensitization to donor WBCs, platelets or plasma proteins.

Common sources: Prior transfusions, previous pregnancies, previous transplants.

Caused from **HLA class I antigens or leucocyte antigens on the WBCs of the donor** that react with the recipient antibody (components with WBCs)—activate complement which releases cytokines.

Signs and Symptoms

- Fever with or without chills, with increase of 1°C to 2°C temperature.
- Most symptoms are mild. With severe reaction, there can be hypotension, cyanosis, tachycardia, tachypnoea, dyspnoea, cough, etc. There can be headache, flushing, anxiety and muscle pain.

Prevention

- Antipyretics are used to treat fever or are given prior to blood transfusion as a preventive measure.
- Discontinue blood transfusion, if the patient has severe reaction.

Allergic Reactions

This is a frequent kind of reaction.

Causes

Exact mechanism for sensitization is not known. Patient is sensitized (usually IgE antibody) to foreign plasma antigens. Commonly caused by transfusion of plasma containing blood components, e.g. FFP, cryoprecipitate and platelet concentrates.

Pathophysiology (Fig. 8.2)

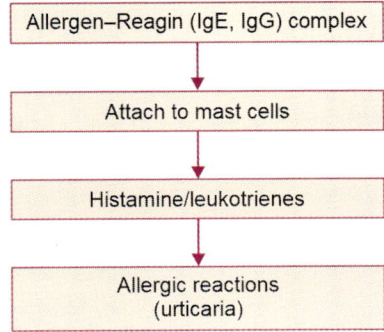

Fig. 8.2: Pathophysiology of allergic reactions

Signs and Symptoms

- Flushing
- Headache
- Itching
- Urticaria
- Rarely, angioedema—epiglottal oedema; bronchial airway constriction, hypotension, dyspnoea and rales.

This is not life-threatening.

Management

- Pre-medicate patient with antihistamines.
- If signs/symptoms are mild and/or transient, restart transfusion after treatment.
- Do **NOT** restart transfusion, if pulmonary symptoms/signs and fever present.

Prevention

Use plasma deficient blood components. Prophylactically treat with antihistamines.

Anaphylactic and Anaphylactoid Reactions

Anaphylaxis can range from mild urticaria to severe shock and death although rare.

These occur at the rate of about 1 per 150,000 patients.

Pathophysiology

Preformed anti-IgA antibodies are present in the recipient's blood with IgA deficiency which reacts with IgA present in the donor plasma.

Signs and Symptoms

Anaphylactic reactions → coughing, dyspnoea, nausea, emesis, bronchospasm, flushing of skin, hypotension, abdominal cramps, diarrhoea, cardiac arrest, shock, and death.

Anaphylactoid (less severe) → urticaria, periorbital swelling, dyspnoea, or perilaryngeal oedema.

Prevention

- Stop transfusion
- Keep IV line open
- Medication: Use epinephrine (vasoconstrictors and bronchodilators) and corticosteroids.
- Use washed RBCs and blood components.
- Transfuse IgA deficient blood.

Acute Haemolytic Transfusion Reactions (AHTRs)

- Most common cause for AHTR is ABO incompatibility (clerical error).
- Incidence: 1:25,000

- As little as 10–15 ml can trigger a reaction.
- Occurs within 24 hours.

Causes

- Transfusion **of incompatible donor RBCs into patient**.
- Usually an ABO incompatibility, most commonly **antibodies of A, B or AB**.
- Red cell destruction due to **complement activation by IgM antibodies**. Antibodies in patient plasma attaches to antigens on donor RBCs causing RBC destruction intravascularly.
- Potent anaphylactotoxins including **C3a and C5a are released, later form membrane attack factor.**
  Table 8.3 shows signs and symptoms of AHTR.

Table 8.3	Signs and symptoms of AHTR
Chills	Fever
Facial flushing	Dyspnoea
Hypotension	Generalized bleeding
Renal failure	Haemoglobinaemia
DIC	Haemoglobinuria
Shock	Nausea
Chest pain	Vomiting
Pain along infusion vein	Back pain

Steps to be taken when a transfusion reaction occurs due to AHTR:

- Stop the transfusion immediately.
- An intravenous line with normal saline should be maintained.
- Obtain vital signs.
- Begin O_2, if pulmonary symptoms are prominent.
- Obtain a new blood sample for repeat ABO compatibility test and for evidence of haemolysis.
- Obtain a urine sample, if the patient can void.
- Obtain a chest X-ray, if pulmonary symptoms are prominent.
- Physician is notified.
- Bedside clerical checks of all forms, labels and patient identification for correctness of the unit and the intended recipient are required.
- The unit and all tubing should be returned to the blood bank, along with post-infusion blood and urine samples.
- Finally, the reaction should be documented in the patient's chart.
- Once these initial measures have beeb implemented, the investigation of the reaction by the transfusion service can proceed.

Management

- Treat hypotension, renal failure, DIC, etc.
- Submit blood samples for blood bank/laboratory tests.
- Avoid, if possible, further transfusions till work-up is complete and/or patient recovers from reaction.
- To prevent renal failure, fluids (saline) are infused along with diuretics to increase urine output.

Transfusion-Related Acute Lung Injury (TRALI)

This occurs in 1 in 5,000 transfusions.

Symptoms occur within 2 hours and may end in 2–4 days, if treated.

Patient displays **acute respiratory insufficiency** with X-ray showing bilateral symmetric **pulmonary oedema.**

Pathophysiology

Donor antibodies activate recipient's WBCs or vice versa which cause damage to blood vessels in lung tissue. Then fluids and proteins leak into alveolar space/interstitium. Mechanism is similar to ARDS. Non-cardiogenic bilateral pulmonary oedema develops (Fig. 8.3).

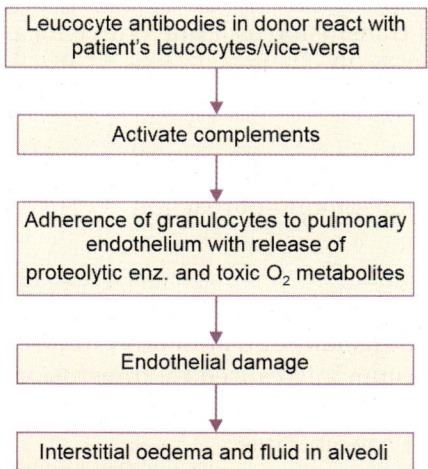

Fig. 8.3: Pathophysiology of TRALI

Signs and Symptoms

- Severe dyspnoea, cyanosis, tachycardia, and hypoxaemia
- Hypotension
- Fever
- Chills

Prevention

- Avoid donations from multiparous women and those who have received multiple transfusions.

- Transfuse washed RBCs from which plasma is removed.
- Platelet units can also be washed, but platelet function is significantly reduced.

Bacterial Contamination

- Does not involve antigen–antibody interactions.
- Results from bacterial contamination of blood products.

Pathophysiology

Bacteria growing in cold and room temperature produce toxins.

Symptoms and Signs

- Acute onset within 30 minutes after transfusion.
- Dryness and flushing of skin.
- Fever, hypotension, shaking chills, muscle pain, vomiting, abdominal cramps, bloody diarrhoea, haemoglobinuria, shock, renal failure, and DIC.

Transfusion-Associated Circulatory Overload (TACO)

Patients at significant risk are:

- Children
- Elderly patients
- Chronic anaemia
- Cardiac disease
- Thalassemia major, sickle cell disease or congenital hemolytic anaemis

Pathophysiology (Fig. 8.4)

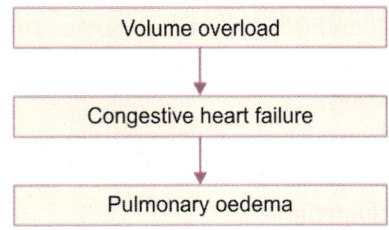

Fig. 8.4: Pathophysiology of TACO

Table 8.4	Symptoms and signs in TACO
Dyspnoea	Chest discomfort
Coughing	Headache
Cyanosis	Restlessness
Orthopnoea	Tachycardia
Hypertension	

Physical and Chemical Haemolysis

Following are the causes:

- Improper storage: Overheating or freezing.
- Improper preperation: Freezing without cryo-protective agent.
- Mechanical stress: Cardiopulmonary bypass pump.
- Simultaneous mixing of blood with drugs/hypotonic (5% dextrose)/hypertonic solutions (50% dextrose).

Metabolic Derangements

- Citrate toxicity
- Hyperkalaemia
- Hypothermia
- Coagulopathy in massive transfusion
- Air embolism

Note:

- These have synergystic effects.
- Blood warmer can prevent hypothermia.
- Slow infusion rate is required.

Delayed Haemolytic Transfusion Reactions (DHTRs)

- DHTRs may not be recognised for weeks or months after transfusion. This is due to anamnestic reaction mediated by IgG antibodies on the following occasions:
  - Patient previously exposed to RBC antigen and has low antibody titer until exposed again.
  - Antibodies to Rh, Kidd, Duffy, and Kell blood groups
- DAT is negative at first, but becomes positive later.
- Tests are performed to identify antibody.
- Patient may be asymptomatic.
- Fever and anaemia 10–14 days after transfusion is due to DHTRs.

Symptoms

- Fever
- Mild jaundice
  These patients must be given antigen negative blood.

Transfusion-Associated Graft-Versus-Host Disease (TA-GVHD)

Patients at risk are:

- Immunocompromised patients
- Newborn and geriatric patients
- Patients with bone marrow transplantation
- Patients on chemotherapy
- Patients with radiation treatment
- Patients who receive relatives blood

Pathophysiology (Fig. 8.5)

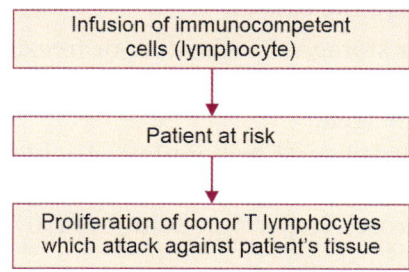

Fig. 8.5: Pathophysiology of TA-GVHD

Signs and Symptoms

- Onset—3 to 30 days after transfusion.
- Clinically significant pancytopenia.
- Other effects include fever, rise in liver enzyme, copious watery diarrhoea, erythematous skin, erythroderma and desquamation.

Prevention

- No adequate therapy available.
- Irradiation of blood components is safer.
- Avoid potential fatalities.
- Avoid relatives blood.
- Rare but fatal condition that has a 90% mortality rate.
- Symptoms appear usually **after about 12 days**.
- Caused by donor lymphocytes, which are transfused into an immunocompromised recipient.
- **Pancytopenia** occurs as a result of the immunologic response.
- Any components that contain T lymphocytes should be irradiated to prevent GVHD.

Post-Transfusion Purpura

- Rare complication
- Rapid onset of thrombocytopenia as a result of anamnestic production of platelet alloantibody.
- Usually occurs in multiparous women who do not have the antigen.

Pathophysiology

Platelet antibody (anti-PL^{A1}) → attach on platelet surface → destruction of platelets by reticuloendothelial system.

Signs and Symptoms

- Purpura and thrombocytopenia occur.

- Occur 1–2 weeks after transfusion.
- The platelet count drops to <10,000/µl.

Iron Overload

- 1 unit of packed red cells has 250 mg of iron.
- Iron that can be removed by the body—1 mg/day.
- Thus, with multiple transfusions, iron accumulates in tissues and causes hemosiderosis.

Post-Transfusion Haemosiderosis

Affected organs: Heart, liver, endocrine glands.

Signs and Symptoms

- Muscle weakness, fatigue, weight loss, mild jaundice, anaemia, mild diabetes, and cardiac arrhythmia.
- Occurs in individuals who receive multiple transfusions.
- Excess iron accumulates in macrophages in various tissues (liver, heart, endocrine glands).
- It appears as dark brown granules in the cells.
- May lead to organ failure.
- Therapy → Iron-chelating agents.
- Prevention → Transfuse with young RBCs.

Transfusion Transmitted Diseases (TTDs)

Blood transfusion can transmit diseases and the list of possible transmitted diseases is given in Table 8.5.

Table 8.5	Transfusion transmitted diseases (TTDs)

Viral infections
- Hepatitis viruses: HBV, HCV
- Retroviruses: HIV
- Herpesviruses: CMV, EBV
- Parvovirus: B19 parvovirus
- Prion: Infectious particle of CJD
- Other viruses: West Nile disease

Bacterial infection
- Gram-negative and Gram-positive bacteria

Syphilis

Lyme disease (borreliosis)

Parasitic infections
- Malaria
- Chaga's disease
- Toxoplasmosis
- Leishmaniasis

SELF-ASSESSMENT EXERCISE

1. **Antigens of ABO blood group RBCs are:**
   A. Carbohydrate in nature
   B. Fats
   C. Haptens
   D. All of the above

2. **Amongst A blood group:**
   A. A_1 is most frequent
   B. A_2 is most frequent
   C. Both A_1 and A_2 equally frequent
   D. A_3 frequent

3. **Major crossmatch, all are true** *except*:
   A. Recipient serum and donor cells mixed
   B. Recipient cells and donor serum mixed
   C. Detects iso-antibodies to donor cells
   D. Must be done on a unit blood to be transfused

4. **Direct Coomb's test detects:**
   A. Antibodies coated on red cells
   B. Antibodies in the serum
   C. Both of the above
   D. None of the above

5. **Febrile transfusion reactions are due to:**
   A. HLA class I antigens on WBCs or platelets
   B. HLA class II antigens
   C. Both of the above
   D. None of the above

6. **AHTRs are due to:**
   A. Complement activation by IgM antibodies
   B. Allergic reaction by plasma proteins
   C. Reaction due to IgG antibodies
   D. All of the above

7. **AHTR, all are true** *except*:
   A. Clerical errors
   B. Errors in patient identification
   C. Wrong blood transfusion to a patient
   D. All of the above

8. **TRALI, all are true** *except*:
   A. Donor antibodies activate recipient's WBCs
   B. Damage to blood vessels of lung tissue
   C. Pulmonary oedema develops
   D. Cardiogenic oedema develops

9. **AB blood group was discovered by:**
   A. Landsteiner
   B. Decastello and Sturli
   C. Virchow
   D. Coomb's

10. **Bombay blood group, all are true** *except*:
    A. Found only in India
    B. Named after Bhende and colleagues
    C. Anti-H antibodies present
    D. 1952 is the year of discovery

Answers

1. A	2. A	3. B	4. A	5. A	6. A	7. D	8. D
9. B	10. A						

General Pathology

Introduction and History of Pathology

INTRODUCTION TO PATHOLOGY

The word pathology is derived from the combination of the words Pathos and Logos. "Pathos" meaning suffering and "Logos" meaning study. It is a scientific study of structure and function of the body tissues in a diseased state.

The three basic components of the study include:

- Etiology
- Pathogenesis
- Structural and functional changes in the tissues.

These changes are studied by gross and microscopic examination along with laboratory investigations.

Unless the pathology of a particular disease is understood, clinicians cannot treat those diseases.

Branches of Pathology

- **Surgical pathology:** This branch of pathology deals with interpretation of biopsies and evaluation of resected specimen. Frozen section is used for rapid diagnosis and enzyme studies.
- **Haematology:** This branch of pathology deals with the study of blood and the blood-forming organs.
- **Cytology:** This branch of pathology deals with study of cells and body fluids.
- **Clinical pathology:** This branch of pathology deals with urine, renal function tests, liver function tests, thyroid functions, etc.
- **Autopsies:** The causes of death are studied in this branch of pathology.

HISTORY OF PATHOLOGY

Documentation of disease begins with Egyptian medicine. The most important sources are the **Edwin**

Smith Papyrus (17th century BC) and **Papyrus Ebers** (around 1550 BC). These are the ancient egyptian written medical documents. There have been many notable individuals throughout history who have contributed a lot to our knowledge of pathology today.

Hippocrates (460–377 BC): He was a Greek physician. He is called the **father of medicine**. He established the basic principles of medicine. His contributions included detailed observations of disease and an understanding of how health is often influenced by external factors.

Cornelius Celsus (25 BC–50 AD): He was a Roman physician, first described the four cardinal signs of inflammation (rubor, calor, tumour and dolor).

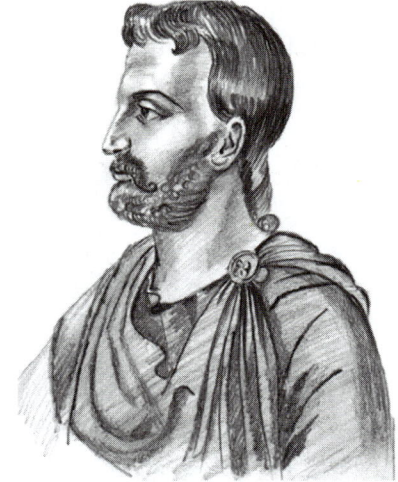

Cornelius Celsus

William Harvey (1578–1657): Established circulation of blood and the function of the heart, also made important observations on the pathology of heart: Ventricular rupture and left-sided hypertrophy in a patient with aortic valve insufficiency.

Giovanni B Morgagni (1682–1771): He was an Italian Anatomist and Pathologist. He was trained the great anatomist Antonio Valsalva. At the age of 24, he wrote his fisrt book "*Adversaria Anatomica*". He conducted 700 postmortums with clinicopathological correlations and described morbid antomy.

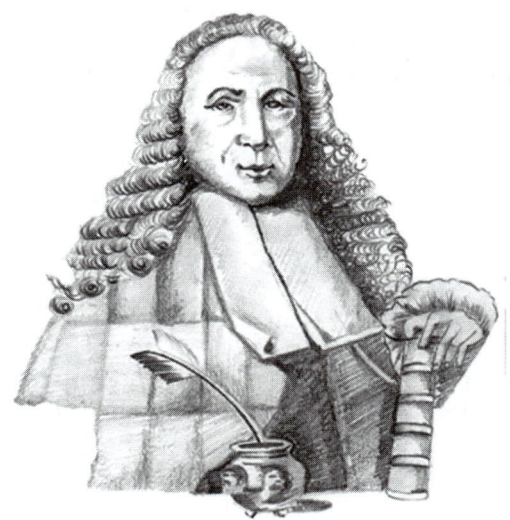

Giovanni B. Morgagni

John Hunter and William Hunter: Described inflammation, defence mechanism and repair mechanism. Also wrote a book on venereal diseases. There is a Huntarian Museum at the Royal College of Physicians and Surgeons and named after Huntarian brothers to appreciate their enormous contribution to science. John Hunter, a famous surgeon, was a Royal Navy Officer. William Hunter was an anatomist and an outstanding obstetrician and his guidance and training made John Hunter famous.

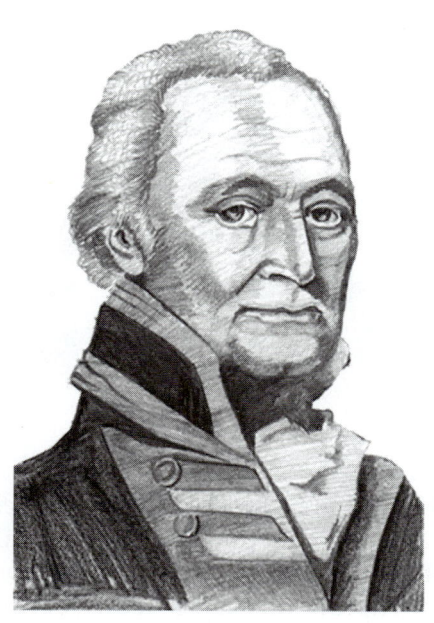

John Hunter

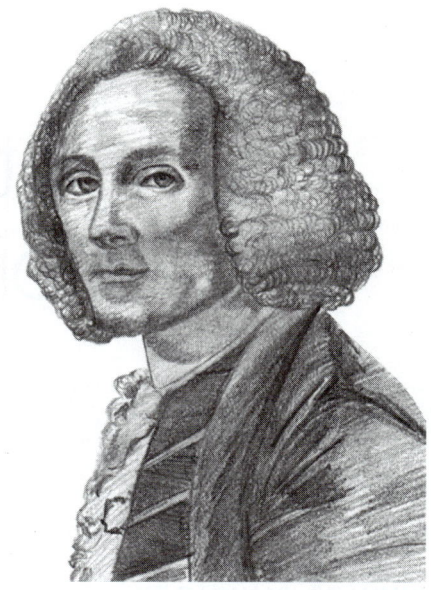

William Hunter

Mathew Baillie: He was a nephew of John and William Hunter. He combined their knowledge and expanded the teaching of morbid anatomy.

Thomas Hodgkin (1798–1866): A general physician with a broad range of interests. Still as a student, he wrote a paper on "uses of spleen" and described the reasons for enlargement of lymph nodes, spleen and liver. At the age of 27, he was appointed as lecturer of Morbid Anatomy at Guys hospital and curator of museum, London. He wrote a treatise on morbid anatomy of mucous and serous membranes.

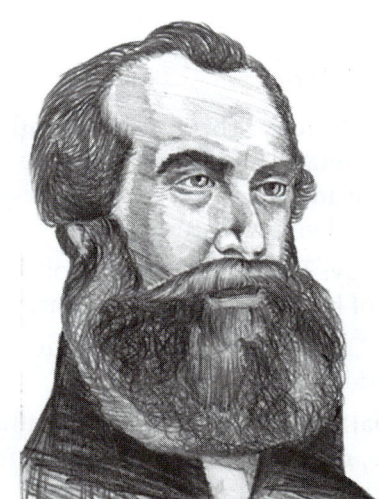

Thomas Hodgkin

Carl Von Rokitansky (1804–1878): He was a Bohemian physician, conducted 30,000 autopsies, described endocarditis, lobar pneumonia, bronchopneumonia, anomalies like Rokitansky Ascoff sinuses and septal defects of heart.

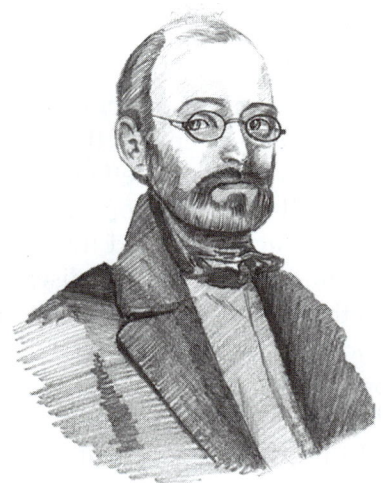

Carl Rokitansky

Rudolf Virchow (1821–1902): Virchow is father of cellular pathology. His most important work *"Die Cellularpathologie"* laid foundation for understanding cell-based disease as opposed to organ-based disease. On his name are Virchow's Method of Autopsy, Virchow Cell and Virchow Triad which are described by him.

Paul Ehrlich (1854–1915): He was a German scientist, discovered mast cells and his prodigious laboratory talent lead to the use of aniline dyes as metachromatic stains.

Friedrich von Recklinghausen (1833–1910): He is remembered for 'multiple neurofibromatosis'. He also did studies on thrombosis, embolism, infarction, degenerations, hemochromatosis, adenomyomata of the uterus, and many other pathologic conditions.

Sternberg and Reed: These two scientists described the RS cells and histopathological changes in Hodgkin disease.

Ludwig Aschoff (1866–1942): Developed the concept of the reticuloendothelial system and described Ascoff cells.

Nikolai Anitschkov (1885–1964): Described the histopathology of the heart, in rheumatic fever.

Paul Klemperer (1884–1964): Introduced the concept of "collagen disease" and described the LE cell phenomenon.

Albert Coons (1912–1978): He is known for revolutionary discoveries of fluorescein-labelled antibodies.

George Kohler (1946–1995): George Kohler was awarded Nobel Prize in physiology in 1984 along with other two scientists for the work on immune system and production of monoclonal antibodies.

Dr. James Holmer Wright: He demonstrated that multiple myeloma is a tumour of plasma cells, that platelets arise from megakaryocytes, that spirochetes can be identified in syphilitic aneurysms of the aorta,

and that neuroblastoma is of nerve cell lineage and contains what became famous as "Homer Wright" rosettes.

George Papanicolaou (1883–1962): He was a pioneer in cytopathology and early cancer detection, and inventor of the "Pap smear". He worked as a physiologist in France and later joined New York University's Cornell Medical School in 1913. Here, he along with Mary Papanicolou worked on vaginal smear changes in menstrual cycle and cancer cell detection in cervical cancer. His scientific treatise was "Atlas of Exfoliative Cytology".

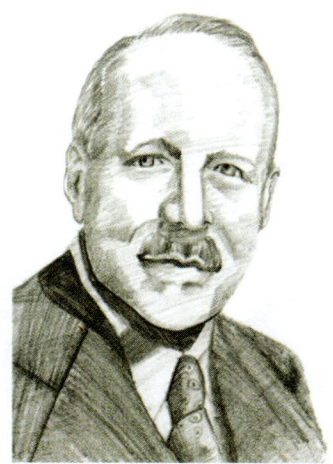

George Papanicolaou

Watson and Crick: Described the structure of DNA and revolutionised genetic study.

Karl Landsteiner (1868–1943): In 1900, Karl Landsteiner (Austrian physician) discovered A, B and O. AB blood group was discovered in the year 1902 by A. Decastello and A. Sturli.

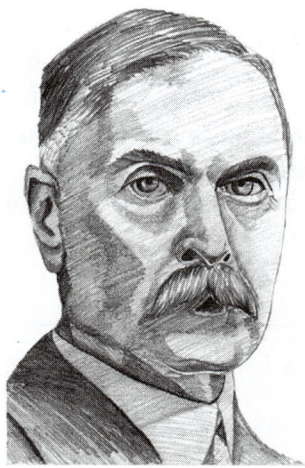

Karl Landsteiner

James Paget (1814–1899): He was a surgical pathologist, prepared catalogue of pathology museum of the Royal College of Surgeons in 1882.

Julium Cohnheim (1839–1884): He was a pathologist from Germany, described migration of leucocytes in inflammation.

Richard Bright (1789–1858): He was a physician from England, described Bright disease.

Gregor Johann Mendel (1822–1884): Experimented on green peas and discovered the fundamental laws of inheritance.

DL Romanowsky (1861–1921): Developed stain to stain blood cells. He used two basic stains methylene blue and eosin.

Barry Marshall and Robin Warren: In 2005, Barry Marshall and Robin Warren were awarded the Nobel Prize in Physiology for their pioneering work on *Helicobacter pylori.*

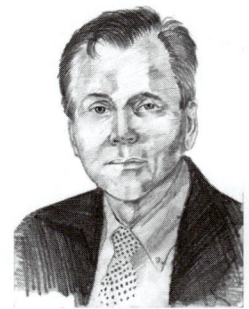 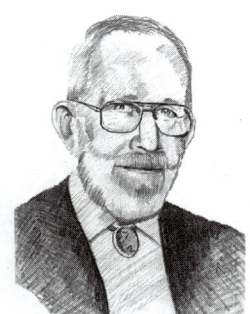

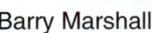
　　Barry Marshall　　　　　　Robin Warren

Role of Pathologist in Diagnosis and Management of Disease

Pathologists are medical specialists, who have considerable skills which enable them to contribute significantly to high quality of efficient and effective health care. The skills they develop because of training first as a medical practitioner and then as a specialist allows them to understand clinical disease processes, diagnostic methods and gives them the specialised ability to report diagnostic tests.

A pathologist plays a crucial role in medical care. Sometimes he or she is the one who first gives the diagnosis and thus, helps the treating physician. The management of patients with disease inflammatory or neoplastic (either benign or malignant) is becoming ever more dependent on a knowledge of the pathology. The pathologist is well versed in diagnosing diseases on histopathology (tissues), haematology (blood), cytology (cells from tissues and fluids) and clinical pathology (urine, etc.), thus helps the clinician in treatment. The pathologist is also helpful in identifying the disease at an early stage of cancer by using pap smears (e.g. carcinoma cervix), fine needle aspiration cytology (palpable and deep seat masses) and using tumour markers.

SELF-ASSESSMENT EXERCISE

1. **Father of modern cellular pathology:**
   A. Rudolf Virchow　　B. Paul Ehrlich
   C. Albert Coons　　　 D. Ascoff

2. **Following scientist is known for his contributions towards staining methods, treatment and chemotherapy:**
   A. Paul Ehrlich　　　 B. Rudolf Virchow
   C. Albert Coons　　　 D. Ascoff

3. **Neurofibromatosis type I disease is also called after scientist:**
   A. von Recklinghausen　B. Paul Ehrlich
   C. Albert Coons　　　　　D. Ascoff

4. **Ludwig Aschoff described:**
   A. Aschoff cells
   B. Rokitansky-Aschoff sinuses
   C. Aschoff sinus
   D. All of the above

5. **All are true for Anitschkow cells *except*:**
   A. Caterpillar cells
   B. They are macrophages
   C. Named after scientist who described
   D. They are lymphocytes

Answers

1. A　　　**2.** A　　　**3.** A　　　**4.** D　　　**5.** D

Cell Injury and Cell Death

CELL INJURY AND CELL DEATH: MECHANISMS

The cells have efficient mechanisms to sustain the effects of injurious agent to some extent. The effects of injury are evident, only when the cell can no more able to maintain the normal homeostasis because of sustained exposure to injurious agent.

Causes of Cell Injury

1. Oxygen deprivation
2. Chemical agents
3. Physical agents
4. Infectious agents
5. Immunological mechanisms
6. Genetic defects
7. Nutritional imbalance
8. Ageing

Types of Cell Injury

The injury can be of following types:
• Reversible cell injury
• Irreversible cell injury

Reversible Cell Injury

If the injurious agent is removed in time, or if the cell can withstand the assault with mild forms of injury, the changes can be reversed and complete structural and functional integrity can be restored. At this stage, the cell has not progressed to severe membrane damage or nuclear damage. For example, if circulation can be re-established within first 20 minutes of myocardial infarction, the fuctional and structural alterations can be reversed back. If the cell is exposed for sublethal injury for a prolonged period, the cell has time to adapt to reversible injury, e.g. exposure of bronchial mucosa to tobacco smoke, the metaplasia of respiratory epithelium to stratified squamous epithelium occurs.

Irreversible Cell Injury

If the injurious agent is of severe nature and not taken off and the damage continues, the cell undergoes irreversible injury, the cell cannot recover and its death occurs. The death can be of two types—necrosis and apoptosis. When damage to membranes is severe, the enzymes leak out lysosomes and digest the cell resulting in necrosis. Apoptosis is characterised by nuclear dissolution without complete loss of membrane integrity. Apoptosis is active, energy dependent mechanism, tightly programmed cell death, whereas necrosis is always pathological process. For details refer to topic on necrosis and apoptosis.

Mechanism of Cell Injury

Cell injury results in functional and biochemical changes. They are mentioned below (Fig. 10.1):
1. ATP depletion
2. Damage to mitochondria
3. Defects in cell membrane permeability
4. Influx of calcium ions
5. Accumulation of oxygen free radicals/reactive oxygen species (ROS)
6. Damage to DNA and proteins

Depletion of ATP

ATP is required for synthetic and other functions of the cell including membrane transport of ions, protein synthesis, lipogenesis, deacetylation and reacetylation reactions of phospholipid turn over. ATP even less than 5 to 15% of normal levels have effect such as (Fig. 10.2):

1. Failure of membrane transport ions–sodium pump with intracellular accumulation of sodium and efflux of potassium causing cell swelling and dilatation of endoplasmic reticulum.

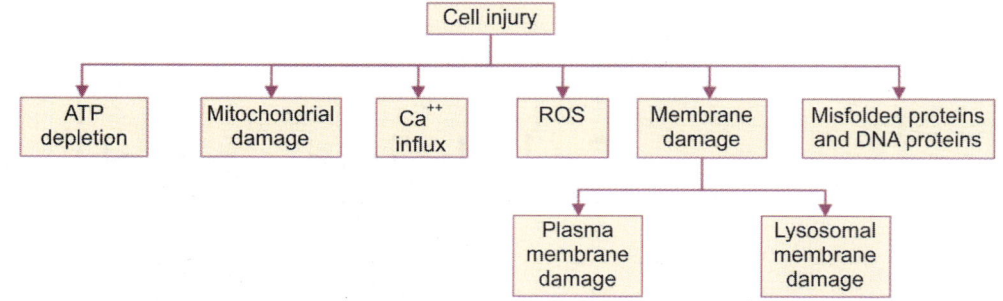

Fig. 10.1: Cell injury: Various effects on cell

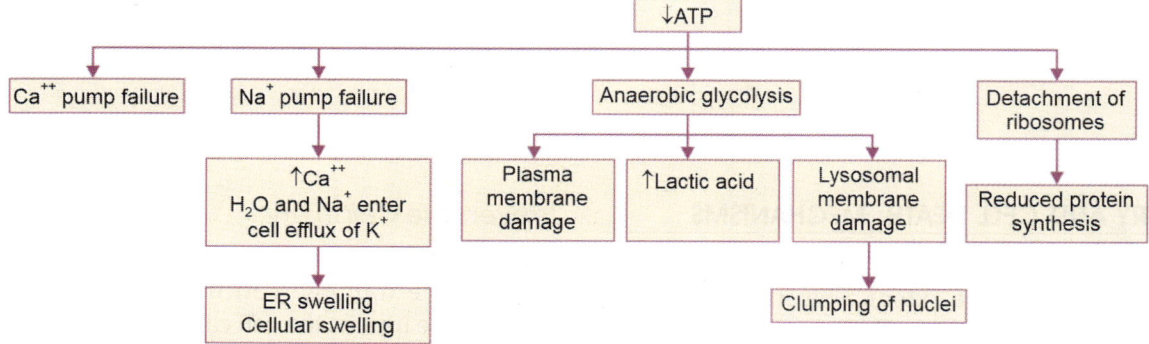

Fig. 10.2: Cell injury: Effects due to reduced ATP

2. Failure of aerobic respiration; anaerobic respiration sets in; glycogen stores are depleted. Lactic acid accumulates with reduction of pH and reduced activity of many cellular enzymes.
3. Failure of calcium pump; influx of calcium activates many enzymes.
4. Disruption of protein synthesis; ribosomes detach from rough endoplasmic reticulum with reduction in protein synthesis.

Damage to Mitochondria

Mitochondria can be damaged by increased cytosolic Ca^{2+}, ROS, hypoxia and all types of injurious stimuli including toxins.

Mitochondrial damage leads to failure of oxidative phosphorylation and progressive depletion of ATP and cell death. Also cytochrome C induced cell death by apoptosis can occur (Fig. 10.3).

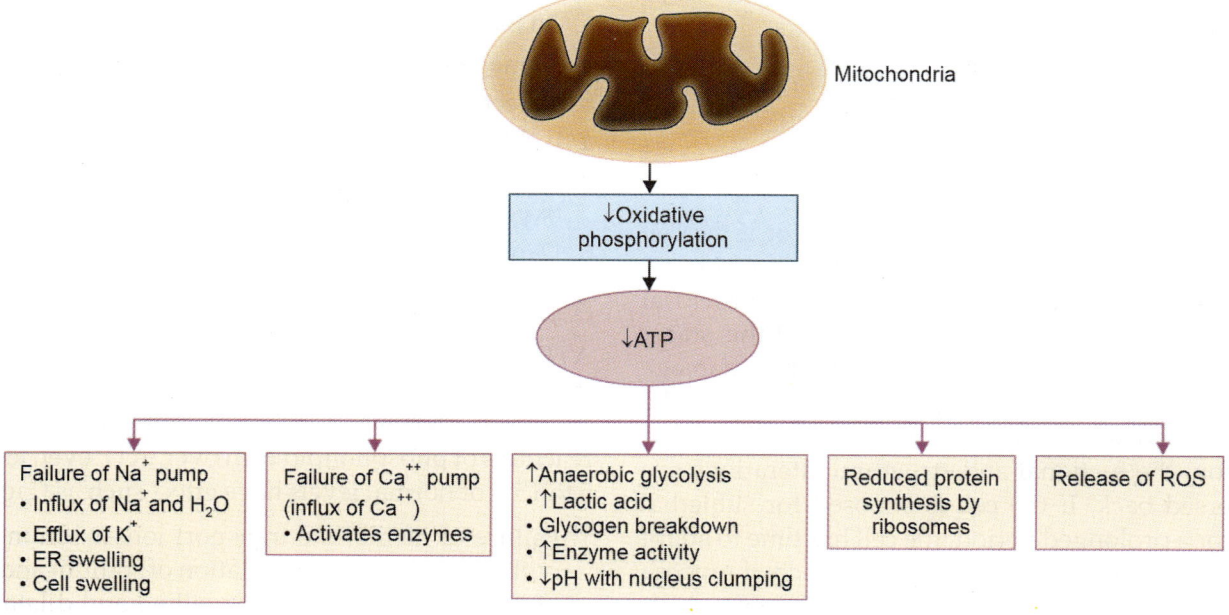

Fig. 10.3: Effects due to damage to mitochondria

Defects in Cell Membrane Permeability

Defects in cell membrane permeability have the following effects:

1. Decreased O_2 and increased cytosolic Ca^{2+} seen in ischaemia leads to activation of proteases.
2. ROS cause injury to cell membrane by lipid peroxidation.
3. Breakdown of membrane phospholipids by activation of endogenous phospholipases by increased cytosolic Ca^{2+}.
4. Lipid breakdown products accumulated in the injured cells cause changes in permeability. The most important cell components affected are:
   i. Damage to mitochondria leads to decreased ATP, necrosis and/or triggers apoptosis.
   ii. Damage to plasma membrane leads to loss of osmotic balance, influx of water and Na^+, loss of K^+, leakage of enzymes, activation of enzymes which leads to enzymatic digestion of cell components and cells undergo necrosis.

Influx of Calcium Ions

Intracytosolic calcium is maintained by ATP dependent calcium transporters at low concentration.

Ischaemia and certain toxins lead to increased cytosolic calcium and following events are expected.

1. Activation of many enzymes
2. Phospholipases breakdown cell membrane
3. Leakage of proteases damage cell membrane and cytoskeleton
4. Endonucleases breakdown DNA
5. Activation of caspases and cell death by apoptosis

Accumulation of Oxygen-Free Radicals/Reactive Oxygen Species (ROS)

Reactive oxygen species (ROS) are oxygen-free radicals having single unpaired electrons in the outer orbit. These are produced during energy generation and removed by cellular defence mechanisms. These are unstable and react with inorganic or organic chemicals. These attack nucleic acid, proteins and lipids. The scavenging systems are ineffective and lead to oxidative stress. Accumulation of free radicals depends on rate of production and removal of ROS (Fig. 10.4).

In mitochondrial metabolism (oxidation reduction reaction), small amount of toxic intermediate species ROS are generated by partial reduction of oxygen. These include superoxide radicals (O_2^-), hydrogen peroxide (H_2O_2) and hydroxyl ions (OH^-). During this process, copper and iron also accept or donate free electrons and catalyse free radical formation as in Fenton reaction (Fig. 10.4).

Radiant energy can hydrolyse water into hydroxyl (OH^-) and hydrogen free molecules (H^+), e.g. UV rays,

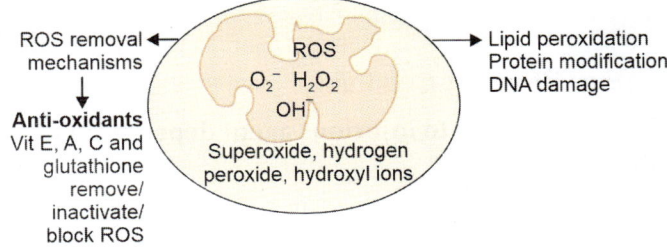

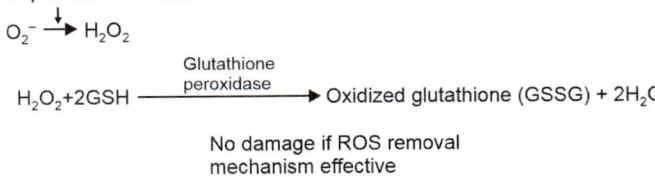

Scavenging systems
catalase acts on $2H_2O_2$ converts to $2H_2O + O_2$
Superoxide dismutase converts

$$O_2^- \xrightarrow{} H_2O_2$$

$$H_2O_2 + 2GSH \xrightarrow{\text{Glutathione peroxidase}} \text{Oxidized glutathione (GSSG)} + 2H_2O$$

No damage if ROS removal mechanism effective

Proteins bind Cu and Fe
Ceruloplasmin binds Cu
Haptoglobin–uptake of extracellular haemoglobin
Ferritin–For Fe^{+++} storage
Lactoferrin–binds Fe^{+++} in leucocytes
Transferrin–binds Fe^{+++} in blood

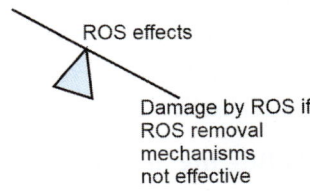

Fig. 10.4: ROS removal mechanisms

X-rays, etc. The enzymatic metabolism of exogenous toxins can produce free radicals, e.g. CCl_4. Nitric oxide, a chemical mediator can act as free radical or can get converted to nitrites which are highly reactive.

Free radicals promote:

1. Lipid peroxidation of membranes
2. Sulfhydroxyl-mediated cross-linking of proteins with loss of enzyme activity and polypeptide fragmentation.
3. DNA fragmentation leading to cell death, aging and malignant transformation.
4. Ageing
5. Malignant transformation

The cells have many mechanisms to remove these free radicals:

1. Superoxide dismutase takes off superoxide which in combination with hydrogen molecule gets converted to H_2O_2 and oxygen.
2. Glutathione peroxidase (GSH) removes the hydroxyl molecules as glutathione gets oxidized.
3. Catalase degrades H_2O_2 to water and oxygen.
4. Endogenous and exogenous antioxidants (vitamin A, E, C and beta-carotenes) block the formation of free radicals.
5. Iron and copper can catalyse the generation of ROS. The reactive metals are reduced once they bind to storage and transport proteins.

Damage to DNA and Proteins

There can be severe damage to DNA and proteins. The cells when severely damaged undergo necrosis or die by apoptosis.

Factors Affecting Cell Injury

The cell response to injurious agent depends on the following factors:

1. Type of injury
2. Duration
3. Severity

Toxins in low doses and for a short time may cause reversible injury, whereas longer duration and larger doses result in irreversible injury and cell death.

The consequences of injurious agent on the injured cell depend upon the following:

1. Type of cells
2. Nutritional status
3. Adaptability
4. Genetic factors

Following are some of the occasions:

1. Cardiac cells die after 20–30 minutes of ischaemia, whereas skeletal muscle can withstand for 2–3 hrs.
2. The nutritional or hormonal status is also important.
3. Genetically determined metabolic variations may differ from individual to individual, e.g. variations in gene encoding cytochrome P-450 may catabolize the toxin at different rates.

Information on Causative Factors

Oxygen Deprivation

Hypoxia or oxygen deficiency reduces aerobic oxidative respiration and is an important cause of cell injury and cell death. Hypoxia can be caused by ischaemia. Oxygen deficiency can also result from inadequate oxygenation of blood as in pneumonia, chronic anaemia or in carbon monoxide poisoning.

Chemical Agents

These can injure cells and derrange osmotic environment. Oxygen at high partial pressure is also directly toxic. These cause damage at cellular level, such as alteration in membrane permeability, disturb osmotic homeostasis, enzymes, cofactors and cause cell injury and cell death.

Air pollutants, insecticides, carbon monoxide, asbestos, ethanol and drugs cause damage in susceptible individuals or when used excessively.

Physical Agents

The physical agents include trauma, temperature changes (e.g. heat stroke and frost bite), radiation, electric shock, changes in atmospheric pressure, etc.

Infectious Agents

These include parasites, microbes, viruses, fungi, rickettsiae, etc. These cause injury to the cells and tissue in different ways.

Immunological Mechanisms

Immune mechanisms although protect us against organisms, they may sometimes can cause tissue injury. Examples of this type of injury are: Rheumatic heart disease, systemic lupus erythematosus, glomerular diseases, etc.

Genetic Defects

Genetic defects are associated with congenital defects, deficiency of important proteins as in in-born errors of metabolism, accumulation damaged DNA, susceptibility of cells to injury by chemicals and environmental insults.

Nutritional Imbalance

Deficiencies and excess of nutrition can predispose to diseases. Infectious diseases are common in protein energy malnutrition patients. Diets rich in animal fat are implicated in development of cancer and atherosclerosis. Obese individuals are prone for type 2 diabetes mellitus and heart diseases.

Ageing

Ageing leads to reduced repair capacity of the tissues and reduced ability to respond to injury.

CELLULAR ADAPTATIONS

Cellular adaptations refer to reversible changes in size, number, phenotype, appearance and metabolic and functional activity of cells due to adverse environmental changes. It can be reversible, if the causative factor is taken off. The cell adapts to the new environment in different ways due to adverse environment.

The basic types of cellular adaptation are:

1. Hyperplasia
2. Hypertrophy
3. Atrophy
4. Metaplasia

Hyperplasia

Definition

Hyperplasia is increase in number of cells in organ or tissue. This type of adaptation occurs in tissues which can undergo division. It does not occur in heart and brain. It can occur along with hypertrophy.

Physiological Causes

1. Hormonal stimulus can cause proliferation of the glands and stromal tissue as it happens in:
   a. Breast during puberty and pregnancy
   b. Uterus in pregnancy
   c. Prostate enlargement called benign prostatic hyperplasia (BPH) or nodular prostatic hyperplasia (NPH)
2. Compensatory hyperplasia which occurs after portion of tissue is resected or diseased, e.g. liver when partially resected, the remaining cells undergo mitoses, which begin as early as 12 hours of resection and restores the liver to its normal size and weight. The stimulus for restoration is polypeptide growth factors released by the remaining normal hepatocytes and non-parenchymal cells of liver. Once the liver attains the normal mass, the proliferation stops by various inhibitors released by the normal cells only.

Pathological Causes

These are caused by hormone or growth factors stimulation.

The examples are:
1. Endometrial hyperplasia due to excess estrogen hormone.
2. Wound healing—proliferation of epithelial cells, fibroblasts and blood vessels in wound healing—the growth factors are produced by WBCs responding to injury and by the cells in the extracellular matrix.
3. Skin epithelium with HPV infection which causes hyperplasia of stratified squamous epithelial cells causing papilloma (viral wart).
4. Skin epithelium as in psoriasis.
5. Pancreatic islet cell hyperplasia in infants of diabetic mothers.

   If the stimulus/growth factor ablates or removed, hyperplasia recedes or disappears.

Hypertrophy

Definition

Hypertrophy is an increase in the size of the cells resulting in increased size of the organs. In hypertrophy, there are no new cells. There is increase in size of the cells with increased amount of structural proteins and organelles. Hypertrophy is an adaptive response in cells incapable of dividing. It can be physiological or pathological and is caused either due to increased demand or by hormonal stimulus. Hyperplasia and hypertrophy can occur together and both of these can lead to enlarged organ.

Physiological Causes

1. **Uterus during pregnancy:** Estrogen stimulates smooth muscle cells to undergo hypertrophy and hyperplasia.
2. **Skeletal muscle of limbs in athletes:** Skeletal muscles undergo hypertrophy due to increased muscle activity.

Pathological Causes

Heart muscles undergo hypertrophy: This is due to increased demand as in hypertension or aortic valve incompetence/stenosis (Fig. 10.5).

Mechanism of Hypertrophy

Hypertrophy involves two types of signals:
1. Mechanical triggers such as stretch
2. Trophic triggers such as activation of adrenergic receptors

   The signals stimulate synthesis of cellular proteins including growth factors and structural proteins and thus can achieve increased performance.

Atrophy

Definition

There is shrinkage in size of the cell due to loss of cell substances. This is called atrophy. When good number of cells are involved, the entire tissue or organ is reduced in size and weight. Along with reduction in size of the cells, the number of the cells may also be reduced. The atrophic cells have diminished function but are not dead.

Causes include:
1. Decreased workload (immobilisation of limb in plaster cast in fracture of limb bones)
2. Loss of innervation
3. Loss of endocrine stimulus
4. Old age (senile atrophy)

Physiological Causes

1. Involution of branchial cleft, thyroglossal duct, and notochord.

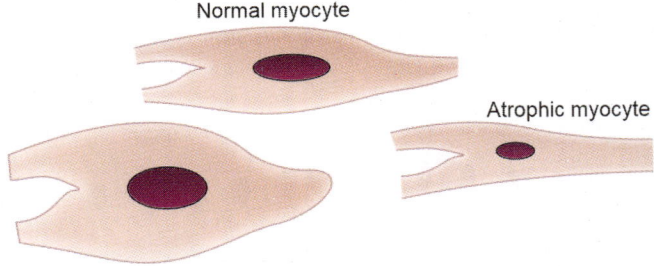

Fig. 10.5: Normal myocyte, hypertrophied myocyte and atrophic myocyte

2. Involution of Wolffian duct and müllerian duct in females and males, respectively.

3. Atrophy of ovary, endometrium after menopause and other tissues in old age.

Pathological Causes

1. Disuse atrophy of limb
2. Loss of innervations
3. Loss of blood supply
4. Pressure atrophy
5. Lack of nutrients
6. Reduced hormones
7. Loss of endocrine stimulation

Mechanism of Atrophy

1. There is reduced protein synthesis due to reduction in metabolic activity.
2. Increased protein degradation by ubiquitin protease pathway.
3. Nutrient deficiency and disuse atrophy may activate ubiquitin ligase.
4. Atrophy is also accompanied by autophagy (self-eating) with vacuoles.
5. There may be production of lipofuscin (wear and tear) pigment, the organs size and weight are not only reduced (Fig. 10.5) but also change to brown colour due to deposition of lipofuscin pigment.

Metaplasia

Definition

Metaplasia is a reversible change in which one adult cell type (epithelial or mesenchymal) is replaced by another adult cell type.

Mechanism of Metaplasia

The cells are sensitive to particular stress and are replaced by another type of cell which can able to withstand the adverse environment.

Metaplasia can be:
1. Epithelial metaplasia
2. Mesenchymal metaplasia

Epithelial Metaplasia

Most common type of epithelial metaplasia is replacement of columnar epithelia by stratified squamous epithelium. Rarely squamous epithelium may be replaced by glandular epithelium (Fig. 10.6).

Following are the examples:

a. Respiratory epithelium (ciliated pseudostratified columnar epithelium) changes to stratified squamous epithelium in habitual cigarette smokers and vitamin A deficiency.

b. Endocervical epithelium may change to stratified squamous epithelium.

c. Ducts of salivary glands with glandular epithelium may undergo metaplasia to stratified squamous epithelium due to chronic irritation by stones.

d. Ducts of pancreatic glands may change to stratified squamous epithelium due to stones.

e. Transitional epithelium of bladder and pelvis of kidney may change to stiatified squamous epithelium due to irritation by renal stones.

f. Endometrial metaplasia may show different types of epithelia.

g. The lower end of oesophagus which is usually lined by stratified squamous epithelium may change to columnar epithelium due to reflux oesophagitis.

Mesenchymal Metaplasia

The fibrous tissue and other types of tissue, such as cartilage, may transform into bone.

The undifferentiated cells transform into other adult mesenchymal cells. Cartilage metaplasia or osseous metaplasia are more common.

1. In old scars, necrotic areas, myositis ossificans foci of bone may develop.

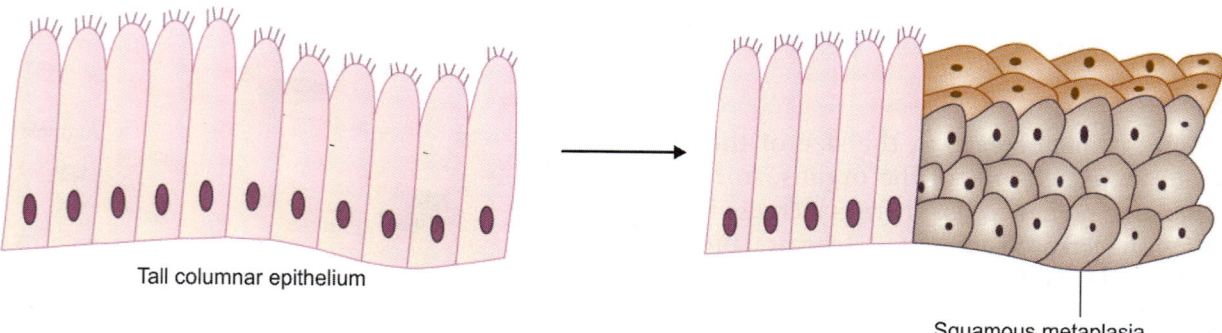

Tall columnar epithelium

Squamous metaplasia

Fig. 10.6: Squamous metaplasia (schematic)

2. Walls of diseased arteries destroyed by injury or inflammation, foci of bone may develop.

3. In laryngeal and bronchial cartilage of old people, cartilage undergo ossification.

4. Fibromas may show osseous metaplasia.

5. Uterine leiomyoma may undergo osseous and mesenchymal metaplasia.

Though the metaplastic epithelium has survival advantages with metaplasia, the important protective mechanisms are lost, such as:

1. Mucus secretion

2. Ciliary clearance of particulate matter as in respiratory tract.

The metaplastic epithelium may predispose to malignant transformation, if it is not reserved back or the causative agent is not removed.

REVERSIBLE CELL INJURY (Degenerations)

Definition

These are retrogressive changes in the cells due to direct action of the injurious agents. The term reversible cell injury or degeneration is used to denote changes in the cell due to sublethal injury. There is no death of the cells. The cell has time to adapt to reversible injury in many ways. If the injury is severe, it leads to cell death.

Types of degeneration include:

  i. Cloudy degeneration
 ii. Hydropic degeneration/vacuolar change
iii. Hyaline change
 iv. Mucoid degeneration
  v. Fatty degeneration
vii. Amyloid degeneration

CLOUDY DEGENERATION

Definition and Other Details

There is accumulation of water in the cells. This is called by different names like cloudy swelling, granular degeneration, albuminous degeneration and parenchymal degeneration. The parenchymal cells affected are rich in mitochondria.

Tissues like renal tubules and muscle are affected. If the injurious agent is taken off, the changes can be reversed.

Causes

• Ischaemia
• Hypoxia

• Poisons: Carbon tetrachloride, phosphorus, mercuric chloride
• Bacterial toxins

Mechanism

Krebs cycle is impaired. There is failure of sodium pump. Sodium enters the cells along with chlorides and thus water accumulates.

Gross: The affected organ is normal in size or enlarged. Weight is increased. Colour is pale because of vascular compression. It is soft in consistency. Cut section bulges outwards.

Microscopy: The cells are swollen, water logged, borders are frayed. Nuclei appear normal. Mitochondria are damaged, appear beaded and cristae are lost. Endoplasmic reticulum shows dilatation of cisternae. Cytoplasm is pale eosinophilic and granular.

Most commonly, the renal tubules are affected. The epithelium shows above changes, lumen appears narrowed.

HYDROPIC DEGENERATION

Definition

This is the extension of changes seen in cloudy degeneration. Thus there is excess accumulation of water within the cytoplasm of the cell. The changes are reversible as long as cell and nuclei are intact. The changes are principally seen in hepatocytes, skin, tubular epithelial cells of kidney, neuronal cells, etc.

Following are the causes of hydropic degeneration in different organs:

a. Liver in infectious hepatitis, carbon tetrachloride and chloroform poisoning

b. Kidney tubules in potassium deficiency

c. Skin blisters as seen in herpes simplex infection, varicella-zoster, smallpox

d. Untreated diabetes mellitus

e. Neural cells in viral infections

Gross: Findings are similar to cloudy degeneration. Affected organ is enlarged, weighs more, pale, soft and cut section bulges outwards.

Microscopy: The cells are ballooned, cytoplasm has water vacuoles. These vacuoles are negative for glycogen and fat stains. Nucleus may be in the centre or pushed to the periphery and may show karyorrhexis and karyolysis.

HYALINE DEGENERATION

Definition

The word hyaline means glassy. It is glassy, amorphous and homogenous material which stains pink/eosinophilic with H and E stain. The origin of hyaline change is not exactly known. This does not refer to any specific substance. It may be physiological or pathological, representing plasma proteins, damaged muscle tissue, connective tissue, secretions, etc.

Physiological conditions with hyaline degeneration are:

   i. Arteries of atrophic uterus
  ii. Colloid in multinodular goitre
 iii. Corpora amylacea in prostate
 iv. Corpora albicans in ovary

Pathological Conditions

Extracellular Hyaline

1. Collagen in:
   a. Old scar tissue
   b. Keloid
   c. Thickened capillaries and vessels
2. Fibroma
3. Vessels in:
   a. Diabetes mellitus
   b. Hypertension
4. KW lesions of kidney in diabetes mellitus
5. Hyalinization of islets of Langerhans in diabetes mellitus

Intracellular Hyaline

1. *Mallory hyaline:* Also called alcoholic hyaline, seen as eosinophilic material in the cytoplasm represents damaged prekeratin intermediate filaments. Commonly seen in fatty change, hepatitis or cirrhosis due to alcohol, Wilson's disease, Indian childhood cirrhosis, primary biliary cirrhosis, non-alcoholic steatohepatitis (NASH), hepatocellular carcinoma, etc.
2. *Councilman bodies:* Seen in yellow fever.
3. *Russell bodies:* These represent immunoglobulins in plasma cells.
4. *Viral hyaline*
5. *Epithelial hyaline:* These are commonly seen in epithelium of the proximal tubules due to excess absorption of plasma proteins.

Zenker's degeneration: Striated muscles of diaphragm, abdomen and thigh show hyaline change in typhoid.

The muscle cells are swollen, loose striations and hyalinized. The nuclei are lost.

MUCOID DEGENERATION

Definition and Other Details

In mucoid degeneration, there is excess accumulation of mucin or mucin-like material. It is mainly because of excess production of glycoproteins or mucoproteins. It can be of epithelial or mesenchymal origin.

Mucoid degenerations due to epithelial origin are as in:

1. Catarrhal rhinitis
2. Hyperplasia of bronchial mucous glands as in asthma.
3. Mucocoele appendix
4. Pseudomyxoma peritonei

Mucoid degenerations due to mesenchymal origin are:

1. Wharton's jelly
2. Fibroma with mucoid/myxoid generation
3. Leiomyoma with mucoid/myxoid degeneration
4. Fibroadenoma
5. Ganglion
6. Myxomatous change in dermis of skin which is seen in myxoedema.
7. Myxomatous degeneration of heart valves as in Marfan's syndrome.

In mesenchymal origin, pools of basophilic material collect along with stellate cells or in connective tissue.

NICE TO KNOW

The changes in the reversible cell depend upon:
1. **Nature of injurious agent:**
  • Its toxicity
  • Concentration
2. **Duration**
3. **Tissue affected:**
  • Liver cells
  • Myofibrils
  • Epithelial cells
4. **Inherent susceptibility of the tissue:**
  • Liver cells in carbon tetrachloride poisoning
  • Renal tubular cells in mercury poisoning
  • Beta cells of pancreas with alloxan drug

FATTY CHANGE

Liver is the common site of fat accumulation as it plays a pivotal role in fat metabolism. Occasionally, fatty change can be also encountered in heart, skeletal muscle, kidney and other organs.

Fatty Change Liver

Definition

Abnormal accumulation of triglycerides within the parenchymal cells is referred to as fatty change. It is also called steatosis. Terms like fatty degeneration, fatty phenarosis and fatty metamorphosis were used earlier. It is most commonly seen in liver as it is a major organ of fat metabolism.

Causes (Etiology)

- Diabetes mellitus
- Congenital hyperlipidaemia
- Alcohol
- Starvation
- Protein calorie malnutrition
- Chronic illness
- Pregnancy
- Hypoxia
- Hepatotoxins—CCl$_4$
- Drugs
- Reye's syndrome

Pathogenesis of Fatty Change

Free fatty acids from fat depots or diet are transported to hepatocytes. In the liver, they are esterified to triglycerides, converted into cholesterol or phospholipids or oxidized to ketone bodies. Some fatty acids are synthesized from acetate also. In association with apoproteins, triglycerides form lipoproteins which enter the circulation. Excess accumulation of triglycerides within the liver may occur from defects in any one of the events from entry of fatty acids to exit of lipoproteins (Fig. 10.7).

Morphological Changes

Gross: The liver is enlarged (mild/moderate/severe enlargement) depending upon the accumulation of fat. The capsule is tense and glistening. The margins are rounded. It is yellowish in colour, greasy to touch, soft in consistency, C/S bulges slightly and weight is increased. In severe fatty change, the liver may weigh 3 to 6 kg (Fig. 10.8).

Microscopy (Figs 10.9 to 10.11): The normal liver architecture is maintained. The characteristic feature is presence of numerous lipid vacuoles in the cytoplasm

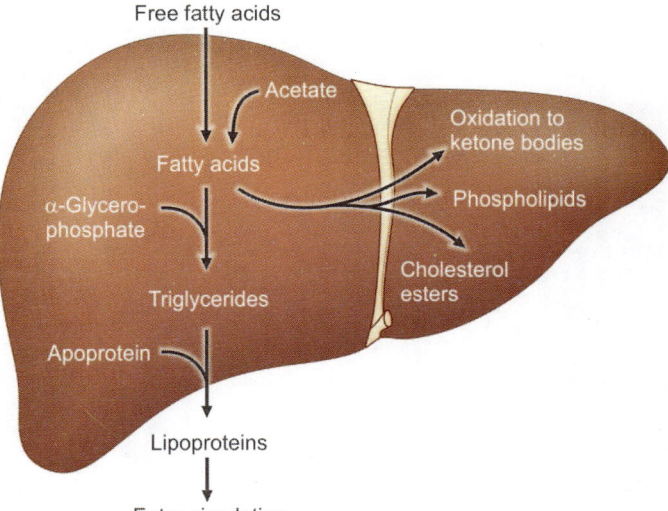

Fig. 10.7: Mechanism of fatty change

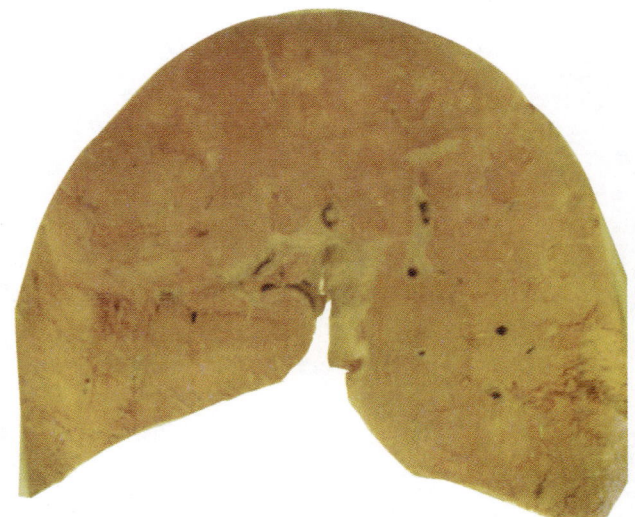

Fig. 10.8: Fatty change liver (gross picture)

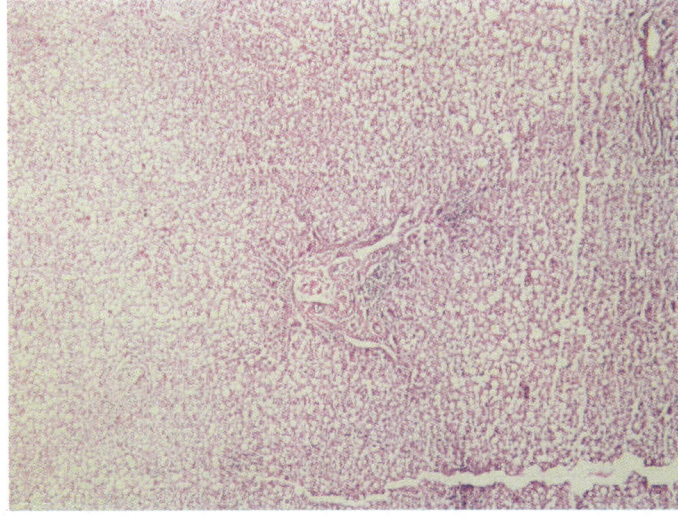

Fig. 10.9: Microphotograph of fatty change liver, note severe fatty change (low magnification)

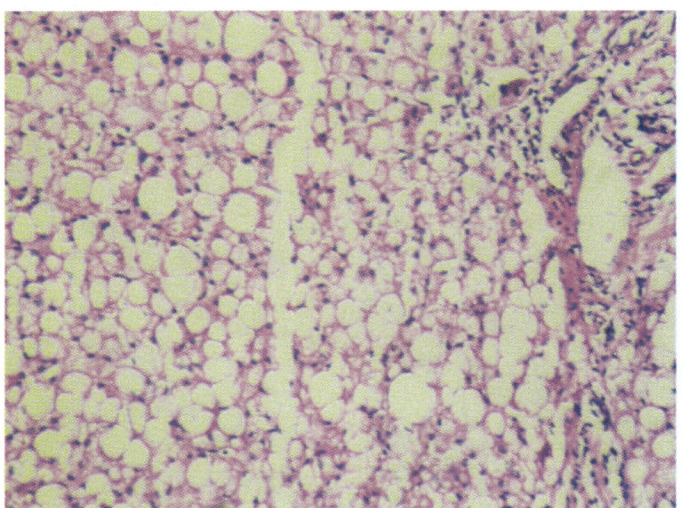

Fig. 10.10: Microphotograph of fatty change liver, note severe fatty change (higher magnification)

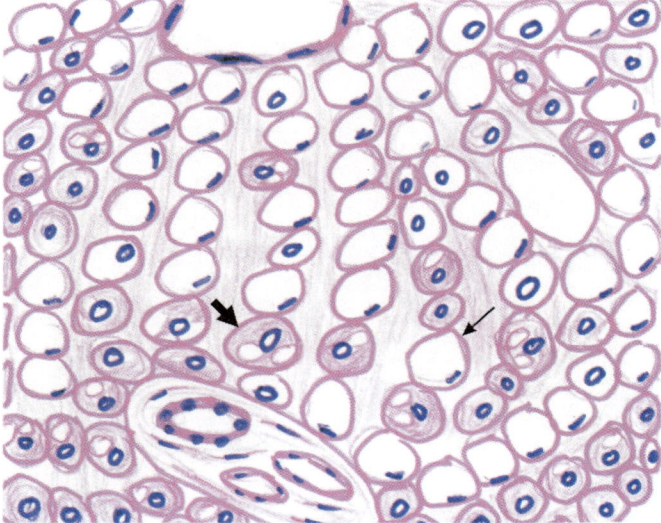

Fig. 10.11: Microscopy of fatty liver, note microvesicular (thick arrow) and macrovesicular (thin arrow) fatty change (schematic)

of hepatocytes. In mild fatty change, small sized fat vacuoles/liposomes are present around the nuclei (microvesicular); later they coalesce and displace the nucleus to the periphery (macrovesicular). The contiguous cells rupture and form fatty cysts.

Stains for Demonstration of Fat

The demonstration of fat can be done by using frozen sections. Some of the fat stains which can be applied are:
   i. Oil red 'O'—fat stains red
  ii. Sudan III/IV—fat stains orange to red
 iii. Osmium tetroxide—with alpha naphthylamine reaction, phospholipids are stain orange red; cholesterol and triglycerides are stained black.
 iv. Neutral fat is stained black with 1% osmic acid in saturated bichlorides or mercury.

Fatty Change Heart

Definition

There is accumulation fat in the cardiac muscle fibres.

Causes of Fatty Change Heart

1. Prolonged moderate hypoxia as seen in severe anaemia results in focal intracellular fat deposits, grossly, this gives yellowish appearance to the affected myocardial fibres and the normal fibres remain darker and red brown. This pattern is referred as 'tigered' or 'thrush breast' effect. It may also occur in myocarditis, coronary arteriosclerosis, starvation, fever, etc.

2. The myocardial fibers are **uniformly and diffusely** affected due to some toxins, e.g. diphtheria. The anaemia is more severe and profound.

AMYLOIDOSIS

Amyloid is an abnormal proteinaceous substance deposited extracellularly in various organs. It is eosinophilic and hyaline-like with H and E stain. The accumulation encroaches and produces pressure atrophy of adjacent cells.

Amyloidosis refers to extracellular protein deposits that have:
1. Common morphological types
2. Affinity for special dyes
3. Characteristic appearance under polarised light

Amyloidosis was first described by Rokitansky in 1842. Virchow named it as amyloid after its starch or cellulose-like nature after staining with iodine and sulphuric acid which turned violet coloured.

Ultrastructure and Physicochemical Nature of Amyloid

Amyloid is fibrillar in nature. Ultrastructurally, it is comprised of non-branching fibrils, polypeptide chains, and these are 7.5 to 10 nm in diameter. These are arranged in beta-pleated sheets. All amyloids have a "p component" (10% of amyloid) which is pentagonal, doughnut-shaped and has complex carbohydrates (glycoproteins) which have given its name amyloid. More than 20 biochemically known distinct forms of amyloid proteins are identified (Fig. 10.12).

Classification of Amyloidosis

Amyloidosis can be classified as:
1. Primary amyloidosis or
2. Secondary amyloidosis

They can also be classified as (Table 10.1):
1. Systemic
2. Localised

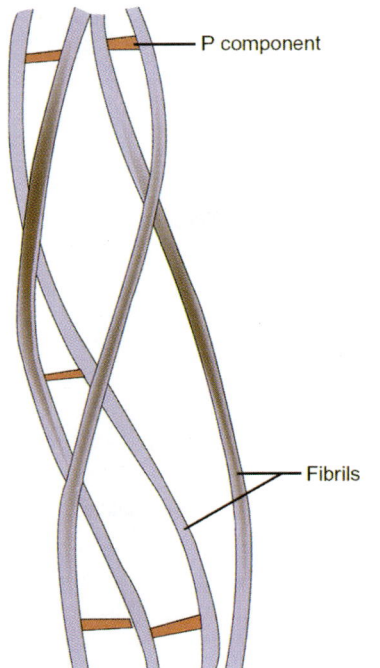

Fig. 10.12: Ultrastructure of amyloid fibrils (schematic)

The most common types are the following:

1. AL (amyloid light chains) protein: It is produced by plasma cells and comprised of immunoglobulin light chains and seen in monoclonal B cell proliferations like:

- Multiple myeloma
- Waldenstrom's macroglobulinaemia
- Lymphomas

2. Amyloid-associated (AA) protein: It is a non-immunoglobulin protein derived from serum precursor protein—SAA (serum amyloid associated) which is synthesized in the liver and defective proteolysis leads to the deposition in conditions like:

- Tuberculosis
- Rheumatoid arthritis
- Carcinomas
- Bronchiectasis
- Other causes like:
  - Dermatomyopathies
  - Crohn's disease
  - Ankylosing spondylitis
  - Lepromatous leprosy

3. A beta amyloid protein: It is found in cerebral lesions in Alzheimer's disease in cerebral plaques and blood vessels.

4. Mutant transthyretin: The mutations of transthyretin that transports thyroxin and retinol aggregates in the form of amyloid deposits. This results in familial amyloid polyneuropathies. It can also develop in the heart in aged people.

5. Beta 2 microglobulin: This protein is present in the serum of patients with renal disease which is retained in circulation as it is not filtered through dialysis membranes.

Mechanism of Amyloidosis

Mechanism of amyloidosis is depicted in Fig. 10.13.

Changes in Different Organs

Amyloidosis of Liver

Gross: The amyloid deposits may be grossly inapparent or may show moderate to marked hepatomegaly. The cut section is waxy.

Microscopy: The amyloid gets deposited in the space of Disse and progressively encroaches on the adjacent hepatocytes and sinusoids. In advanced stages, it has pressure atrophy features with disappearance of hepatocytes. Vascular involvement is frequent (Figs 10.14 and 10.15).

Amyloidosis of Spleen

Gross: The amyloid deposits may be grossly inapparent or may show moderate to marked splenomegaly.

Table 10.1	Classification with precursor proteins and clinical setting in amyloidosis	
Amyloid protein	**Protein precursor**	**Clinical setting**
Systemic/generalized		
AL	Kappa or lamda chains	Multiple myeoloma, plasma cell dyscrasias
AA	ApoSAA	Chronic inflammations, certain neoplasia, hereditary conditions, familial mediterranean fever
Localised		
A beta amyloid	A beta protein	Alzheimer's disease and blood vessels
Mutant transthyretin (ATTR)	Transthretin	Familial amyloid polyneuropathies and heart in aged people
ABeta2 microglobulin	Beta 2 microglobulin	Renal dialysis
ACal	(pro) calcitonin	Medullary carcinoma thyroid
PrPs	Plasma membrane protein	Prion disease

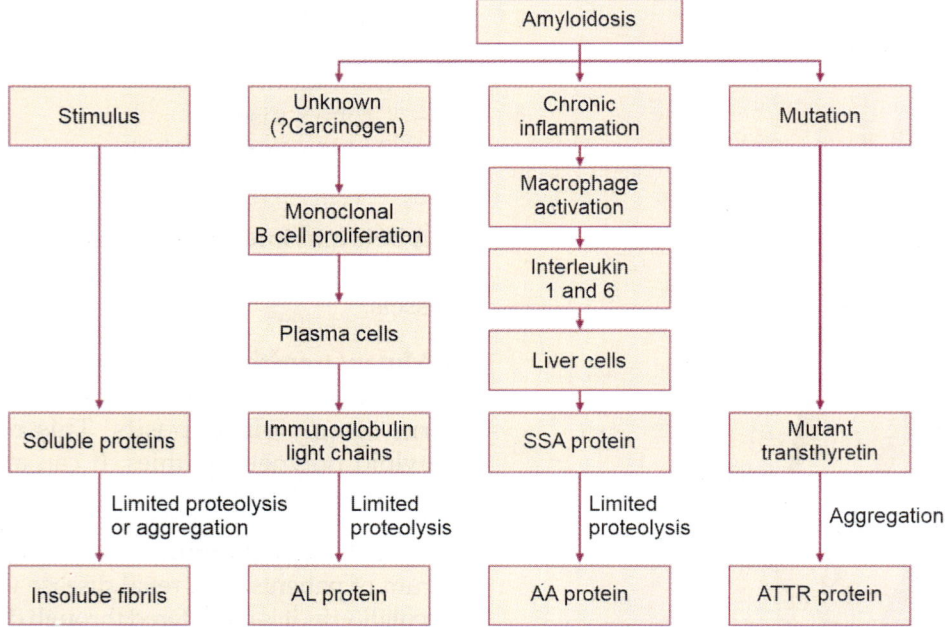

Fig. 10.13: Flowchart for mechanism of amyloidosis

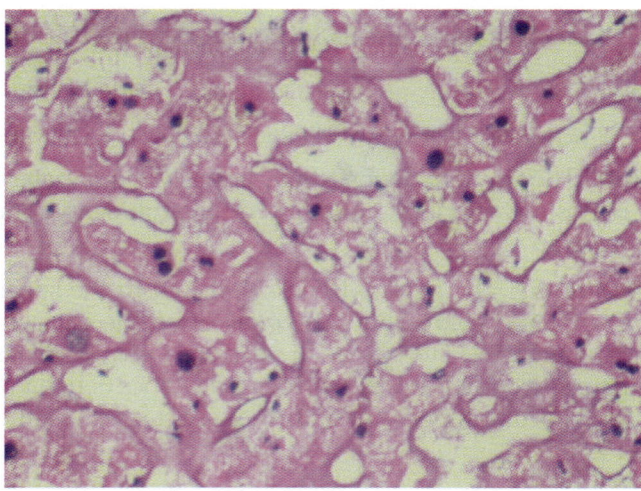

Fig. 10.14: Microphotograph of amyloidosis liver

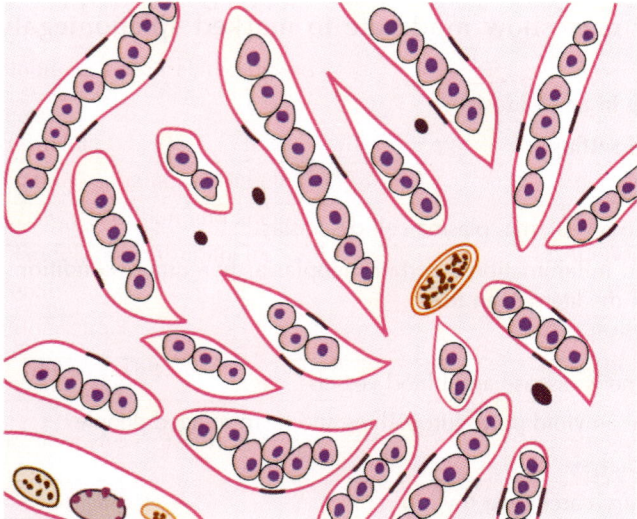

Fig. 10.15: Microscopy in amyloidosis liver (schematic)

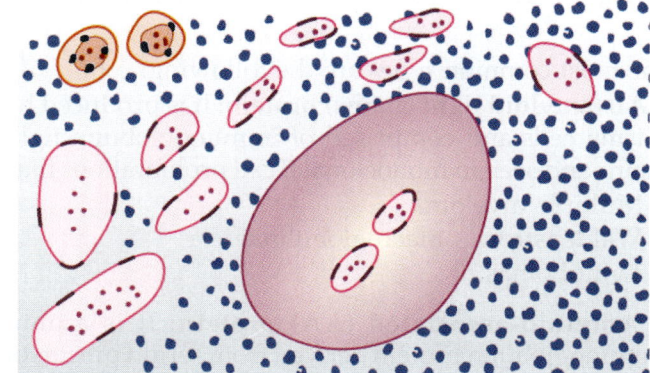

Fig. 10.16: Microscopy of amyloidosis spleen (sago spleen) (schematic)

Deposits in malpighian corpuscle may present as sago spleen (tapioca-like granules) and deposits in red pulp (sinusoids) give the appearance of lardaceous spleen (large map-like areas). The cut section is waxy.

Microscopy

Sago spleen (Fig. 10.16): The amyloid deposits are limited to the splenic follicles (in the vessel and may replace the follicle).

Lardaceous spleen: The amyloid spares the follicles but involves the walls of the splenic sinusoids and connective tissue framework of the red pulp.

Amyloidosis of Kidney

This is the serious form of organ involvement. The renal amyloidosis is the major cause of death.

Gross: The kidney may appear normal in size and colour. It may be enlarged and waxy. In advanced cases,

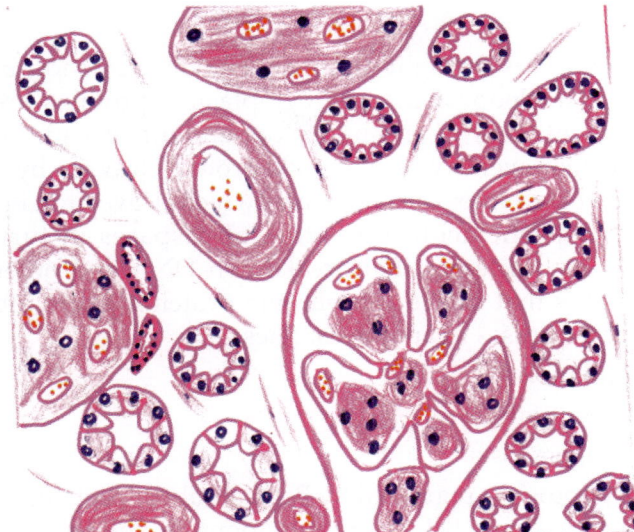

Fig. 10.17: Microscopy in amyloidosis kidney (schematic)

it may be shrunken and contracted owing to the vascular narrowing induced by amyloid deposits within the arterial and arteriolar walls.

Microscopy: The amyloid gets deposited in the glomeruli, interstitium, peritubular tissue, arteries and arterioles. In the glomeruli, the amyloid is deposited in the glomerular basement membrane and in the mesangial matrix (Fig. 10.17).

Demonstration and Stains for Amyloid

1. **H and E stain:** Amyloid stains homogenous and pale pink.
2. **PAS stain:** Amyloid stains magenta pink.
3. **Van Gieson:** Amyloid stains yellow to yellow brown.
4. **Iodine (Gram's or Lugol's):** Amyloid stains mahogany brown turning to blue or violet with application of **dilute sulphuric acid.**
5. **Metachromatic stains (e.g. 1% methyl violet, 1% toluidine blue):** Amyloid stains pink, other tissues stain violet.
6. **Congo red:** Amyloid stains orange.
7. **Congo red with polarisation:** Apple green birefringence.
8. **X-ray diffraction:** Cross beta pleat structure.
9. **Fluorescence with thioflavin T and S.**

APOPTOSIS

The body is good at maintaining a constant number of cells. So there are mechanisms for ensuring excess and unwanted cells in the body to be removed, when appropriate.

There are two mechanisms to remove unwanted cells and these are:

1. Apoptosis meaning suicide is a programmed cell death.
2. Necrosis meaning killing, undergoes decay and destruction.

Definition

Apoptosis is a process that helps to eliminate unwanted cells by an internally programmed series of events. The process is tightly regulated and the cells are destined to die.

In the human body, good numbers of cells are produced every second by mitosis and a similar number die by apoptosis. There is activation of enzymes capable of degrading the cells, its nuclear DNA, and nuclear and cytoplasmic proteins. Fragments of the apoptotic cells break off giving the appearance that is termed as "apoptosis" or "falling off". The plasma membrane of an apoptotic cell remains intact, the membrane is altered and it is phagocytosed. The cell is rapidly cleared off, before the contents are leaked off and thus this process does not elicit inflammation.

Causes of Apoptosis

These can be physiological or pathological.

Physiological Causes

1. During development, removal of excess cells during embryogenesis including implantation, organogenesis, involution and metamorphosis
   a. During limb formation, separate digits evolve.
   b. Ablation of cells which are no longer needed (tadpole).
2. To maintain cell population in tissues with high turnover of cells, such as skin and intestinal crypt epithelium so as to maintain constant number.
3. To eliminate immune immature lymphocytes in bone marrow and autoreactive T cells.
4. Hormone-dependent involution in tissues such as endometrium while shedding during menstrual cycle, ovary during postmenopausal period, regression of breasts after weaning period, etc.

Pathological Causes

1. Apoptosis mechanism tries to eliminate potentially harmful cells.
2. It helps in deletion of damaged/dangerous cells.
3. It removes cells damaged by virus.
4. It eliminates cells with DNA damage by radiation, cytotoxic agents, genetically altered cells (mutated cells), etc.
5. It causes cell death in tumours.

6. Pathological atrophy after duct obstruction as in pancreas, parotid gland and kidney.

Morphology of Cells in Apoptosis

1. Shrinkage of cells.
2. Condensation of nuclear chromatin peripherally under nuclear membrane.
3. Formation of apoptotic bodies by fragmentation of the cells and nuclei. The fragments remain membrane bound and contain cell organelles with or without nuclear fragments.
4. Phagocytosis of apoptotic bodies by phagocytes.
5. Unlike necrosis, apoptosis is not accompanied by inflammatory reaction (Fig. 10.18 and Table 10.2).

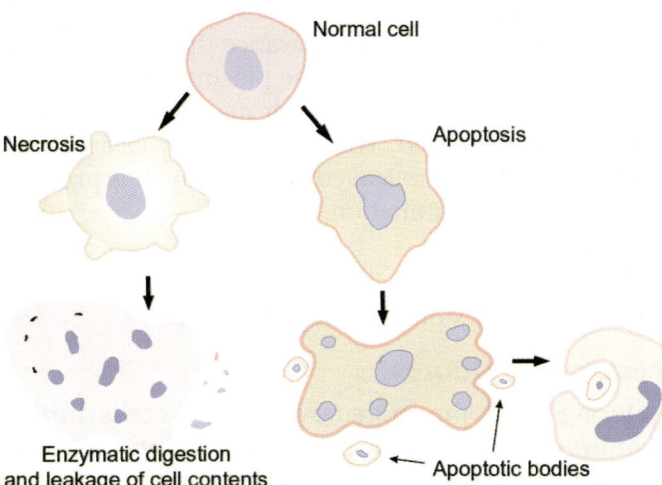

Fig. 10.18: Necrosis and apoptosis

Table 10.2	Differences between necrosis and apoptosis
Necrosis	**Apoptosis**
Detrimental	Beneficial
Pathological	Physiological/pathological
Groups of cells affected	Single cells affected
Effects	**Effects**
Cellular swelling	Cellular condensation
Membranes are broken	Membranes remain intact
Leakage of lysozymes	No leakage
ATP is depleted	Requires ATP
Specific proteases not activated	Specific proteases activated
Cell lyses, eliciting an inflammatory reaction	Cell is phagocytosed, no tissue reaction
DNA fragmentation is random	Ladder-like DNA fragmentation
In vivo, whole area of the tissue is affected	In vivo, individual cells appear affected

Mechanism of Apoptosis

Apoptosis is brought about by enzymatic action in which nucleoproteins and cytoplasmic proteins are fragmented. It is an energy-dependent cascade of molecular events which include protein cleavage by a group of enzymes called caspases which cleave proteins after aspartic acid. Activation of caspases in turn activates nucleases that breakdown DNA and other enzymes that cleave cytoplasmic proteins. There are three processes in apoptosis. These are:

1. Initiation
2. Execution
3. Phagocytosis

Apoptosis is regulated by Bcl-2 family of proteins of which Bcl-2 and Bcl-XL are anti-apoptotic and Bak and Bax are pro-apoptotic molecules. These molecules regulate extrinsic and intrinsic pathway mechanisms (Fig. 10.19). There are two pathways in initiation of apoptosis. These are:

1. Extrinsic pathway
2. Intrinsic pathway.

Similar execution and phagocytosis process follow the initiation by whichever pathway.

1. Extrinsic Pathway (Death Receptor Pathway)

Many cells express death receptors that promote apoptosis. Most of these are members of tumour necrosis receptor family, e.g. TNFR1 receptor and Fas (CD95). The Fas ligand (FasL) is expressed on activated T lymphocytes.

Steps

1. The activated T lymphocytes having FasL recognize Fas expressing targets. The Fas molecule as it cross-links with FasL or TNFR on cell membrane binds to TNF expressing cells, adaptor proteins and cytosolic part of death domain gets activated.
2. This activates initiator caspase 8. This further activates other caspases 9, 10, 12.
3. Executioner caspases like caspase 2, 3, 6, 7 are activated.
4. Cytoplasmic and nuclear proteins are broken down by executioner caspases.
5. The apoptotic bodies are engulfed by the macrophages.
6. Undergo degradation.

2. Intrinsic Pathway (Mitochondrial Pathway)

Mitochondria contain several proteins capable of inducing apoptosis which include cytochrome C and inhibitors of apoptosis.

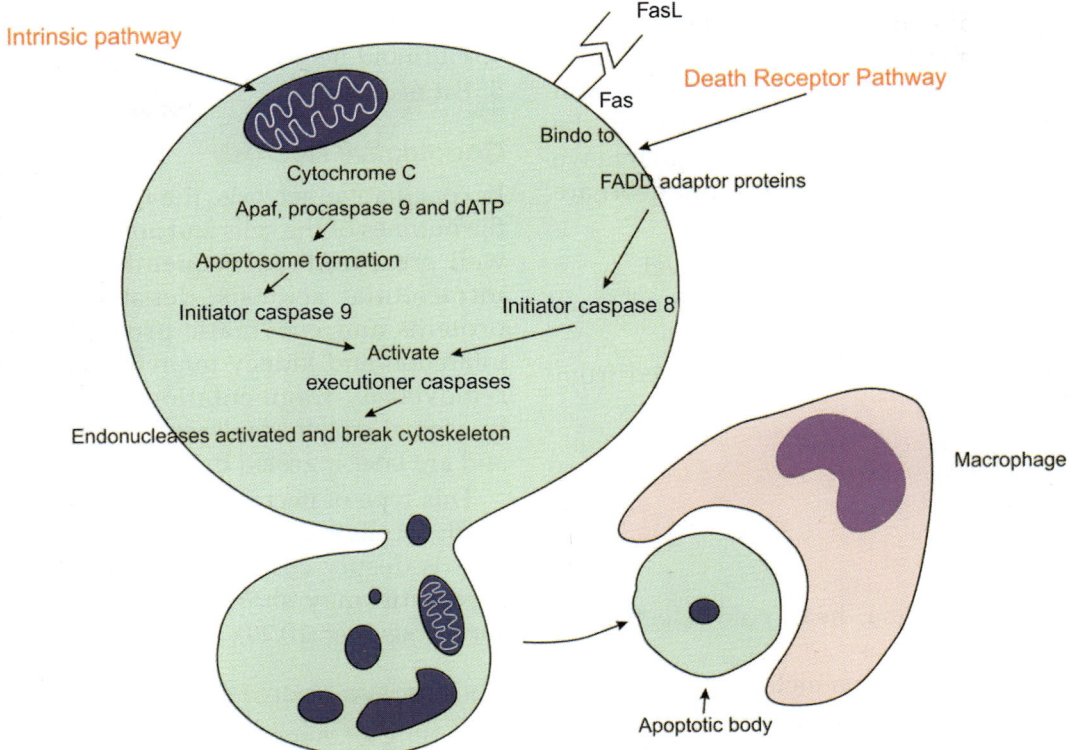

Fig. 10.19: Mechanism of apoptosis by extrinsic and intrinsic pathways

Steps

1. Following cellular stress, the pro-apoptotic proteins from cytosol relocate to the surface of the mito-chondria where the anti-apoptotic proteins are located.

2. This interaction between pro- and anti-apoptotic proteins disrupts the normal function of the anti-apoptotic Bcl-2 proteins and can lead to the formation of pores in the mitochondria and the release of cytochrome C and other pro-apoptotic molecules from the intermembrane space.

3. The release of cytochrome C from the mitochondria is an important event in the induction of apoptosis. Once cytochrome C has been released into the cytosol, it is able to interact with apoptosome protein-activating factor 1 (Apaf-1), procaspase 9 and dATP, together form an apoptosome.

4. Apoptosome formation leads to activation of initiator pro-caspase 9, block the action of caspase inhibitors.

5. Further activates executioner caspases 3 and 7 which breakdown cytoskeleton and nuclear proteins.

6. The apoptotic bodies are engulfed by the macro-phages.

7. Undergo degradation.

Following are the pro-apoptotic and anti-apoptotic factors:

Anti-apoptotic	Pro-apoptotic
Bcl-2	Bax
Bcl-XL	Bad
Bcl-W	Bid
Mcl-1	Bik
	Bak

NECROSIS

Definition

It is a spectrum of morphological changes that follow cell death in living tissue, largely resulting from progressive degradative action of enzymes on lethally injured cells. The damage caused is irreversible. The word necrosis is derived from a Greek word "*nekros*" meaning corpse.

A gross and histologic correlate of cell death or necrosis occurs in a setting of irreversible exogenous or endogenous injury.

Mechanism of Necrosis

In necrotic cells, the cell membrane is not intact and thus the contents of the cell leak out. The morphological appearance of necrosis is a result of two processes:

1. Enzymic digestion of the cell
2. Denaturation of the proteins.

The enzymes which digest the cells are derived from dying cells themselves or from the lysosomes of the cells recruited by the inflammatory process to remove the dead or dying cells. The dead cells and debri are removed by phagocytosis.

Thus in necrosis, the following words are used.

- **Autolysis:** Catalytic enzymes are derived from lysosomes of dead cells itself.
- **Heterolysis:** Catalytic enzymes are derived from immigrant leucocytes

Causes

1. Exogenous stimuli
2. Ischaemia
3. Chemical injury
4. Physical agents—trauma, heat, cold, electricity, ionizing radiation
5. Poisons—toxins, endogenous metabolic products
6. Dietary deficiencies—methionine and thiamine

Necrotic cells show the following changes:

1. Cytoplasmic changes:
   i. *Increased eosinophilia:* This is due to loss of RNA material and accumulation of lactic acid due to anaerobic respiration.
   ii. *Glassy homogenous appearance:* This is due to loss of glycogen.
   iii. *Cytoplasmic vacuolations:* This is because of digestion of organelles and cytoplasm appears "moth eaten".
   iv. *Calcification of dead cells:* This is due to dystrophic calcification.

2. Nuclear changes indicating cell death are of three patterns:
   i. Karyolysis
   ii. Pyknosis
   iii. Karyorrhexis

- In *karyolysis*, there is dissolution of nuclear mass, which has shadowy outlines and this is due to the action of DNases on DNA material.
- In *pyknosis*, the nucleus progressively shrinks, becomes like a small wrinkled mass of tightly packed chromatin.
- In *karyorrhexis* (Greek word meaning bursting), the nucleus is broken into fragments. This is explained on the basis of rupture of nuclear membrane and spillage of nucleic acid in the cytoplasm. Usually, pyknotic cells undergo karyorrhexis.

Types of Necrosis

1. Coagulative necrosis
2. Liquefactive necrosis
3. Caseous necrosis
4. Fibrinoid necrosis
5. Fat necrosis

Coagulative Necrosis

In coagulative necrosis, the tissue shortly after death, the outlines of the cells and architecture of the tissue is well preserved. Subsequently, there is increase in intracellular acidosis, denaturation of structural proteins and enzymatic proteins, e.g. myocardial infarction and kidney infarcts. The necrotic cells are removed by fragmentation of cells by proteolytic lysosomal enzymes released by immigrant leucocytes and are later ingested by these leucocytes.

This type of necrosis is characteristic in all hypoxic death of cells except in brain. The cytoplasm of necrotic cells is deeply eosinophilic than usual. The nuclear chromatin may show: Pyknosis, karyorrhexis and karyolysis (Fig. 10.20).

Liquefactive Necrosis

This type of necrosis is characteristically seen in infarction of brain, fungal and bacterial infections. These pathological entities constitute powerful stimuli for the accumulation of inflammatory cells. Whatever is the pathogenesis, there will be complete digestion of dead cells by the hydrolytic enzymes.

The end result is transformation of tissue into a liquid viscous mass or abscess cavity. The solid tissue is converted into a cavity filled with liquid material (Fig. 10.21).

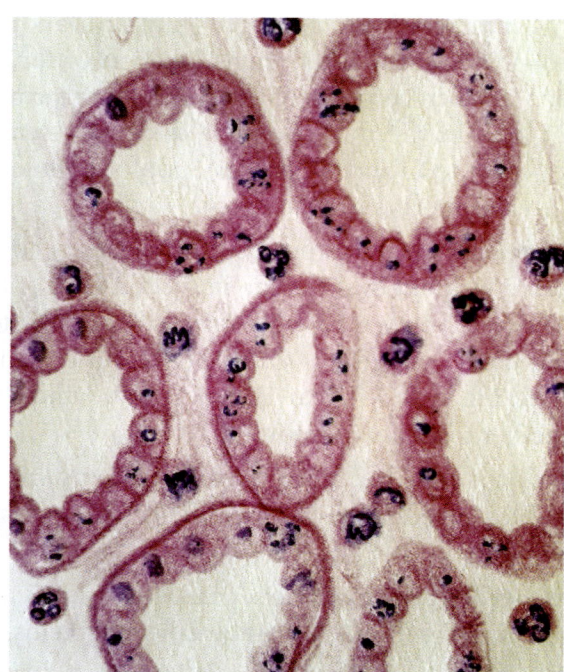

Fig. 10.20: Coagulative necrosis. Note tomb-stone appearance (outlines of cells in renal tubules seen) and nuclear changes (schematic)

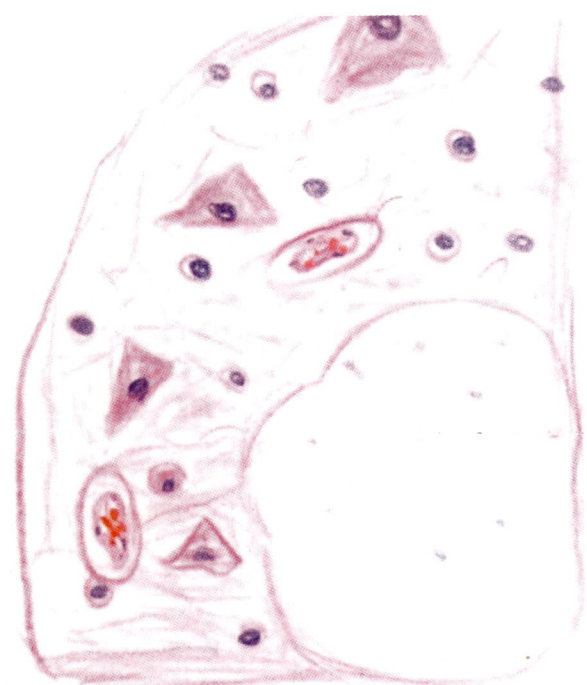

Fig. 10.21: Liquefactive necrosis of brain. Note cavity formation (schematic)

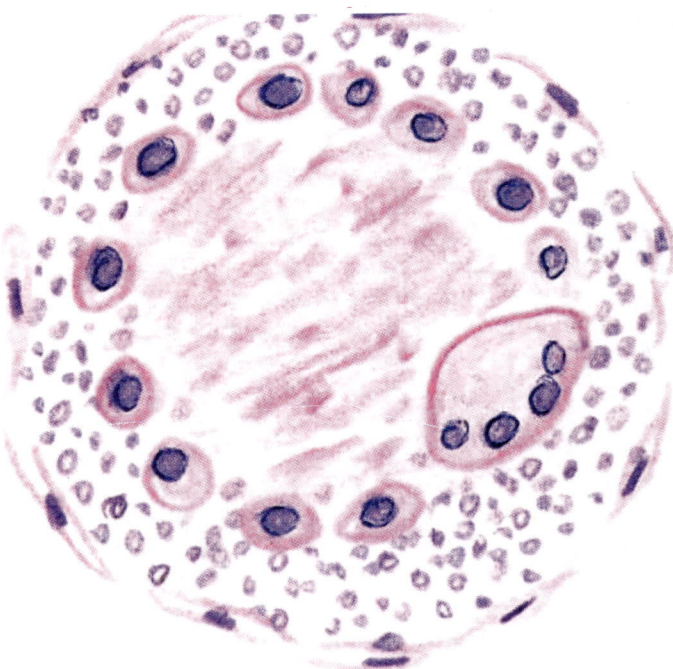

Fig. 10.22: Caseous necrosis. Note necrosis surrounded by epithelioid cells, Langhan type of giant cells and mantle of lymphocytes (schematic)

If the process is initiated by acute inflammation, the material is creamy yellow due to dead WBCs and degenerating cells, e.g. gangrenous necrosis.

Caseous Necrosis

This is distinctive form of necrosis and is encountered in tuberculosis. This type of necrosis is due to the toxic effects of mycobacterial cell wall which has mycolic acid and glycolipids.

The necrotic cells fail to retain their cellular outlines as in coagulative necrosis or do not disappear by lysis as in liquefactive necrosis. The dead cells persist as granular eosinophilic debris. It is a combination of coagulative and liquefactive necrosis.

Gross: The necrotic area is soft, grey white and cheesy.

Microscopy (Fig. 10.22): The tissue architecture is destroyed. Necrotic focus appears as amorphous granular debris composed of fragmented cells enclosed with in a distinctive inflammatory granulomatous reaction.

Fibrinoid Necrosis

It is a special form of necrosis seen in immune-mediated reaction. It is mainly seen in the wall of the blood vessels.

There is deposition of antigen–antibody complexes along with fibrin material which has been leaked from the lumen of the vessel giving the appearance of pink/eosinophilic amorphous material on H and E stain. Hence named fibrinoid, meaning fibrin-like, e.g. vessel walls in polyarteritis nodosa (PAN) (Fig. 10.23).

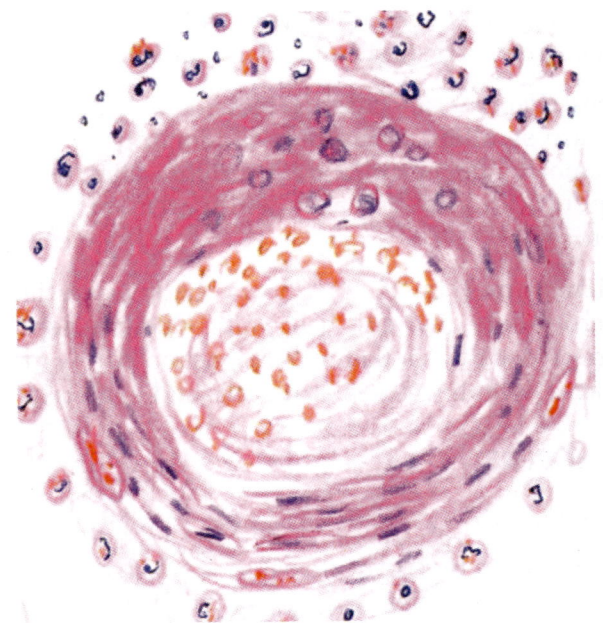

Fig. 10.23: Fibrinoid necrosis. Note eosinophilic fibrinoid material (schematic)

Fat Necrosis

This is due to release of activated pancreatic lipases, amylases and proteases into substance of pancreas and peritoneal cavity. Activated pancreatic lipases and proteases escape from acinar cells and ducts. These enzymes liquefy fat cell membranes; hydrolyse triglyceride esters within the fat cells to fatty acids. The released free fatty acids combine with calcium to

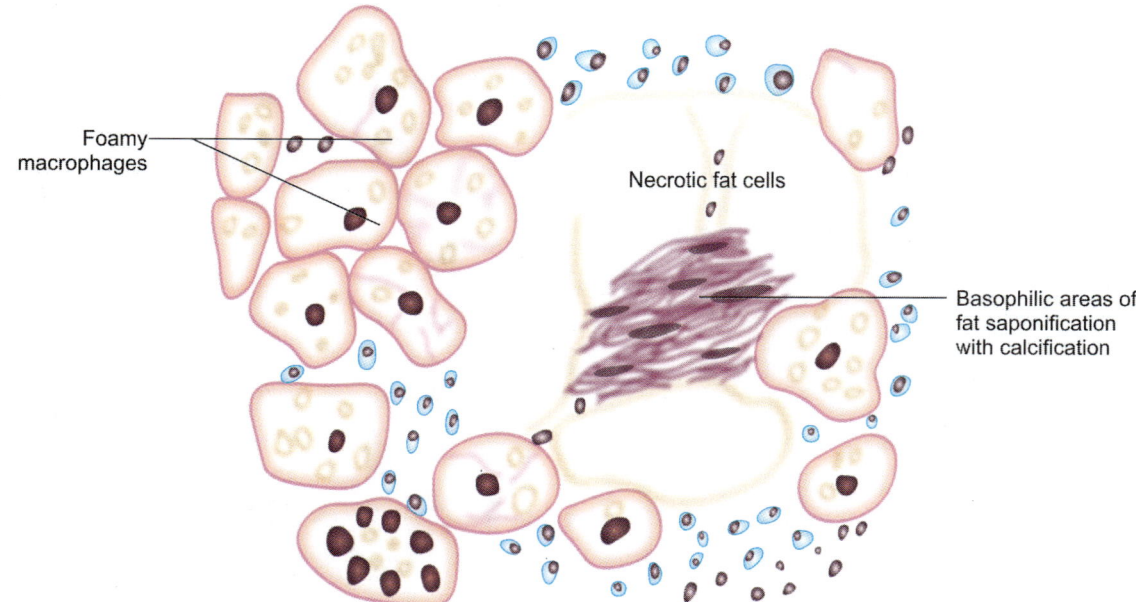

Foamy macrophages

Necrotic fat cells

Basophilic areas of fat saponification with calcification

Fig. 10.24: Fat necrosis. Note necrotic fat cells, inflammatory cells and calcification (schematic)

produce chalky white areas (fat saponification). This appears as amorphous basophilic deposits. Fat necrosis of abdominal mesentery and omental fat is commonly associated with pancreatic injuries or acute pancreatitis. It can be also observed in trauma to breast fat tissue or subcutaneous fat tissue due to inflammatory response.

Gross: Pancreas and affected mesenteric and peritoneal fat are swollen, indurated, oedematous and show haemorrhagic/necrotic areas, bright yellow areas of saponification and chalky white areas of calcification.

Microscopy (Fig. 10.24): Shows shadowy outline of necrotic fat cells with basophilic calcium deposits, surrounded by an inflammatory reaction (foamy macrophages, lymphocytes, plasma cells and giant cells).

GANGRENE

Definition

Gangrene is a form of death of tissue which results from severe hypoxic injury along with necrosis and may be associated with superadded putrefaction.

Causes

1. Blockage of arteries due to atherosclerosis of vessels or emboli
2. Blockage of venous supply
3. Vessels in diabetes mellitus with arteriosclerosis/atherosclerosis
4. Raynaud's disease
5. Thromboangiitis obliterans (TAO)/Beurger's disease
6. Ergot alkaloids

Types

1. Dry gangrene
2. Wet gangrene
3. Gas gangrene

Dry Gangrene

The tissue undergoes basically coagulative necrosis.

Cause for dry gangrene: The common causes include atherosclerosis, TAO, Raynaud's disease, trauma and ergot alkaloids. Usually, artery is blocked without affecting the venous return, and the artery is pulseless, e.g. gangrene of extremities and toes and fingers.

Gross: The affected part is dry, shrunken, mummified, and skin is wrinkled. The colour of the affected organ changes to dark brown or black due to formation of iron sulphide (Fig. 10.25).

Relase of hydrogen sulphide combines with iron from haemoglobin of broken RBCs and forms iron sulphide which is brown in colour.

The spread of dry gangrene is slow. There is clear line of demarcation between the affected tissue and normal tissue.

Microscopy: Cells show coagulative necrosis with smudging of tissue and there is granulation tissue at line of separation.

Moist Gangrene/Wet Gangrene

There is liquifactive necrosis. Along with ischaemia, bacterial infection supervenes as secondary complication. Thus, in wet gangrene, the organisms are present. The infection spreads proximally and unless controlled, death may occur due to sepsis and toxaemia. There is no clear line between affected and normal tissue.

Table 10.3	Differences between dry and wet gangrene	
Features	Dry gangrene	Wet gangrene
Site	Common in limbs	Common in bowel and tissue affected with *Clostridia* organisms
Mechanism	Thrombus or emboli are arterial origin	Thrombus or emboli are venous origin and toxins produce necrosis
Type of necrosis	Mainly coagulative necrosis	Mainly liquefactive necrosis along with coagulative necrosis
Gross	Dry, shrunken and black due to formation of iron sulphide	Moist, soft, swollen, crepitent and dark
Putrefaction	Limited	Marked
Line of demarkation	Present	Absent
Bacteria	Absent	Present
Prognosis	Good	Poor, toxaemia

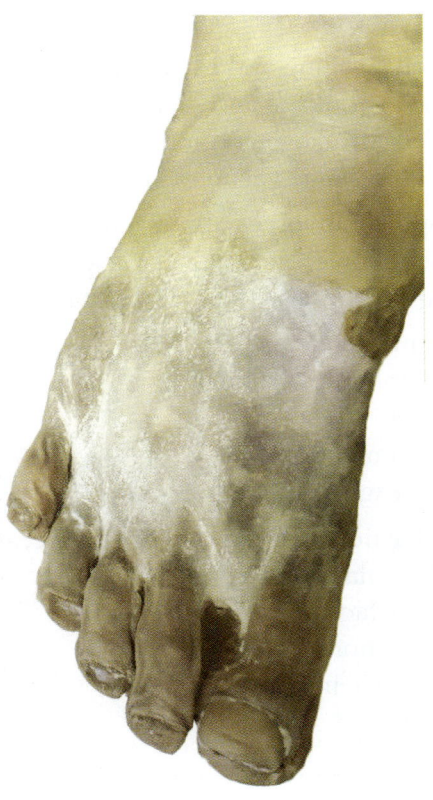

Fig. 10.25: Specimen showing dry gangrene

Wet gangrene develops rapidly due to blockage of venous flow, affected organ is congested with favourable condition for bacterial growth. This type of gangrene develops rapidly.

Causes
1. Veins with thrombosis or embolism
2. Blockage of vessels in diabetes mellitus

For example: Diabetic foot, bedsores, gangrene occurring in moist tissues like bowel, lung, etc.

Gross: Organ is soft, swollen, putrid, rotten, dark and pulseless.

Microscopy: Tissue is congested, intense inflammatory infiltration and shows liquefactive necrosis.

Differences between dry and wet gangrene are given in Table 10.3.

Gas Gangrene

This is a form of wet gangrene seen with soil contaminated wounds during accidents, with compound fractures or trauma with external soft tissue injury.

Cause: Bacteria like *Cl. perfringens* or *Cl. welchii.*

These are anaerobic spore-forming organisms. These produce toxins causing death of muscle cells, extensive haemolysis of RBCs, haemolytic anaemia, haemoglobinuria and renal failure.

There is formation of hydrogen sulphide gas which is responsible for formation of blebs and crepitus in the parenchyma of these affected organs. The toxins produce profound systemic effects along with extensive necrosis and oedema.

Gross morphology: Affected part is swollen, oedematous, painful, crepitant, later becomes dark and foul smelling.

Microscopically: Muscle fibres undergo coagulative necrosis with liquefaction, large number of organisms can be identified. Capillary and venous thrombi are common.

SELF-ASSESSMENT EXERCISE

1. **Lysozymes with undigested debris are called:**
   A. Residual body
   B. Rice body
   C. Councilman body
   D. Russell body

2. **Pinocytosis is:**
   A. Exocytosis
   B. Endocytosis
   C. Coming out of vessel wall
   D. Moving towards injurious agent

3. **Amyloid protein in chronic infections is:**
   A. Abeta protein
   B. Beta 2 microglobulin
   C. AL protein
   D. SAA protein

4. **A patient of haemodialysis will have which amyloid protein?**
   A. Abeta protein
   B. Beta 2 microglobulin
   C. AL protein
   D. SAA protein

5. **Intracellular and extracellular homogenous substance is:**
   A. Amyloid
   B. Hyaline
   C. Calcium
   D. Iron

6. **Tigered effect of myocardium is seen in:**
   A. Prolonged ischaemia
   B. Profound ischaemia
   C. Myocardial infarction
   D. Myocarditis

7. **Fat can be demonstrated by:**
   A. HE section
   B. Frozen section with oil red O
   C. MGG stain
   D. Paraffin section with oil red O

8. **CD95 is a marker for:**
   A. Apoptosis by extrinsic pathway
   B. Apoptosis by intrinsic pathway
   C. Necrosis
   D. Surface receptor to recognize pathogen

9. **Apoptosis is due to activation of:**
   A. Caspases
   B. Catalase
   C. Lipase
   D. Elastase

10. **DNA ladder in gel electrophoresis is seen in:**
    A. Apoptosis
    B. Sickle cell anaemia
    C. Thalassaemia
    D. Haemolytic anaemia

11. **Apoptosis is distinguished from necrosis by the following:**
    A. Cell swelling and inflammation
    B. Cell shrinkage and no inflammation
    C. Cell shrinkage and inflammation
    D. Cytoplasmic vacuoles and inflammation

12. **Apoptosis involves all *except*:**
    A. Bcl-2 molecules
    B. Caspases
    C. Apaf1
    D. Elastases

13. **Sign of apoptosis:**
    A. Membrane blebbing
    B. ROS
    C. Inflammation
    D. Leakage of lysozymes

14. **Similarities between cerebral infarct and abscess:**
    A. Coagulative necrosis
    B. Liquefactive necrosis
    C. Caseation necrosis
    D. Embolic in nature

Answers

1. A	2. B	3. D	4. B	5. B	6. A	7. B	8. A
9. A	10. A	11. B	12. D	13. A	14. B		

Inflammation

DEFINITION, CAUSATIVE AGENTS AND CARDINAL SIGNS

Definition

Inflammation is reaction of a living tissue to an injurious agent. Inflammation tries to eliminate, dilute or neutralize the harmful agents.

Causative Agents

1. Infections—bacteria, viruses, fungi, parasites
2. Trauma
3. Physical agents—heat, cold, pressure effects, radiation, mechanical injury
4. Chemical—drugs, toxins, alkali and acids
5. Immunological disorders—hypersensitivity reactions, autoimmunity, immunodeficiency states, etc.
6. Genetic and metabolic disorders, e.g. gout, diabetes, etc.
7. Tissue necrosis
8. Foreign bodies

Cardinal Signs

The cardinal signs were named by the Roman scientist Celsus. They are:
- **Rubor** (redness)
- **Tumour** (swelling)
- **Calor** (heat)
- **Dolor** (pain)
- Virchow added the 5th cardinal sign which is function laesa (loss of function).

Inflammation is divied into acute and chronic depending upon duration, virulence of organisms and other changes.

CHANGES IN ACUTE INFLAMMATION

In acute inflammation, initially there will be vascular changes followed by cellular changes.

VASCULAR CHANGES (Fig. 11.1)

Changes in Vascular Flow and Caliber

The changes in the vessels begin soon after the injury or infection. The rate of development depends on the nature and severity of injurious agent.

Soon after the injury, there is transient vasoconstriction lasting for a few seconds, after this there is arteriolar vasodilatation, resulting in engorgement of the arterioles, capillaries and venules. There is increased blood flow which is responsible for redness (rubor), and warmth (calor or erythema).

Increased Vascular Permeability

Increased vascular permeability begins in early phase of inflammation. Arterioles, capillaries and venules show dilatation. There is increased vascular flow which

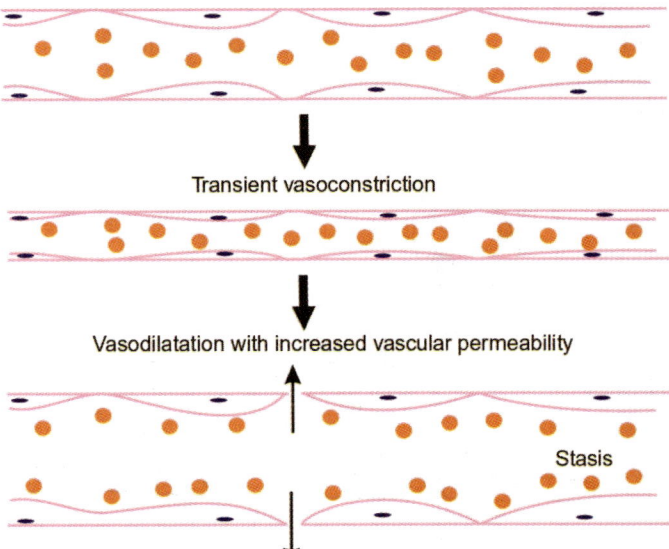

Transient vasoconstriction

Vasodilatation with increased vascular permeability

Stasis

Fig. 11.1: Vascular changes (changes in vascular flow and caliber and increased vascular permeability) (schematic)

leads to increased hydrostatic pressure resulting in movement of plasma out of the vessels (Fig. 11.1).

The vessels show increased vascular permeability, protein-rich fluid moves out into extracellular space causing oedema (tumour or swelling is a cardinal sign due to oedema fluid). Initially this is transudate, later it becomes exudate as white blood cells move out of the vessel. Several chemical mediators and mechanisms will contribute to the increased vascular permeability.

Because of loss of fluid, the red cell concentration increases with increased viscosity of blood. Thus there is slowing of blood flow and stasis occurs. The stasis is depicted microscopically as dilated arterioles, capillaries and venules, packed with RBCs.

Mechanism of Leaky Endothelium

Following factors may be responsible for leaky endothelium.

1. Endothelial gaps in venules due to:
   a. Contraction of endothelial cells by chemical mediators like histamine, bradykinins and leucotrienes.
   b. Re-organization of cytoskeleton of endothelial cells by chemical mediators like IL-1, TNF-α and IFN-γ.
2. Direct endothelial injury as in necrosis of the cells, burns and bacterial infections.
3. Delayed prolonged leakage due to direct injury: Usually leakage starts after 2 to 12 hours and lasts for hours to days. This occurs in thermal injury, radiation UV rays and bacterial toxins.
4. Leucocyte-mediated injury: This is mainly due to oxygen radicals and proteolytic enzymes. Target organs for this type of injury are lungs and kidneys.
5. Increased transcytosis across the endothelium.
6. Leakage from new blood vessels. (Newly formed capillaries are leaky.)

The vascular permeability is a dynamic event. The vasoactive amines from plasma and cellular origin are generated at the site of injury. These mediators bind to specific receptors on vascular endothelium and smooth muscle cells causing vasoconstriction and vasodilatation. These mediators bring about contraction of the endothelial cells and gap is created between the endothelial cells. The contractile proteins of the endothelium are stimulated by chemical mediators causing contraction of the endothelial cells. With vasodilatation, there is increase in blood flow and hydrostatic pressure at the site of injury.

Chemical Mediators of Increased Permeability

Acting immediately and transiently are histamine, bradykinin, serotonin, NO, leucotriene B4 and platelet activating factor (PAF).

Causes: Heat, cold, UV rays, X-rays, bacterial toxins, chemicals, etc. Some of these bring about delayed and prolonged vascular permeability.

CELLULAR CHANGES

Early phase of inflammation, for the first 24 hours neutrophils are the cells which try to eliminate the injurious agent. Later by 48 to 72 hours macrophages and other cells will play role in inflammation.

The cellular events in inflammation are as below.

1. Margination, rolling, pavementation, adhesion and transmigration (Fig. 11.2)
2. Chemotaxis
3. Phagocytosis

Margination

Leucocytes from axial flow move towards plasmatic flow due to stasis. Margination is peripheral positioning of leucocytes on the endothelial cells from the axial flow.

Rolling and Pavementation

Subsequently, rows of leucocytes tumble along the endothelium in a process called rolling. Leucocytes

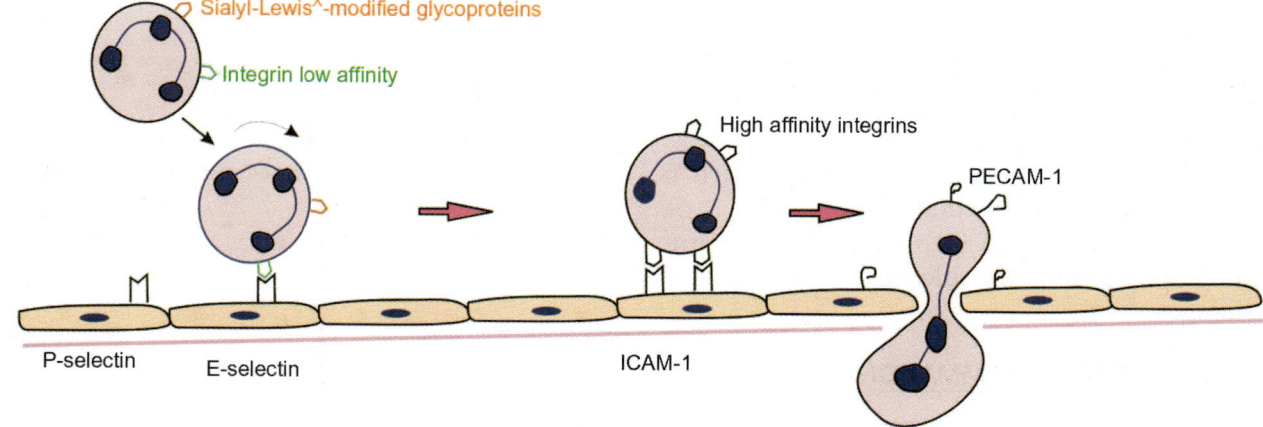

Fig. 11.2: Cellular events: Margination, rolling, pavementation, adhesion and transmigration

adhere to the vascular endothelium and become activated. The adhesion molecules are involved in bringing the adhesion of leucocytes to the endothelium. **For rolling, selectin family of adhesion molecules plays a role.** These are weak and cause transient adhesion and this makes them roll.

Selectin Family

This family of adhesion molecules includes:
1. P-selectins on platelets and endothelial cells
2. E-selectins on endothelial cells
3. L-selectins on leucocytes

These are transmembrane glycoproteins and have lectin-binding domain. These selectins are activated by TNF, leucotriene B4, C5a, histamine and thrombin.

P-selectins are stored in Weibel-Palade bodies of endothelial cells and alpha granules of platelets. On stimulation, they are rapidly transported to the cell surface and bind to sialyl- Lewis^X carbohydrate ligand of leucocytes. E-selectins are normally on endothelial cells, and are induced by inflammation by chemical mediators. L-selectins are mainly expressed on leucocytes. In time, the white blood cells are lined up on the endothelial cells and this appearance is called **pavementation.**

Adhesion

Firm adhesion of leucocytes is brought about by adhesion molecules mediated by integrins which are transmembrane heterodimeric glycoproteins and have alpha and beta chains. These function as cell surface receptors. These are normally expressed on leucocyte plasma membrane in a low affinity form. When leucocytes are activated by chemokines, the integrins undergo conformational changes and get converted into high affinity form. At the same time, TNF, IL-1 and endotoxins activate ligands on endothelial cells (LFA1 and VLA-4) for integrins. These are:
1. ICAM-1 (intercellular adhesion molecule which binds to LFA-1 (lymphocyte function associated molecule 1).
2. MAC-1(membrane attack complex 1) which binds to VLA-4 (very late activation molecule 4).
3. VCAM-1 (vascular cell adhesion molecule 1) which binds to VLA-4.

Now, leucocytes firmly adhere to the endothelial cells and undergo transmigration through the vessel wall.

Transmigration

Leucocytes escape from the vessels in between the endothelial cells, by active movement and their extending pseudopodia helps them to come out of the vessels. PECAM-1 (platelet endothelial cell adhesion molecule 1), also called CD31, is an adhesion molecule expressed both on leucocytes and endothelial cells, helps in traversing through the endothelium. After traversing the endothelium, the leucocytes cross the basement membrane by focally degrading with the help of collagenases secreted by the leucocytes. Along with leucocytes, RBCs also come out passively. This is called transmigration of leucocytes.

Chemotaxis

The movement of leucocytes along a chemical gradient is called **chemotaxis.** This is unidirectional movement of leucocytes from vascular channels towards the site of inflammation.

The chemotactic factors for leucocytes are:
a. Components of complement system—C5a
b. Bacterial products particularly peptides with N-formylmethionine terminal amino acids and some lipids.
c. Chemokines: Cytokines especially from chemokine family(IL-8)
d. Products of the lipoxygenase family particularly leucotriene B4 (LTB4)

Chemotactic molecules bind to the specific receptors on the leucocytes. This mediates G-protein-mediated signal transduction. There is increased production cytosolic calcium, which triggers the assembly of cyto-skeletal contractile proteins necessary for movement. Leucocytes move by extending pseudopodia and actin filaments help in forward movement near the leading edge of the pseudopodia.

Neutrophils predominate in the inflammatory infiltrate in the first 6 to 24 hours and by next 48–72 hrs are replaced by monocytes and other chronic inflammatory cells.

Chemokines: In Greek, "*kinos*" means movement. Chemokines are chemoattractant cytokines released by many cells at the site of inflammation. These attract leucocytes to the site of inflammation. Chemoattractant for neutrophils is Interleukin-8 (IL-8), for monocyte is monocyte chemotactic protein 1 (MCP-1). These are members of CXC and CC chemokine families, respectively.

Chemokines are classified into four main subgroups. These are CXC, CC, CX3C and XC. All these proteins exert their biological effects by interacting with chemokine receptors found on the target cells.

Leucocyte activation: Leucocytes are attracted to the site of infection. They must be activated to perform their function. The stimuli for activation include microbes, products of necrotic material and several chemical mediators. Leucocytes on their surface express different

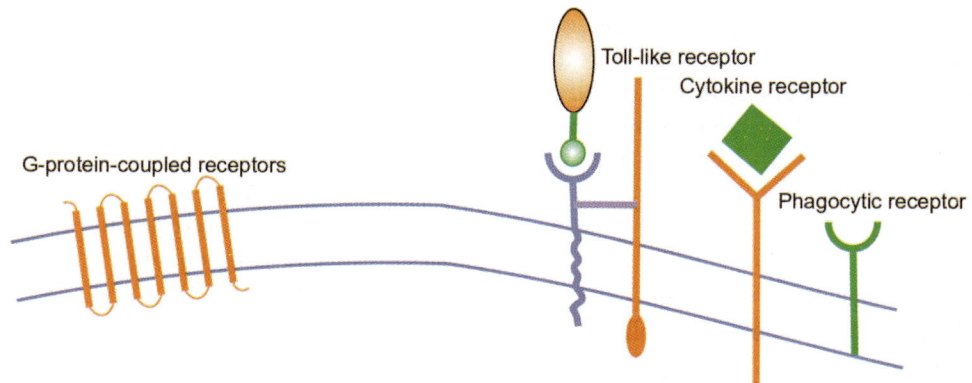

Fig. 11.3: Leucocyte surface receptors: G-protein-coupled receptors, toll-like receptor and cytokine receptors are shown (schematic)

kinds of receptors which help them to sense the presence of injurious agent, may be bacteria, virus, fungi, etc. These include toll-like receptors (TLRs) (Fig. 11.3).

Phagocytosis

After the step of chemotaxis, the pathogen has to be phagocytosed. Phagocytosis involves three different, but interrelated steps (Fig. 11.4). These are:
1. Recognition and attachment
2. Engulfment
3. Killing and degradation

Recognition and Attachment

Recognition of the injurious agent by the leucocytes is through the following:
1. Mannose receptors present on leucocytes recognise mannose molecules on microbes
2. Scavenger receptors present on macrophages recognise bacteria
3. Macrophage integrins
4. Opsonised bacteria
5. Toll receptors recognise Toll proteins on microbes (pattern recognition receptors).

For leucocytes to attach to the injurious agent, it has to be coated with certain substances/proteins called **opsonins.** The important opsonins are:
1. Fc portion of immunoglobulin G class
2. Complement C3b is an important complement molecule, when bound to the antigen on the pathogen, is recognised by the phagocytes. These are present in the blood or produced as a reaction to microbes.
3. Lectins are carbohydrate-binding proteins, which are present in the plasma membrane. These bind to the cell wall of pathogen and act as opsonins.

The leucocytes have surface receptors for these opsonins.

Engulfment

Binding of opsonised particles triggers the process of engulfment. During this process, extension of cytoplasm flow around the object engulfed, eventually resulting in complete closure of the particle by the cytoplasm. This is phagosome; the organism is covered by cytoplasmic membrane. For degradative action by the leucocyte, the phagosome has to combine with lysosomes, thus forming phagolysosome, in which degradative enzymes are present.

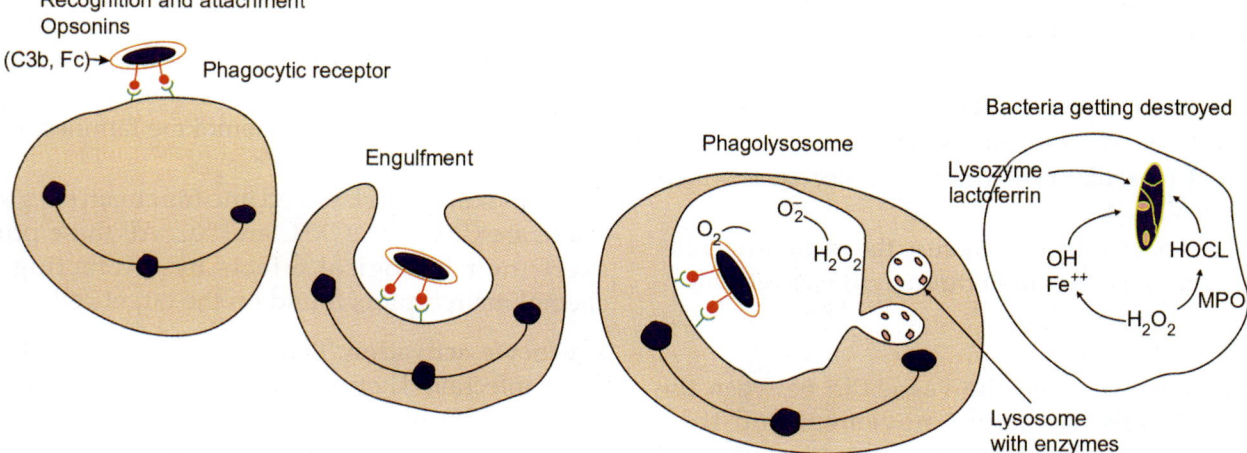

Fig. 11.4: Recognition, attachment, engulfment, phagocytosis and killing (schematic)

Killing and Degradation

The steps in killing and degradation are production of microbicidal substances which are present within the lysosomes and fusion of these lysosomes with phagosome. Thus the ingested particle is exposed to destructive mechanism of leucocytes.

The microbicidal substances may be produced by:
- Myeloperoxidase independent mechanisms:
  1. Reactive oxygen species (ROS)
  2. Leucocyte granules
- Myeloperoxidase dependent mechanisms

Myeloperoxidase independent mechanisms: These mechanisms do not require the myeloperoxidase enzyme. The two important mechanisms in this are:

1. The phagocytosis stimulates an oxidative burst characterized by sudden increase in oxygen consumption with production of **reactive oxygen species (ROS)** and these are **superoxide anion (O_2^-), hydrogen peroxide (H_2O_2) and hydroxyl radical (OH).**

   The oxygen metabolites are generated due to activation of NADPH oxidase which oxidizes NADPH and converts oxygen to superoxide ions. Superoxide is converted to H_2O_2. The ROS can destroy the microbes. Superoxide, H_2O_2, hydroxyl ions are not sufficient to kill the pathogen. After the action is over, superoxide dismutase can catalyse superoxide ions to either ordinary O_2 or H_2O_2 which is broken down to H_2O and O_2 molecules. After the oxidative burst, H_2O_2 is broken down to water and O_2 by catalase and other ROS are degraded.

   The dead microbes are degraded by the action of lysosomal acid hydrolases, the most important being elastase.

2. Also, the **leucocyte granules** have **bactericidal permeability increasing protein** causing activation of phospholipases and degradation of phospholipid membrane. Lysozymes degrade bacterial wall oligosaccharides. **Major basic protein** present in the granules of the eosinophils is cytotoxic to parasites.

Other antimicrobials in leucocyte granules:
- Lactoferrin
- Defensins (punch holes in membranes)

Myeloperoxidase dependent mechanisms: Lysosomes contain myeloperoxidase enzyme (MPO) which converts H_2O_2 in presence of Cl^- ions to HOCl (hypochlorous acid). The H_2O_2-MPO-halide system is the most powerful oxidant and an antimicrobial agent. This is the major bactericidal agent. HOCl also activates collagenase and other enzymes released neutrophils and inactivates alpha-1 antitrypsin.

CHEMICAL MEDIATORS

These originate from the cells or plasma. They are in precursor form and later get activated. They are synthesized *de novo*. Chemical mediator production is triggered by microbial products or host proteins. They perform their activity by binding to the receptors on the target cells. One mediator can stimulate release of other mediators by target cells with opposing activities. The mediators can act on few or one target cell types, having different cell types. Once activated or released, they are short lived. They get decayed/inactivated/scavenged/inhibited. There are checks and balances to control their synthesis, function and time of action.

The chemical mediators are:
- *Cell derived:*
  1. Vasoactive amines
  2. Lysosomal component
  3. Platelet activating factor
  4. Cytokines
  5. NO and O_2 metabolites
  6. Arachidonic acid metabolites
- *Plasma derived:*
  1. The kinin system
  2. The clotting system
  3. The fibrinolytic system
  4. The complement system

Cell-derived Chemical Mediators (Table 11.1)

Vasoactive Amines

These are histamine and serotonin.

Histamine: It is released by mast cells, basophils, and platelets. Preformed histamine is released with stimuli, such as:
1. Physical agents: Trauma, heat and cold
2. Immune reactions: IgE antibodies binding to Fc receptors on mast cells, C3a and C5a, histamine-releasing proteins from leucocytes, neuropeptides (substance P), cytokines (IL-1 and IL-8).

Effects: Dilatation of arterioles, increased vascular permeability, induce contraction of venular endothelium, constriction of large arteries and activation of endothelium.

Serotonin (5-hydroxytryptamine): This is produced by platelets, enterochromaffin cells and mast cells. Platelets in contact with collagen, thrombin and antigen–antibody complexes are stimuli for preformed serotonin release. Platelet-activating factor from mast cells also causes platelet aggregation and release of serotonin.

Effects: Similar to histamine.

Lysosomal Components

Specific granules	Azurophilic granules
Lactoferrin	Myeloperoxidase
Lysozyme	Lysozyme
Alkaline phoshphatase	Cationic proteins
Plasminogen activator	Acid hydrolases
	Elastases
	Collagenase
	Phospholipase

Platelet Activating Factor

This is a phospholipid-derived chemical mediator. This causes:
1. Platelet stimulation
2. Vasoconstriction
3. Bronchospasm
4. In low concentrations, it causes: Vasodilatation, increased vascular permeability (100–10000 times powerful)
5. Increased leucocyte adhesion
6. Increased chemotaxis
7. Degranulation
8. Oxidative burst

Cytokines

These are produced from various cells including activated lymphocytes and macrophages.

IL-1 and TNF causes:
1. Endothelium: Induction and synthesis of adhesion molecules, procoagulant and anticoagulant properties
2. Release of acute phase reactants
3. Fibroblast proliferation
4. Fever

NO and O$_2$ Metabolites

Nitric oxide: This is released from endothelial cells, macrophages and neurons and has the following functions:
1. Vascular smooth muscle relaxation
2. Vasodilatation
3. Reduces platelet aggregation
4. Antimicrobial action

Oxygen-derived free radicals: These are superoxide, hydrogen peroxide and OH molecules and these have following effects:
1. Endothelial damage
2. Increased vascular permeability
3. Inactivate antiproteases
4. Injury to cells

Table 11.1	Summary of chemical mediators in inflammation
Chemical mediator	**Effect**
Histamine and serotonin	Increased vascular permeability, vasodilatation
TNF, LB4, C5a, histamine and thrombin	Selectin activation
TNF, IL-1, chemokines	Integrins: Firm adhesion molecules
C5a, bacterial products, Cytokine—IL-8, LTB4	Chemotaxis
C3a and C5a	Opsonisation
PAF	Platelet stimulation, vasoconstriction, bronchospasm, adhesion, chemotaxis, oxidative burst. In low concentration: Vasodilatation, increased vascclar permeability
Cytokines (IL1, TNF)	Adhesion molecules, release of acute phase reactants, fibroblast proliferation
ROS	Increased vascular permeability, inactivate anti-proteases, injury to cells
NO and O$_2$ metabolites	Vascular smooth muscle relaxation, vasodilatation
PGI$_2$/prostacyclin	Vasodilatation, inhibits platelets
Thromboxane A2	Vasoconstriction, platelet aggregation
PG$_2$, PGE$_2$	Vasodilatation, increased vascular permeability
5-HETE	Chemotaxis
LTC4, LTD4 and LTE4	Vasoconstriction, brochospasm and increases vascular permeability of venules

Arachidonic Acid Metabolites

These are 20-carbon polyunsaturated fatty acids derived from diet or cell membrane which are released by activated cellular phospholipases (Fig. 11.5).

There are two pathways:
1. Cyclo-oxygenase pathway: Prostaglandins, thromboxane.
2. Lipoxygenase pathway: Leukotrienes, lipoxins.

Amongst arachidonic acid metabolites, following are the important chemical mediators.
- **In cyclo-oxygenase pathway:**
  1. Prostacyclin (PGI$_2$): Vasodilatation and inhibits platelets.
  2. Thromboxane A2: Vasoconstriction and platelet aggregation
  3. PG$_2$ and PGE$_2$: Vasodilatation and increased vascular permeability
     COX-1, and COX-2 inhibitors, aspirin and indomethacine can inhibit cyclo-oxygenase pathway.

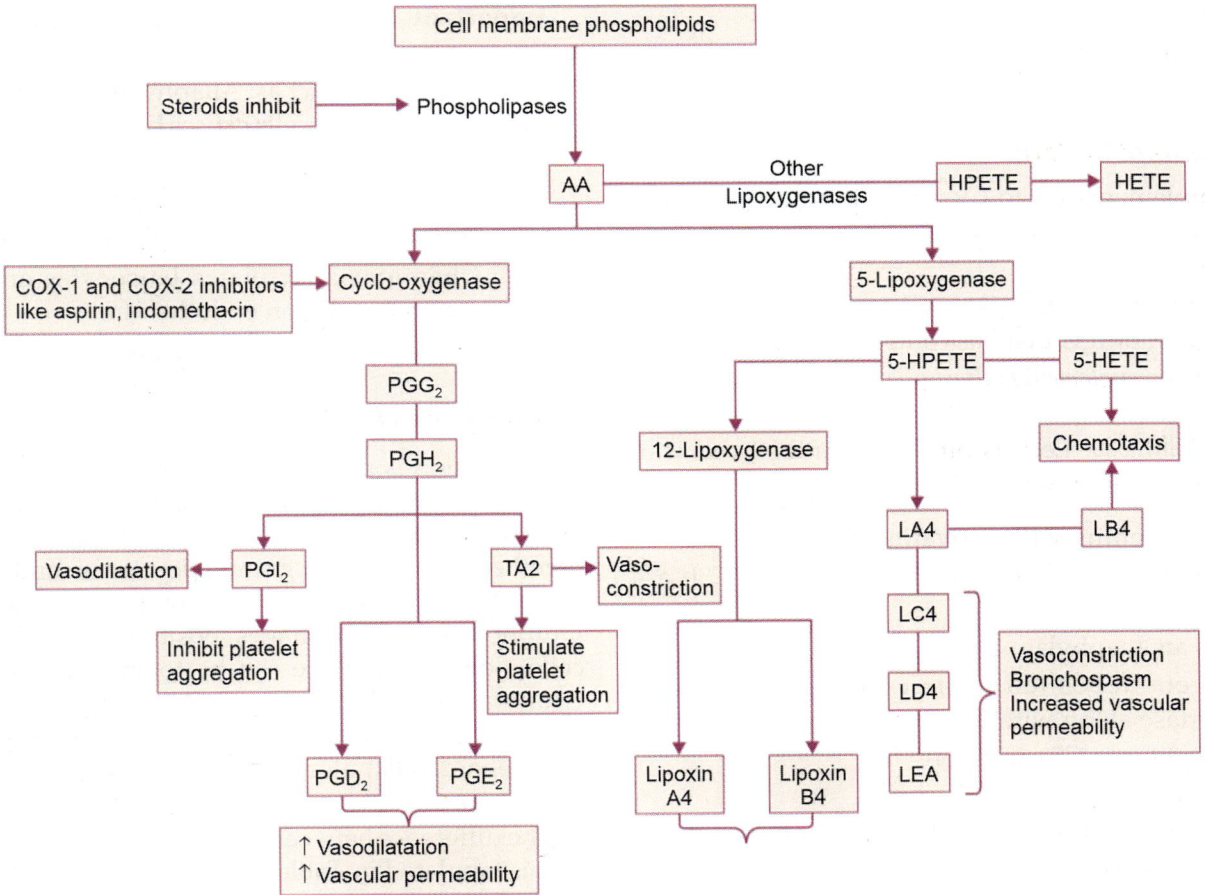

Fig. 11.5: Production of arachidonic acid metabolites (AA: Arachidonic acid, 5-HPETE: 5-hydroperoxyeicosatetraenoic acid, 5-HETE: 5-hydroxyeicosatetraenoic acid, PG: Prostaglandin, PGI₂: Prostacyclin)

- **In lipoxygenase pathway:**
  1. 5-Hydroxyeicosatetraenoic acid (5-HETE): Chemotactic to neutrophils
  2. LTB4: Potent chemotactic agent
  3. LTC4, LTD4 and LTE4: Vasoconstriction, brochospasm and increase vascular permeability of venules.

Plasma-Derived Chemical Mediators

Kinin System

Kinins are vasoactive peptides derived from kininogens by the action of kallikreins. Bradykinin increases vascular permeability, causes vasodilatation, smooth muscle contraction and pain. The immediate effects of kinins are due to B_1 and B_2 receptors. The action is short lived and degraded by kinases. These amplify the inflammatory response by stimulating additional mediators like TNF alpha, interleukins and nitric oxide.

Clotting System

Thrombin activates platelet-activating receptors (PARs) and has major role in platelet activation during clotting.

Hageman factor (Factor XII) is activated which triggers conversion of plasminogen to plasmin, pre-kallikrein to kallikrein, activates alternate complement pathway and coagulation system (Fig. 11.6).

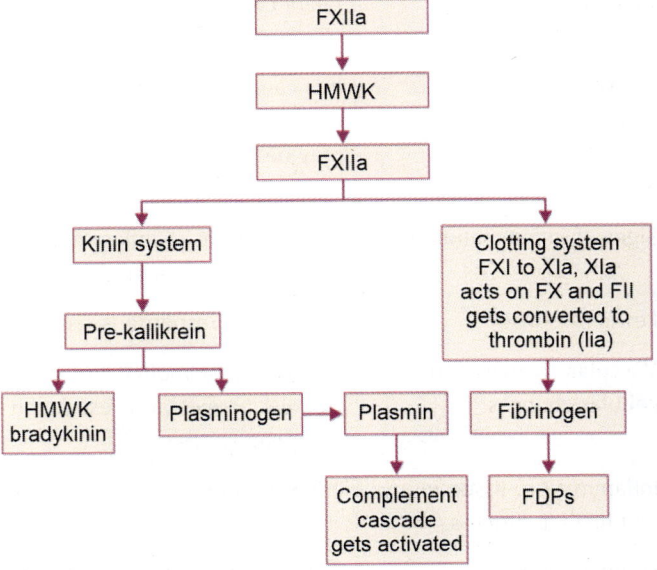

Fig. 11.6: Chemical mediators, due to activation of FXII in inflammation

Fibrinolytic System

Plasmin causes fibrinolysis and fibrin degradation products are formed.

Complement System

The complements C1 to C9 are in inactive form. The critical step is activation of C3. This occurs by three pathways.

1. *Classical complement pathway:* Triggered by fixation of C1 to IgM or IgG that has combined with antigen.
2. *Alternate complement pathway:* Triggered by microbial molecules.
3. *Lectin pathway:* Lectins bind to microbial cell wall carbohydrates and directly activates C1.

Events happening with activation of C3:

1. By the action of C3 convertase, C3a and C3b are formed.
2. C3a is an anaphylatoxin.
3. C3b gets deposited on microbes and form C5 convertase along with C4b and C2a.
4. C5 is split into C5a and C5b.
5. C5a is an anaphylatoxin.
6. C5b along with C6 to C9 forms membrane attack complex (MAC).

Important mediators in complement activation pathway are:

1. C3a, C5a and C4a act as: Anaphylatoxins, histamine released from mast cells causes bronchoconstriction, vasodilatation and oedema.
2. C3a and C5a increase vascular permeability.
3. C3b, C4b and C5b: Opsonisation and phagocytosis.
4. C5a: Chemotaxis, activates leucocytes and their adhesion molecules on endothelium.
5. C5b-9 MAC complex on cell membrane: Cell lysis.

CHRONIC INFLAMMATION

Inflammation is prolonged for long duration, may be because the organisms still remain, or organisms are less virulent. Tissue injury and repair mechanisms occur together. There can be granulation tissue and fibrosis areas. The important cells of chronic inflammation are lymphocytes, macrophages, eosinophils and plasma cells. Sometimes there can be foamy macrophages. Granulomatous inflammation is a type of chronic inflammation wherein the modified macrophages (epithelioid cells) along with lymphocytes and giant cells are present.

The difference between acute and chronic inflammation is tabulated in Table 11.2.

Table 11.2	Differences between acute and chronic inflammation	
	Acute inflammatiom	**Chronic inflammatiom**
Duration of inflammation	Short duration	Prolonged duration—weeks to months to years
Type of inflammatory cells	Neutrophils are the main inflammatory cells	Lymphocytes and plasma cells are the main inflammatory cells
Including giant cells	Giant cells are not seen	Giant cells are seen, e.g. foreign body giant cells, Langhans giant cells, Touton giant cells
Cause	It is caused by trauma, infectious agents with organisms of high virulence, injury caused may be severe	It is caused by irritant substances and granulomatous infections. Occurs due to persistent and less virulent microbes (as seen in TB, leprosy, etc.), autoimmune or allergic diseases
Signs of inflammation	Classical signs of inflammation are seen—pain, redness, heat and swelling	Classical signs of inflammation are not seen
Lewis response	Lewis triple response is seen	Lewis triple response is not seen
Vascular changes and cellular changes	Consists of haemodynamic changes, increased vascular permeability, exudation of leucocytes and phagocytosis	Infiltration with mononuclear cells and formation of granulomas Oedema and vascular changes less predominant
Inflammation, tissue injury and healing process	Inflammation and tissue injury only occur	Inflammation, tissue injury and healing occur simultaneously
Systemic effects	Systemic manifestations are fever, leucocytosis, shock, DIC, metabolic abnormalities	Systemic manifestations are less pronounced

GRANULOMATOUS INFLAMMATION

Definition

Granulomatous inflammation is a distinctive type of chronic inflammation characterised by focal collection of epithelioid cells (modified macrophages), giant cells and mantle of lymphocytes.

Pathogenesis of Granuloma Formation

There is phago-cytosis by macrophages and giant cells. This reaction towards inert substance or foreign body. Sometimes persistent microbe or microbial antigens can induce T cell-mediated immune response.

In chronic granulomatous disease, there is absence of NADPH oxidase. Catalase positive organisms do not produce H_2O_2. Even oxygen independent mechanisms do not work. Thus, organisms which gain entry into the body, cannot be killed and these patients are host for variety of infectious diseases.

Pathogenesis of Granuloma Formations in Tuberculosis

Tubercle bacilli do not produce exotoxin or endotoxin. Its surface glycolipid has a cord factor which prevents fusion of phagosome with lysosome of macrophages is responsible for granuloma formation.

LAM heteropolysaccharide of bacilli induces macrophage to produce: (a) TNF-α—fever, weight loss, tissue damage; and (b) IL-10—suppresses T cell population.

Hypersensitivity is induced by immunogenic 65 kDA mycobacterial heat shock protein which plays role in immune reaction.

M. tuberculosis typically leads to the development of delayed hypersensitivity to mycobacterial antigens. The antigen presenting cells (macrophages) produce IL-12 and stimulate the T lymphocytes by about 3 weeks. These T cells release IFN-γ which creates an inhospitable acidic environment for the bacteria; also stimulates production of NO and free O_2 radicals and causes oxidative destruction of the bacilli. IFN-γ also inturn activates the macrophages, these release TNF-α mediators which lead to formation of epithelioid cells and granuloma formation (Fig. 11.7).

In 2–6 weeks of infection: Delayed hypersensitivity reaction will set in. Direct toxicity of bacteria to macrophage, TNF alpha and hydrolytic enzymes, procoagulant factors secreted by macrophages are responsible for ischaemia and thrombosis. Caseation necrosis creates an acidic environment with less oxygen. Bacteria cannot grow and thus infection is controlled.

Causes

Causes of granulomatous diseases are shown in Table 11.3.

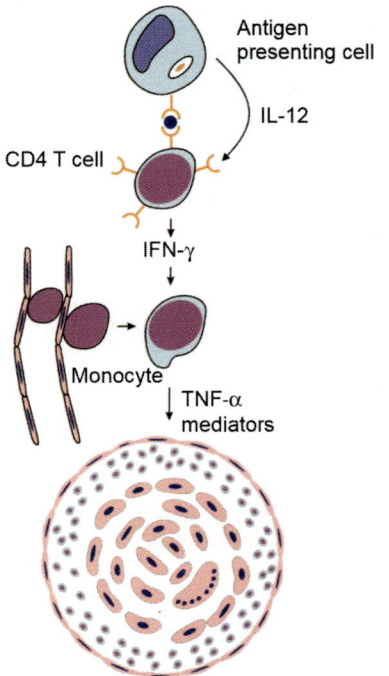

Fig. 11.7: Mechanism of granuloma formation

Table 11.3	Causes of granulomatous diseases[12]
Bacterial infections: Mycobacteria	Mycobacterial tuberculosis Atypical mycobacteria Leprosy
Bacterial infections: Gram-negative/positive bacillus	Cat-scratch disease Brucellosis, actinomycosis, nocardiosis
Fungi	Cryptococcosis, histoplasmosis, aspergillosis, sporotrichosis, etc.
Parasites	Schistosomiasis, leishmaniasis, (worms, larvae, eggs)
Spirochetes	Syphilis, pinta, yaws
Viruses	Measles, mumps, etc.
Materials that don't get digested	Endogenous like keratin, necrotic bone, cholesterol, sodium urate Exogenous—talc, silica, suture material, oils
Specific chemicals	Berylliosis
Unknown mechanism	Crohn's Sarcoidoisis Wegener's granulomatosis Chronic granulomatous disease of childhood
Drugs	Hepatic granulomas due to allopurinol, phenyl butazone, sulfonamides

Tuberculous granuloma: There can be initially non-caseating granulomas and later caseating granulomas develop.

The classical microscopic picture is that the granulomas have central area of caseation necrosis surrounded by epithelioid cells, Langhans type of giant cells and surrounding this is a mantle of lymphocytes.

Leprosy: In tuberculoid leprosy, there will be non-caseating granulomas.

Syphilis: There is a gumma with good number of plasma cells, histiocytes and lymphocytes. The centre may be necrotic without loss of cellular outer layer.

Cat-scratch disease: There will be granulomas, containing central granular debris, neutrophils, and giant cells.

NICE TO KNOW

Toll-Like Receptors

These are transmembrane proteins; the extra-cytoplasmic domain has leucine-rich repeats and cysteine. The first member of this family was identified as Toll, the mutations of which disrupted the establishment of dorsoventral polarity in Drosophilia melanogaster embryos. Human TLRs are homologs to TLR of Drosophilia. To date 10 TLRs are identified that belong to the TLR family. TLRs help in innate immunity, recognize microbial determinants and helps to set in motion the humoral and cellular mechanism for defence against pathogens.

Leucocytes express many types of Toll-like receptors which identify Toll proteins present on the microbes. These TLRs are present on neutrophils, macrophages, natural killer cells, epithelial cells and endothelial cells. Most important amongst these TLRs is TLR4 which can bind LPS binding proteins on microbes and activate potent cytokines like IL-1 and TNF.

Other Toll-Like Receptors

- TLR2 recognises bacterial LAM, BPL, and PGN following their initial interaction with CD14.
- TLR5 activation occurs following interaction with bacterial flagellin.
- TLRs 1, 2, 4, 5 and 6 are located on the cell surface and other TLRs are located in the cytoplasm.
- TLRs 3, 7, 8 and 9 are activated by viruses.
- TLRs 7 and 8 are activated by imidoquinoline compounds and many others.

MORPHOLOGICAL PATTERNS OF INFLAMMATION

The vascular changes, leucocyte infiltrate, severity of reaction, its specific causes, particular tissue and site involved introduce morphological variations in the basic pattern. Many patterns are recognised which vary in morphology and clinical condition.

Serous inflammation: This is characterised by outpouring of thin fluid which may be derived from plasma or epithelial secretions particularly involves epithelial cells, mesothelial cells and skin. This type of inflammation is seen in:

1. Skin in burns and viral infections
2. Pericardial, pleural and peritoneal effusions

Fibrinous inflammation: With severe injuries, there is increased vascular permeability and fibrinogen passes through the vessels. The fibrin is deposited into extra-vascular spaces. In H and E sections, fibrin appears as eosinophilic mesh. This inflammation is characteristic in inflammations lining body cavities like meninges, pericardium and pleura. This may be resolved by fibrinolysis and clearing by macrophages, resolve completely assuming original features or undergoes fibrosis. Conversion to scar tissue is called organization which leads to thickening and adhesions.

Suppurative or purulent inflammation: This is characterised by production of large amounts of pus or purulent exudate consisting of neutrophils, necrotic debris, and oedema fluid. Certain bacteria are responsible for this type of inflammation, e.g. staphylococci. The classic features can be appreciated in acute suppurative appendicitis and acute pyogenic meningitis.

Abscess: It is a localized collection of pus within a part of tissue because of an inflammatory process, e.g. liver abscess and lung abscess.

Gangrene: Gangrene is localized death, necrosis or decomposition of body tissue resulting because of obstruction to circulatory system or due to bacterial infection.

Ulcer: There is a local defect or breach in the continuity or excavation of the surface epithelium or organ which is produced by sloughing of the cells. This is seen in:

1. Ulcers of mouth, stomach, intestine and genito-urinary tract.
2. In older people, subcutaneous inflammation of lower extremities occurs because of circulatory disturbances.

DIFFERENT TYPES OF GIANT CELLS

1. Langerhans type of giant cell (tuberculosis).
2. Foreign body giant cell (chronic infection associated foreign body).
3. RS cell (Hodgkin's disease)
4. Touton giant cell (xanthogranuloma)
5. Osteoclastic giant cell (normal bone, osteoclastoma)
6. Tumour giant cell (high grade malignant tumours)
7. Warthin-Finkeldey giant cell (measles and viral infection).

SELF-ASSESSMENT EXERCISE

1. **True for bradykinin:**
   A. Causes increased vascular permeability
   B. Causes vasodilatation
   C. It is an inflammatory chemical mediator
   D. All of the above

2. **Opsonins are:**
   A. Receptor-mediated endocytosis
   B. Respiratory burst
   C. Fc portion of IgG and C3b
   D. Binding of adhesion molecules

3. **Cytokines which produce fever are all *except*:**
   A. TNF   B. IL-1
   C. IL-6   D. IL-8

4. **Migration (emigration) of leucocyte from vessel was described by:**
   A. Mechnikoff   B. John Hunter
   C. Celsus   D. Cohnheim

5. **Diapedesis requires:**
   A. Integrin   B. Selectin
   C. Lamanin   D. PECAM

6. **Following do not belong to selectin family *except*:**
   A. P-selectin   B. E-selectin
   C. L-selectin   D. A-selectin

7. **Functio laesa cardinal sign was given by:**
   A. Celsus   B. Morgagni
   C. Virchow   D. Rokitansky

8. **Delayed prolonged leakage from vessels due to direct injury to endothelium occurs in:**
   A. ROS   B. Thermal injury
   C. Young capillaries D. Transcytosis

9. **Ligand for E-selectin:**
   A. High affinity integrins
   B. PECAM
   C. Sialyl Lewis X modified glycoprotein
   D. None

10. **E-selectin and P-selectin binding with their ligand helps:**
    A. Adhesion   B. Transmigration
    C. Rolling   D. Chemotaxis

11. **MPO dependent mechanisms, all are correct *except*:**
    A. Produce HOCl
    B. Powerful killing mechanism
    C. Activate collagenase
    D. Activates alpha-1 AT

12. **All are correct for arachidonic acids *except*:**
    A. Component of cell membrane phospholipids
    B. Can be derived from diet
    C. Can be acted by COX and 5-lipoxygenase
    D. These are C10 polyunsaturated fatty acids

13. **All are true for PAF *except*:**
    A. Platelet aggregation
    B. Bronchodilatation
    C. Increased vascular permeability
    D. Released by activation of G protein-coupled reaction

14. **Epithelioid cell formation in tuberculosis is due to:**
    A. Release of TNF   B. Release of IFN gamma
    C. Release of IL-12   D. T cells

15. **TLRs in inflammation, all the following are true *except*:**
    A. Pattern recognition receptors
    B. Recognise microbes
    C. Can bind carbohydrates
    D. Part of innate immunity

Answers

1. D	2. C	3. D	4. D	5. D	6. D	7. C	8. B
9. C	10. C	11. D	12. D	13. B	14. A	15. C	

Regeneration and Repair

Wound healing is referred to restoration of the lost tissue with its function after an injury. Tissue undergoes repair:

1. It may be by process of epithelial regeneration, or
2. By connective tissue (scar/fibrosis) formation

NORMAL CELL CYCLE

The cell cycle has four phases: G_1, S, G_2 and M phase. The whole cell cycle lasts for about 18 hours (Fig. 12.1).

Gap 1 (G_1) phase: This is pre-DNA synthetic phase. The time is variable and short in mitotically active cells. One-third of the time is taken by this phase and usually lasts for 6–12 hours or sometimes may be more (up to 100 hours). In this phase, the cells grow in size and synthesize mRNA and proteins which are required for DNA synthesis. Sufficient nucleotides and amino acids must be present in order to synthesize mRNA and proteins. The temperature should be maintained at 37°C in humans.

DNA synthesis phase (S phase): DNA synthetic phase lasts for 6–8 hrs. This is again for a short period.

Gap 2 (G_2) phase: This is pre-mitosis phase, lasts for 2–4 hrs.

Mitosis (M) phase: This is mitosis phase, and lasts for a short time (usually 1 hour).

The period between two cycles is called interphase. Ki-67 depicts mitotically active cells. After mitotic phase, many cells re-enter G_1 phase, may become quiescent or resting cells. This is called G_0 phase. These cells may be permanent cells, which may not return to G_1 phase or some retain the ability to enter G_1 phase when appropriate stimuli are present (stable cells). Cells in late-G_2 and M phase are radiosensitive.

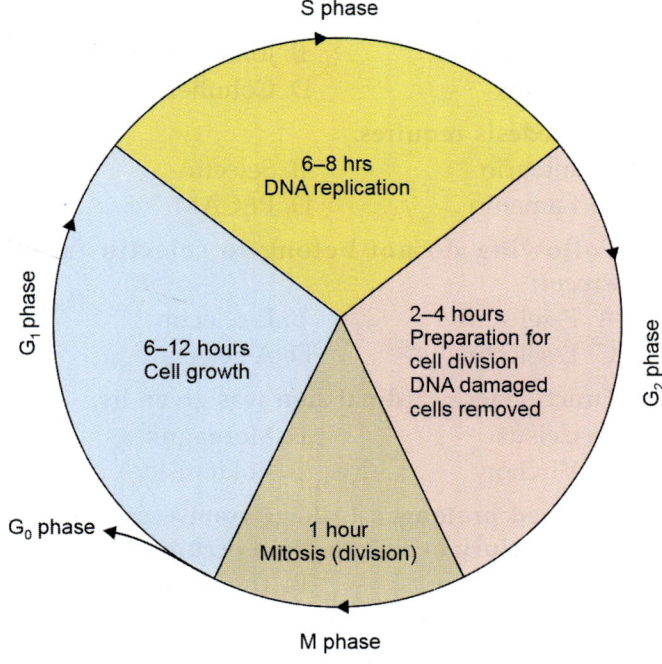

Fig. 12.1: Cell cycle

Check Point Controls in Cell Cycle (Fig. 12.2)

1. **G_1/S cell cycle check point:** Cyclin-dependent kinases (CDKs) monitor phosphorylation of cyclins. CDKs control this check at G_1/S cycle. Cyclins D and E are involved, RB gene and P53 (guardian of genes), CDK inhibitors play important role in G_1/S check points.

   These checks ensure that damaged DNA is repaired and determine whether cells should enter S phase. Until repair of damaged gene is done, cell cycle is slowed down, if not repaired or cell undergoes elimination by apoptosis.

2. **S to G_2 check points:** This check point **ensures** that the DNA has been replicated and is undamaged and permits the cells to undergo M phase.

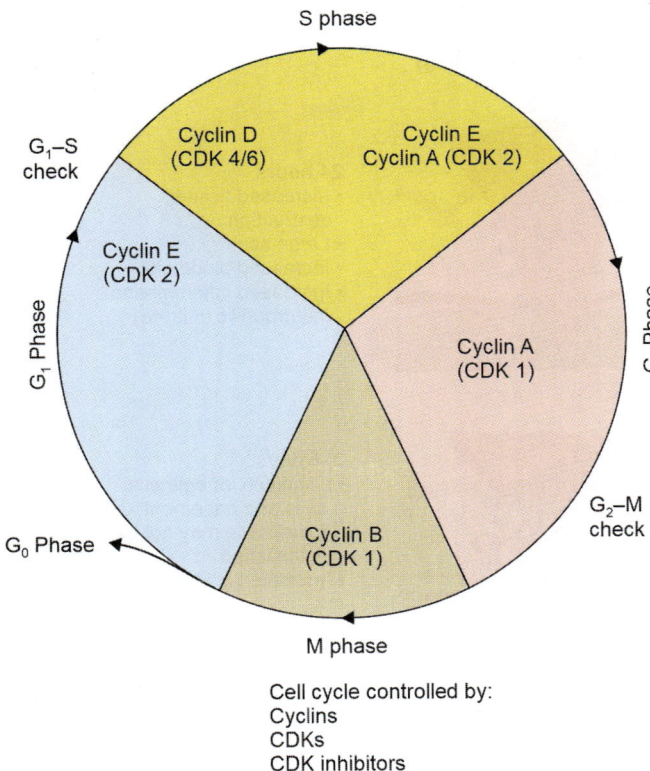

Cell cycle controlled by:
Cyclins
CDKs
CDK inhibitors

Fig. 12.2: Cell cycle with various check points

3. **G$_2$ to mitosis check point:** This is controlled by cyclins, CDKs, cytokines, various growth factors and adhesion molecules.

Other cyclins and CDKs regulate S to G$_2$ and G$_2$ to M transitions.

CUTANEOUS WOUND HEALING

Cutaneous wound healing involves epithelial regeneration and formation of connective tissue.

These are of two types (Fig. 12.3):
1. Wound healing by **first intention (primary union)**
2. Wound healing by **second intention (secondary union).**

Wound Healing by First Intention (Primary Union)

The best example for wound healing by first intention is clean, uninfected surgical incision healing, which is approximated by sutures. The incision causes disruption of epithelial basement membrane and death of relatively few epithelial and connective tissue cells.

Steps of Wound Healing by First Intention

1. **Initial effect:** Immediately after incision, there is **bleeding with formation of fibrin clot (haematoma formation) and above this scab forms**.

2. **Within 24 hrs, neutrophils appear at the incision margin.** The neutrophils migrate towards the fibrin clot. There is hyperaemia. The inflammatory cells remove clot and debris, if any.

3. **The epithelial cells (basal cells) at the cut edge show increased mitotic activity within 24–48 hrs.** Epithelial cells migrate from edges and lost cells are restored. The continuity of the cells and basement membrane is established. Thus, the thin layer of epidermis covers the surface below the clot and thus fills the gap.

4. **By 3rd day, neutrophils are replaced by macrophages and granulation tissue is formed** in the incision space. Epithelial cell proliferation continues to restore normal thickness.

5. **By day 5, epidermis recovers normal thickness.** Granulation tissue completely fills the incisional space and neovascularisation reaches its peak; collagen fibres are more abundant and bridge the incision.

6. **By the 2nd week, there is continued collagen accumulation, deposition and regression of vascular channels. The leucocyte infiltration, oedema, and vascularity are reduced.** Scab becomes loose and falls off. A thin scar is formed.

7. **By the end of first month, the tensile strength of the wound increases.** The connective tissue is devoid of inflammatory cells and surface is covered by normal epidermis.

Wound Healing by Second Intention (Secondary Union)

Wound healing by second intention defers from wound healing by first intention.
1. The tissue destruction is more and edges are ragged. The edges cannot be approximated due to extensive loss of tissue.
2. As bleeding is heavy, large clot or haematoma formation is present, which is rich in fibrin and fibronectin. Scab formed is also more. This type of wound occurs in road traffic accidents or injury by blunt instruments.
3. Inflammation is more intense, necrotic debris and exudate formed is more, which is lysed by enzymes released by leucocytes or by phagocytosis.
4. Epithelial cells migrate to replace the dead cells within a few days.
5. Larger amount of granulation tissue is formed to fill the large defect.
6. A large amount of collagen is laid down.
7. In 4–6 weeks, there is wound contraction, large skin defects are reduced to 5–10% of their original size by wound contraction. Contractile smooth muscle cells (myofibroblasts) play role in wound contraction.

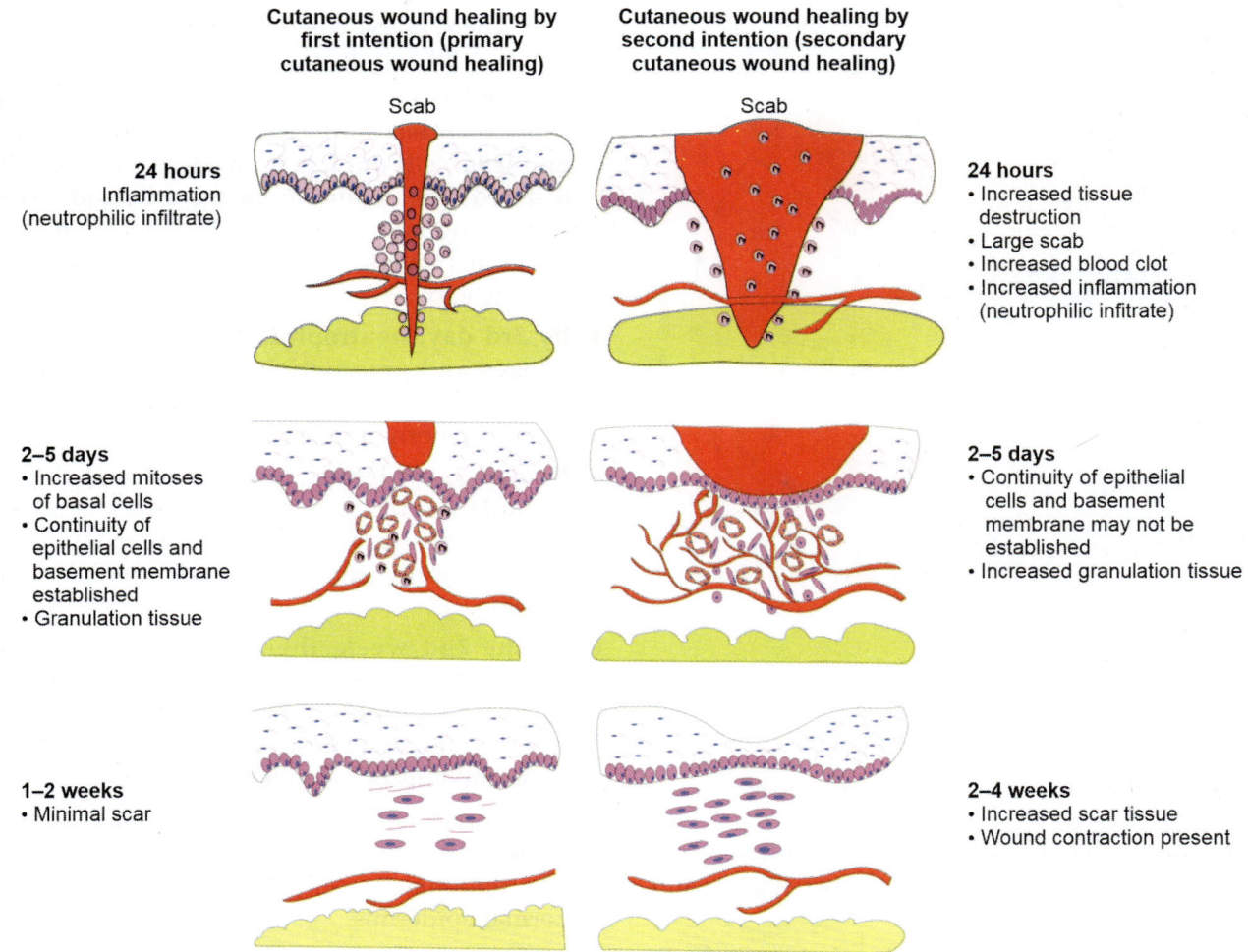

Fig. 12.3: Wound healing by first and second intention

Factors Influencing Wound Healing

Local Factors

1. Location of wound on joints and bones.
2. Intervening tissue or foreign body have necrotic debris
3. Type of tissue
4. Mechanical variables local pressure, movement.
5. Wound dehiscence
6. Infection
7. Growth factors: **PDGF** and **EGF** help in cell division and proliferation of cells. Fibroblast growth factor helps in angiogenesis and fibrosis.

General Factors (Systemic Factors)

1. Age: Older the age delay in healing.
2. Nutrition status: Vitamin C deficiency, lack of zinc and protein energy malnutrition cases have delayed wound healing.
3. Blood supply: Atherosclerosed blood vessels and tissues with less blood supply have delayed wound healing.

4. Exogenous corticosteroids/increased gluco-cortico-steroids retards wound healing by inhibiting collagen and protein synthesis and also have anti-inflammatory effects.
5. Diabetes and some haematological disorders: Diabetes has decreased phagocytic and chemotactic activity of inflammatory cells. Agranulocytosis leads to susceptibility of infection. Coagulation disorders like haemophilia, von Willebrand disease and genetic defects like Ehlers-Danlos disease have impaired wound healing.
6. Radiation energy: Ultraviolet rays, and X-rays in small doses stimulate wound healing, whereas large doses delay healing.
7. Smoking delays healing
8. Environmental temperature: Wound healing is slow in cold weather.

Complications of Wound Healing

1. Infection
2. Wound dehiscence
3. Exuberant granulation tissue or proud flesh

4. Keloid and hypertrophic scar formation
5. Wound contraction formation: Burn scar

FRACTURE BONE HEALING

Lamellar bone is composed of haversian system. It has good strength compared to the woven bone. Woven bone is immature bone, later gets remodelled to lamellar bone. Bone is covered by periosteum. With fracture, there is discontinuity of bone [may be simple, compound, comminuted (into small pieces)].

Types of Bone Fractures

1. **Simple fracture:** In this, the overlying skin is intact. The bone is into two pieces.
2. **Compound fracture:** Exposure of bone through injured skin and soft tissue.
3. **Greenstick fracture:** Partial fracture of bone.
4. **Pathological fracture:** The deseased bone breaks under normal conditions.
5. **Comminuted fractures:** Bone is broken into pieces.

Healing of Fracture Bone (Simple Fracture)

In some bones, the integrity of periostium is very important, as it ensures blood supply and osteogenic cells to the healing process. Hence, pre-requisite for healing is adequate blood supply and also mechanical stability (Fig. 12.4).

Steps of Healing

1. **Haematoma formation:** With fracture of bone, the endosteum and periosteum are stripped off. The soft tissue also may be injured. The intraosseous vessels and vessels from periosteum and surrounding tissue are ruptured. These bleed and form a haematoma, which holds the two ends of bones and serves as a scaffold for formation of granulation tissue, which forms subsequently.
2. **Inflammatory reaction:** At the end of 24 hours, inflammatory reaction sets in. The inflammatory cells remove small fragments of dead bone and resorb the clot.
3. **Granulation tissue formation:** There is proliferation of mesenchymal stem cells from periosteum and endosteum and neovascularisation. In 2–5 days, granulation tissue is formed.
4. **Provisional callus formation** (procallus/soft tissue callus/callus composed of cartilage and woven bone): After 6th day, woven bone formation begins at the periphery of the clot. The cartilage cells migrate into granulation tissue and undergo enchondral ossification. Pluripotent stem cells at the edges of

24 hours: Haematoma formation
Inflammatory reaction

2–5 days: Granulation tissue

6 days onwards: Procallus
Woven bone forms with the help
of chondrocytes and osteoblasts

By 3 weeks: Lamellar bone formation
Woven bone is replaced by lamellar bone

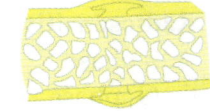

Remodelling: Excess of lamellar bone
is removed and attains shape as before

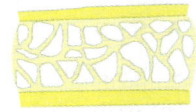

Fig. 12.4: Fracture bone healing (schematic)

bone and from soft tissue form osteoblasts and synthesize woven bone.
5. **Callus formation:** By around 3 weeks, woven bone is replaced by lamellar bone. The capillaries and osteoclasts invade the woven bone and osteoblasts lay down lamellar bone with haversian system.
6. **Remodelling:** Excess bone formed is removed by osteoclasts and bone attains normal shape.

Factors Influencing Fracture Bone Healing

Local Factors

1. Immobilization of fractured bone in plaster cast: Healing faster.
2. Inadequate opposition (mal-alignment) of fracture ends of bone: Delays healing.
3. Type of fracture: Simple fracture heals faster whereas intra-articular fracture is slow.
4. Infection: Delays healing.
5. Blood supply: Atherosclerotic vessels and other vascular diseases delay healing.
6. Pre-existing bone disease: Osteoporosis delays healing.
7. With severe injury, fractured ends with interposed soft tissue, foreign body and fragments of bone: Healing is delayed.

General/Systemic Factors

1. Age: In younger age (children and young adults), healing is faster.
2. Nutrition: Proteins and carbohydrates are necessary for healing. Vitamin C helps in bone healing.
3. Hormones: Growth hormones, thyroid hormones, and calcitonin play significant role in healing.
4. Genetic factors: Patients with TLR4 mutations have delay in healing which makes the patient prone for infections.
5. Diabetes mellitus: Delays healing.
6. Coagulation disorders: Delay healing.
7. Drugs: Corticosteroids delay healing.

Complications

1. Slow union/delayed/non-union/fibrous union.
2. Spread of infection to bone
3. Injury to soft tissue
4. Injury to underlying vital organs
5. Injury to joints
6. Myositis ossificans
7. Fat embolism

SELF-ASSESSMENT EXERCISE

1. **Radiosensitive stage of cell cycle is:**
   A. S phase   B. G_1 phase
   C. G_0 phase   D. M phase

2. **Radiosensitive stage of cell cycle is:**
   A. S phase   B. G_1 phase
   C. G_0 phase   D. Late G_2 phase

3. **Interphase is:**
   A. Period between G_1 and S phase
   B. Period between S and G_2 phase
   C. Period between two cycles
   D. Period between G_2 and M phase

4. **Longest phase of the cell cycle is:**
   A. G_2 B. S
   C. M   D. G_1

5. **Regarding G_1-S check, which is untrue?**
   A. Ensures damaged DNA repaired
   B. Damaged cells undergo apoptosis
   C. Damaged cells do not undergo division
   D. Dependent on cyclins which are discovered by Coons

6. **Wound healing by primary intention, which is untrue?**
   A. 24 hrs neutrophils appear at incision site
   B. Epithelial cells migrate from the edges by 48 hrs

   C. Wound healing is faster in patients with mutations of TLRs.
   D. By day 5 epidermis recovers normal thickness

7. **Fracture bone healing is delayed in:**
   A. Vitamin A
   B. Vitamin B_{12}
   C. Folic acid
   D. Deficiency of vitamin C

8. **Vitamin C required in wound healing for:**
   A. Synthesis of hydroxyproline and hydroxylysine
   B. Synthesis of myofibrils
   C. Prevents infection
   D. Required re-epithelialisation

9. **Hydroxyproline stabilizes:**
   A. Triple helix of collagen
   B. Synthesis of myofibrils
   C. Prevents infection
   D. Required re-epithelialisation

10. **Hydroxylysine is necessary for:**
    A. Formation of intermolecular crosslinks in collagen synthesis
    B. Synthesis of myofibrils
    C. Prevents infection
    D. Required re-epithelialisation

Answers

1. D	2. D	3. C	4. D	5. D	6. C	7. D	8. A
9. A	10. A						

Haemodynamic Disorders

CHRONIC VENOUS CONGESTION

Hyperaemia and congestion indicate local increase of volume of blood in a particular tissue.

* Hyperaemia is an active tissue process, and
* Congestion is a passive process resulting from impaired venous return from the tissue.

Long-standing congestion is called **chronic passive congestion or chronic venous congestion (CVC)**.

The stasis of poorly oxygenated blood causes chronic hypoxia, which causes:

* Degeneration, and
* Death of parenchymal cells.

Chronic Venous Congestion of Lung

Chronic venous congestion of lung is encountered whenever there is elevated left atrial pressure and consequent elevated pulmonary venous pressure. Long-standing chronic venous congestion can lead to fibrosis and haemosiderin-laden macrophages giving rise to **"brown induration lung"**.

The common conditions include:

1. Congestive cardiac failure
2. Left-sided heart failure
3. Mitral stenosis

Gross: The lungs are heavy and reddish brown coloured. The vessels are engorged. In long-standing cases, the lungs are firm in consistency, brownish and reduced in size (Fig. 13.1).

Microscopy: The septa are widened and the vessels are tortuous and congested. The alveolar spaces contain numerous haemosiderin-laden macrophages **(heart failure cells)**. In late stages, the septa are thickened fibrotic with deposition of haemosiderin pigment (brown induration) (Fig. 13.2).

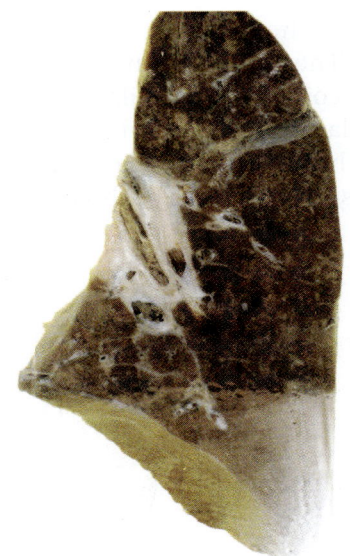

Fig. 13.1: CVC lung (gross picture)

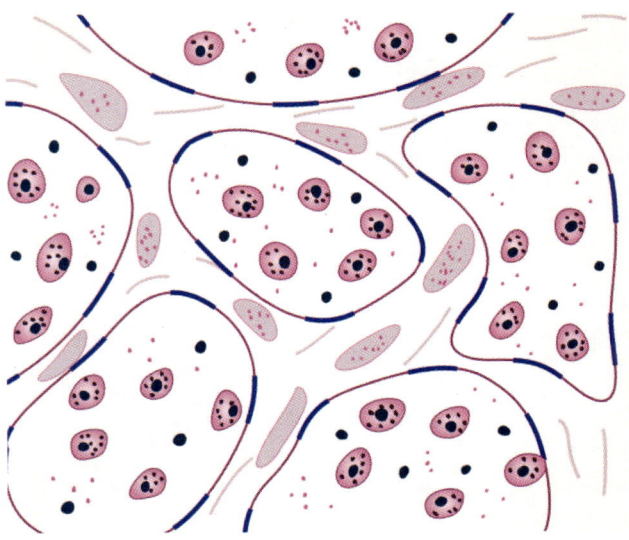

Fig. 13.2: Microscopy of CVC lung (schematic)

Chronic Venous Congestion of Liver

Chronic venous congestion of liver is usually seen in patients with:

1. Right-sided heart failure
2. Obstruction to the inferior vena cava, or
3. Obstruction to hepatic vein as in cirrhosis

Long-standing chronic venous congestion of liver can progress to hepatic fibrosis followed by cirrhotic changes termed as '**cardiac cirrhosis'**.

Gross: The liver is congested and enlarged. The cut section shows pale and dark areas **(nutmeg appearance)**. The red/dark areas are the regions around the central vein and the surrounding sinusoids. The pale areas represent the cells with fatty change around the portal triad (Fig. 13.3).

Microscopy: The normal liver architecture is maintained. The central vein and the surrounding sinusoids are congested and dilated. There is evidence of centrilobular necrosis showing loss of hepatocytes with areas of haemorrhage. In late stages, there may be hepatic fibrosis and cardiac cirrhosis (Fig. 13.4).

Chronic Venous Congestion of Spleen

The causes for chronic venous congestion of spleen are:

1. Right-sided heart failure as in cor pulmonale, tricuspid/pulmonary valvular disease, or
2. Following left-sided heart failure.
3. Portal vein and splenic vein thrombosis.
4. Cirrhosis
5. It can also occur secondary to obstruction of intra-hepatic or extrahepatic disorders those impinge on portal vein and splenic vein.

Gross: In passive congestion, the spleen is enlarged, weighs more and may show fibrosiderotic calcified areas (Gamna-Gandy bodies) (Fig. 13.5).

Microscopy: The sinusoids of the red pulp are dilated with areas of haemorrhage. The white pulp is reduced. In late stages, there is fibrosis with haemosiderin-laden macrophages and calcification (Figs 13.6 and 13.7).

Rupture of dilated and congested capillaries can cause haemorrhage, haemosiderin-laden macrophages followed by fibrosis and in some organs calcification occurs as seen in spleen producing **Gamna-Gandy bodies (siderofibrotic calcific nodules).**

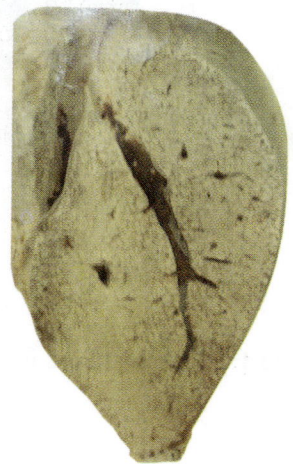

Fig. 13.3: CVC liver (gross picture)

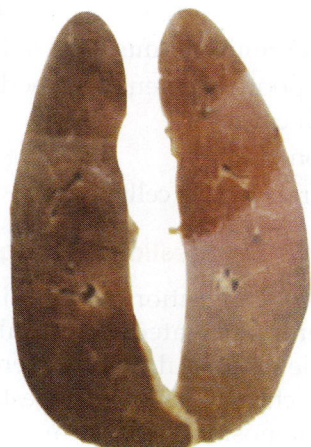

Fig. 13.5: CVC spleen (gross picture)

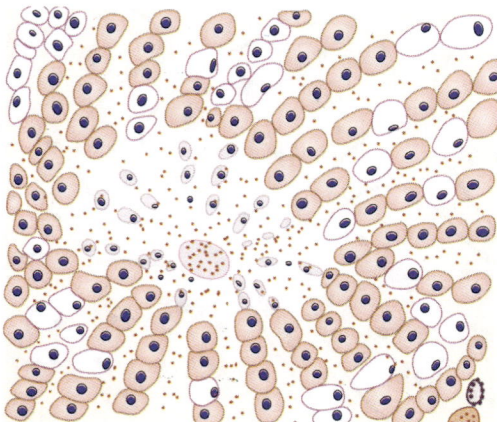

Fig. 13.4: Microscopy of CVC liver (schematic)

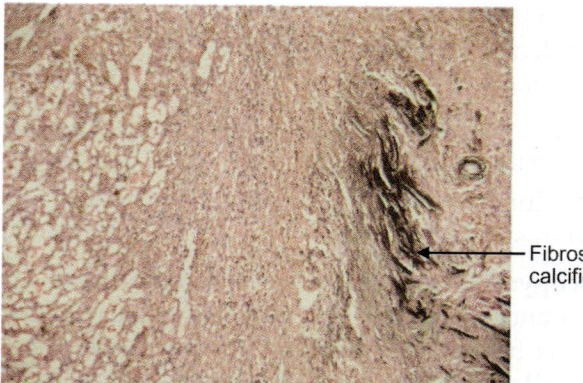

Fibrosiderotic calcified area

Fig. 13.6: Microphotograph of CVC spleen, note congestion with Gamna-Gandy bodies

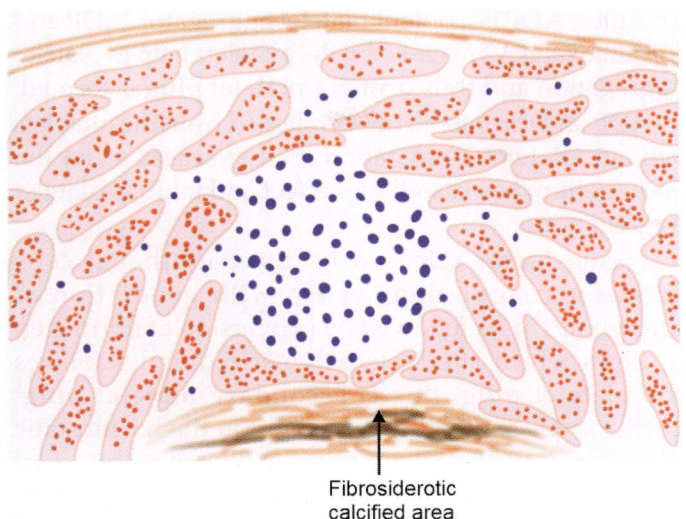

Fig. 13.7: Microphotograph of CVC spleen (schematic)

THROMBOSIS

Definition

Formation of solid mass from the constituents of blood is thrombosis. The mass formed is called thrombus.

Predisposing Factors (Virchow's Triad)

Predisposing factors (Virchow's triad) for thrombosis are the following (Fig. 13.8):
1. Abnormalities of the vessel wall
2. Abnormalities of the blood flow (stasis or turbulence)
3. Abnormalities in blood coagulation (hypercoagulable states): Thrombosis, antiphospholipid antibody syndrome, SLE, factor V Leiden, antithrombin III deficiency or secondary to bed rest, tissue damage and malignancy. Any one of these may lead to thrombus.

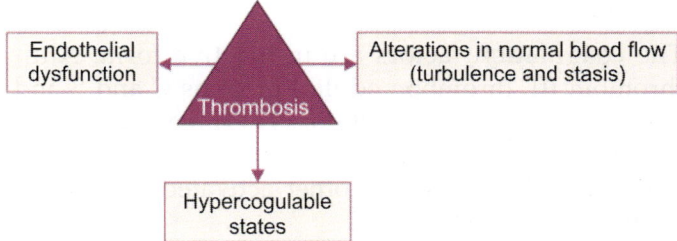

Fig. 13.8: Virchow's triad, the main causes of thrombosis

Before going into the pathogenesis, let us discuss the factors involved in normal haemostasis.

NORMAL HAEMOSTASIS

The blood in our body is maintained in fluid state by tightly regulated processes. This is normal haemostasis. The endothelial cells, platelets, coagulation factors play role in this event.

Endothelium

The endothelium modulates normal haemostasis. It has prothrombotic and antithrombotic properties which are tabulated in Table 13.1. With balance between the two, the blood is maintained in fluid state.

Platelets

Platelets play a crucial role in normal haemostasis. They have alpha granules and dense bodies. The alpha granules have fibrinogen, fibronectin, FV, FVIII, PDGR and TGFα. The dense bodies have ADP, ATP, ionized calcium, histamine, serotonin, and epinephrine. The details regarding the major role of platelets are discussed in sequence of events in haemostasis.

Table 13.1	Prothrombotic and antithrombotic properties of endothelium	
Antithrombotic properties	**Prothrombotic properties**

1. **Antiplatelet effect:**
  a. Non-activated platelets do not adhere to endothelium, endothelium acts as barrier
  b. PGI$_2$, NO and ADPase (produced by endothelium) prevent platelet activation, aggregation and adhesion
 	
2. **Anticoagulant properties:**
  a. Heparin-like molecules activate antithrombin III which binds thrombin and inactivates enzymes of coagulation system
  b. Thrombomodulin binds thrombin which activates protein C which is a anticoagulant (potent inhibitor of Va and VIIIa)
  c. Tissue factor pathway inhibitors
3. **Fibrinolytic properties:** Endothelium synthesizes t-PA which lysis fibrin
	1. **Von Willebrand factor** produced by endothelium enhances binding of platelets to ECM
	2. **ADP** is potent platelet aggregator
	3. **Tissue factor** produced by endothelium, it activates extrinsic clotting pathway
	4. **Plasminogen activator inhibitors** (PAI)

Coagulation System

The coagulation factors are in inactive form. Anti-thrombin III, thrombomodulin, proteins C and S and tissue factor pathway inhibitor (TFPI) have important role in haemostasis. Antithrombins (e.g. antithrombin III) reduce thrombin, and other activated coagulated factors (IXa, Xa, XIa, XIIa).

Fibrin formed gets dissolved by fibrinolysis which is accomplished by plasmin which breaks fibrin to FDPs and D-dimer. Plasmin is generated by plasminogen. Tissue plasminogen activator (t-PA) is synthesized by endothelial cells which activates plasminogen to plasmin.

The sequence of events in haemostasis:

1. Vasoconstriction followed by vasodilatation
2. Endothelial injury
3. Platelet adhesion to subendothelial ECM/collagen and activation
4. Aggregation of platelets—primary haemostatic plug
5. Secondary haemostatic plug

After injury to the endothelium, there is vasoconstriction followed by vasodilatation. The platelets adhere to the subendothelial collagen (ECM) by GPIb receptors present on the platelets, vWF acts as a bridge between the two. The platelets undergo release reaction with degranulation releasing calcium and ADP from dense granules. ADP is a potent platelet aggregator. ADP and thromboxane A2 released by the platelets help in platelet aggregation and thus **primary platelet plug** is formed.

ADP and thromboxane A2 released from the platelets activate platelet aggregation. PGI$_2$ released from the endothelium has vasodilator effect and inhibits platelet aggregation.

Tissue factor released by the endothelial cells activates coagulation system with generation of thrombin. This is followed by conversion of fibrinogen to fibrin which later gets polymerized and stabilizes the platelet plug, this is **secondary platelet plug**. Erythrocytes and WBCs are caught in the haemostatic plug. Fibrin and platelets adhere to each other by cross-linkage via GPIIb/ IIIa receptors on the platelets which binds to fibrin (Fig. 13.9).

Pathogenesis of Thrombosis

The defects in any of the factors can cause thrombosis like endothelial injury, alterations in blood flow or hypercoagulabity of blood (Fig. 13.10). These three factors are discussed below.

Endothelial Injury

This is the major cause of thrombosis. Endothelial cells are activated by injury, infection, plasma mediators and cytokines. The prothrombotic properties are activated

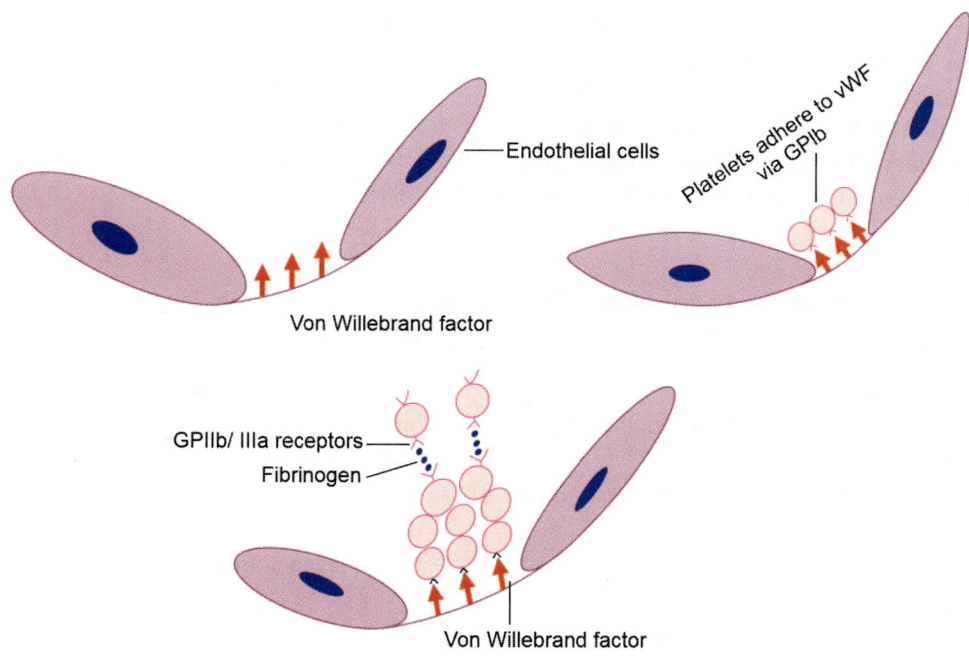

Activated platelets release ADP and thromboxane A2
These are potent aggregators and form primary platelet plug

Tissue factor released by endothelium generates thrombin, converts fibrinogen to fibrin which gets stabilised and this is secondary platelet plug

Fig. 13.9: The role of platelets in pathogenesis of thrombosis

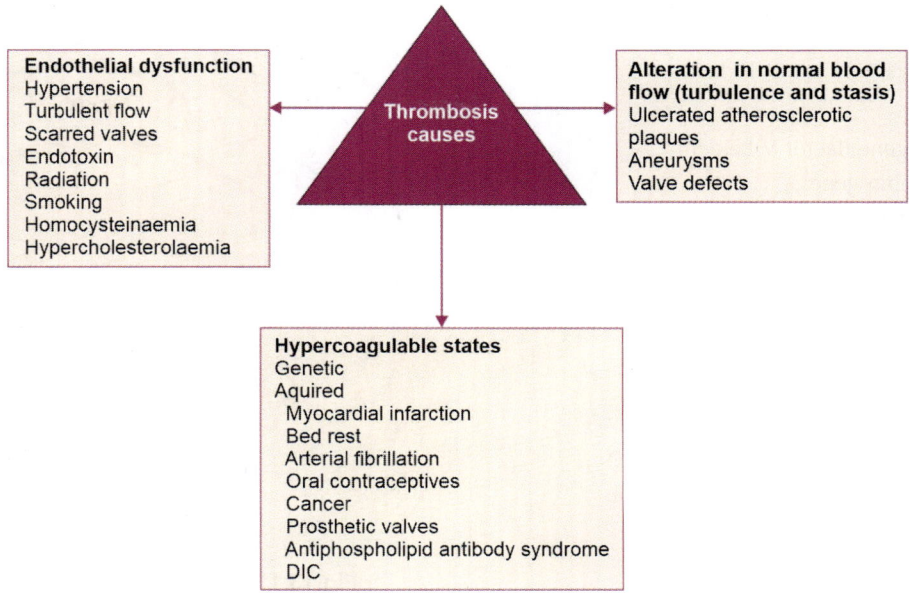

Fig. 13.10: Different causes of thrombosis

and antithrombotic functions are reduced. This is particularly important in thrombosis occurring in heart and arteries.

The slowing of blood reduces the inflow of fresh blood and inhibitors of coagulation factors and stasis brings about adhesion of platelets to the endothelium. Thus, thrombosis is more common in chambers of heart after myocardial infarction in blood vessels with ulcerated atherosclerotic plaques and in vasculitis.

With injury (dysfunction) to endothelium or loss of endothelial cells, there is release of greater amounts of procoagulant factors and reduced antithrombotic factors.

1. The ECM is exposed to which platelets adhere via vWF.
2. There is adhesion of platelets by thromboxane A2.
3. There is downregulation of thrombomodulin with sustained activation of thrombin.
4. There is depletion of PGI_2 and plasminogen activation inhibitors released by endothelium.
5. There is release of tissue factor.

Significant endothelial dysfunction can be seen with hypertension, turbulent flow over damaged or scarred valves or by action of endotoxins. Radiation, smoking, homocysteinaemia and hypercholesterolaemia may play role in endothelial dysfunction.

Alterations in Normal Blood Flow
(Stasis and Turbulence)

Turbulence causes endothelial injury and endothelial dysfunction. Turbulence also causes stasis.

The examples which cause turbulence and stasis are:

1. Ulcerated atherosclerotic plaque
2. Aneurysms
3. Valve defects

Turbulence and stasis bring about the following changes:

1. Disrupts the laminar flow, brings platelets in contact with endothelium.
2. Prevents dilution of activated clotting factors by preventing flow of fresh blood.
3. Prevents inflow of inhibitors and permits building of thrombus.
4. Promotes endothelial cell activation resulting in thrombosis and leucocyte adhesion.

With turbulence (e.g. as in atheroma) and stasis/hyperviscosity of flow of blood, there is loss of endothelial cells and subendothelial collagen is exposed leading to platelet aggregation. The coagulation cascade sets in with fibrin meshwork formation in which RBCs and WBCs are trapped. The platelets, followed by fibrin with entrapped WBCs and RBCs form alternate layers, this is called **'lines of Zahn'**.

Hypercoagulability of Blood

Hypercoagulability is a less frequent cause of thrombosis. Table 13.2 shows hypercoagulable states.

The common causes are:

1. In Leiden mutations, the activated factor V (Va) cannot be cleaved by protein C.
2. Mutations of prothromin and antithrombin III, proteins C and S are the common causes in hypercoagulability.

Gross: Thrombus is firmly attached to the vessel, occluding or non-occluding, with lines of Zahn which are alternating pale and dark areas (pale areas representing platelets, dark areas representing RBC rich layer with fibrin and WBCs). These are arterial thrombi,

Table 13.2	Hypercoagulable states

Primary (genetic)

Common
- Mutation in factor V gene (factor V Leiden)
- Mutation in prothrombin gene
- Mutation in methyltetrahydrofolate gene

Rare
- Antithrombin III deficiency
- Protein C deficiency
- Protein S deficiency

Very rare
- Fibrinolysis defects

Secondary (acquired)

Most common causes for thrombosis
- Prolonged bed rest or immobilisation
- Myocardial infarction
- Atrial fibrillation
- Tissue damage (surgery, fracture, burns)
- Cancer
- Prosthetic cardiac valves
- Disseminated intravascular coagulation
- Heparin-induced thrombocytopenia
- Antiphospholipid antibody syndrome (lupus anticoagulant syndrome)

Less common causes for thrombosis
- Cardiomyopathy
- Nephrotic syndrome
- Hyperestrogenic states (pregnancy)
- Oral contraceptive use
- Sickle cell anaemia
- Smoking

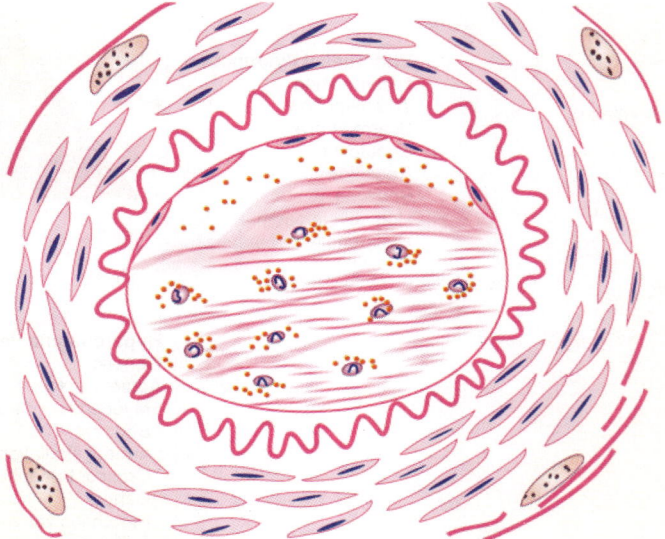

Fig.13.11: Microscopy of thrombus (schematic)

which develop in flowing blood. Venous thrombi form in a sluggish flow and are red due to more trapping of RBCs.

Microscopy: Shows platelet aggregates and RBCs and WBCs cought in fibrin (Fig. 13.11).

Venous thrombosis is usually due to damaged valves (trauma, stasis and occlusion). Immobilised patients are at higher risk of deep vein thrombosis.

Clinical effects:
- Infarction
- Strokes
- Thrombophlebitis migrans occurs in a previously normal vessel. Thrombosis appears and disappears with changing site.

Fate of Thrombus (Fig. 13.12)

1. Propagation: Eventually causes vessel block.

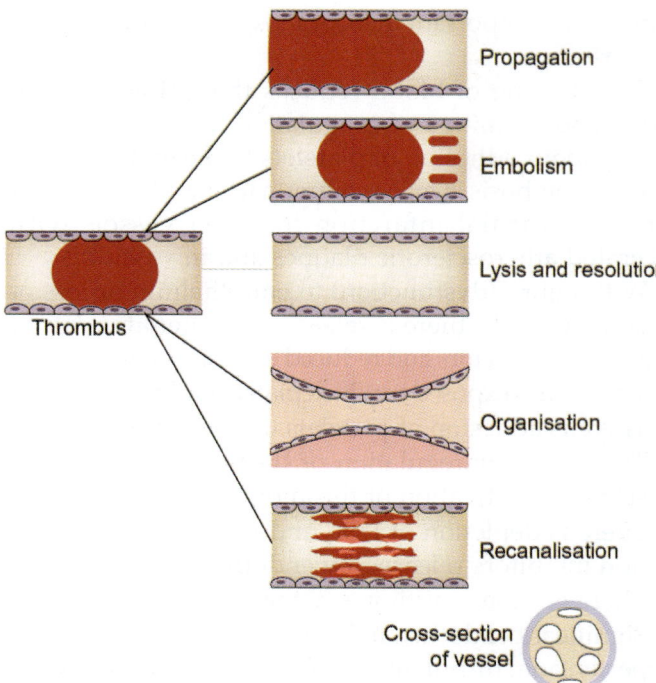

Fig. 13.12: Fate of thrombosis

2. Embolisation: Thrombus dislodges a fragment and causes infarcts elsewhere.

3. Dissolution: Removed by fibrinolytic mechanism and blood circulation is re-established.

4. Organisation and recanalisation: Induce inflammation and fibrosis (organisation) or may recanalise or re-establish some degree of flow of blood.

Differences between thrombus (antemortem clot) and postmortem clot are given in Table 13.3.

Table 13.3	Differences between thrombus (antemortem clot) and postmortem clot	
	Thrombus (antemortem clot)	**Postmortem clot**
Colour	Pale	Gelatinous mass, **dark red (current jelly)** or lower red with upper yellow **(chicken fat)**
Cause	Endothelial injury	Stagnation
Attachment	Firmly attached to the vessel wall	Not attached
Consistency	Dry	Moist
Surface	Granular, rough	Smooth, glistening
Endothelial surface	Damaged, rough	Smooth, intact
Organisation	Partially organised	Not organised
Lines of Zahn	Laminated	Absent, homogenous

EMBOLISM

Definition

An embolism is a detached intravascular solid or liquid or gaseous mass that is carried by bloodstream to a site distant from its point of origin.

Classification

The emboli can be classified as:

1. Depending upon the type of the tissue
   a. Commonest form: From dislodged thrombus (thromboembolism). About 99% of emboli are thrombotic in origin.
   b. Rare forms:
      i. Fat embolism
      ii. Air embolism
      iii. Amniotic fluid
      iv. Atherosclerotic plaque contents (cholesterol)
      v. Tumour fragments
      vi. Bone marrow tissue
      vii. Foreign bodies such as bullets, parasites.
2. Emboli can be:
   a. Solid: Tumour, atherosclerotic plaque contents, parasites, foreign body
   b. Liquid: Amniotic fluid, fat globules
   c. Gaseous: Air, nitrogen
3. Emboli can be:
   a. Sterile
   b. Infected
4. Depending on the flow of bloods:
   a. Paradoxical
   b. Retrograde
5. Depending on the site of origin:
   a. Cardiac
   b. Arterial
   c. Venous
   d. Lymphatic

Important Emboli

1. Embolus arising from lower leg vessels causes pulmonary embolism.
2. Embolus arising from left ventricular wall causes system embolism.
3. Embolus of bone marrow due to fractured bone causes fat embolism.
4. Embolus comprised of amniotic fluid causes amniotic fluid embolism.
5. Embolus comprised of air or nitrogen causes air embolism (decompression sickness).

Effects of Embolism

1. Depending upon the site of origin, the emboli may lodge anywhere in the vascular flow, too small to permit further passage.
2. Emboli results in partial or complete blockage of vascular circulation, the consequences of which are:
   a. Ischaemia
   b. Infarction of the downstream tissue supplied by that vessel after the site of blockage.

THROMBOEMBOLISM

Thromboembolism most often occurs in arterial system. The consequence of systematic thromboembolism depends upon the size of the emboli and the vessel which they obstruct.

Amongst the systemic thromboembolism:

1. 80% arise from cardiac mural wall. About two-thirds of these are associated with myocardial infarction.
2. Rest may arise from:
   a. Aneurysm
   b. Ulcerated atherosclerotic plaques, or
   c. Valvular vegetations as in bacterial endocarditis.

3. Small fraction of emboli may originate in veins and pass to the arterial side through defects in heart (paradoxical emboli) such as: (i) Foramen ovale, (ii) ventriculoarterial septal defects like ASD and VSD.

Arterial emboli travel to any site in the systemic circulation. These systemic emboli can harm the organs depending upon where they cause block. Some of the important organs are given below.
1. Emboli of brain can do most damage.
2. Large emboli may lodge at bifurcation of aorta.
3. Small emboli may lodge anywhere in limbs, digits, toes, kidneys or spleen. These can cause infarcts or later followed by scars and some may be asymptomatic. Emboli of superior mesenteric artery can cause infarction of small intestine which can lead to perforation and peritonitis.

Organs which suffer the most from systemic thromboembolism are:
1. *Brain*—strokes causing infarction, haemorrhage and hemiplegia.
2. *Intestine*—manifest as acute abdomen with infarction, ulceration, perforation and peritonitis.
3. *Kidney*—infarcts of entire kidney or small infarcts which are later converted to scars.
4. *Heart*—emboli of coronary artery lead to myocardial infarction.

Other instances of systemic thromboembolism are:
1. Patients on bed rest may develop venous thrombosis, may cross to arterial side with congenital heart defects.
2. Hypercoagulability conditions (oral contraceptive pills)
3. Genetic mutations of coagulation factors
4. Acquired causes of hypercoagulability conditions
5. Autoimmunity can activate platelets which induce thrombosis
6. Hyperviscocity conditions, e.g. polycythemia vera
7. Dehydration
8. Sickle cell anaemia

PULMONARY EMBOLISM

Causes

Causes of pulmonary embolism are:
a. 95% of the instances originate from leg veins as in bedridden patients, varicose veins, and pulmonary hypertension.
b. Rest of them arise from pelvic veins.
c. Few from intracranial venous sinuses.
d. Rarely pulmonary embolism can be due to arterial emboli through arteriovenous communications.

Effects due to Pulmonary Embolism

The emboli get detached from the primary site, enter the venous drainage, right side of the heart and then enter the lungs through pulmonary circulation (Fig. 13.13).
1. The effects depend upon the size of emboli. Most of the pulmonary emboli (60–80%) are small emboli and may go unnoticed, may remain silent or may be lysed in the lung or get organized and may cause small respiratory deficiency.
2. Emboli in small-sized vessels will cause pulmonary hypertension and may not cause lung infarct as lung has dual blood supply and intact bronchial arterial circulation continues to supply the affected area. However, when bronchial arterial circulation is compromised, or in a context of chronic heart failure, the blockage in pulmonary circulation causes infarcts. Commonly, multiple small emboli are seen impacting the vessels of lower lobe of lungs.
3. Many small emboli, over a period of time, can cause pulmonary hypertension and right heart failure.
4. Large emboli may cause acute respiratory and cardiac dysfunction (acute cor pulmonale) when 60% or more of pulmonary circulation is obstructed by embolism. This causes chest pain, shortness of breath. There is ischaemia and infarction of the lung tissue due to occlusion of the vessel. There may be changes in heart with ECG changes of right heart failure.

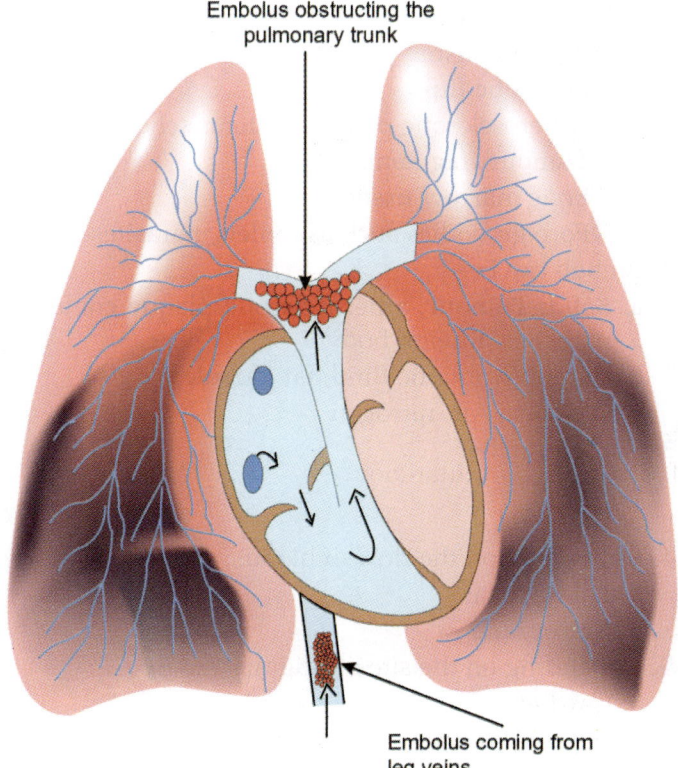

Embolus obstructing the pulmonary trunk

Embolus coming from leg veins

Fig. 13.13: Effects of saddle pulmonary embolism (diagrammatic)

5. Large pulmonary emboli blocking the main trunk of the pulmonary artery (saddle embolus) impacting across the bifurcation may cause sudden death. The embolus may be seen in right ventricle also.

Paradoxical Embolus

This is also called '**crossed embolus**' (Fig. 13.14) passed from vein to artery or right side of heart to left side of heart as in patent foramen ovale, atrial septal defect and ventriculoseptal defect.

Once the embolism is in systemic circulation, it can cause strokes (cerebrovascular accidents). Thus, even a small defect in the heart has to be closed in these patients.

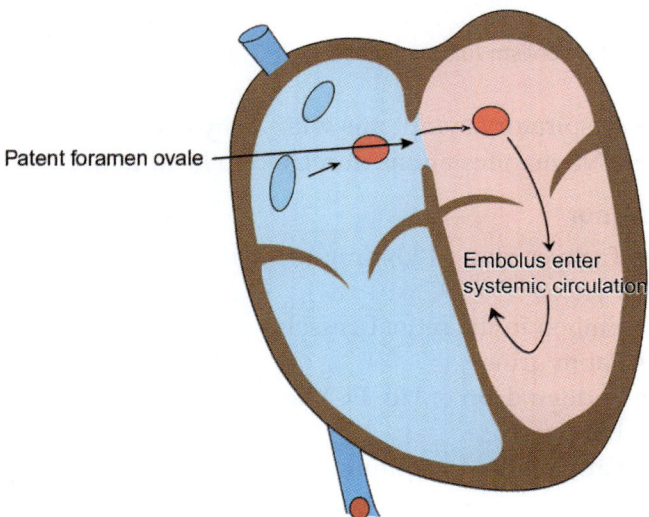

Embolus from leg vessels enters systemic circulation through patent foramen ovale or arterial septal defect

Fig. 13.14: Crossed embolus (diagrammatic)

Consequences of Pulmonary Infarction

a. Sudden death
b. Acute respiratory failure/cardiac failure/acute cor pulmonale
c. Pulmonary infarction
d. Pulmonary haemorrhage
e. Pulmonary hypertension
f. Resolution of infarction

FAT EMBOLISM

Causes

Causes for fat embolism are the following: Fat globules from the following can enter the circulation.
1. *Trauma-related causes:*
   • After fracture of bones (from fatty marrow from fracture bone and usually from fracture of long bones).
   • Severe burn
   • Liposuction
   • Orthopaedic procedures
   • Bone marrow harvesting and transplant
   • Extensive soft tissue injury
2. *Non-trauma-related causes:* Pancreatitis, diabetes mellitus, osteomyelitis, panniculitis, etc.

Fat enters circulation in 90% of the skeletal injuries. Only in 10% of the patients, it is fatal and experience clinical signs and symptoms of fat embolism and is termed as "**fat embolism syndrome**". The syndrome appears in 24–72 hours of the injury. It is characterised by triad of following:
1. Respiratory changes: These are first to appear. There is pulmonary insufficiency with features like ARDS and diffuse opacity of lungs on chest X-ray.
2. Neurological symptoms
3. Petechial rash due to thrombocytopenia

Patients will have anaemia, tachycardia, tachypnoea, dyspnoea, hypoxaemia, neurological symptoms like irritability and restlessness followed by delirium and coma, renal impairment and petechiae.

Pathogenesis

Fat embolism involves mechanical obstruction and biochemical injury. Fat microemboli enter and obstruct pulmonary and also systemic arterial circulation. The cerebral microvasculature and renal vasculature occlusion is aggravated by platelet and erythrocyte aggregation. This pathogenesis is also accentuated by injury to the endothelium due to release of free fatty acids from the fat globules leading to endothelial injury, disseminated intravascular coagulation, platelet activation, pulmonary haemorrhage and oedema and inflammatory cell recruitment (Figs 13.15 and 13.16).

Microscopy

Lung shows acute respiratory distress syndrome (ARDS) features. Fat globules are seen in the microvasculature, haemorrhage and oedema.

Brain shows cerebral oedema, small haemorrhages and occasional microinfarcts. Fat globules may be seen in the microvasculature.

Kidneys: Microinfarcts and fat globules may be seen in the microvasculature.

In fat embolism, demonstration of fat globules in the vasculature of lung, brain and other organs requires frozen sections followed by staining with special stains like Congo red, Sudan black, Sudan red, etc. which confirms the diagnosis.

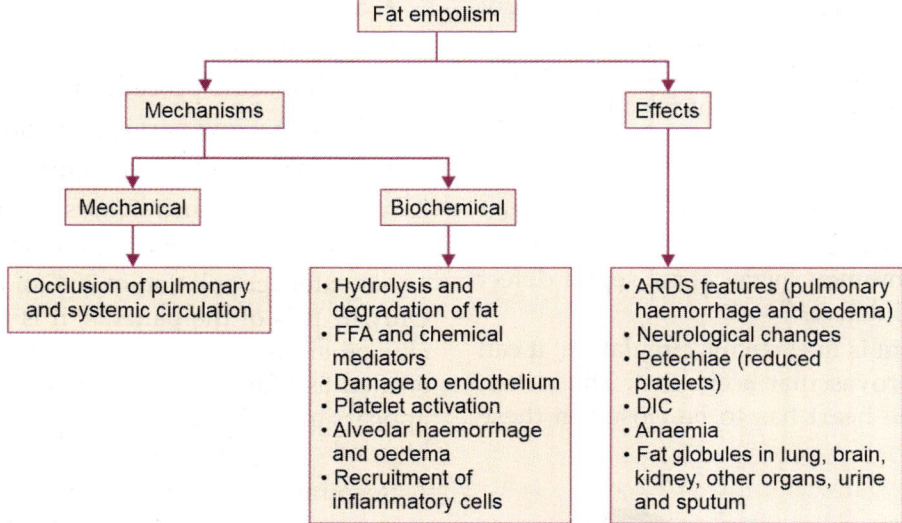

Fig. 13.15: Mechanism and effects of fat embolism (diagrammatic)

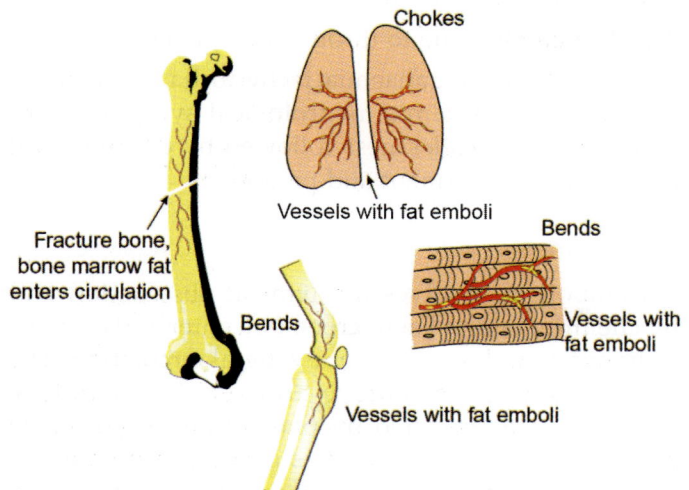

Fig. 13.16: Mechanism and pathology of fat embolism (diagrammatic)

NICE TO KNOW

Diagnosis of Fat Embolism

1. Clinical findings: Pulmonary, neurological manifestations, petechiae.
2. Biochemical values: Hb—reduced, PCV—reduced, platelet count—reduced, serum calcium—reduced and ESR—raised.

Criteria for Diagnosis

Gurd's criteria: At least 1 major and 4 minor criteria to be present.

Gurd's Criteria

Major

- Petechiae

- Respiratory symptoms with X-ray changes
- CNS manifestations unrelated to head injury

Minor

- Tachycardia: >120/minute
- Pyrexia >39.4°C
- Emboli in the retinal vessels
- Fat in urine
- Sudden drop of Hb, PCV and platelet count
- ESR increase
- Fat globules in sputum

AIR (GAS) EMBOLISM

Air or gas bubbles within the circulation can mechanically obstruct the vascular flow and cause infarction and necrosis. Gas bubbles can enter vein or artery or can be crossed from venous to arterial side with presence of right-to-left shunts (patent foramen ovale, atrial septal defects). Arterial gas emboli are serious and cause blockage of blood supply to central nervous system, heart, lungs and other vital organs.

Gas bubbles in pulmonary veins can enter systemic circulation or venous emboli as in iatrogenic causes (neurosurgical and otolaryngological procedures), dissolved gases coming out as gas bubbles on depressurization in decompression sickness which overwhelms the filtering capacity of pulmonary capillaries and enter systemic circulation.

Air can enter the circulation in following situations:
1. Chest wall injury
2. Caisson's disease (decompression sickness)
3. Obstetric procedures
4. Orthopaedic procedures
5. Open heart surgeries
6. Intravenous drip

7. Haemodialysis treatment
8. Barotrauma from mechanical ventilation

Small amount of air is of little consequences, but 5 ml/kg of air can damage the tissue with shock and cardiac arrest. About 0.5 ml in coronaries (left anterior descending branch) can cause cardiac problems and about 2–3 ml air into cerebral circulation can be fatal.

Mechanism

These are due to mechanical obstruction of the vascular flow or due to rupture or compression of tissues or activation of coagulation and inflammatory cascade.

Effects

Following can be signs and symptoms:
1. Related to CNS manifestations: Altered mental status, hemiparesis, focal motor and sensory deficits, seizures, ischaemic stroke with loss of consciousness. The neurological symptoms occur within minutes, apnoea and death
2. Pulmonary manifestations: Difficulty in breathing or respiratory failure
3. Coronary artery blockage: Chest pain with arrhythmias, myocardial infarction, cardiac arrest
4. Cyanosis
5. Low blood pressure
6. GIT: Abdominal pain and bowel ischaemia
7. Renal: Haematuria, proteinuria and renal failure
8. Uterine bleeding

Caisson's Disease

Scuba, deep divers, and underwater construction workers (tunnelers) are at risk of air embolism.

Underwater, these individuals breathe air (combination of gases oxygen, nitrogen and sometimes helium) with high pressure. Increasing amounts of gas particularly nitrogen gets dissolved in blood and tissues. If these individuals ascend slowly (depressurize), gas is slowly released from blood and exhaled. However, if the ascent is too rapid, nitrogen/helium bubbles out of the blood to form gas embolism.

In acute form (Type I), gas embolism, which is one of the leading causes of death in diving—the gas bubbles in the vessels of skeletal muscles and joints, causes severe pain (bends) around knee and legs. Abdominal pain, vomiting, dizziness, general malaise, fatigue and headache are common features. In lungs, these bubbles in vasculature cause pulmonary oedema, haemorrhage and focal atelectasis with emphysema leading to respiratory distress called the chokes.

In chronic form (Type II), there is infarction and necrosis of tissues including brain and joints. Persistence of gas emboli in bone leads to multiple foci of ischaemic necrosis. Head of femur, tibia and humerus are commonly affected due to small vessel obstruction which leads to bends and chokes. In neurological manifestations, there can be damage to spinal cord, paraplegia, loss of bladder control, memory loss, ataxia and visual and speech disturbances. Pulmonary manifestations include chest pain, dyspnoea, cough, haemoptysis, right ventricular flow obstructiuon, and circulatory collapse. Neurological complications are more common than the pulmonary ones (Fig. 13.17).

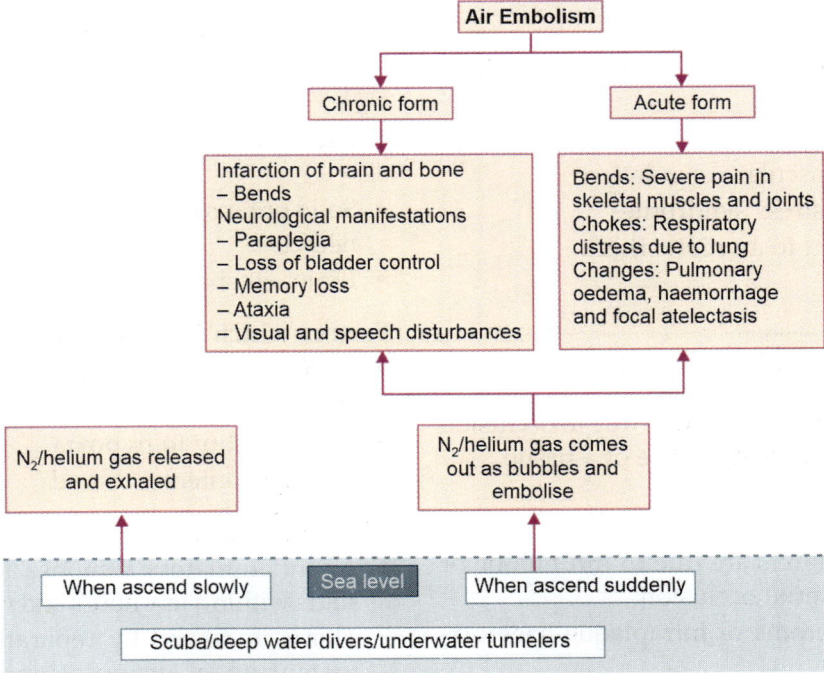

Fig. 13.17: Mechanism and effects of air embolism in Caisson's disease

AMNIOTIC FLUID EMBOLISM

Amniotic fluid embolism is a rare but catastrophic maternal complication during childbirth.

About 1:50000 deliveries have this complication. It has mortality rate of 20–40%.

Pathogenesis

Contents of the amniotic fluid enter mother's circulation due to tear of placental membrane and rupture of uterine and/or cervical vessels. In half of these patients, disseminated intravascular coagulation (DIC) occurs due to thrombogenic substance, i.e. thromboplastin/tissue factor in amniotic fluid.

Clinical Features

These patients can have the following clinical features.
1. Sudden respiratory distress with dyspnoea, cyanosis and marked pedal oedema.
2. Hypotensive shock.
3. Seizures, convulsions, coma and death.
4. Features of disseminated intravascular coagulation.

Microscopy of Organs in Amniotic Fluid Embolism

1. Lungs show oedema and diffuse alveolar damage.
2. Pulmonary circulation contains fetal squamous cells, lanugo hairs, fat from vernix caseosa, mucin derived from fetal respiratory tract and gastro-intestinal tract.
3. Fibrin thrombi are present in DIC.

Cause of Death in Amniotic Fluid Embolism

This is due to:
1. Mechanical obstruction of vessels leading to pulmonary oedema
2. Haemorrhage
3. Disseminated intravascular coagulation
4. Acute respiratory distress syndrome
5. Anaphylactic reaction to amniotic fluid.

INFARCTION

Definition

Infarct is an area of ischaemic necrosis due to occlusion of **arterial supply or venous drainage** of a tissue.

Causes

- About 99% of the infarcts are due to thrombotic or embolic events of arterial occlusion.
- Complication of atheroma or intraplaque haemorrhage.
- Occasionally, it can be because vasospasm.

- Compression of vessel due to tumour or tumour-like lesion, oedema or entrapment as in hernial sac.
- Twisting of pedical having vessels (testicular and ovarian torsion) and bowel volvulus.
- Traumatic vessel rupture.

Types of Infarct

Infarcts are classified as: Red infarcts and white infarcts.
- **Red infarcts are seen in:**
  1. Venous obstruction (ovarian or testicular torsion).
  2. Loose tissues such as lung which allows collection of blood.
  3. Tissues with dual circulation (lung and small intestine).
  4. Tissues with sluggish venous outflow.
  5. Arterial occlusion followed by re-established flow.
- **White infarcts occur in:** Solid organs like heart, spleen, kidney due to arterial obstruction with limitation of haemorrhage that can seep into areas of necrosis.

Infarcts can be:

- **Septic infarcts:** Bacterial vegetations which are embolised and bacteria seed into area of infarction.
- **Bland infarcts:** These infarcts do not have bacteria in the occluded thrombus or emboli.

Infarcts are **wedge-/fan-shaped, the occluded vessel is at the apex and periphery of the organ forms the base.** The base with serosal surface can have fibrinous exudate. Initially infarcted zone is poorly defined and with time it becomes well defined by narrow rim of congestion and inflammation at the edge of the infarction adjacent to normal tissue.

Histopathological Characters of Infarct

The features vary with tissue and organ involved, such as:
- Solid organs like heart, lung, spleen have coagulative necrosis.
- Brain, etc. have colliquative necrosis.

Factors which influence development of infarct are:
- Nature of vascular supply
- Rate of development of occlusion
- Vulnerability to hypoxia
- Oxygen content of blood

The histological findings:
1. An inflammatory response at the margins of infarct starts within a few hours and well defined by 1–2 days.
2. This is followed by reparative phenomenon with formation of granulation tissue which is later replaced by scar.

MYOCARDIAL INFARCTION (MI)

Gross Findings (Figs 13.18 to 13.20)

The gross findings depending upon the duration of infarct are as follows:

0–4 hours	**There are no gross changes during this time.** To detect the infarct during this time, immerse a piece of heart tissue in a solution of **TTC (triphenyltetrazolium chloride)**. The necrosed area will be pale as dehydrogenase enzyme is depleted, while the normal myocardium stains brick red.
4–12 hours	There is a dark mottling of necrosed tissue (due to stagnated/trapped blood).

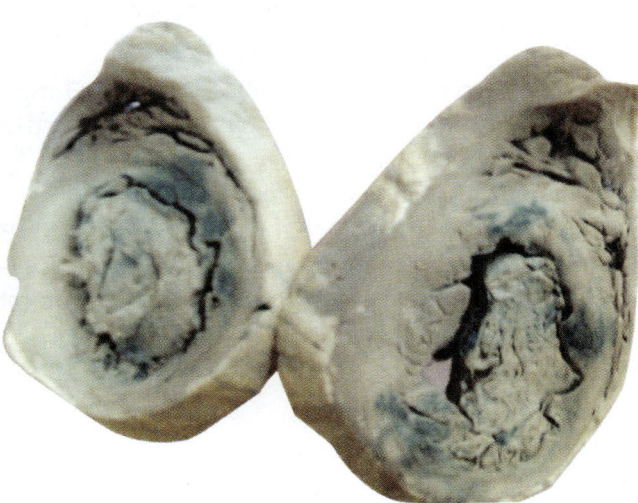

Fig. 13.18: Myocardial infarction, recent (gross picture)

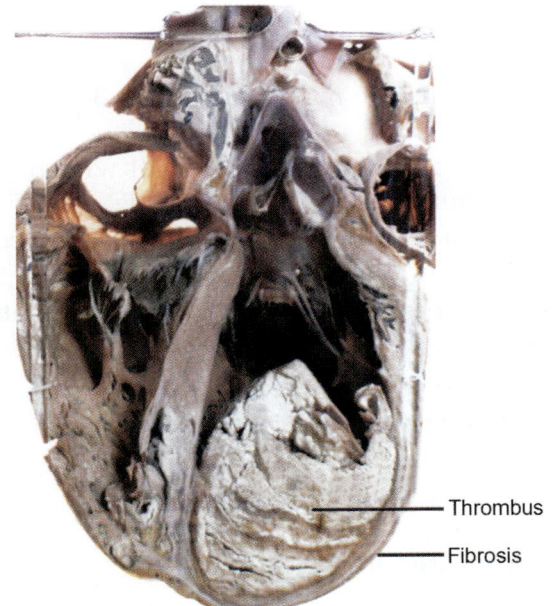

Fig. 13.19: Myocardial infarction, healed with mural thrombus (gross picture)

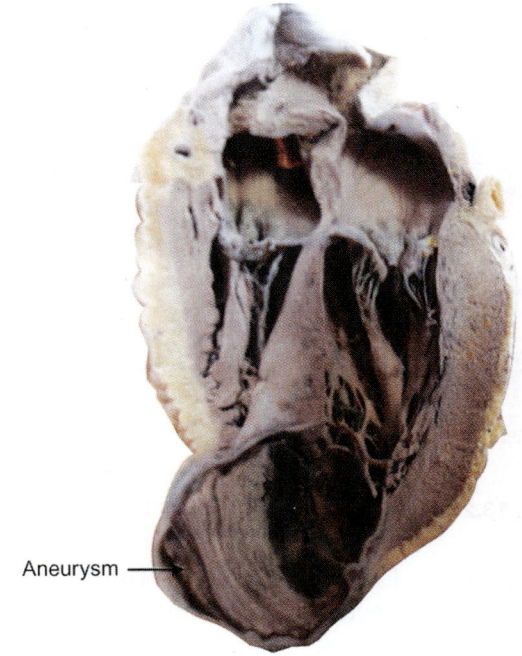

Fig. 13.20: Myocardial infarction, healed with aneurysm formation (gross picture)

1–3 days	The necrosed area has yellow-tan-coloured centre with mottling.
3–7 days	The necrosed area is yellow-tan coloured with soft consistency and has hyperaemic border. The hyperaemic border is due to the formation of granulation tissue.
7–10 days	The necrosed area is yellow-tan-coloured with soft centre with reddish margins.
10–14 days	The necrosed area has red grey margins as granulation tissue is replaced **by collagen.**
2–8 weeks	During this period, the necrosed tissue is replaced by grey scar.
>2 months	The necrosed area is completely replaced by scar tissue.

Microscopic Findings (Fig. 13.21)

The microscopic findings depending upon the duration of infarct are as follows:

4–12 hours	There is oedema and haemorrhage. There are wavy fibres at the periphery, because of the forceful systolic tugs by viable fibres, adjacent to non-contractile necrosed fibres. There is vacuolar degeneration at the margins of the infarct.

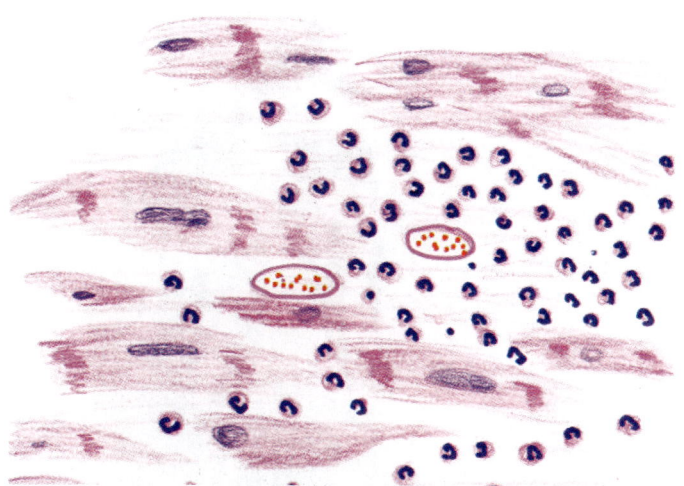

Fig. 13.21: Microscopy of myocardial infarct (schematic)

12–24 hours	During this time, there is ongoing necrosis, pyknosis of the nuclei and contractile band necrosis.
	There will be myocyte hypereosinophilia.
	The neutrophils start appearing in the infarcted zone.
1–3 days	During this period, the neutrophils increase in number.
	The myocardial fibres show coagulative necrosis with loss of nuclei and striations.
3–7 days	The neutrophils decrease in number and the other inflammatory cells make their appearance.
7–10 days	There is phagocytosis of dead cells with formation of granulation tissue at the margins.
10–14 days	Granulation tissue formation continues with laying down of collagen.
2–8 weeks	There is collagen tissue with decreased cellularity
>2 months	The infarcted area is replaced by scar.

Laboratory Investigations

Laboratory investigations in a case of myocardial infarction are as follows:

i. **Cardiac troponin T and I:** These are normally not detected. In acute MI, the levels of both **troponin T and I rise by 2–4 hours and peak levels are reached by 12–16 hours and remain elevated for 7–10 days and later return to normal.**

ii. **Creatinine kinase (CK):** This is an enzyme concentrated in brain, myocardium and skeletal muscle. It is composed of M and B dimers. The isoenzyme CK-MM is predominantly localized to skeletal muscle and heart; CK-BB is localized to lungs, brain and many other tissues.

However, **CK-MB is principally from myocardium** although variable amounts are found in skeletal muscle. In myocardial infarction, **the levels of CK-MB rise by 2–4 hours, peak levels are reached by 24 hours and return to normal by 72 hours. The ratio of CK-MB2 to CK-MB1 more than 1.7 is suggestive of acute myocardial infarction.**

iii. **The plasma myoglobin** is increased in 2 hours and remains increased for 7–12 hours (levels are more than 85 ng/ml).

iv. **The LDH levels** are increased; **LDH1 peaks by 48–72 hours and remains elevated for 10–14 days. The level of LDH1 more than LDH2 predicts the risk of myocardial infarction.**

v. **The C-reactive protein (CRP):** More than 3 mg/l is associated with higher risk of myocardial infarction in angina patients.

vi. **Transient leucocytosis** in first 1–3 days.

vii. **Plasma levels of B type natriuretic peptide (BNP) and N terminal fragment of its prohormone (NT–pro-BNP)** increase according to the size of infarct.

Complications

1. Contractile dysfunction
2. Arrhythmias:
   - Sinus bradycardia
   - Heart block
   - Tachycardia
   - Ventricular premature contraction or ventricular tachycardia
   - Ventricular fibrillation
3. Myocardial rupture may occur during 3–7 days of infarction:
   - Rupture of ventricular free wall with hemopericardium and cardiac tamponade
   - Rupture of ventricular septum with new ventriculoseptal defect and left-to-right shunts
   - Papillary muscle rupture with mitral regurgitation
4. Pericarditis
5. Infarct expansion
6. Mural thrombus and thromboembolism
7. Ventricular aneurysm
8. Papillary muscle dysfunction

PULMONARY/LUNG INFARCTION

Pulmonary infarct occurs mainly due to venous thrombi. 95% of venous thrombi are from leg veins and pelvic veins and occur with bed rest.

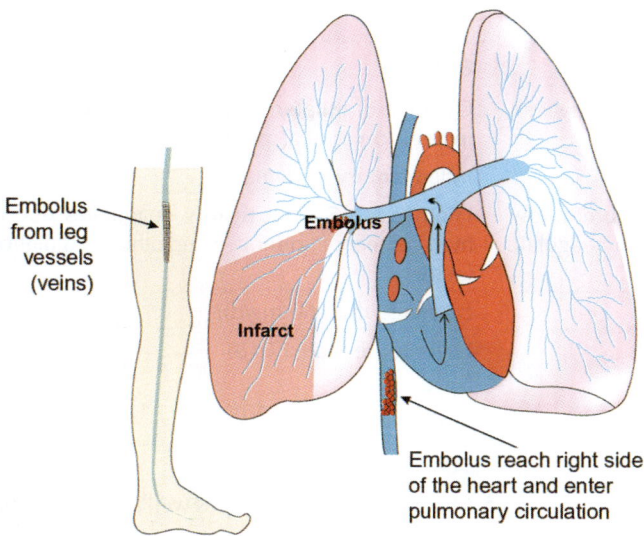

Fig. 13.22: Infarction lung (schematic)

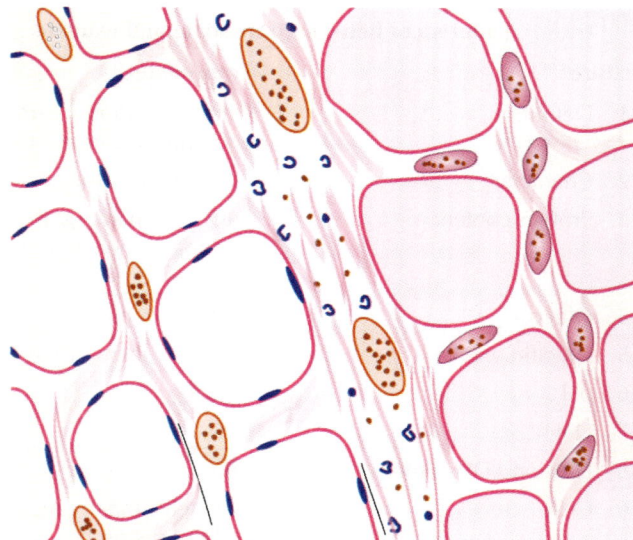

Fig. 13.24: Microscopy of lung infarction (schematic)

Pathogenesis

The effects depend upon the size of the embolus, and cardiopulmonary status. The lungs get blood supply from pulmonary arteries and also by bronchial arteries. If one circulation is sufficient enough to maintain the oxygen supply, the the blockage by thrombus in the other circulation will not cause changes of infarction. The changes of infarction are evident, only with compromise in cardiac function or bronchial circulation or underventilated due to pulmonary disease and blockage of pulmonary circulation with a thromboembolism (Fig. 13.22).

Pathology

Gross: The infarcts are wedge-shaped apex towards the blockage of vessel near the hilum and broader area towards the pleura (Fig. 13.23).

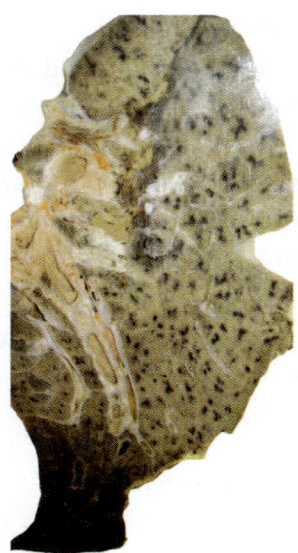

Fig. 13.23: Infarction lung (gross picture)

Pulmonary infarcts are classically haemorrhagic, appear reddish blue and raised from the cut surface. The underlying pleura shows fibrinous pleuritis. Eventually colour changes to reddish brown with lysis of RBCs and deposition of hemosiderin pigment.

Microscopy: Shows infarcted area with coagulative necrosis, inflammatory zone and normal adjacent lung parenchyma (Fig. 13.24).

OEDEMA

Definition

The term oedema refers to increased fluid accumulation in the interstitial tissue or intercellular compartment (extracellular or extravascular).

Approximately 60–75% of body weight is water. 50% of this water is in intracellular compartment, 20% is in interstitial compartment and 5% is in intravasular compartment.

There is continuous exchange of fluid between the tissue and blood. At arterial end, some fluid is lost but returns back at venous capillary level. To maintain this, hydrostatic pressure and oncotic pressure are the two factors which control the rate and direction of fluid movement.

The fluid accumulated in body cavities are termed differently as below depending on the site of accumulation.

1. Abdominal cavity: Ascites
2. Pleural cavity: Pleural effusion
3. Pericardial cavity: Pericadial effusion or hydropericardium
4. CSF pathway excess fluid collection: Hydrocephalus

Table 13.4 shows differences between transudate and exudate.

Table 13.4	Differences between transudate and exudate	
Feature	Transudate	Exudate
1. Definition	Filtrate of blood plasma without changes in endothelial permeability	Oedema of inflamed tissue associated with increased vascular permeability
2. Character	Non-inflammatory oedema	Inflammatory oedema
3. Protein content	Low (less than 1 g/dl); mainly albumin, low fibrinogen; hence no tendency to coagulate	High (2.5–3.5 g/dl), readily coagulates due to high content of fibrinogen and other coagulation factors
4. Glucose	Same as in plasma	Low (less than 60 mg/dl)
5. Specific gravity	Low (less than 1.015)	High (more than 1.018)
6. pH	>7.3	<7.3
7. LDH	Low	High
8. Effusion LDH/serum LDH ratio	<0.6	>0.6
9. Cells	Few cells, mainly mesothelial cells and cellular debris	Many cells, inflammatory as well as parenchymal
10. Examples	Oedema in congestive cardiac failure	Purulent exudate such as pus

Classification of Oedema

1. According to distribution of fluid:
- Localised oedema
- Generalised oedema (anasarca)

2. According to causes:

Increased hydrostatic pressure
- Impaired venous return
  - Congestive heart failure
  - Constrictive pericarditis
  - Cirrhosis
  - Venous obstruction or compression
    - Thrombosis
    - External pressure (e.g. mass compressing vessels)
    - Lower extremity inactivity with prolonged standing
- Arteriolar dilatation
  - Heat
  - Inflammation
  - Neurohumoral dysregulation
  - Hypervolaemia (sodium retention)

Reduced plasma osmotic pressure
- Hypoproteinaemia
  - Protein-losing glomerulopathies (nephrotic syndrome)
  - Cirrhosis (ascites)
  - Malnutrition
  - Protein-losing gastroenteropathy

Lymphatic obstruction
- Inflammation
- Neoplasms/cancer
- Post-surgical lymphoedema
- Postirradiation

Sodium retention
- Excessive salt intake with renal insufficiency
- Increased tubular reabsorption of sodium
  - Renal hypoperfusion
  - Increased renin–angiotensin–aldosterone secretion

Increased vascular permeability
- Inflammation
  - Burns
  - ARDS

3. According to gravity of oedema:
- Pitting
- Non-pitting

The oedema fluid can be transudate or exudate.

The differences between transdute and exudates are given in Table 13.4.

Pathophysiology of Oedema

The formation and retention of fluid depends on filtration and resorption of fluid at the level of capillaries (Starling's law).

The following factors play role in formation of oedema:
1. Hydrostatic pressure
2. Oncotic prssure
3. Lymphatic drainage

Apart from these three factors, the other factors which play role in oedema formation are:
 i. Malnutrition (Kwashiorkar)
 ii. Increased capillary permeability
 iii. Sodium and water retention
 iv. Tissue factors
 v. Atrial natriuretic peptide
 vi. Renin–angiotensin system

In normal health, at arteriolar end, hydrostatic pressure is more than the oncotic pressure, hence the fluid passes into interstitium. At venular end, the oncotic pressure is more than the hydrostatic pressure, hence fluid returns to capillary bed. Still some fluid remains in the interstitium. This fluid in the interstitium and proteins diffused into interstitium are carried by lymph vessels. Thus obstruction of the lymphatic vessels causes oedema.

Thus, increased capillary hydrostatic pressure, decreased oncotic pressure and lymphatics play role in formation of oedema (Fig. 13.25).

Hydrostatic Pressure

The normal hydrostatic pressure is 32 mm Hg at the arteriolar end of the capillary, and 12 mm Hg at the venular end.

Hydrostatic pressure (capillary pressure) forces the fluid from blood, pass into the tissues through the capillary wall.

Increased hydrostatic pressure pushes out large quantities of fluid into the interstitial tissue and all of this cannot be drained back with the oncotic pressure at the venular end or by the lymphatics and fluid accumulates into the interstitial tissue. Some of the examples due to increased hydrostatic pressure are given below.
1. Cardiac oedema (congestive heart failure)
2. Ascites in portal vein obstruction
3. Pregnancy
4. Deep vein thrombosis
5. Pulmonary oedema

Accumulation of excess oedema fluid due to elevated hydrostatic pressure is also called hydrostatic oedema.

Oncotic Pressure

The plasma proteins (especially albumin) are responsible for the oncotic pressure and oncotic pressure tries to keep the fluid in the capillary and tend to draw fluid inside the vessel from the interstitial tissue. The oncotic pressure of the capillary is 28 mm Hg with albumin contributing to 22 mm Hg of this oncotic pressure.

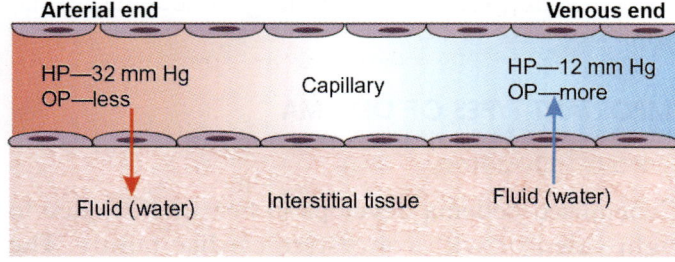

Fig. 13.25: Oedema formation (schematic) (OP—oncotic pressure, HP—hydrostatic pressure)

In hypoalbuminaemia, reduced plasma proteins in the blood causes reduced oncotic pressure which leads to oedema formation and this is mainly because of reduced inward movement of the interstitial fluid at the venular end. The examples due to reduced oncotic pressure are given below.
1. *Liver disorders:* Common liver causes include cirrhosis of liver and alcoholic liver disease. It is usually seen with ascites. There is decreased albumin synthesis in liver in alcoholic liver disease. Some proteins are excreted in faeces due to portal hypertension. Aldosterone breakdown in liver decreases, thus leading to secondary hyperaldosteronism.
2. *Protein-losing kidney diseases:* Protein loss in glomerular diseasess.
3. *Protein-losing enteropathies:* Protein loss in intestinal diseases.
4. *Starvation:* Proteins are broken down.

Lymphatic Drainage

Normally some amount of fluid in the interstitial tissue which has escaped from the arterial end of the capillary is drained through the lymphatics. With blockage or iatrogenic causes, oedema develops. Some of the examples are as mentioned below.
1. *Post-mastectomy lymphoedema:* The oedema develops due to removal of axillary lymph nodes in radical mastectomy for carcinoma breast.
2. *Peau d'orange appearance in breast carcinoma:* This is due to obstruction of the lymphatics due to tumour cells in carcinoma breast.
3. *Filariasis:* Inflammation and obstruction by filariasis (*Wuchereria bancrofti*) results in lymphoedema of scrotum and oedema of lower limbs.
4. Radiation
5. Infections
6. *Milroy's disease:* This is hereditary lymphoedema due to abnormal development of vascular channels.
7. *Other causes:* Increase in capillary pressure, reduced oncotic pressure, disruption of endothelial barrier function and lymphatics, all in combination or individually may be responsible for oedema formation.

Malnutrition (Kwashiorkor)

This is due to low serum proteins and suppose to have similar pathophysiology as in Finnish congenital nephrotic syndrome. The defect is in component of glomerular filtration barrier especially nephrin and podocin.

Increased Capillary Permeability

The normal vessels allow some amount of free flow of fluid and minimal passage of crystalloids through the intact endothelium. However, when endothelium is injured by various mechanisms like toxins, anoxia, smoking, certain drugs, release of chemical mediators like in infections and allergic conditions, the vascular endothelium becomes more leaky and protein-rich fluid escapes forming oedema. Thus, raises the effective interstitial colloid pressure thereby reducing the effective colloid osmotic pressure gradient. Some examples are given below. It can be localized or generalized.

Localised oedema is seen in:
1. Acute respiratory distress syndrome.
2. Inflammation: There is release of mediators which increase vascular permeability, vasodilatation and induce cellular phenomena of inflammation. There is relaxation of smooth muscle of vessel wall and precapillary sphincters which reduce upstream resistance and increases capillary pressure. Plasma-rich fluid oozes out with interstitial fluid volume, pressure and tissue colloid osmotic pressure.
3. Angioneurotic oedema.

Generalised oedema as in:
1. Burns
2. Allergy
3. Anaphylaxis
4. Anoxia

Sodium and Water Retention

About 80% of the sodium excreted in glomerular filtrate is reabsorbed by the distal convoluted tubules which are under the influence renin–aldosterone mechanism. With hyponatraemia (causes like diarrhoea, vomiting, diuretic use, Addison's disease, salt wasting nephritis syndrome of inappropriate antidiuretic hormone, glucocorticoid deficiency, hypothyroidism, heart failure and renal failure), renin is stimulated and end product aldosterone release increases sodium absorption. Along with sodium, water is also absorbed. Angiotensin II stimulates ADH release which re-absorbs water from DCT again contributing to oedema. There are osmo-receptors in hypothalamus which sense the levels of sodium and water in the body.

Increase in sodium absorbs more water, thus increases the intravascular hydrostatic pressure and at the same time this reduces plasma oncotic pressure. Thus, at arterial end, large amounts of fluid will be lost which cannot return back at venular end and oedema sets in.

Tissue Factors

The oncotic pressure in the tissue is very negligible to counteract the effects of plasma oncotic pressure and capillary hydrostatic pressure. However, when hydrostatic pressure is more and with inadequate removal of fluid by lymphatics, in this situation, there will be elevation of tissue oncotic pressure. Hence, with loose subcutaneous tissues such as eyelid and external genitalia, oedema formation is earliest to occur.

Atrial Natriuretic Peptide

Atrial natriuretic peptide (ANP) is secreted by the secretory granules from the atrial muscle tissue. Secretion is stimulated by atrial enlargement (when plasma volume increases). It has functions opposite of ADH, increases diuresis and sodium excretion in urine, causes vasodilatation and inhibits renin and angiotensin release.

Renin–Angiotensin–Aldosterone System

This system regulates blood pressure, fluid balance and electrolyte metabolism. Angiotensin which is synthesized in the liver is a substrate for renin, an arterial enzyme. Renin is in inactive form and gets converted to active form by juxtaglomerular cells in the kidney. Renin converts angiotensin to angiotensin I which later gets converted to angiotensin II by angiotensin-converting enzyme (ACE) found in lungs. Angiotensin II increases blood pressure by causing vasoconstriction, inhibits renin release and stimulates aldosterone with sodium and water retention. Angiotensin II also stimulates antidiuretic hormone (ADH also called vasopressin) secretion from the posterior lobe of the pituitary gland which acts on distal convoluted tubules and collecting ducts.

Aldosterone

This is the mineralocorticoid hormone produced by zona glomerulosa of adrenal cortex, acts on kidney. It increases reabsorption of sodium by distal convoluted tubule.

Antidiuretic Hormone

It is produced from posterior lobe of pituitary gland and increases reabsorption of water by distal and collecting tubule contributing to oedema formation.

IMPORTANT TYPES OF OEDEMA

Cardiac Oedema

Generalised oedema develops in heart failure due to right-sided or with congestive cardiac failure. The common causes of heart failure are already mentioned above.

Mechanism (Fig. 13.26)

1. There is reduced cardiac output and hypoperfusion stimulates renin–angiotensin–aldosterone mechanism which initiates ADH release resulting in sodium and water retention and oedema formation.
2. The other mechanism for oedema formation in cardiac oedema is increased hydrostatic pressure leading to passive congestion in the veins and capillaries as heart is not able to function.
3. Retention of tissue metabolites, increases tissue osmotic pressure and causes oedema.

In cardiac oedema, the organs show chronic venous congestion changes as blood stagnates due to failing heart especially lungs, liver, spleen **(for details please refer to topic on CVC).**

Oedema due to Hypoalbuminaemia

Mechanism

Hypoalbuminaemia reduces effective colloid osmotic pressure gradient and thus efflux of fluid into the interstitial tissue.

This type of oedema is seen in patients with protein energy malnutrition.

Renal Oedema

Generalised oedema occurs when kidney function is affected.

Mechanism (Fig. 13.27)

1. Renal hypoperfusion stimulates renin–angiotensin–aldosterone response and ADH release which conserves water and absorbs sodium and water, thus oedema develops.

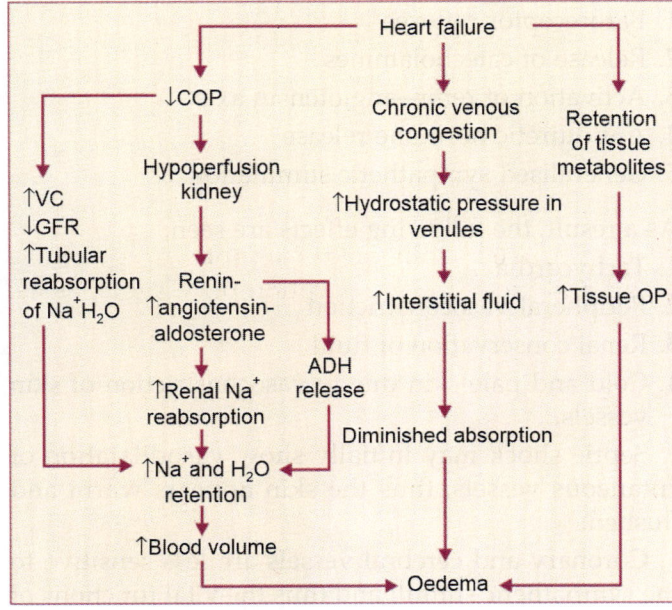

Fig. 13.26: Mechanism of cardiac oedema

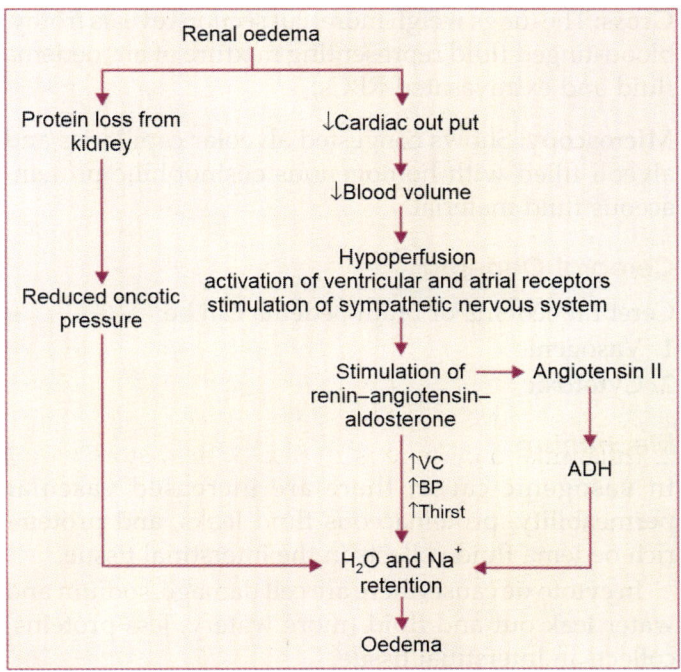

Fig. 13.27: Mechanism of renal oedema

2. Increased glomerular capillary permeability to proteins, protein loss leading to hypoalbuminaemia.

Decreased colloidal pressure, decreased blood volume and stimulation of renin–angiotensin–aldosterone response and ADH release which conserves water and absorbs sodium and thus causing oedema.

Oedema due to Increased Venous Pressure

Elevation in arterial or venous pressure increases capillary pressure which favours enhanced capillary filtration. There is increased interstitial fluid pressure, reduced tissue osmotic pressure as fluid is poor in proteins. Thus this oedema is mainly transudate.

Pulmonary Oedema

Mechanism

Pulmonary oedema can develop as a result of increased hydrostatic pressure in the capillaries or as a result of injury to the endothelium of the capillaries as in inflammation of lungs. The hydrostatic pressure of the pulmonary capillaries is much lower compared to the capillaries in other areas. It is 10 mm Hg. As plasma oncotic pressure prevents escape of fluid generally oedema does not occur in lungs.

In heart failure due to mitral stenosis, mitral regurgitation, pulmonary vein obstruction, there is elevation of hydrostatic pressure in the pulmonary veins. This disturbs the plasma oncotic pressure and hydrostatic pressure balance and oedema develops, initially in the lung interstitial tissue around the capillaries and subsequently in the alveoli also.

Gross: The lungs weigh more, cut section reveals frothy, blood-tinged fluid representing mixture of air, oedema fluid and extravasated RBCs.

Microscopy: Shows congested alveolar capillaries and alveoli filled with homogenous eosinophilic protein-aceous fluid material.

Cerebral Oedema

Cerebral oedema or brain oedema can be:
1. Vasogenic
2. Cytotoxic

Mechanism

In vasogenic cause, there are increased vascular permeability, proteinaceous fluid leaks, and protein-rich oedema fluid collects in the interstitial tissue.

In cytotoxic cause, there are cell damage, sodium and water leak out and fluid (more watery, less proteins) collects in interstitial tissue.

Gross: Brain oedema may be localised as in infarcts, abscesses or neoplasms. It may be generalised as in cases of encephalitis, hypertension, or obstruction to venous blood flow to brain.

Microscopy: In generalised oedema, brain is swollen with sulci being narrow, gyri are flattened with impressions of overlying skull.

Oedema due to Endocrine Pathology

This is seen in the following conditions:
- Myxoedema
- Premenstrual oedema
- Pregnancy

Mechanism

Oedema due to endocrine pathology is mainly because of:
1. Accumulation of connective tissue components, proteins and mucopolysaccharides.
2. There may accumulation of glycosaminoglycans, hyaluronic acid and chondroitin sulphate.

In myxoedema, there is deposition of mucopoly-saccharides due to stimulation of fibroblasts. There is high negative interstitial fliud pressure because of enhanced elastic recoil of the extracellular matrix and intravascular fluid oozes out.

SHOCK

Definition

Shock is a state of life-threatening systemic hypo-perfusion, with inadequate or impaired tissue perfusion and cellular hypoxia caused either by reduced cardiac output or by reduced effective circulatory blood volume.

Shock may initially have reversible tissue injury; persistence of shock eventually causes irreversible tissue injury and may be fatal causing death of the patient.

The important types of shock are:
- Cardiogenic shock
- Hypovolemic shock
- Septic shock

The other types are:
- Neurogenic shock
- Anaphylactic shock

Before we discuss about the pathogenesis of shock of different types, let us have a glance at stages of shock.

Stages of Shock

1. **Non-progressive stage (compensated stage)** during which the body's compensatory mechanisms are able to maintain some degree of tissue perfusion.
2. **Progressive stage (decompensated stage)** in which the body's compensatory mechanisms fail to maintain tissue perfusion with onset of worsening circulatory and metabolic imbalances.
3. **Irreversible stage** where body has tissue and cellular damage, which is so massive that even if the haemodynamic defects are corrected, the survival is not possible.

In non-progressive stage, various neurohumoral mechanisms maintain cardiac output and blood pressure which are as below:
1. Baroreceptor reflexes
2. Release of catecholamines
3. Activation of renin–angiotensin axis
4. Antidiuretic hormone release
5. Generalised sympathetic stimulation

As a result, the following effects are seen:
1. Tachycardia
2. Peripheral vasoconstriction
3. Renal conservation of fluid
4. Cold and pale skin due to vasoconstriction of skin vessels.

Septic shock may initially show vasodilatation of cutaneous vessels, thus the skin appears warm and flushed.

Coronary and cerebral vessels are less sensitive to the sympathetic stimuli and thus the vital functions of heart and brain are still unaffected.

If the underlying causes are not corrected, shock passes into progressive phase. The following changes are seen with progressive phase:

1. The tissues suffer hypoxia.
2. Persistence of oxygen deficiency causes stoppage of aerobic respiration.
3. Anaerobic glycolysis sets in with excessive production of lactic acid.
4. The metabolic lactic acidosis lowers tissue pH and slows down vasomotor response.
5. The arterioles dilate and blood pools in microcirculation. With these effects, cardiac output is reduced.
6. The endothelial cells undergo anoxic injury and subsequently disseminated intravascular coagulation develops.

If the progressive phase is not corrected, eventually enters into irreversible stage. The cellular and tissue injuries are so severe that the changes cannot be reversed and survival is not possible even if haemodynamic effects are corrected. The following changes are seen with irreversible stage:

1. There is widespread cell injury with lysosomal enzyme leakage which further aggravates the shock stage.
2. Myocardial contractile function worsens because of nitric oxide release.
3. Ischaemic bowel may allow intestinal flora to enter circulation, and endotoxic shock may be superimposed.
4. The kidney suffers ischaemic acute tubular necrosis.
5. Death supervenes.

CARDIOGENIC SHOCK

This results from failure of cardiac function. The heart cannot pump enough blood to meet the metabolic demands of the body due to inadequate tissue perfusion.

Causes

The causes of this can be:

Loss of Contractility

- Acute myocardial infarction: This is the major cause of cardiogenic shock.
- Arrhythmias
- Loss of critical mass of left ventricle
- Rignt ventricular pump failure
- Left ventricular aneurysm
- End-stage cardiomyopathy
- Acute myocarditis

- Toxic global left ventricular dysfunction
- Dysrhythmias/heart blocks

Mechanical Impairment of Blood Flow

- Valvular disease
- Aortic dissection
- Ventricular septal wall rupture
- Massive pulmonary embolus
- Pericardial tamponade

Pathogenesis of Cardiogenic Shock

Whatever the etiology, the following mechanisms will contribute to cardiogenic shock (Fig. 13.28).

1. There is decreased cardiac output (COP) and decreased stroke volume. This causes hypotension and decreased coronary pressure leading to myocardial ischaemia.
2. Reduced COP stimulates catecholamine release which increases contractility and peripheral blood flow, but also increases myocardial oxygen demand which further reduces cardiac output and causes tissue hypoperfusion.
3. With reduced COP, renin–angiotensin–ADH axis is stimulated which causes vasoconstriction and conserves sodium and water from kidneys. This increases cardiac volume, COP, and atrial pressure. These mechanism increases load on the heart and again adds to tissue hypoperfusion.
4. Reduced COP stimulates SIRS (systemic inflammatory response syndrome) causing GI tract ischaemia and intestinal bacteria proliferate and cytokines like IL-6 and TNF-α, NO, and O_2 free radicals are released. This adds to tissue hypoperfusion and pulmonary oedema and other organ injury.
5. Decreased tissue perfusion leads to:
   i. Heart failure
   ii. Anaerobic glycolysis releasing pyruvate and lactate leading to metabolic acidosis.
   iii. Renal failure adds to metabolic acidosis
   iv. Metabolic acidosis causes peripheral pooling of blood.
   v. Vasodilatation, peripheral pooling of blood which further adds to decreased cardiac output and hypoperfusion.
   vi. End result is metabolic acidosis, heart failure, pulmonary oedema and renal failure.

Following are the clinical features:
- Hypoperfusion (oliguria, cyanosis, cool extremities)
- Tachycardia
- Altered mental status
- Ultimately develop systolic hypotension, systolic BP below 90 mm Hg. Pulse is weak and thready.

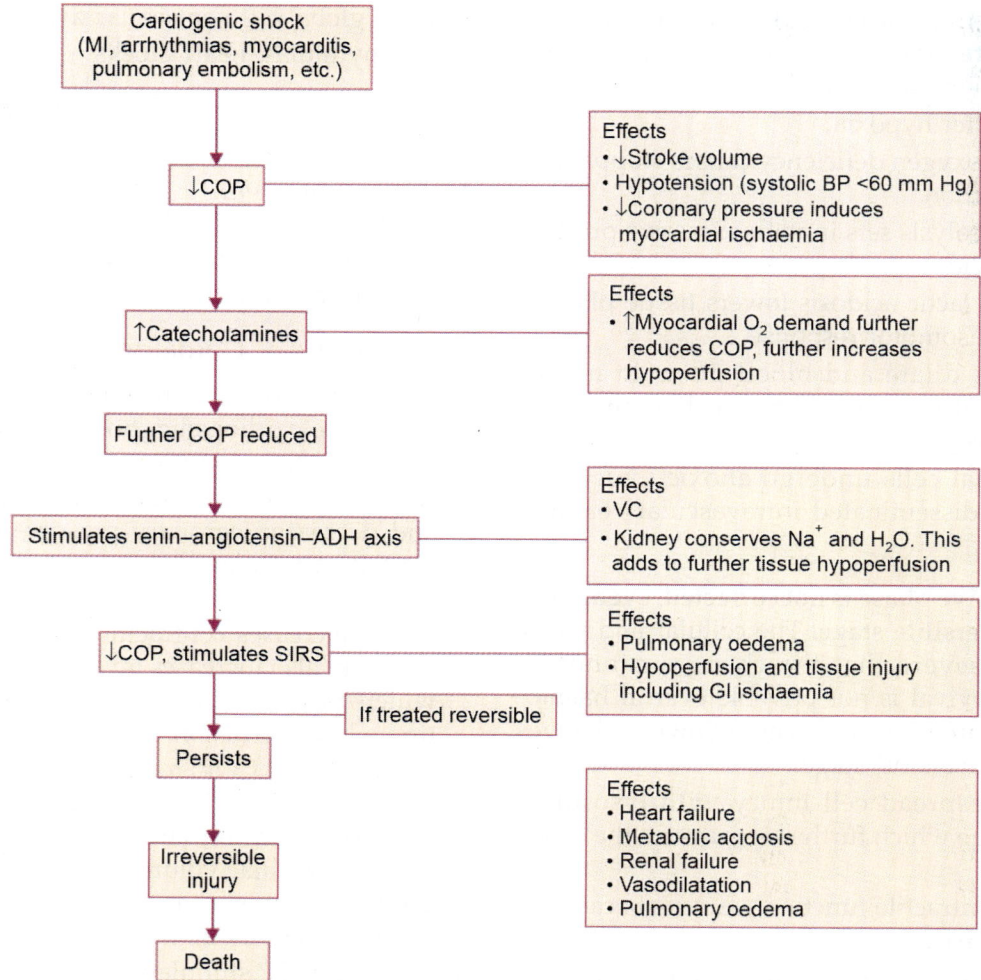

Fig. 13.28: Mechanism and effects of cardiogenic shock

HYPOVOLAEMIC SHOCK

This results from loss of blood or plasma volume.

The causes of this can be:

- Haemorrhage
- Fluid loss from severe burns, trauma, vomiting, diarrhoea.

Pathogenesis of Hypovolaemic Shock

In hypovolaemic shock which is also called haemorrhagic shock, there is decreased blood volume, due to fluid loss; there is decreased cardiac output and arterial pressure. The compensatory mechanisms are activated to restore the arterial pressure and blood volume back to normal (Fig. 13.29).

The compensatory mechanisms include:

1. *Baroreceptor stimulation:* Arterial and cardiopulmonary baroreceptors sense fall in blood pressure, activate sympathetic system to stimulate heart and constrict blood vessels.

2. *Chemoreceptor stimulation with systemic acidosis:* This mechanism tries to increase blood pressure and regulate respiratory rate.

3. *Sympathetic adrenergic system stimulated with release of catecholamines:* Causes vasoconstriction and heart is stimulated to increase COP. Heart and brain get sufficient blood as it is redistributed from GIT, renal, musculoskeletal and other tissues.

4. *Renin–angiotensin–ADH mechanism activated:* Vasoconstriction and conserve sodium and water.

5. *Activation of thirst centres*

The decompensatory mechanisms include: As arterial pressure cannot be restored and cannot perfuse vital organs, irreversible shock and death occurs and following factors contribute.

1. *Impaired coronary flow resulting from hypotension* leads to myocardial ischaemia, acidosis and depress cardiac function and cause arrhythmias.

2. *Sympathetic escape* with accumulation of metabolic vasodilator substances, impair sympathetic mediated vasoconstriction which leads to loss of vascular tone,

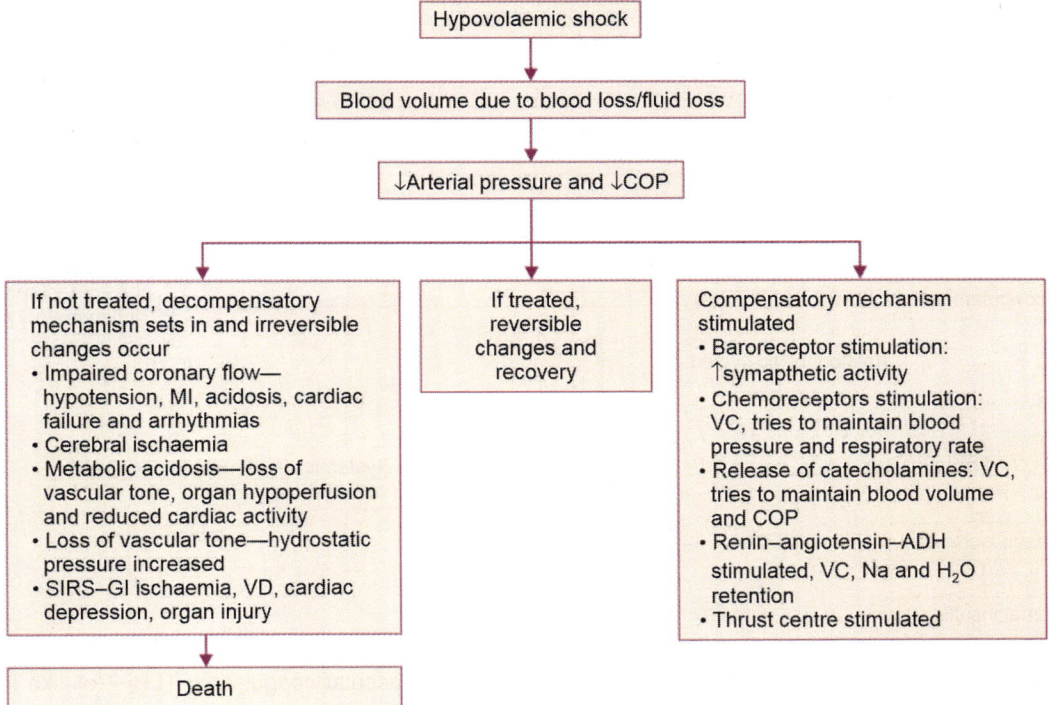

Fig. 13.29: Mechanism and effects of hypovolaemic shock

hypotension and organ hypoperfusion. Loss of capillary tone increases hydrostatic pressure and reduces plasma volume.

3. *Cerebral ischaemia:* Causes loss of sympathetic outflow from ischaemic adrenal medulla, causes VD which reduces arterial pressure and induces cerebral ischaemia.

4. *Metabolic acidosis* depresses cardiac muscles and vascular tone which further reduce arterial pressure.

5. *SIRS (systemic inflammatory response syndrome)* causing GI tract ischaemia, may play role in vaso-dilatation, cardiac depression and organ injury.

SEPTIC SHOCK

Septic shock most commonly occurs in gram-negative bacterial infections (endotoxic shock).

Gram-positive organisms and fungal infections may also cause septic shock.

Pathogenesis of Septic Shock (Fig. 13.30)

Septic shock ranks the first amongst causes of death due to shock.

The causes of septic syndromes are increasing, and can be attributed to:

1. Improved life support for high-risk patients
2. Increased invasive procedures
3. Increased number of immunocompromised hosts possibly secondary to chemotherapy, immuno-suppression and HIV infection.

Most cases of septic shock are due to endotoxin producing gram-negative organisms and hence termed as endotoxic shock. The cell wall of gram-negative bacilli have lipopolysaccharides (LPS) consisting of toxic fatty acid core.

The free fatty acids released by these bacteria attach to LPS-binding protein and this complex binds to specific receptor (CD14) on monocytes, macrophages, neutrophils and vascular endothelial cells.

The LPS now gets recognized by TLR-4, which results in release of IL-1 and TNF. These cytokines in turn release IL-6, IL-8, and IL-10 from other inflammatory cells and endothelium. These cytokines enhance local inflammatory response and clearance of infection. LPS directly activates complement system. With severe infections and higher levels of LPS, there is release of NO and PAF. Systemic effects of TNF and IL-1 are responsible for fever, acute phase reactants and increased number of neutrophils. With still higher levels of LPS, due to action of IL-6, IL-8 NO and PAF, pro-coagulant activity of endothelium is stimulated and these also produce vasodilatation, increased vascular permeability and hypoperfusion. Myocardial pump failure and DIC induces further hypotension.

With higher levels of LPS, the following changes occur:

1. There is vasodilatation.
2. Decreased myocardial contractility.
3. Widespread endothelial injury and activation of endothelial cells leading to leucocyte adhesion and diffuse alveolar capillary damage in lung.

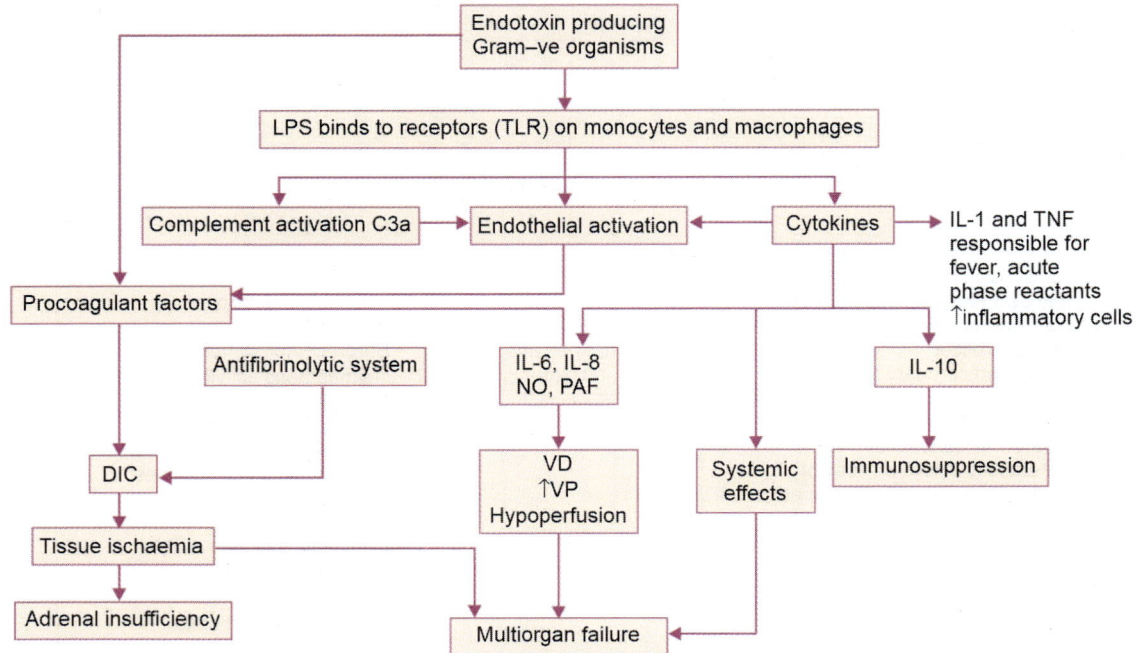

Fig. 13.30: Pathogenesis of septic shock (DIC—Disseminated intravascular coagulation; TLR—Toll-like receptor)

4. Activation of coagulation system and DIC can occur.
5. Hypoperfusion resulting from combined effect of widespread vasodilatation, myocardial pump failure and DIC causes multiorgan failure which affects liver, kidneys, CNS and other organs.

Neurogenic shock: It may occur in a setting of an anaesthetic accident, spinal cord injury as a result of loss of vascular tone and peripheral pooling of blood.

Anaphylactic shock: It is caused by hypersensitivity reaction. There is severe and widespread vasodilatation which leads to tissue hypoperfusion and tissue anoxia.

ORGAN CHANGES IN SHOCK

The changes in tissues are mainly by hypoxic injury due to hypoperfusion and microvascular thrombosis. As shock is characterised by failure of many organs, the cellular changes may appear in any tissues. The changes are particularly evident in brain, heart, kidneys, adrenal glands and GI tract.

Adrenal gland shows changes seen in stress, such as cortical cell lipid depletion. The cells are metabolically active which use stored lipids for synthesis of steroid hormones. There may be focal or massive haemorrhage.

Kidneys show acute **tubular necrosis. Fibrin thrombi** are evident in any tissue, but readily visualised in **glomeruli.**

GIT may show **acute stress ulcers (Curling's ulcer), focal mucosal haemorrhage and necrosis.**

Lungs are less commonly affected in hypovolaemic shock as they are resistant to hypoxic shock. It may show interstitial pneumonitis and oedema. Septic shock may show diffuse alveolar damage (shock lung).

Heart may show subendocardial haemorrhage, patchy myocardial necrosis, and contractile band necrosis.

Brain may show neuronal damage and haemorrhage.

SELF-ASSESSMENT EXERCISE

1. **All are true about blood coagulation *except*:**
   A. Factor X is a part of both intrinsic and extrinsic pathways
   B. Extrinsic pathway is activated by contact of plasma with negatively charged surfaces
   C. Calcium is very important for coagulation
   D. Intrinsic pathway can be activated *in vitro*

2. **Oedema in nephritic syndrome is due to:**
   A. Na^+ and water restriction
   B. Increased venous pressure
   C. Decreased serum albumin
   D. Decreased fibrinogen

3. **Vitamin K dependent clotting factors are:**
   A. IX, X   B. I, V
   C. VII, VIII   D. I, VIII

4. **All of the following are anticoagulant substances *except*:**
   A. Antithrombin III   B. Proteins
   C. PGI_2 D. NO

5. **Which of the following is not involved in local haemostasis?**
   A. Fibrinogen   B. Calcium
   C. Vitamin K   D. Collagen

6. **Which of the following factors is not synthesized in liver?**
   A. II   B. VII
   C. IX   D. vWF

7. **Fat embolism is commonly seen in:**
   A. Head injuries   B. Long bone fractures
   C. Drowning   D. Hanging

8. **Pale infarct is seen in all *except*:**
   A. Lungs   B. Spleen
   C. Kidney   D. Heart

9. **Virchow's triad includes all *except*:**
   A. Injury to vein
   B. Venous thrombosis
   C. Venous stasis
   D. Hypercoagulability of blood

10. **Necrosis with putrefaction is called:**
    A. Desiccation
    B. Gangrene
    C. Liquefaction
    D. Coagulative necrosis

11. **The initiating mechanism in endotoxic shock is:**
    A. Peripheral vasodilatation
    B. Endothelial injury
    C. Increased vascular permeability
    D. Reduced cardiac output

12. **Which is a feature of DIC?**
    A. Normal prothrombin time
    B. Reduced plasma fibrinogen
    C. Normal platelet count
    D. Normal clotting time

Answers

1. B	2. C	3. A	4. B	5. C	6. D	7. B	8. A
9. B	10. B	11. B	12. B				

Infectious Diseases

TUBERCULOSIS

M. tuberculosis is responsible for most of the cases of tuberculosis. *M. bovis* is rare but still present in countries where consumption of pasteurized milk is not practiced.

Mode of spread: Congenital, direct inoculation, ingestion (tonsils and GIT), droplet infection, and pharyngeal mucosa.

Epidemiology: Malnutrition, poverty, crowding, chronic debilitating illness, elderly patients with weakened immunity, patients with AIDS, lack of medical care are prone for tuberculosis.

Occupation: Exposure to dust and silica.

Tuberculosis infection also depends upon:
1. Racial and ethnic origin
2. Virulence of the organisms and
3. Dose of tuberculous bacillus

Pathogenesis: Please refer to topic on "inflammation".

Primary Tuberculosis

Ghon's complex: It has three components: (1) Ghon's focus: This is 1–1.5 cm in size, grey-white-colored, opaque, consolidated, and is a circumscribed area in the lung parenchyma. Usually, it is present in lower portion of the upper lobe or upper portion of the lower or middle lobe, (2) lymphangitis, and (3) lymphadenitis.

Fate of primary focus: Shrinkage (fibrosis), calcification, ossification, can harbour bacilli for years.

Secondary Tuberculosis

Morphological types of secondary tuberculosis are:
• Fibrocaseous tuberculosis
• Fibrocaseous cavitatory tuberculosis
• Miliary tuberculosis
• Tuberculous pneumonia

Organs involved: Bone marrow, eye, lymph nodes, liver, spleen, kidneys, adrenals, prostate, seminal vesicles, fallopian tubes, endometrium, meninges, etc. are common tissues affected in tuberculosis. Apical tuberculosis on X-ray is called **Simon's focus.**

Note: For details refer to topic on respiratoty system.

Lab diagnosis:
1. Ziehl-Neelsen staining
2. Auromine–rhodomine fluorescent staining
3. TB antibodies (IgG and IgM)
4. LAM antibodies

Gross (Fig. 14.1): The lymph nodes are enlarged, matted and soft in consistency. Cut section shows areas of caseation necrosis (cheese-like material).

Microscopy (Figs 14.2 and 14.3): The normal lymph node architecture is effaced and replaced by granulomas

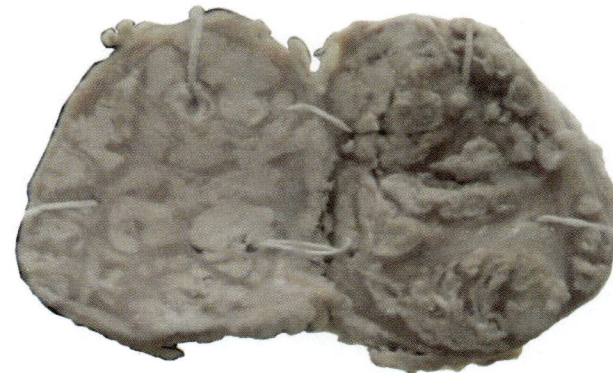

Fig. 14.1: Lymph node with areas of caseation necrosis (gross picture)

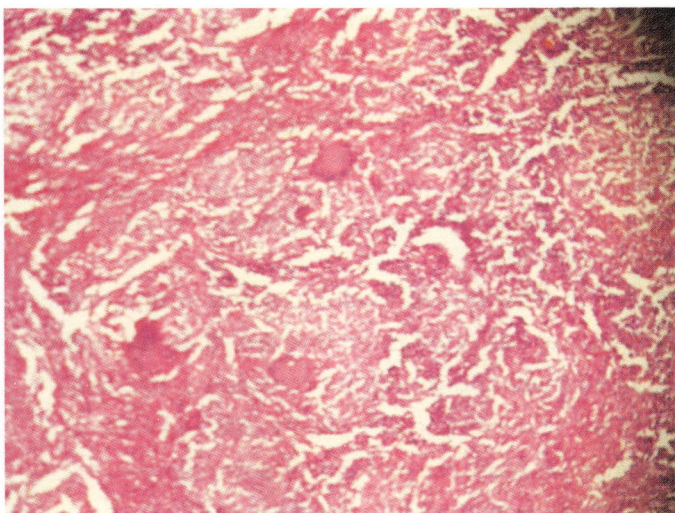

Fig. 14.2: Microphotograph of granuloma in tuberculosis. Note necrosis, epithelioid cells and giant cells

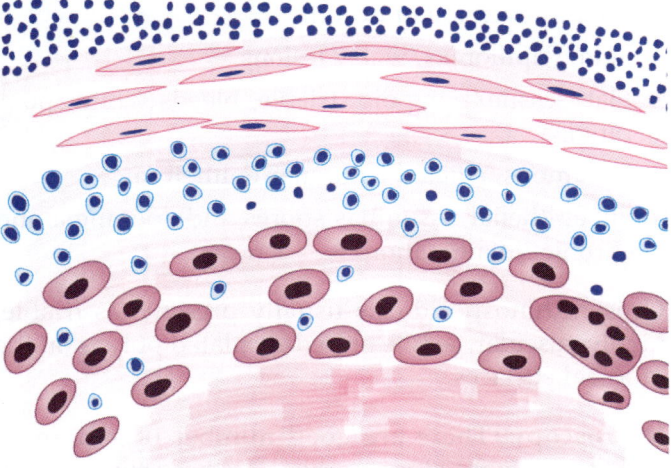

Fig. 14.3: Microscopy in tuberculosis (schematic)

which are comprised of central necrosis surrounded by epithelioid cells and Langhans type of giant cells with a mantle of lymphocytes. Fibrosis is present surrounding these cells.

ACTINOMYCOSIS[13]

It is a type of chronic suppurative inflammation. The classical forms are cervicofacial, abdominal and thoracic actinomycosis. The infection is caused by *A. israelii*; other species such as *A. viscosus*, *A. odontolyticus* and *A. naeslundii* rarely produce the disease. The chronic suppurative inflammation is associated with multiple abscesses along with sinuses.

Morphology of the Organisms

The organisms belong to higher bacteria, arranged in the form of delicate branching intertwined hyphae.

They are Gram-positive, non-acid-fast, PAS+ and GMS+. They are strict anaerobes and are difficult to culture.

They are commensals in the following sites: Oral cavity, tonsillar crypts, teeth, tarter, GIT and vaginal flora. They become pathogenic with devitalized tissue.

There are three forms of actinomycosis: (1) Cervicofacial, (2) thoracic, and (3) abdominal.

1. *Cervicofacial actinomycosis:* In this, gingiva and soft tissue are swollen and indurated, later abscess is formed. There is woody swelling at angle of the jaw. There can be osteomyelitis, periostitis and and overlying skin has sinus tracts. It lasts for months and years unless treated.

2. *Thoracic actinomycosis:* It involves lungs with subdiaphragmatic abscesses and pulmopleural fistulas.

3. *Abdominal actinomycosis:* It affects appendix and colon with peritonitis, involves adjacent intestinal loops, retroperitoneal tissue, anterior abdominal wall and may spread to liver.

With use of intrauterine contraceptive devices (IUCDs), organs like uterus, cervix, fallopian tube, ovary, adjacent viscera may be affected by actinomycosis.

Gross: The infection produces microabscesses with formation of sinus tracts. The colonies of organisms appear as sulphur granules on gross inspection (Fig. 14.4).

Microscopy: There are microabscesses with central suppurative necrosis. The centre of the microabscess has the colony of organisms. The organisms show intertwined radial filaments; the periphery of these filaments is capped by eosinophilic clubs. Good number of neutrophils, histiocytes, plasma cells and lymphocytes are seen around the suppurative necrosis. Adjacent to this area, granulation tissue and fibrosis are present (Figs 14.5 and 14.6).

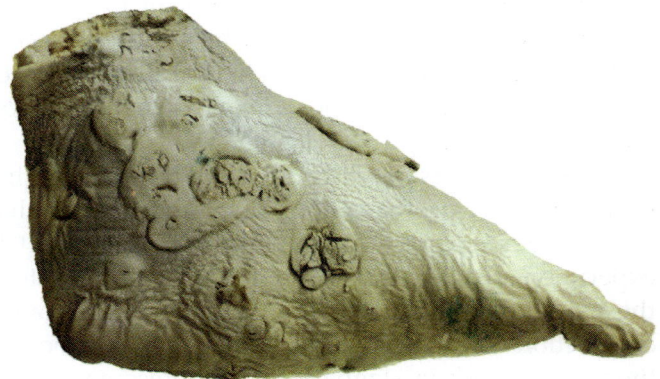

Fig. 14.4: Actinomycosis, note sinus openings (gross picture)

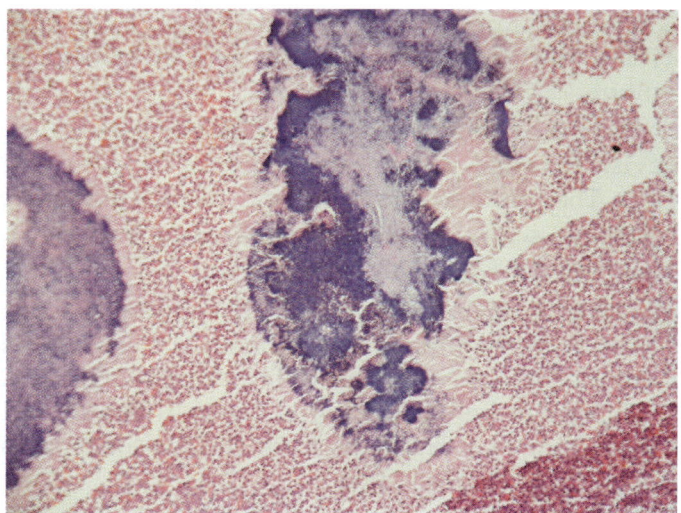

Fig.14.5: Microphotograph of actinomycosis

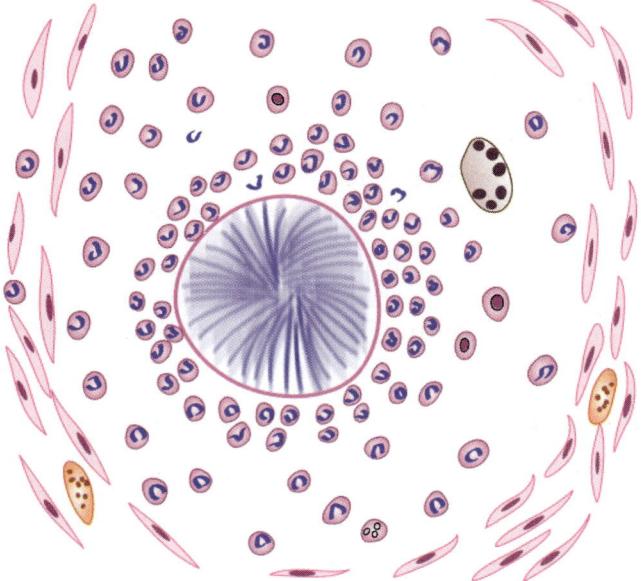

Fig. 14.6: Actinomycosis—note colony of organisms (schematic)

RHINOSPORIDIOSIS[13]

Rhinosporidiosis is a chronic granulomatous disease characterised by production of polyps or hyperplasia of mucous membrane surfaces. The etiological agent is ***Rhinosporidium seeberi.*** The commonest sites involved are mucosa of nose, nasopharynx and soft palate.

Seeber (1900) first described this infection. It was first grouped under protozoa and later into fungus. It has neither been grown in culture nor transmitted experimentally. The mature spore (8–12 μ) presents in the sporangia can infect the human beings. The source of infection is water. Swimmers in swimming pools or those who work in stagnant water pools can get the infection. The spore undergoes different stages of

maturation like: Early trophocyte has central nucleus with distinct nucleolus. The cell wall is laminated and consists of chitinous membrane incorporating neutral polysaccharides. In later stages, the cell undergoes nuclear divisions, can have numerous nuclei surrounded by cytoplasm and develops into sporangia (350 μ). The chitinous wall ruptures releasing spores and the cycle continues.

- It is more common in children and young adults.
- Males are affected more frequent than the females.
- Swimmers and divers are commonly affected.
- It is a water-borne disease, by infected water.
- Mucosa: Nose, nasopharynx, soft palate—74%
  - Conjunctiva and lacrimal sac—26%
  - Larynx, penis, rectum, vagina and skin

  Nose: Painless, itching, mucoid discharge

  Eye: Foreign body sensation, lacrimation, photophobia, eversion of eyelid.

  Skin: Papillomas/warty lesions
- Flat/sessile/polypoid, friable, bleeds white spots, pinkish
- Squamous/ciliated columnar epithelium
- Subepithelial tissue has spores and sporangia and chronic inflammation.

Gross: Rhinosporidiosis usually presents as friable, highly vascular, sessile or pedunculated polyps on the mucosal surfaces.

Microscopy: There are good number of sporangia in varying stages of maturation. As these mature, they have spores. Some of the sporangia may rupture and there is a chronic inflammation at the rupture site (Fig. 14.7).

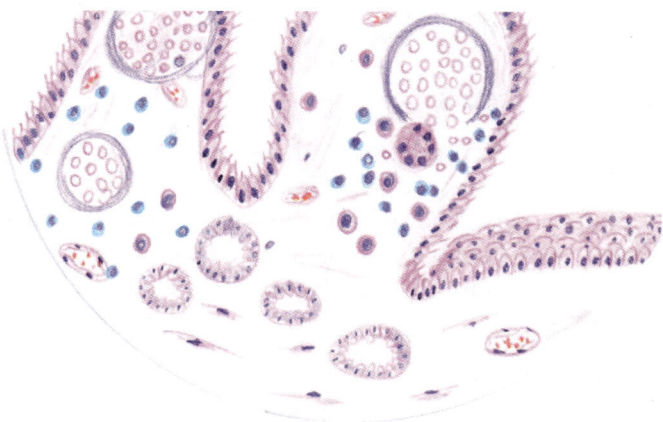

Fig. 14.7: Microscopy in rhinosporidiosis. Stroma shows chronic inflammation (schematic)

RHINOSCLEROMA

Rhinoscleroma affects the upper respiratory tract. It is a chronic granulomatous disease caused by bacteria *Klebsiella rhinoscleromatis*. It is a Gram-negative, encapsulated rod-shaped diplococci. It is a tropical disease, endemic in Africa and central Asia.

- Nose is involved in 95 to 100% of the cases. It also affects nasopharynx, larynx, trachea, and bronchi.

- Females are more commonly affected than the males.

- **Three stages:**

  1. *Catarrhal/atrophic stage:* There is non-specific rhinitis which progresses to purulent fetid rhinorrhoea and crusting. This lasts for weeks to months.

  2. *Granulomatous stage:* Mucosa becomes bluish red with development of nodules and polyps. Epistaxes, nasal deformity, and destruction of nasal cartilage are noted. There may be obstruction of various degrees.

  3. *Sclerotic stage:* There is sclerosis and fibrosis.

- Microscopy shows pseudoepithelial hyperplasia. Subepithelial tissue has chronic inflammatory cells, vacuolated histiocytes containing organisms (Mikulicz cells), plasma cells, plasma cells with Russell bodies and lymphocytes (Figs 14.8 and 14.9).

- Tetracyclin and ciprofloxacin are effective.

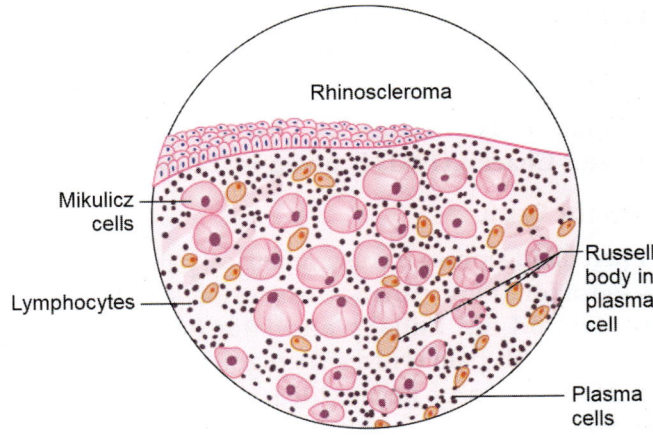

Fig. 14.9: Microscopy of rhinoscleroma. Note Mikulicz cells, plasma cells and plasma cells with Russell body (schematic)

LEPROSY

Leprosy is a slowly progressive chronic inflammatory disease caused by *M. leprae* affecting the skin and the peripheral nerves. It is a slowly progressive and cripples, mutilates and disfigures the person. Hansen (1872), Boeck and Danielssen were the scientists who worked on leprosy.

Organism information:
- Extra- and intracellular, cigar-shaped bundles, straight or curved.
- With 5% H_2SO_4 weakly acid-fast.
- Cooler parts (34–36°C): Skin, peripheral nerves, eye, upper airways, face, ear, wrists, elbow, knees and buttocks.
- Glycolipid and glycoprotein of bacilli—elicit hypersensitivity reaction.

Experimental animals: Armadillo, mice, rats.

Sources: Wounds, cut wounds and discharges, cloths and articles used by the patients.

13 days multiplication time.

Incubation period: 2–20 years.

Mode of spread: Droplets, contacts, breast milk.

Classifications

There are various classifications. According to the classification **by Ridley and Jopling,** there are five types of leprosy. They are:
1. Tuberculoid leprosy (TT)
2. Borderline tuberculoid leprosy (BT)
3. Borderline borderline leprosy (BB)
4. Borderline lepromatous leprosy (BL)
5. Lepromatous leprosy (LL).

Madrid (1953) classification:
1. Lepromatous leprosy
2. Tuberculoid leprosy
3. Dimorphous leprosy
4. Indeterminate leprosy (I)

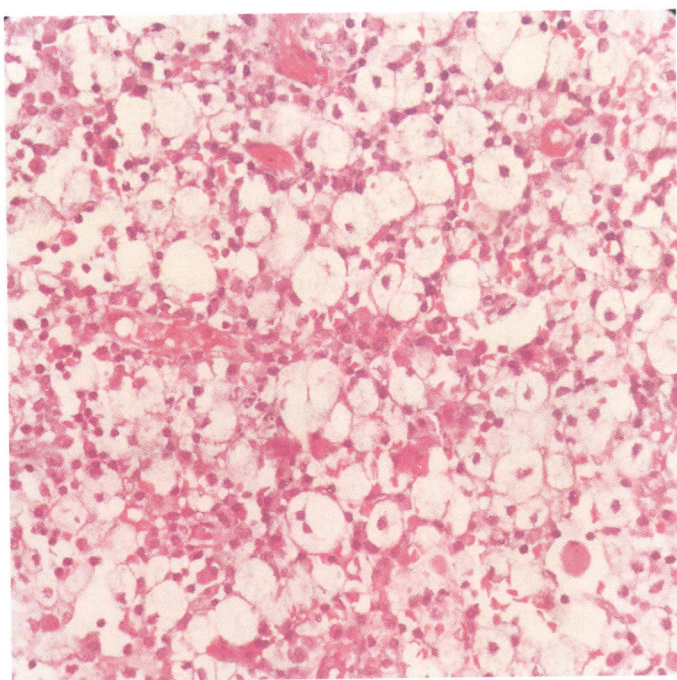

Fig. 14.8: Microscopy, rhinoscleroma, note Mikulicz cells

WHO classifies based on bacterial load as:
1. Paucibacillary (includes I,TT, BT types)
2. Multibacillary (includes BB, BL, LL types)

Indian Classification by Dharmendra (1955) and Job and Chacko (1981) is given in Table 14.1.

Clinical Features

Tuberculoid leprosy has asymmetrical patches with loss of sensation (hypoesthetic or anaesthetic). The patches are flat and red initially and later have pigmented margins with pale centres (depigmented). Because of the destruction of nerve, there may be skin ulcers, paralysis of eyelids, keratitis, corneal ulceration, etc.

- Lepromatous leprosy patients have symmetrical hypoesthetic patches with plenty of bacilli in the tissues such as skin, Schwann cells, endoneural and perineural macrophages. Patient can have hypo-pigmented, erythematous macules/papules, nodules, plaques, diffuse borders, symmetrical, confluent lesions.
- Tuberculoid leprosy (TT) has asymmetrical patches with loss of sensation (hypoesthetic and anaesthetic patches). The patches are flat and red (erythematous lesions) initially and later have pigmented margins with pale centres (depigmented or hypopigmented). They have sharply defined borders. Because of destruction of nerve, there may be skin ulcers, paralysis of eyelids, keratitis, corneal ulcers, etc.

Microscopy

In tuberculoid leprosy, the epithelium is within normal limits. The dermis shows granulomas around the skin appendages, nerves and vessels. The granulomas closely resemble those granulomas found in tuberculosis except for necrosis. The absence of bacteria suggests T cell immunity (Figs 14.10 and 14.11).

In case of lepromatous leprosy, the epidermis is thinned out. The dermis shows sheets of foamy macrophages which are lipid laden-macrophages with masses of acid-fast bacilli in their cytoplasm (Figs 14.12 and 14.13).

Differences between tuberculoid leprosy and lepromatous leprosy are depicted in Table 14.2.

Table 14.1	Indian classification of leprosy
Dharmendra	**Job and Chacko**
1. Lepromatous	1. Lepromatous
2. Tuberculoid	2. Tuberculoid
3. Maculoanaesthetic	3. Borderline tuberculoid
4. Borderline	4. Borderline lepromatous
5. Polyneuritic	5. Polyneuritic
6. Indeterminate	6. Indeterminate

Table 14.2	Difference between tuberculoid leprosy and lepromatous leprosy		
1	Cell-mediated immunity	Good	Poor
2	Cell response	Good Th1 cell response with production of IL-2 and interferon gamma	Th1 response weak
3	Microbial burden (bacillary index)	Less or absent (paucibacillary)	Plenty (multibacillary)
4	Histology	Granulomas with plenty of lymphocytes	No or less lymphocytes with lipid-laden foamy macrophages with globi of bacteria
5	Nerve involvement	Asymmetric involvement of peripheral nerves	Symmetrical involvement
6	Skin lesions	Depigmented pale centres with hyper-pigmented bordres	Nodules, papules and macules with leonine facies
7	Trauma due to atrophy of muscle and anaesthesia due to nerve destruction	Prone for injuries	Prone for injuries, chronic ulcers, paralysis, autoamputation, etc.

The bacilli can be demonstrated with special stains like **Wade-Fite or Fite-Faraco stain on tissues or Ziehl-Neelsen technique** on smears.

Bacterial index (BI) is the numerical index of density of bacilli in a smear or biopsy. Table 14.3 shows BI and average number of bacilli in oil immersion field.

Lepramin test is done to know the level of immunity and it has two reactions:
1. Fernandez reaction
2. Mitsuda reaction

About 0.1 ml of lepramin reagent (obtained from experimentally inoculated armadillos) is injected intradermally, on the forearm and the **Fernandez reaction is read after 48–72 hours**. It is positive in TL with increased reaction of skin and nerve lesion. It is negative in LL and BL types.

Table 14.3	Bacterial index in leprosy
BI	**Average no. of lepra bacilli in oil immersion field**
0	0/100 fields
1+	1–10/100 fields
2+	1–10/10 fields
3+	1–10/ field
4+	10–100/field
5+	100–1000/field
6+	>1000/field

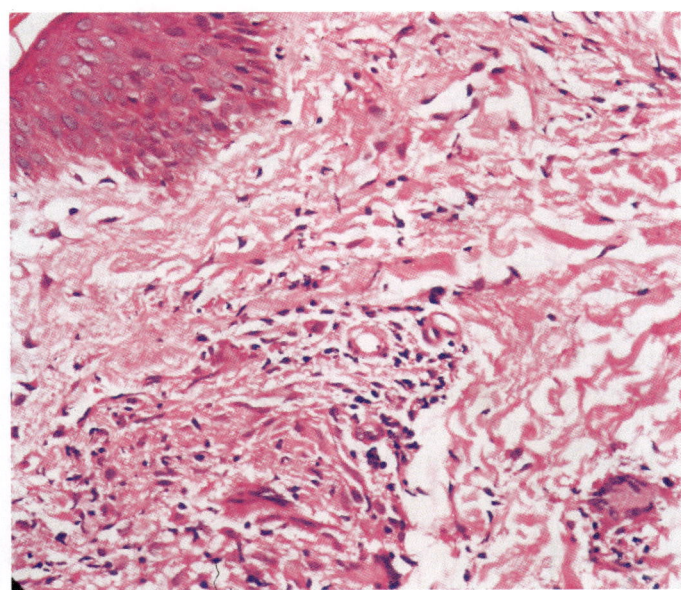

Fig. 14.10: Microphotograph of tuberculoid leprosy

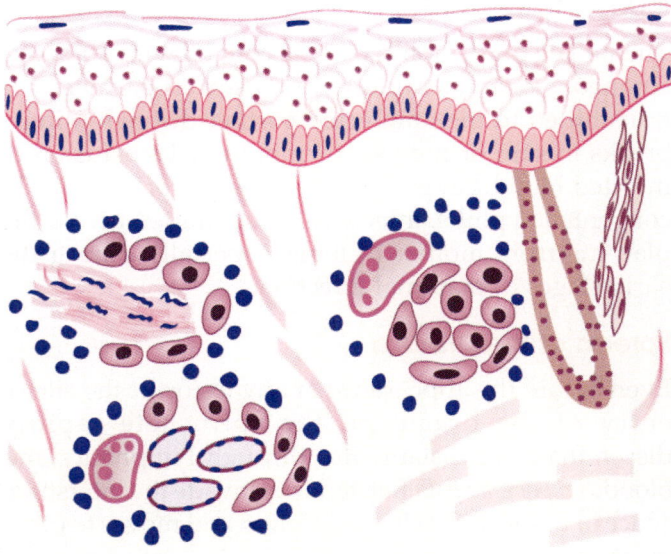

Fig. 14.11: Microscopy in tuberculoid leprosy (schematic)

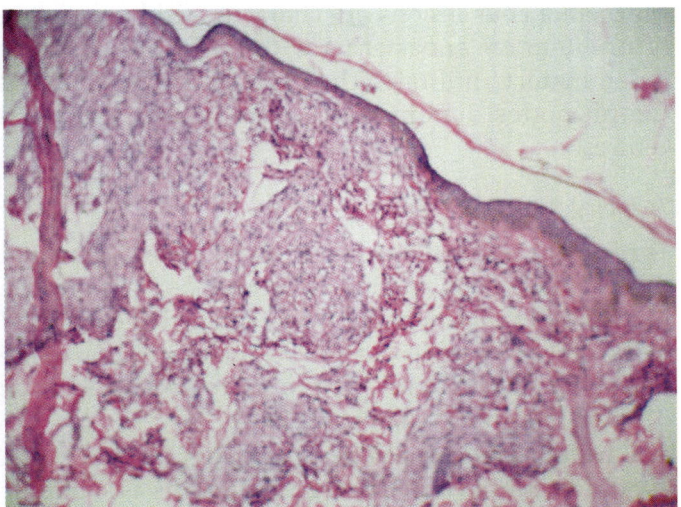

Fig. 14.12: Microphotograph of lepromatous leprosy

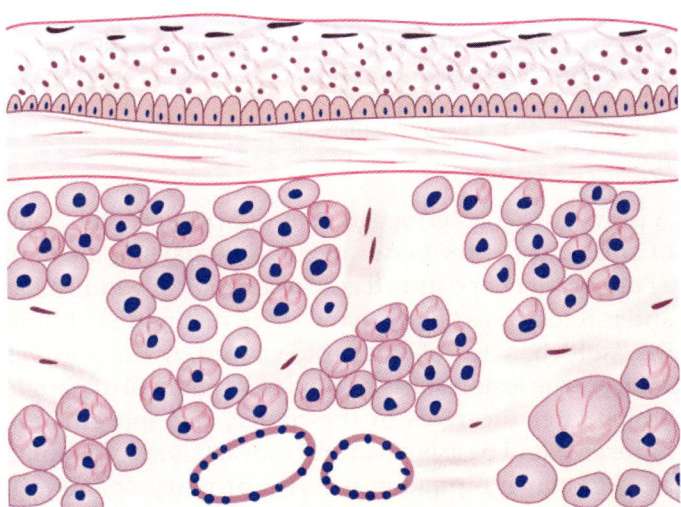

Fig. 14.13: Microscopy in lepromatous leprosy (schematic)

Mitsuda reaction is read after 3–4 weeks and it is positive in TT and BT and negative in LL patients.

SYPHILIS

Syphilis is a chronic venereal disease caused by the spirochete *Treponema pallidum.* The word syphilis is derived from Greek mythology, a boy named Syphilus was cursed by Greek God Apollo with this disease.

Epidemiology

It was first recognized in epidemic form in Europe in 16th century and was called Great Pox. In United States, the numbers of cases are on a rise. African Americans are affected 30 times more than Whites. Male homosexuals are at greater risk for acquiring syphilis.

Organism

Treponema pallidum is a fastidious Gram-negative organism. The only natural host is man. It is a spiral filament measuring around 10 μ. It is actively motile in fresh preparations. The name spirochete is derived from Greek term 'coiled hair'. It can be demonstrated by dark-ground illumination, silver impregnation techniques, fluorescent microscopy, and nucleic acid amplification techniques by PCR.

Virulence Factor

The outer membrane proteins are associated with adherence to the surface of the host cells, the spirochetes produce hyaluronidase which facilitate perivascular infiltration. The organism is coated with fibronectin which protects it against phagocytosis.

Mode of Transmission

The usual source of infection is contact with an active cutaneous or mucosal lesion in a sexual partner. It is transmitted to the uninfected partner through minute breaks in skin or mucous membranes. Transfusion of infected blood can lead to transmission of syphilis. In congenital syphilis, infection is transmitted across the placenta from mother to fetus, especially during the early stages of maternal infection.

Spread of the Disease

Even before the appearance of any lesion at the site of entry of the organism, the spirochete rapidly disseminates to distant sites through lymphatics and blood. *Treponema pallidum* tends to invade the interstitial space of tissue at the site of infection and moves to other location. The disease can be divided into primary, secondary and tertiary stages in adult patients. During the course of the disease, two types of antibodies are formed: Antibodies to specific treponemal antigens and those that crossreact with host constituents. These antibodies are detected in the serological tests for syphilis.

Stages of the Disease (Fig. 14.14)

Primary Syphilis

A primary lesion, termed as *chancre,* appears at the point of spirochete entry between 9 and 90 days (a mean of 21 days) after exposure. It is characteristically indurated and is referred as "hard chancre", to distinguish it from the "soft chancre" of chancroid caused by *Haemophilus ducreyi.* The lesion starts as a painless small firm papule which later ulcerates in the centre. The margins are indurated and base is clean and moist. It is accompanied by regional lymphadenitis. The primary chancre in males is usually on the penis, whereas in females there may develop multiple chancres in vagina or the uterine cervix. The primary chancre resolves without scarring. Antibody tests are positive after the appearance of chancre. The organism can be demonstrated by dark-ground illumination and immunofluorescence from the material scraped from the ulcer base. Regional lymph nodes are enlarged but painless. The chancre resolves spontaneously in 4–6 weeks without therapy and 25% of the untreated patients develop secondary syphilis.

Histology of syphilitic ulcer: The ulcer reveals proliferative endarteritis and inflammatory infiltrate rich in plasma cells along with lymphocytes and macrophages.

Secondary Syphilis

The chancre in primary lesion may resolve by 2 months that is the time when the lesions of secondary syphilis appear. The manifestation of this stage typically includes generalized lymph node enlargement and mucocutaneous lesions. The skin lesions may be maculopapular, scaly, or pustular. Spirochetes are abundant in these mucocutaneous lesions and hence are very contagious. Involvement of palm and sole of feet is seen. In areas like anogenital region, inner thighs, and axilla, typical broad-based lesions appear which are called condylomata lata. The lesions resolve over several weeks (generally 6 weeks) to months without treatment and finally entering into early latent phase. Lesions may recur anytime during this phase. The early latent phase lasts for around one year. The untreated patients enter into an asymptomatic late latent phase, although about 25% of the patients can have relapses. Other manifestations in secondary syphilis include iritis, hepatitis, renal diseases, CNS, bone, etc. Both non-treponemal and anti-treponemal antibody tests are positive throughout the stage and the organism can be demonstrated in the mucocutaneous lesions.

Histology of the lesions in secondary syphilis: Mucocutaneous lesions are characterized by presence of proliferative endarteritis with lymphoplasmacytic inflammatory infiltrate. The examination of enlarged lymph nodes demonstrates hyperplastic germinal centres.

Tertiary Syphilis

Tertiary stage develops in one-third of the untreated cases, after a latent period of around 5–20 years. The lesions of tertiary syphilis are less infective compared to the other two stages, therefore, demonstration of the spirochete is difficult. The manifestations can be divided into three major categories:

a. **Cardiovascular syphilis:** It accounts for more than 80% of cases in tertiary stage. It presents as syphilitic aortitis. It mainly involves aortic root and arch. The wall of the involved aorta is weakened and gets dilated to form syphilitic aneurysm due to endarteritis of vasa vasorum, scarring of the media and loss of elasticity. These patients commonly die of heart failure induced by aortic valve incompetence.

b. **Neurosyphilis:** It accounts for less than 10% cases of tertiary syphilis. There is increased frequency of concomitant HIV infection. It may manifest as:

i. Meningovascular neurosyphilis affecting the meninges, usually involving the base of the brain with obliterative endarteritis.

ii. Parenchymal involvement by the spirochete results in paretic neurosyphilis leading to neuronal loss and proliferation of microglial cells leading to general paresis of the insane (GPI).

iii. Tabes dorsalis results from damage to the sensory nerves in the dorsal roots, that produces impaired joint position sense, leading to skin and joint

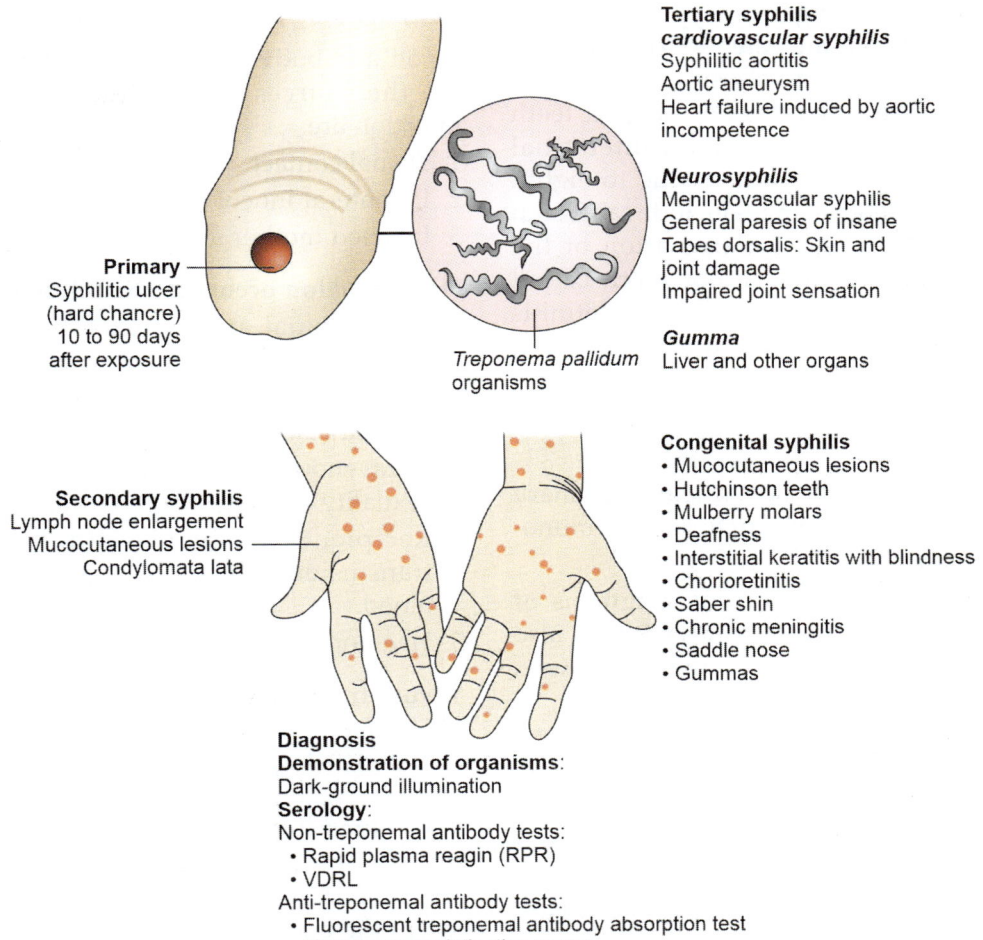

Tertiary syphilis
cardiovascular syphilis
Syphilitic aortitis
Aortic aneurysm
Heart failure induced by aortic
incompetence

Neurosyphilis
Meningovascular syphilis
General paresis of insane
Tabes dorsalis: Skin and
joint damage
Impaired joint sensation

Gumma
Liver and other organs

Primary
Syphilitic ulcer
(hard chancre)
10 to 90 days
after exposure

Treponema pallidum
organisms

Congenital syphilis
• Mucocutaneous lesions
• Hutchinson teeth
• Mulberry molars
• Deafness
• Interstitial keratitis with blindness
• Chorioretinitis
• Saber shin
• Chronic meningitis
• Saddle nose
• Gummas

Secondary syphilis
Lymph node enlargement
Mucocutaneous lesions
Condylomata lata

Diagnosis
Demonstration of organisms:
Dark-ground illumination
Serology:
Non-treponemal antibody tests:
 • Rapid plasma reagin (RPR)
 • VDRL
Anti-treponemal antibody tests:
 • Fluorescent treponemal antibody absorption test
 • Microhaem agglutination assay

Fig. 14.14: Changes in different stages of syphilis

damage, called as "Charcot joints". Argyll-Robertson pupil may be present in both tabes dorsalis and GPI. This is caused by lesion in midbrain due to which pupil constricts during accommodation (near vision) but does not react to light.

c. **Gumma:** It is an uncommon form characterised by development of painless solitary, localized, rubbery lesions with central necrosis called *gumma*, the lesion probably related to delayed hypersensitivity. Gummas most commonly occur in bone, skin, liver, testis and mucous membranes of upper airway and mouth, but any organ may be affected. Spirochetes are rarely demonstrated in these gummas. Histologically, the gummas show central coagulative necrosis surrounded by a zone of palisaded macrophages with many plasma cells, a few giant cells, fibroblast and lymphocytes.

Congenital Syphilis

The fetus acquires *Treponema pallidum* infection across the placenta from an infected mother anytime during pregnancy. The transmission is greater during the early stages of the disease when the burden of organism is more. During pregnancy, the manifestation of the disease is subtle and, therefore, routine serological testing is mandatory. The manifestation in infected fetus includes stillbirth, infantile syphilis or late congenital syphilis.

The stillborn fetus shows hepatomegaly with extra-medullary haematopoiesis and portal tract inflammation, bone abnormalities like epiphysitis and periostitis with occasional bone resorption and fibrosis of the flat bones of the skull. There is pancreatic fibrosis and pneumonitis seen in lungs being firm and pale (pneumonia alba). Spirochetes are readily demonstrated in tissue sections. The placenta in such cases is enlarged, pale and oedematous. Microscopic examination shows proliferative endarteritis.

The fetus born alive with the infection is referred as infantile syphilis. These newborns manifest the disease at birth or within first few months of life. They manifest with chronic rhinitis and mucocutaneous lesions similar to the adults with secondary syphilis. Other visceral and skeletal changes resemble with those seen in stillborn infants already mentioned.

The untreated cases of congenital syphilis of more than two years of duration are categorized as late or tardive congenital syphilis. The classical Hutchinson triad seen in these cases includes peg-shaped teeth called Hutchinson teeth seen at birth, interstitial keratitis with blindness and deafness due to eighth cranial nerve damage. Other changes include saber shin deformity caused by chronic inflammation of the periosteum of tibia, deformed molar teeth called mulberry molars, chronic meningitis, chorioretinitis and saddle nose deformity due to gummas on nasal bone and cartilage.

Diagnosis of Syphilis

1. Direct demonstration of the spirochete in primary syphilis by dark-ground illumination or immuno-fluorescence microscopy.
2. Serology remains the mainstay of diagnosis of syphilis. Polymerase chain reaction (PCR) has also been developed for detection of the spirochete. Serological tests are divided into two:
   i. *Non-treponemal antibody tests:* These measure the antibody to host tissue, cardiolipin, which is also present in treponemal cell wall. These antibodies are detected by the rapid plasma reagin (RPR) and venereal disease research laboratory (VDRL) tests. These tests are negative in early stages of disease and strongly positive in the secondary phase of infection but may revert to negative during the tertiary phase.
   ii. *Anti-treponemal antibody tests:* This includes fluorescent treponemal antibody absorption test and microhaemagglutination assay for *Treponema pallidum* antibodies. These tests become positive within 4–6 weeks of infection but remain positive for indefinite period even after treatment is completed. They are not recommended as screening test due to the false positive result. The tests are strongly positive in all cases of secondary syphilis.

The serological tests may be exaggerated, delayed or even absent in syphilitic patients with concomitant HIV infection.

AQUIRED IMMUNODEFICIENCY SYNDROME

Aquired immunodeficiency syndrome (AIDS) is a retroviral disease caused by virus called human immunodeficiency virus (HIV). It is characterised by depletion of CD4+ T lymphocytes and profound immunodepression leading to immunosuppression and as a result opportunistic infections, secondary neoplasms, and neurological manifestations.

Epidemiology

Blood and body fluids containing virus-infected cells are the sources of infection. The major routes of infection are:

1. Sexual contact
2. Parenteral inoculation
3. Infected mother to their child

HIV infection occurs in the following settings:

1. Homosexual and bisexual males constitute the largest group to be infected.
2. Heterosexual group with high-risk behaviour is the next largest group to be infected.
3. Intravenous drug abusers with no history of homo-sexuality are target population.
4. Recipients of blood and blood component transfusion, who have received the HIV-infected blood.
5. Haemophiliacs who receive factors VIII and IX.

Sexual transmission: More than 75% of the cases of HIV infections globally are by this sexual route. In Unitated States, it is attributed to both homosexual and bisexual male contacts, the vast majority of sexually transmitted infection globally are due to heterosexual activity. The HIV is present in the semen, in the seminal plasma and within the mononuclear cells. The virus enters the body through lacerations and abrasions in mucosa. In addition to male-to-male and male-to-female transmission, HIV is present in vaginal and cervical cells and disease can spread from females-to-males too. HIV is also common among sexually transmitted diseases, as presumably the inflammatory cells can harbour the virus. Syphilis, chanchroid, herpes simplex virus, gonorrhoea and Chlamydia act as cofactors for HIV infection.

Parenteral transmission: Parenteral HIV transmission is documented in the following settings:

1. IV drug abusers
2. Haemophiliacs receiving factor VIII and factor IX.
3. Recipients of blood and blood products

In IV drug abusers, HIV infection occurs through sharing of needles, syringes or other instruments contaminated with HIV containing blood. Transmission of HIV with blood and blood product recipients was common before 1985. Strict vigilance by Drug and Cosmetic Act and improved technologies to detect the organism have reduced incidence of HIV infection by this route.

Mother-to-child transmission: This type of vertical infection is the major cause of paediatric AIDS. Trans-placental spread, intrapartum during delivery and ingestion of HIV-infected mothers breast milk are three major routes for paediatric HIV.

Etiology

AIDS is caused by HIV, a human retrovirus of Lentivirus family. The two forms are HIV1 and HIV2. Amongst these two, HIV1 is the commonest type associated with HIV in most of the countries.

Structure of HIV (Fig. 14.15)

HIV-1 virion is spherical and contain electron-dense cone-shaped core, this is surrounded by a double-layered lipid envelope.

The virus core contains capsid proteins p24, p7, p9 and p17.

Inside the core, there are:

1. Two copies of RNA and the enzymes
2. Reverse transcriptase
3. Protease
4. Integrase

p24 is the most detected core antigen to diagnose HIV infection. The bilayered envelope has gp120 and gp41 glycoproteins. The genome contains *gag, pol* and *env* genes which code for various viral proteins. There are several other genes like *tat, rev, vif, nef, vpr* and *vpn* also are present. The RNA is copied into DNA by reverse transcriptase enzyme. The DNA copy gets integrated into host DNA using viral enzyme integrase to form provirus.

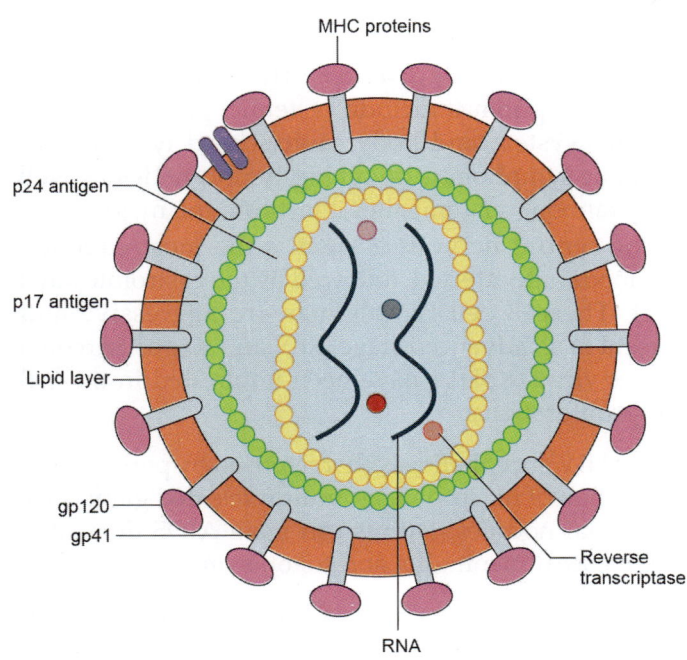

Fig. 14.15: Structure of HIV

Pathogenesis

1. The envelope glycoprotein gp120 attaches to CD4 receptor of host T cells.
2. gp41 helps to promote fusion of the viral envelope with host plasma membrane. Viral genome enters the host T cells.
3. The reverse transcriptase enzyme copies viral DNA into double-stranded DNA.
4. Viral DNA enters nucleus, and gets integrated into host DNA.
5. RNA transcripts produce early genes necessary for virus replication. These get assembled and bud from the cell surface.

Natural History of HIV Infection

This has three phases: These are as given below.

1. Acute phase (initial)
2. Chronic phase (middle)
3. Crisis phase (final)

Acute phase (initial phase) is the initial response of an immunocompetent adult to the HIV infection. This is self-limited, develops in 50–70% of the patients and usually after 3–6 weeks after the infection. This has non-specific symptoms like sore throat, myalgia, fever, rash, and sometimes aseptic meningitis. In this phase, there is viral proliferation in lymphoid tissues and macrophages with reduction of CD4 counts and viremia. In 3 to 17 weeks, seroconversion occurs and virus-specific CD8+ T cells develop.

In chronic phase (middle phase), the immune system is still intact. There is continued HIV replication which lasts for several years in lymphoid organs. Patients are either **asymptomatic or develop persistent lymphadenopathy** and have minor opportunistic infections such as thrush or herpes zoster.

The extensive viral load is associated with continued loss of CD4+ T cells. Initially, CD T+ count is within normal range, however, later starts falling. The number of surviving CD4+ T cells infected with HIV increases and host defense declines. Persistent lymphadenopathy, constitutoinal symptoms (fever, fatigue and rash) reflect immune system decompensation, increased viral proliferation and onset of crisis stage.

The crisis phase (final phase) has breakdown of immune mechanisms, marked viremia, and stage of clinical disease.

In this stage, patients have the following features:

1. Fever more than 1 month
2. Fatigue
3. Weight loss

4. Diarrhoea

5. CD4+ cell count is less than 500 cells/μl.

AIDS Defining Conditions

After variable interval patients develop serious opportunistic infections, secondary neoplasms, and neurological manifestations and the patient is said to have full blown AIDS. The CD4+ cell counts will be less than or equal to 200/μl and this is what CDC defines this condition, even if AIDS defining conditions are not present.

Clinical Features

As already mentioned, a patient of AIDS will present with diarrhoea, generalized lymphadenopathy, opportunistic infections, neurological desease and secondary neoplasms.

Pathology in HIV

HIV infects multiple organs. Opportunistic infections are very common in AIDS. Table 14.4 shows the list of infections.

AIDS Consequences

HIV affects many organs. The morphological changes in HIV are non-specific, may cause some lesions or lesions can be attributed to opportunistic infections in brain, lungs, kidneys and intestine (Fig. 14.16).

Lymph node: In the early stages, lymph nodes reveal a marked follicular hyperplasia due to polyclonal B cell proliferation. The germinal centers merge with the

Table 14.4	AIDS—defining opportunistic infections

1. Protozoal and helminthic infections
a. Cryptosporidiosis or isosporidiosis (enteritis)
b. Toxoplasmosis (pneumonia or CNS infection)

2. Fungal infections
a. Pneumocystosis (pneumonia or disseminated infection)
b. Candidiasis (esophageal, tracheal, or pulmonary)
c. Cryptococcosis (CNS infection)
d. Coccidioidomycosis (disseminated)
e. Histoplasmosis (disseminated)

3. Bacterial infections
a. Mycobacteriosis (atypical, disseminated or extrapulmonary; *M. tuberculosis*, pulmonary or extrapulmonary)
b. Nocardiosis (pneumonia, meningitis, disseminated)
c. *Salmonella* infections (disseminate)

4. Viral infections
a. Cytomegalovirus (pulmonary, intestinal, retinitis, or CNS infections)
b. Herpes simplex virus (localized or disseminated)
c. Varicella-zoster virus (localized or disseminated)
d. Progressive multifocal leukoencephalopathy

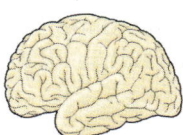

Brain
AIDS dementia
Cryptococcal meningitis
Toxoplasmosis

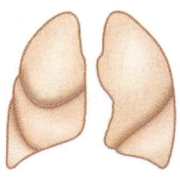

Lungs
Pneumonia
Pneumocystis carinii
CMV
Mycobacterial TB
Mycobacterium avium intracellulare

Mucocutaneous lesions
Herpes infection
Candidiasis

Skin
HPV
Molluscum
Kaposi sarcoma

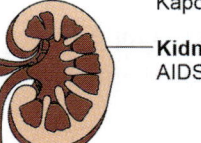

Kidneys
AIDS nephropathy

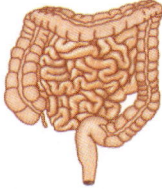

Intestine
Protozoal diseases:
Cryptosporidium
Isospora belli
Giardiasis
Bacterial: Mycobacteria
Viruses: CMV

Fig. 14.16: Pathology of AIDS

interfollicular area as the mantle zones are thin. In advanced disease, lymph nodes become small and atrophic due to follicular cell depletion. But in majority of cases, node harbours opportunistic infections due to profound immunosuppression. Axillary, inguinal, and posterior cervical nodes are most commonly involved. Spleen and thymus also show similar features. Non-Hodgkin and Hodgkin lymphomas may occur.

Lymphoproliferative disorders: Three groups of AIDS-related lymphomas include systemic, primary central nervous system and body cavity-based lymphomas. Systemic lymphomas involving lymph nodes as well as extranodal, visceral sites constitute the majority.

The central nervous system is the most common extranodal site affected, followed by the gastrointestinal tract. These B cell lymphomas are aggressive and present in an advanced stage. EBV and Kaposi sarcoma herpes virus (KSHV) have been implicated in these B cell proliferations.

Brain: HIV encephalitis is characterised by perivascular infiltration of macrophages, multinucleated giant cells, microglial nodules. Patints can have AIDS dementia, cryptococcal meningitis and toxoplasmosis.

Lungs: Lungs show pneumonia, infection by *Pneumocystis carinii*, cytomegalovirus (CMV), *Mycobacterium tuberculosis* and *Mycobacterium avium intracellulare* organisms.

GIT: Patients have diarrhoea. The organisms infecting are protozoal, bacterial and viral diseases. Protozoal infections include: *Cryptosporidium, Isospora belli* and *Giardia lamblia*. Mycobacterial and CMV infections are common.

Mucocutaneous lesions: Herpes and candidial infections are common.

Skin: Infection by human papillomavirus (HPV) and molluscum contagiosum are common. Kaposi sarcoma can occur in these patients.

Kaposi sarcoma is a malignant vascular tumour, the most common neoplasm in patients with AIDS. Kaposi sarcoma is caused by the *Kaposi sarcoma herpesvirus* (KSHV), also called *human herpesvirus 8* (HHV8) and HIV acts as a cofactor. In HIV-infected individuals, the tumour is usually widespread, affecting the skin, mucous membranes, gastrointestinal tract, lymph nodes, and lungs. Tumours have endothelium-lined channels and vascular spaces admixed with spindle-shaped cells.

Kidneys: AIDS nephropathy occurs in these HIV infected patients.

TYPHOID FEVER

Enteric fever is caused by *Salmonella typhi* and *Salmonella paratyphi*. Typhoid fever is acute illness caused by S. Typhi. In endemic areas, *S. typhi* infection is common, whereas *S. paratyphi* is common among travellers. Children and adolescents are commonly affected. Humans are the only natural reservoirs and infection is transmitted via contaminated food or water, especially dairy products and shell fish. Infection spreads by direct contact with faeces and urine. Gall-bladder colonization occurs in chronic carriers and is associated with gallstones and biliary scarring.

Typhoid Mary, a cook, was carrier of typhoid, infected many people through food.

Pathogenesis

S. typhi survives in gastric acid and invades small intestinal mucosa, prominently ileal mucosa in areas overlying Peyer's patches. Here organisms are engulfed by macrophages. Dissemination occurs via lymphatics and blood vessels, leading to reactive hyperplasia of lymphoid tissues throughout the body. Macrophages stimulate IL-1 and TNF production, resulting in fever, malaise and wasting.

Morphology

In the ileum, infection causes marked lymphoid hyperplasia. In certain cases, capillary thrombosis leads to necrosis of mucosa overlying Peyer's patches. Thus the characteristic longitudinal oval ulcers oriented along long axis of intestine are formed. Base of the ulcer is filled with black necrotic tissue. Mesenteric lymph nodes are also enlarged. On microscopy, mucosal ulceration with accumulation of neutrophils, macrophages with ingested bacteria, red blood cells (erythrophagocytosis)and nuclear debris in the superficial lamina propria. Lymphocytes and plasma cells infiltrate are also seen in the lamina propria.

The spleen is enlarged and soft, with prominent phagocyte hyperplasia. Liver, spleen, bone marrow and lymph nodes may show macrophage aggregates called typhoid nodules.

Clinical Features

An *incubation period* of 10–14 days is observed. Patient suffers with anorexia, nausea, vomiting, abdominal pain, bloody diarrhoea, fever in *phase of bacteremia and febrile illness*occuring over 1 week. If patient does not receive treatment, *phase of Fastigium* (1 week) with sustained step ladder type high fever, gastrointestinal bleeding, abdominal tenderness continues. Erythematous maculopapular rashes over chest and abdomen, hepatosplenomegaly may occur. In the *phase of lysis* (1 week), toxic symptoms gradually recede, but gastrointestinal ulcer, bleeding, perforation and peritonitis can occur in this phase. In *convalescence phase*, gradual recovery over a few weeks to months occurs. Relapse and systemic dissemination to CNS, heart, lungs and gallbladder can occur. Sickle cell disease patients are particularly susceptible to salmonella osteomyelitis.

Blood cultures are positive in most patients during the first week of febrile phase. Neutropenia is present. Stool culture positive during bacteraemia (second and third week). Widal test is positive from end of first week till fourth week. Antibiotic treatment will prevent further disease progression. Death occurs in 10–20% cases, mainly due to secondary complications like pneumonia.

DIARRHOEA AND DYSENTRY
(Infectious Enterocolitis)

In underdeveloped countries and in infants, infectious diarrhoea can be lethal. After bacterial colonization, bacterial toxins and enteric hormones lead to increase in intestinal secretion.

Toxigenic diarrhoea: Organisms produce diarrhoea by secreting toxins, e.g. *Vibrio cholerae*, toxigenic strains of *E. coli*. Organism remains on mucosal surface, without invading and damaging mucosa and secretes toxin. Fluid secretion into lumen causes watery diarrhoea. Upper intestinal tract commonly involved.

Invasive diarrhoea: Organisms directly invade the intestinal mucosa causing diarrhoea. Increased prostaglandin synthesis and poor fluid resorption from the damaged mucosa lead to diarrhoea, e.g. *Shigella, Salmonella, E.coli* certain strains, *Yersinia, Campylobacter.* Distal ileum and colon involved. Brief description of some is given below.

CHOLERA

Cholera is one of the common causes of diarrhoea in India. It is caused by Gram-negative bacteria *Vibrio cholerae,* transmitted by contaminated drinking water and food. *V. parahaemolyticus* is the common cause of seafood-associated gastroenteritis in North America.

Bacteria multiply in the small intestinal mucosa without invading it. A *preformed enterotoxin,* cholera toxin, binds to the intestinal epithelium. After endocytosis, stimulates adenylate cyclase, increases intracellular cAMP and releases chloride ions into the lumen. This causes secretion of bicarbonate, sodium and water, leading to massive diarrhoea. Chloride and sodium absorption are also inhibited by cAMP.

Most exposed individuals are asymptomatic or develop only mild diarrhoea. In severe disease, there is an abrupt onset of watery diarrhoea and vomiting following an incubation period of 1 to 5 days. The stools are streaked with mucus, resemble rice water and may have fishy odour. Severe diarrhoea leads to dehydration, hypotension, anuria, shock and death within 24 hours of onset of symptoms, if untreated. Treatment includes timely fluid replacement. Oral rehydration will often suffice. Symptoms subside in 3 to 6 days. Cholera infection confers protection against recurrent infection. Vaccines are available but with limited efficacy.

Vibrio parahaemolyticus: A Gram-negative bacteria causing acute gastroenteritis in marine and coastal waters. It is associated with consumption of inadequately cooked seafood.

CAMPYLOBACTER ENTEROCOLITIS

Campylobacter jejuni is the most common cause of bacterial diarrhoea in developed countries. It causes traveller's diarrhoea. Acute self-limited illness usually associated with ingestion of improperly cooked chicken, unpasteurized milk or contaminated water. Bacteria inhabit cow, sheep, chicken, dog. Spread by person-to-person contact via feco-oral route. Ingested *C. jejuni* multiply in the upper small bowel. Bacterium adheres, colonises, invades mucosa and elaborates various cytotoxins causing epithelial damage and dysentery.

Superficial enterocolitis involving terminal ileum and colon is seen. Epithelial necrosis and acute inflammatory infiltrate are seen involving crypts (cryptitis and crypt abscess). Severe cases may cause ulcers with dense inflammatory exudate forming pseudomembrane. Symptoms vary from profuse watery stools to dysentery, which resolve in 5 to 7 days. Diagnosis is by stool culture. Campylobacter entocolitis has been associated with Guillain-Barre syndrome.

SHIGELLOSIS

Shigella is an unencapsulated, non-motile, anaerobe, accounting for one of the most common causes of bloody diarrhoea. Humans are the only reservoir. *Shigella* are highly transmissible by the fecal-oral route or via contaminated water and food. Most *Shigella* infections and deaths occur in children under 5 years of age. In the intestine, organisms proliferate intracellularly in microfold epithelial cells, are phagocytosed by macrophages in lamina propria, in which they induce apoptosis. Shiga toxin causes host cell damage and causes watery diarrhoea by interfering with fluid resorption. Shigellosis involves left colon and ileum, characterised by haemorrhagic ulcerated mucosa and sometimes with pseudomembranes. Ulcers are located on tip of mucosal folds and perpendicular to long axis of colon.

Clinically, disease presents as diarrhoea, fever and abdominal pain, progresses to dysentery after 6 days. Symptoms may persist up to a month. In a few cases, waxing and waning diarrhoea may mimic ulcerative colitis. Stool culture confirms the infection. Rarely infection can progress to complications like *Reiter syndrome,* affecting mainly HLA-B27 positive males causing a triad of sterile arthritis, urethritis and conjunctivitis. *Shigella dysenteriae* serotype 1, which secretes Shiga toxin, can lead to haemolytic uraemic syndrome.

YERSINIA

GI infections caused by Gram-negative bacteria *Y. enterocolitica* and *Y. pseudotuberculosis* are common in Europe and North America, frequently associated with ingestion of inadequately cooked foods especially pork, raw milk, and contaminated water. Organisms are found in feces of wild and domestic animals. Yersinia invade M cells or absorptive cells, use bacterial adhesion proteins and encode an iron uptake system that mediates iron capture and transport. In *Yersinia,* iron enhances virulence and stimulates systemic dissemination, thus risk of sepsis is greater in haemolytic anaemia or hemochromatosis.

Yersinia infections preferentially involve the ileum, appendix, and right colon, result in Peyer's patch hyperplasia and bowel wall thickening. Apthous ulcers and neutrophilic infiltrate and rarely granulomas develop. Patient presents with abdominal pain, fever and diarrhoea. Pharyngitis, arthralgia, and erythema nodosum may also occur. Bacteria can be detected in stool culture.

ESCHERICHIA COLI

Escherichia coli are Gram-negative bacilli that colonize the GI tract. A few strains are pathogenic and include enterotoxigenic *E. coli* (ETEC), enterohaemorrhagic *E. coli* (EHEC), enteroinvasive *E. coli* (EIEC), and entero-aggregative *E. coli* (EAEC). ETEC produces traveller's diarrhoea and spread via contaminated food or water. Children younger than 2 years of age are particularly susceptible. EHEC is associated with the consumption of inadequately cooked ground beef, contaminated milk and vegetables. It causes large outbreaks, bloody diarrhoea and haemolytic-uraemic syndrome.

WHIPPLE DISEASE

Whipple disease is a rare, chronic disease involving multiple organs, caused by Gram-positive *Actinomycete*, called *Tropheryma whippelii*. It can be associated with malabsorption, lymphadenopathy, and arthritis. Clinical presentation includes a triad of *diarrhoea, weight loss, and malabsorption*. Organism-laden macrophages accumulate within the small intestinal lamina propria and mesenteric lymph nodes. Lymphatic transport is impaired and malabsorption occurs.

Morphology

Villi of small intestine are flattened and thickened. There is accumulation of distended, foamy macrophages in the lamina propria. The macrophages are filled with PAS (periodic acid-Schiff stain) positive cytoplasmic granules representing partly digested bacteria. Bacteria-laden macrophages can also accumulate within mesenteric lymph nodes, synovial membranes of affected joints, cardiac valves and brain.

VIRAL INFECTIONS

Affects mainly infants and young children. Common causes are rotavirus, adenovirus and norovirus infections. Clinically, presents as vomiting, watery diarrhoea and abdominal pain.

PARASITIC INFECTIONS

Parasitic infections can cause chronic or recurrent enteritis. *Ascaris, Strongyloides, Ankylostoma* (hookworms), *Enterobius vermicularis* (pinworm), *Giardia lamblia, Cryptosporidium* are the common causes of parasitic infections of intestinal tract.

AMOEBIASIS

Infection of colon caused by *Entamoeba histolytica*, which spreads by faecal-oral transmission. *E. histolytica* cysts colonize the epithelium of the intestine and release *trophozoites*. Amoebiasis most frequently involves the caecum and ascending colon. A flask-shaped ulcer is formed with a narrow neck and broad base. On colonic biopsy, amoebic trophozoites which resemble macrophages in appearance, are found on ulcer exudate and crater.

Amoebic liver abscess develops when parasites embolise to liver through splanchnic vessels. Abscesses persist even after the acute intestinal illness has passed and may spread to the lung and the heart by direct extension from the liver. Abscess may exceed 10 cm in diameter, contain necrotic brown odourless anchovy paste material. Individuals with amoebiasis may present with abdominal pain, bloody diarrhoea or weight loss.

SELF-ASSESSMENT EXERCISE

1. **People with following are prone for infections due antibody deficiency:**
   A. Wiskott-Aldrich syndrome
   B. ADA deficiency
   C. X-linked agammaglobulinaemia
   D. Glanzmann thrombasthenia

2. **Warthin-Finkedley cells are seen in:**
   A. Rubella
   B. Measles
   C. Chickenpox virus infection
   D. HIV infection

3. **Tuberculosis is an example of:**
   A. Pandemic
   B. Prodemic
   C. Endemic
   D. Epidemic

4. **World annual incidence of cholera cases is:**
   A. 1–2 lakhs   B. 1–3 lakhs
   C. 1–5 lakhs   D. 3–5 millions

5. **Tuberculosis is an example of:**
   A. Type I HS   B. Type II HS
   C. Type III HS   D. Type IV HS

Answers

1. B   2. B   3. C   4. D   5. D

Pathological Calcification

Definition

It is abnormal deposition of calcium salts in tissues along with smaller amounts of iron, magnesium, and other minerals in tissues other than bone and enamel. It occurs in wide variety of disease states.

Types

When the deposits occur in dead or dying/degenerating tissues, the process is called **dystrophic calcification**. The calcium metabolism and serum calcium levels are normal in this type of calcification.

When the deposit of calcium salts occurs in normal tissues it is called **metastatic calcification.** The serum levels of calcium are increased in this type of calcification. This reflects abnormal calcium metabolism with hypercalcaemia.

DYSTROPHIC CALCIFICATION

This is seen in areas of cell injury, degenerated or dying tissue and in necrosis of any type and seen with following situations:

1. Calcification seen in advanced atherosclerosis
2. Calcification in caseation necrosis
3. Calcification which develops due to ageing
4. Calcification on damaged heart valves as in rheumatic heart diseases
5. Abscess wall
6. Fat necrosis
7. Gamna-Gandy bodies
8. Areas of infarct
9. Phleboliths of thrombi: Phlebolith in pelvis can be confused with stones in the ureters
10. Dead parasites like filariasis
11. Toxoplasma: Intracerebral calcification (dystrophic calcification) may occur in toxoplasmosis.
12. Old scars
13. Monckeberg's calcification
14. Leiomyomas
15. Psammoma bodies: Lamellated concentric calcified structures can be seen in papillary carcinoma thyroid, serous carcinoma ovary, psammomatous meningioma, mesothelioma, etc.
16. Senile degenerative changes of cartilage

The calcification process involves steps like:
1. Initiation, and
2. Propagation.

Both these steps can be intracellular and extracellular and final product is formation of crystalline calcium phosphate. In initiation stage, cell injury causes damage to cell membrane and release phospholipids. The phosphate ions are released by the action of phosphatases. These combine with calcium. Calcium and phosphates accumulate in mitochondria and extracellular matrix vesicles. Intracellular calcium deposits start initially in damaged mitochondria. Extracellular deposits of calcium start in membrane bound vesicles known as matrix vesicles by its affinity for membrane phospholipids.

After initiation, crystallization occurs. This crystallization process depends upon the concentration of calcium and phosphates in the extracellular matrix.

Gross findings: Calcification is seen as white granules or clumps and felt as gritty deposits while sectioning.

Microscopic findings: In tissue sections stained with H and E stain, calcification is seen as basophilic deposits, intracellularly and extracellularly in the tissues. With time, heterotrophic bone formation may be seen in calcified tissue.

METASTATIC CALCIFICATION

Metastatic calcification occurs in normal tissues with increased calcium levels in blood.

The major causes for hypercalcaemia are:
1. Increased secretion of parathyroid hormone.
2. Increased bone catabolism as in multiple myeloma.
3. Vitamin D-related disorders.
4. Renal failure: Phosphate retention leads to secondary hyperparathyroidism.
5. Excessive mobilization of calcium ion from the bone.
6. Excessive absorption of calcium from the gut: Milk-alkali syndrome—caused by excessive oral intake of calcium in the form of milk and administration of calcium carbonate in the treatment of peptic ulcer.
7. Hypercalcaemia of infancy.

Metastatic calcification can be seen all over the body. The deposits are commonly seen in lung, kidney and gastric mucosa. These deposits may not generally cause clinical dysfunction. However, massive deposits in kidney, known as nephrocalcinosis, is associated with kidney dysfunction. Metastatic pulmonary calcification is a common complication of multiple myeloma.

Metastatic calcification most commonly occurs in following tissues:
1. Lungs
2. Kidney
3. Stomach
4. Blood vessels
5. Cornea
6. Synovium of joint

Pathophysiology

Occur due to excessive binding of inorganic phosphate ions with calcium ions, which are elevated due to underlying metabolic derangement. This leads to formation of precipitate of calcium phosphate at the preferential sites. This process can be reversible.

SELF-ASSESSMENT EXERCISE

1. **Metastatic calcification occurs in:**
   A. Hyperparathyroidism
   B. Necrosis
   C. Damaged valves
   D. Atherosclerotic plaques
2. **Dumb-bell-shaped deposition of calcium seen in:**
   A. Silicosis
   B. Asbestosis
   C. Coal workers pneumoconiosis
   D. Anthrocosis
3. **Dystrophic calcification occurs in:**
   A. Renal failure
   B. Vitamin D intoxication
   C. Hyperparathyroidism
   D. Myositis ossificans
4. **Pathological calcification seen in:**
   A. Scleroderma
   B. Lichen planus
   C. Dystrophic epidermolysis bullosa
   D. SLE
5. **Dystrophic calcification in necrosis is seen in all except:**
   A. Tuberculosis
   B. Abscess wall
   C. Monkeburg's
   D. Milk alkali syndrome
6. **All are true of calcium homeostasis except:**
   A. Bone
   B. Renal filtration and absorption
   C. Intestinal absorption
   D. Synthesis by liver
7. **All are true with high levels of calcium except:**
   A. Suppress PTH
   B. Increases active form vitamin D
   C. Decrease the activity of renal 1 alpha hydroxylase
   D. Decreases synthesis of vitamin D

Answers

1. A   2. B   3. D   4. A   5. D   6. D   7. B

Pigment Disorders

Pigments are coloured substances present in the tissues. They are exogenous or endogenous in origin.

EXOGENOUS PIGMENTS

Exogenous pigments can be:

  I. Inhaled
 II. Ingested
III. Injected

Inhaled Pigments

1. Anthracosis, in which exogenous excess carbon pigment from pollutant air from urban areas is deposited in lungs. Heavy accumulation may lead to emphysema or fibroblast reaction as in coal workers pneumoconiosis.
2. Inhalation of coal dust, as in coal workers' pneumoconiosis.

Injected Pigments

Tattoo marks: India ink, cinnabar and carbon are introduced in the dermis in the process of tattooing, the pigment is taken up by the macrophages and lies permanently in the connective tissue.

Ingested Pigments

Chronic ingestion of certain metals which may produce pigmentation, e.g. argyria is chronic ingestion of silver compounds and results in brownish pigmentation of the skin, bowel, and kidney.

ENDOGENOUS PIGMENTS

1. Lipofuscin
2. Melanin
3. Derivatives of haemoglobin

Lipofuscin

Lipofuscin is a wear and tear pigment. It is brownish, granular and intracellular in nature. It accumulates in the organs like heart, liver, brain, etc. This occurs in tissues in old age or with atrophic changes.

Lipofuscin represents complexes of lipid and protein catalysed from peroxidation of polyunsaturated lipids of cell membranes. It is a marker of free radical injury.

This pigment, when in large amounts, imparts brown colour to the tissue and is called brown atrophy and commonly seen in atrophic organs.

Melanin

It is endogenous, brown-black pigment produced by melanocytes and dendritic cells. Tyrosine is converted to dihydroxyphenylalanine by oxidative action of tyrosinase enzyme. It is non-haemoglobin-derived pigment normally present in the hair, skin, etc.

The various disorders of melanin pigmentation include:

1. *Generalised hyperpigmentation:* Addison's disease of skin, skin areas exposed to sun light and buccal mucosa.
2. *Focal hyperpigmentation:* Melanosis coli which has pigmentation of mucosa of colon.
3. *Generalised hypopigmentation (albinism):* These patients have blonde hair, poor vision, severe photophobia.
4. *Localised hypopigmentation (vitiligo):* Hypopigmentation can be of the skin and mucous membrane and mucocutaneous junctions. The condition may be of familial or with autoimmune pathophysiology.

Melanin-like Pigments

1. Ochronosis
2. Dubin-Johnson syndrome

1. **Ochronosis:** This was for the first time described by Virchow in the year 1865. **Ocher** meaning yellowish in colour. This is seen in alkaptonuria, which is a autosomal recessive disease with deficiency of enzyme, homogentic acid oxidase.

   In this, there is accumulation of homogentisic acid which imparts yellowish/bluish black colour to the tissues. Homogentisic acid is deposited in tissues like cartilage, bones, skin knee joint tissues and appear yellow to black in colour.

2. **Dubin-Johnson syndrome:** It is an autosomal recessive form of hereditary conjugated hyper-bilirubinaemia. The hepatocytes contain melanin-like pigment which is due to mutation of canalicular multiple drug resistant protein 2/ABCC2 gene located on chromosome 10, which mediates efflux of bilirubin glucuronide and other conjugated anions from hepatocye to the bile canaliculi.

Haemoglobin-Derived Pigments

These pigments are haemosiderin, acid hematin, bilirubin, biliverdin and porphyrins.

Haemosiderin

It is haemoglobin-derived pigment. It is granular, golden-yellow-coloured pigment accumulates in tissues when there is excess breakdown of red blood cells and stored especially within mononuclear phagocytes of bone marrow, spleen and liver. Haemosiderin is complex of ferritin and denatured proteins. It is iron with apoferritin stored in tissues. In excess, it disturbs the function of the cells. Haemosiderin accumulation can be localised or generalised.

It can be stained by Prussian blue or Perl's stain. Small amounts of haemosiderin are stored in macro-phages in bone marrow, spleen and liver.

Haemochromatosis

Excess deposition of iron damages the cells and cause irreversible changes. Toxicity in iron excess is because of its propensity to form oxygen radicals that damages the cells.

Biliverdin and Bilirubin

Biliverdine and bilirubin are breakdown products of haemoglobin. Biliverdine is green tetrapyloric bile pigment, a product of haem catabolism.

Biliverdine with action of biliverdine reductase is converted to bilirubin which is yellow-coloured product. This later gets converted urobilin a yellow-coloured substance which is excreted in urine.

Stercobilin is brown-coloured substance and excreted in stools.

Haemozoin

Haemozoin is a haemoprotein-derived crystalline, brown birefringent pigment containing haem iron in ferric form in acidic medium. It is formed in the digestive vacuole of the *Plasmodium* species as a product of haemoglobin catabolism. This demarcates the transition of ring form to schizoint stage. This can be stained with Romonwosky stains (Giemsa, Wright, etc.) and methylene blue stain.

SELF-ASSESSMENT EXERCISE

1. **Prussian blue reaction done for:**
   A. Copper   B. Iron
   C. Silver   D. Magnesium

2. **Ochronosis is deposition of:**
   A. Iron   B. Copper
   C. Homogentisic acid   D. Magnesium

3. **Systemic deposition of iron is:**
   A. Albinism   B. Haemosiderosis
   C. Ochronosis   D. Anthrocosis

4. **Golden yellow pigment is:**
   A. Homogentisic acid
   B. Haemosiderin
   C. Haemoglobin
   D. Bilirubin

5. **Lipofuscin is:**
   A. Black   B. Red
   C. Yellow brown   D. Green

Answers

1. B   2. C   3. B   4. B   5. C

Environmental Pathology

The health and environment are interconnected to each other. The word "environment" not only consists of outdoor, indoor and occupational environments but also the one's own personal environment. The first three components are composed of air, water and food. The personal environment is based on the personal habits such as consumption of high fat diet, alcohol, and tobacco in any form (chewing, smoking, etc.). Environmental diseases are referred to those conditions that are caused due to exposure to agents in outdoor, indoor and occupational and personal environments including those secondary to nutritional deficiencies. Those diseases caused due to exposure to agents in workplace alone are termed as occupational diseases. The examples for environmental diseases that can be mentioned and brought to the notice of the public are:

1. **Methylmercury contamination (Minamata disease) of Minamata Bay in Japan:** Methylmercury is the industrial waste. Water with methylmercury from the Chisso Corporation's chemical factory, contaminated Minamata Bay which continued from 1932 to 1968. Eating fish from this bay with high concentration of mercury caused mercury poisoning.

2. **Exposure to dioxin in Seveso, Italy in 1976:** The factory produced trichlorophenol (TCP), a chemical used in deodorants and in antibacterial soaps that doctors use before performing surgery. There was a rupture of a pressure disc in a reaction vessel at the small chemical manufacturing plant. It released extremely toxic compound 2,3,7,8-tetrachloro-dibenzo-p-dioxin (TCDD) or dioxin, into the air. This caused Chloracne a severe skin disorder in humans and killed many birds and animals.

3. **Leakage of methyl isocyanate gas in Bhopal, India in 1984:** On December 2nd night and 3rd early morning hours in 1984, the Union Carbide Pesticide Plant leaked toxic gas methyl isocyanate (cyanide poisoning) exposing 500000 people to this gas and Government of Madhya Pradesh confirmed death toll to be 3,787 people due to choking, circulatory collapse and pulmonary oedema. This is the world's worst industrial disaster.

4. **Dioxin released from trash incinerator:** Dioxin and Furans are released from incineration of garbage, these are toxic and since 1990, the guidelines for emission have been tightened in some of the countries like Australia and European countries.

5. **President of Ukraine (Victor Yushchenko) suffered dioxin toxicity:** He was poisoned shortly before he swept to power in the 2004.

6. **Intentional contamination of Tokyo subways by organophosphorus pesticide in 1995:** The toxicity effects are due to the inhibition of acetylcholinesterase in the nervous system, resulting in respiratory, myocardial and neuromuscular transmission impairment.

7. **A chemical plant in China** released more than 100 tons of benzene, and aniline nitrobenzene into the river Songhua in the 2005, November 13th. This endangered water supply and influenced life of millions of people.

8. **Fukushima nuclear melting following tsunami in 2011:** This was initiated primarily by the tsunami following the Tôhoku earthquake on 11 March 2011. The active reactors automatically shut down their sustained fission reactions. The tsunami disabled the emergency generators that would have provided power to control and operate the pumps necessary to cool the reactors.

ALCOHOLISM

Alcohol in small to medium amounts is not dangerous and has a few health benefits. However, excessive consumption has health hazards. Drugs such as cocaine and heroin have been given more attention when it comes to drug abuse, but alcohol abuse is more widespread and deep rooted. In USA, almost one-third of the population is either mild to moderate alcoholics and many of them are alcohol-dependent or addicts. Apart from direct toxic effects of the alcohol and associated diseases, alcohol is responsible for accidents, psychiatric problems, homicides and suicides. Alcohol is also responsible for 1.8 million deaths per year world-wide approximately accounting for 3.2% of all deaths.

Alcohol Metabolism (Fig. 17.1)

A concentration of 30 mg/dl in the blood characterizes the legal definition of drunken driving in India. This concentration can be achieved by consuming 3 standard drinks containing either 450 ml of wine, 360 ml of beer, or 150 ml of 80 proof distilled spirits. At 200 mg/dl drowsiness occurs and at 300 mg/dl stupor occurs and even higher level may lead to coma and respiratory arrest. Once consumed, ethanol is rapidly absorbed unaltered in the stomach and small intestine. After absorption, ethanol gets distributed to all the tissues and secretions of the body and the levels in the tissue are directly proportionate to the blood levels. Unaltered ethanol (about 10%) is excreted from the urine, sweat and breath and even this excretion is influenced by its levels in the blood. Excretion through breath forms the basis for breath test used by law agencies in drunken driving. The blood ethanol level is influenced by its rate of metabolism. A chronic alcoholic will tolerate ethanol levels up to 700 mg/dl. Other factors influencing the effects of ethanol are age, sex, body fat, etc.

The maximum amount of alcohol is absorbed from the gastric mucosa and the mucosa of small intestine. There are three pathways involved in its further metabolism. Major pathway involves the action of alcohol dehydrogenase (cytosol) and acetaldehyde dehydrogenase (mitochondria) ultimately leading to formation of carbon dioxide and water with intermediate products such as acetaldehyde and acetic acid. The minor pathways involve cytochrome p-450 pathway (microsomes) and catalase pathway (peroxisomes).

The intermediate products are toxic in nature and are involved in disrupting the metabolic pathways. Few and most importants are mentioned below.

- Acetaldehyde is responsible for most of the acute toxicity related to alcohol and also for the development of cancers.
- Fatty liver in alcoholics is secondary to unavailability of nicotinamide adenine dinucleotide (NAD) that is getting used up during oxidation process of ethanol. NAD is necessary for conversion of lactic acid to pyruvate. Lactic acidosis is commonly seen in most of the alcoholics.
- Lipopolysaccharides are released from intestinal Gram-negative bacterial flora that stimulate the macrophages and Kupffer cells to produce tumour necrosis factor, ultimately leading to liver cell injury.
- Reactive oxygen species are accumulated in the liver when ethanol is metabolized by microsomal P-450 cytochrome oxidase pathway. This leads to lipid peroxidation of cell membranes and results in cell injury.

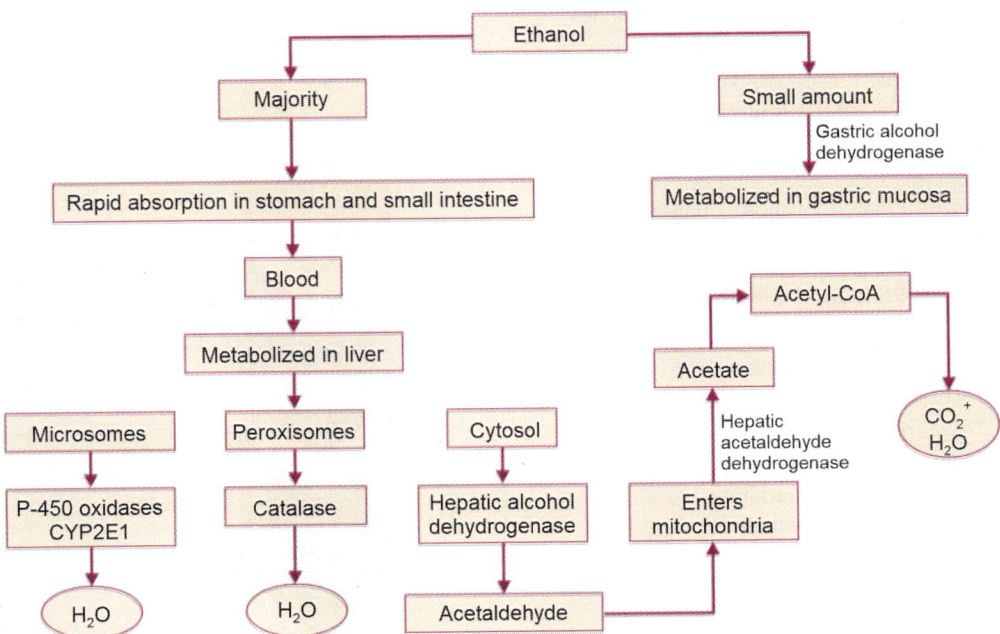

Fig. 17.1: Metabolism of alcohol

Acute Alcoholism

In acute toxicity of alcohol, central nervous system is affected primarily apart from liver and gastric mucosa. Ethanol is a CNS depressant and reduces the cerebral cortical activity. This change is generally reversible. If the alcohol level increases, then the limbic system is affected and ultimately affecting the brainstem reticular formation. Later, there are disturbances in the motor and intellectual behaviour ultimately affecting the neurons and medulla. Respiratory arrest occurs when the respiratory centres are affected in the brain. Alcohol releases cytokines which cause liver cell injury leading to fatty change. Acute gastritis and gastric ulcer are commonly encountered.

Chronic Alcoholism

Virtually any organ can be affected in chronic alcoholism; however, liver, stomach, CNS and pancreas are primarily affected. Chronic alcoholism is associated with increased morbidity and reduced lifespan. Table 17.1 lists the most important ones.

Table 17.1	Pathological changes of different organs with alcoholism
Liver	Fatty liver Alcohol hepatitis Alcoholic cirrhosis with portal hypertension Hepatocellular carcinoma
Stomach	Acute erosive gastritis Gastric ulcer Esophageal varices
Nutritional	Malnutrition Vitamin B complex deficiencies
Thiamine deficiency	Peripheral neuropathy Wernicke-Korsakoff syndrome Cerebral atrophy Cerebellar degeneration Optic neuropathy
Cardiovascular system	Dilated cardiomyopathy Reduced HDL levels (heavy alcohol consumption) Coronary artery disease
Pancreas	Acute pancreatitis Chronic pancreatitis
Pregnancy	Fetal alcohol syndrome Microcephaly Mental retardation Growth retardation Facial abnormalities
Cancers	Oral cavity Esophagus Liver Breast

TOBACCO AND ITS HEALTH HAZARDS

Tobacco in any form such as cigarette, snuff, chewing tobacco, etc. is considered the most common exogenous agent for carcinogenesis in humans especially in development of lung and oral cancer. Tobacco can be of cigarette smoking or smokeless. It can even be second hand smoke in individuals who are not smoking but exposed to its inhalation from environment. The cancer risk in these second hand smokers is also proven to be high. Cigarette smoking is not only associated with increased incidence of cancers, but also in increasing the cardiovascular diseases and respiratory diseases such as chronic bronchitis (Fig. 17.2).

Certain facts about cigarette smoking are mentioned below:

- The leading countries with highest population of cigarette smokers are China (30%), India (10%), Indonesia, Russia, the United States, Japan, Brazil, Bangladesh, Germany, and Turkey.
- Smoking is considered the most preventable cause of death.
- The non-smokers live longer than the smokers.

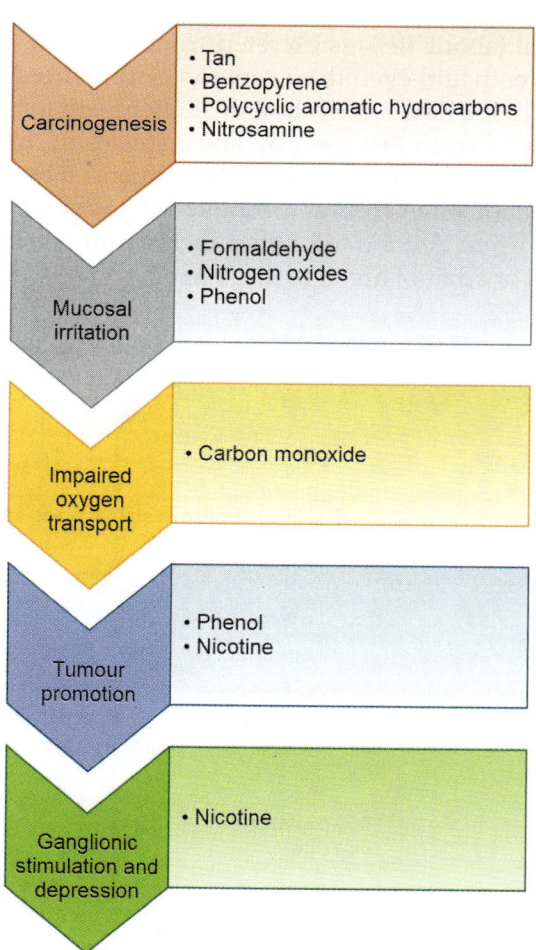

Fig. 17.2: Effects of tobacco and its metabolites

- Delay in the age at which smoking is initiated is associated with reduced risk of cancer development in future.
- The risk of developing lung cancers is reduced by 21% within 5 years, if the individual stops smoking. However, the excess risk compared to the non-smokers lasts up to 30 years.
- The risk of cardiovascular diseases also reduces markedly after cessation of smoking.

There are more than 2000 substances in tobacco and more than 60 substances have been identified as potential carcinogens. Nicotine in tobacco, which is not the direct cause of all the tobacco-related manifestations, is an addictive which makes cessation of smoking habit difficult. It goes and binds the receptors in brain which releases catecholamines into the blood and hence smoking is related to tachycardia, hypertension and increased cardiac output (Table 17.2).

Lung is a major organ that is affected primarily by tobacco and its metabolites. It causes various diseases such as emphysema, chronic bronchitis and lung cancer. Smoking increases the risk of developing lung cancer and the risk is directly proportional to the intensity of exposure and it is expressed in pack years. One pack year means one pack smoked every day for a year. Smoking also multiplies the risk of development of cancers by other carcinogens. Carcinogenic effect of smoking increases with alcohol in various types of cancers (Fig. 17.3).

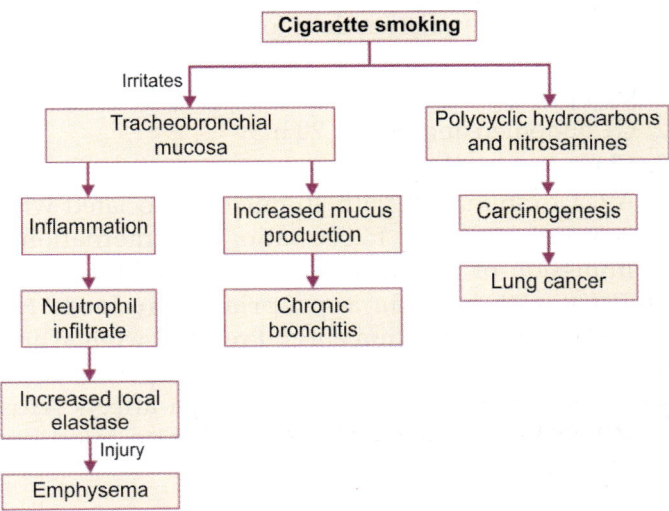

Fig. 17.3: Effects of smoking on lung

Passive Smoking

Tobacco is injurious whether it is inhaled actively or passively. The passive smokers are at increased risk for developing lung cancer, coronary atherosclerosis and fatal myocardial infarction and the incidence of cardiac related mortality is significantly high in the West and been on rise in developing countries like India. In nonsmokers, nicotine is converted to cotinine which can be estimated in their blood.

RADIATION

Radiation units are Curie(Ci), Gray (Gy), Rad, Rem and Sievert (Sv). One rad equals to 0.01 Gy. This produces energy of 100 erg per gram of matter. Rad is replaced by Gy in international system of units (SI) but still used in US. Rem and Sievert are used for neutrons and alpha particle energy. One Sievert equals to 100 rem. Doses below 1mSv produce minimal effects and >100 mSv have serious effects and can produce leukaemia, lymphoma and solid tumours.

Radiation energy can be:
1. Non-ionising radiation
2. Ionising radiation

Non-ionising radiation includes: Ultraviolet rays, infrared rays, microwave and sound waves.

Ionising radiation includes:
a. X-rays
b. Gamma rays
c. High energy neutrons
d. Alpha particles, e.g. uranium, radium, polonium
e. Beta particles, e.g. tritium, carbon-14, strontium-90

Ionising radiation has been used in:
a. Cancer treatment
b. Diagnostic imaging
c. Therapeutic and diagnostic radioisotopes

Table 17.2	Organ systems and diseases caused by tobacco
Organ system	**Diseases caused due to tobacco effect**
Respiratory system	Emphysema Chronic bronchitis Chronic obstructive pulmonary disease Lung carcinomas Laryngeal carcinomas
Cardiovascular system	Atherosclerosis Myocardial infarct
Gastrointestinal and hepatobiliary systems	Peptic ulcer disease Cancers of the lip, mouth, pharynx, oesophagus Carcinoma pancreas
Urinary system	Bladder carcinoma Renal cell carcinoma
Female genital tract	Cervical cancer
Pregnancy	Spontaneous abortion Preterm birth Intrauterine growth retardation

The effective radiation dose for diagnostic purposes is as below:

1. CT abdomen: 10 mSv
2. CT abdomen and pelvis: 20 mSv
3. Chest X-ray: 0.1 mSv

A CT examination with 10 mSv is associated with increase of cancer in 1:2000 ratio. The International Commission of Radiation Protection (ICRP) has set objectives to provide appropriate standards for protection from radiation effect. Pregnant women and individuals below the age of 18 are not permitted to work in radiologic work, as radiation affects fetus causing abnormalities and gonads causing infertility and sterility.

Adverse Effects of Ionising Radiation

1. Ionising radiation has direct and indirect effects. Direct effects affect the DNA of the cell while indirect effects affect through dissociation of water into H and OH ions which react with DNA.
2. Radiation effects depend upon:
   a. Area exposed,
   b. Cells affected,
   c. Cell sensitivity, and
   d. Individual sensitivity.
3. Short-term effects: Radiation effects appear in minutes, days or months. This is termed as acute radiation syndrome. Dose of 100–200 rads produce fatigue and weakness. Dose of 400–600 rads is lethal.
4. Long-term effects: This is non-lethal. Appear after years, decades or in next generation.

Tissue Affected in Radiation Injury

1. Radiations, directly or indirectly, injure cells, directly acting on DNA or indirectly through free radical OH ions released by dissociation of water.
2. Rapidly dividing cells such as germ cells, bone marrow cells, lymphoid cells, epithelial cells of gastrointestinal tract, skin and hair are very sensitive.
3. Muscle, bone, brain and connective tissue are less sensitive.
4. Ionising radiation can cause vascular damage with vasculitis, ischaemic necrosis followed by fibrosis.
5. DNA damage may get repaired, or undergo mutation and carcinogenesis with neoplastic transformation or kill the cells.

Morphology

The cells surviving radiant energy damage may show following changes (Fig. 17.4):

Nuclear and DNA changes:

1. Nuclear enlargement

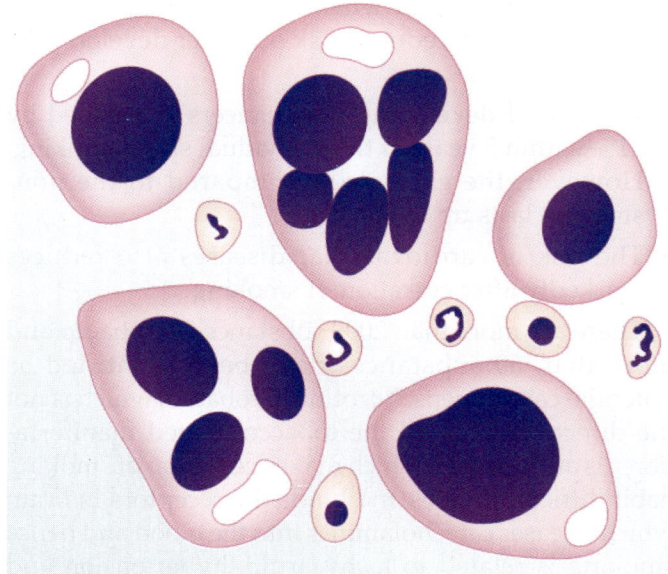

Fig. 17.4: Cell changes in radiation, note multinucleation, enlarged nuclei and cytoplasmic vacuoles

2. Condensation and clumping of chromatin
3. Apoptosis
4. Formation of giant cells, pleomorphic nuclei or more than one nuclei.
5. Extremely high doses of radiant energy causes cell death, nuclear pyknosis and lysis

Cytoplasmic changes:

a. Cytoplasmic vacuolization
b. Cytoplasmic swelling
c. Mitochondrial distortion
d. Degeneration of endoplasmic reticulum
e. Plasma membrane breaks with focal defects

Vascular changes: The vessels show dilatation, swelling and vacuolation of endothelial cells, necrosis and dissolution of venules and capillaries. Vessels may show rupture and thrombosis. Later, endothelial cell proliferation, thickening of the intima with narrowing and obliteration of vessels are the frequent findings.

AIR POLLUTION

Air pollution has significant morbidity and mortality particularly in individuals with pulmonary and cardiac disease.

The effects can be due to:

- Indoor air pollution
- Outdoor air pollution

Indoor Air Pollution

Exposure to indoor air pollution is an important environmental problem. The levels of pollutants often are greater indoor than outdoors. Wood smoke, bio-aerosols, Radon—a byproduct of uranium, and formaldehyde are common amongst air pollutants.

Radon, a radioactive substance, is widely present in the soils and houses. The average level of indoor level of radon is 1.3 pCi/l and outdoor it is 0.4 pCi/l, this has risk of lung cancer.

Formaldehyde is released through biomass combustion and decomposition and eruption of volcanoes.

Bioaerosols may be found indoor as well outdoor environment and these cause:

1. Biomass smoke: Fuel from wood (CO, NO_2, O_3, organic compounds and PM). This alters the oxidative stress, and alters protease and antiprotease balance causing lung diseases. Like COPDs.
2. Infectious diseases due to microbial agents particularly Legionnaires disease and viral pneumonia.
3. Infection by moulds and fungi.
4. Pet dander and dust mites can cause skin irritation and eye irritation.
5. Hypersensitivity reactions.
6. Water, soil and plants are the routes of outdoor pollutants.
7. Industries involved in animal products such as wool contaminated with anthracic bacillus and its spores can cause anthrax disease.

Outdoor Air Pollution

The ambient air in industrialized nations can have mixture of gaseous and particulate pollutants.

Environmental protection agency monitors allowable levels of CO, SO_2, O_3, NO_2, lead and particulate matter, collectively these are known as smog. SO_2 can destroy vegetation and all are hazardous to health mainly to respiratory tract (breathing problems, asthma, bronchitis, etc.).

The ozone layer in the stratosphere protects us from UV rays from sunlight and thinned out during these days increasing the risk of skin malignancies. In recent years, ozone concentration has been increasing at an alarming rate by chlorofluorocarbon gases used in air-conditioners, refrigerators, etc., thus increasing the temperature.

Particulate matter (solid and liquid aerosols suspended in the atmosphere) of less than 10 μ size in environment has morbidities and mortalities related to lung and cardiovascular diseases. Solid particulate matter is dust and liquid particulate matter is mist.

Sources: Oil fired power plants, burning of fossil fuels such as coal, petroleum and diesel from automobiles. These produce two-thirds of the carbon dioxide and one-half of the hydrocarbons and nitrous oxides. Automobiles exhaust leaded gas and particulate lead. Electrical power plants produce sulphur dioxide.

Carbon Monoxide

Carbon monoxide (CO) is a colourless and odourless gas which has high affinity for haemoglobin forming carboxyhaemoglobin which causes asphyxia and central nervous system depression.

Sources: Burning of cigarettes, furnaces, automobile engines and barbeques.

Individuals working in following are at risk:

1. Tunnels
2. Garages
3. Highway toll booths with high automobile fumes

Increased concentration of CO causes:

1. Central nervous system depression
2. Flu-like syndrome
3. Impaired vision
4. Co-ordination problems
5. Dizziness
6. Headache
7. Still higher levels: Loss of consciousness and death
8. Acute inhalation causes cherry red skin and liquid blood.

Other Air Pollutants

1. **Polycyclic hydrocarbons:** Polycyclic hydrocarbons released from fossil fuels (coal, oil, natural gas, gasoline) cause lung cancer and bladder cancer. CO_2 is a good indicator of fossil fuel burnt.
2. **Organochlorines** include: Dichlorodiphenyltrichloroethane (DDT), lindane, aldrin, dieldrin, dioxin and polychlorinated biphenyls (PCBs)—these cause skin cancers and male infertility.
3. **Vinyl chloride** is used in making polyvinyl chloride pipes, wire coatings, automotive parts, plastic kitchen ware, etc. Acute exposure to this gas leads central nervous system effects like dizziness, drowsiness, headache and loss of conciousness. Liver angiosarcoma is the common cancer caused by chronic exposure..
4. **Polychlorinated biophenols and dioxin** which is 2, 3, 7, 8 tetrachlorbenzene-p-dioxin (TCDD) is used in bleaching wood pulp, incinerating garbage and metal smelting. These cause skin disorders.

Food and water plastic containers having bisphenol A (BPA) are used in synthesis of polycarbonate which causes angiosarcoma.

PNEUMOCONIOSIS

Factors like duration of exposure, burden of inhaled particles, size of the particles, nature of inhaled particles, concomitant diseases, additional habits like smoking, etc. influence the disease process. Various types occupational lung diseases due to inorganic and organic dusts are known. Following are some of the diseases.

Coal workers pneumoconiosis: Lung disease develops from inhalation of coal dust from coal mining. This has two forms: Simple coal workers pneumoconiosis and progressive massive fibrosis. Some patients of pneumoconiosis may present with rheumatoid arthritis which is termed as Caplan's syndrome. Anthrocosis develops in urban dwellers due to atmospheric pollution. There is excess accumulation of carbon dust in these individuals.

Silicosis: Silicon dioxide, also termed as silica is inhaled by people engaged working with silaceous rocks or its sand. Silica dust is cytotoxic and fibrogenic. Sometimes may present with Caplan's syndrome.

Asbestosis: Asbestosis causes pleural effusion, fibrosis of visceral pleura, pleural plaques, bronchogenic carcinoma and mesothelioma. Amphibole fibres of asbestosis, especially crocidolite, are associated with above pathology. These are straight, stiff and rigid fibres. The serpentine fibres of asbestosis are mostly used for commercial purposes. Most common of these is crysolite. These fibres are curly, and flexible.

Other mineral dusts: Beryliosis and iron oxide are the mineral dust causing lung diseases.

Organic substances producing lung diseases: Mouldy hay (farmers lung), Bagasse (bagassosis) from pulp of sugarcane, cotton and other fibre dust (byssinosis), bird droppings (bird breeders lung), mushroom compost dust (mushroom workers lung) malt dust (malt workers lung), etc.

For details on above topics, kindly refer to Chapter on Occupational Lung Diseases/Pneumoconiosis.

PRINTING CHEMICALS

Potentially toxic agents used in the printing industry include organic solvents, mineral oils, pigments, resins, lead, and paper dust.

Sources

1. Inhalation and dermal contact with the solvents in inks, thinners, clean-up materials, and so forth.
2. Solvent exposure in offset establishments includes white spirits, methylene chloride, isopropanol, 1,1,1-trichloroethane, ethanol, and trichloroethylene.

Effects

Acute exposure to toxic chemicals in printing causes dizziness, drowsiness, eye irritation, headache, light-headedness, nausea/vomiting, shortness of breath, cough, chest tightness, exacerbation of asthma, skin allergy, etc. The effects are more in the workers dealing with printing process than the other workers.

With repeated and chronic exposure to these toxic substances causes skin, liver, kidney, reproductive, and nervous system damage, and increased risk for melanoma, lung cancer, bladder cancer, cancers of the buccal cavity, pharynx and pancreas.

HEAVY METAL POISONING (Lead, Mercury, Arsenic and Cadmium)

Lead

Lead binds to sulfhydryl groups of protein and interferes with calcium metabolism, decreases haemoglobin synthesis and has effects on growth, hearing, IQ level, neurological, skeletal and renal system. Lead is more hazardous to children.

Sources

Motor vehicles, industries, gasoline, paints/spray painting/flaking of paints especially in old houses, mining, foundries, batteries, tin can, car radiation and mining. Concentration of lead >10 µg/dl causes chronic effects. Blood levels ≥45 µg/dl causes lead poisoning.

Effects

1. Lead is absorbed in bone and teeth.
2. Lead line on gums and bones which is blue-purplish-coloured is also called Burton line after the London based physician Henry Burton who described this.
3. Depression of central nervous system.
4. Peripheral nerve function impaired.
5. Suppresses haemoglobin synthesis and causes anaemia.

Mercury (Hg)

Mercury binds to proteins and damages central nervous system and kidneys. Mercury is converted to methyl-mercury by bacteria, which inturn is consumed through water by sea habitats.

Sources

1. **Industries using mercury:** Electrical equipments preparing batteries and semiconductors, barometers, medical equipment like thermometer and sphygmo-manometer, paints and paper industry. Consuming fish with high concentration of methylmercury as industrial waste left to water source can cause mercury poisoning.

2. Vapour from dental amalgams (mixture of mercury, silver, tin and copper)
3. Volcanos
4. Forest fires
5. Fossils fuels
6. Power plants

Cadmium

This is recently developed health hazard.

Sources

1. Ni-cadmium batteries, plating
2. Plastics
3. Byproduct of zinc, lead and copper exhaustion
4. It is a chemical of low melting point.

The waste produced by the sources has been disposed as house hold waste. Cadmium found in soil and water, shell fish and mushroom food is a source of contamination.

Effects

Kidney damage and lung damage with obstructive lung diseases.

Arsenic (As)

This is found naturally in soil and water.

Other Sources

Wood preservative, herbicide, agricultural pesticides. Bangladesh, Chile and China have large concentration in water. Arsenic trioxide, sodium arsenic and arsenic trichloride are the toxic forms.

Effects

1. Excess amounts interfere with mitochondrial oxidative function and functions of variety of proteins.
2. Toxic effects are on gastrointestinal tract, central nervous system and cardiovascular system. Long-term effect causes skin lesions like carcinoma.

CLIMATE CHANGE

Effects of environmental temperature are:
1. Burns
2. Hyperthermia
3. Heat cramps
4. Heat exhaustion
5. Heat stroke
6. Hypothermia

Climate change can also produce:
1. Volcanos
2. Tornadoes
3. Hurricane

NOISE POLLUTION

Noise pollution affects health and behaviour. The effect depends upon the loudness and frequency of sound. Sound more than 30 decibels is called noise. More than 180 decibels causes death.

Sources

1. Natural sources: Thunder storm, lightening, tornado, cyclones, volcanic eruptions, earthquakes and land slides.
2. Human sources: Industries, transport, population overgrowth.
3. Vehicular noises: Vehicles, crackers and loud-speakers.
4. Commercial activities: Dyeing, printing, repairing cars and grinding.
5. Domestic noise: TV, radio, instruments of various types.
6. Construction activities
7. Noisy hospitals
8. Fireworks

Effects

1. Deafness and rupture of eardrum
2. Irritability
3. Studies affected
4. Increased heart rate
5. Increase of cholesterol
6. Neurological diseases
7. Hypertension
8. Dizziness and exhaustion
9. Hinders sleep and causes insomnia

SELF-ASSESSMENT EXERCISE

1. **Lead poisoning is indicated by:**
   A. MHA
   B. Basophilic stippling
   C. Wrist drop
   D. All of the above

2. **Minamata disease is caused by exposure to:**
   A. Cadmium
   B. Mercury
   C. Arsenic
   D. Zinc

3. **Drowsiness by acute alcohol abuse occurs at blood levels of:**
   A. 200 mg/dl
   B. 300 mg/dl
   C. 400 mg/dl
   D. 500 mg/dl

4. **Fetal alcohol syndrome does not include:**
   A. Microcephaly
   B. Growth retardation
   C. CVS anomaly
   D. Facial defects

5. **Chronic arsenic poisoning does not cause which of the following?**
   A. Basal cell carcinoma
   B. Squamous cell carcinoma
   C. Melanoma
   D. Lung cancer

6. **Itai-itai disease in Japan was caused by:**
   A. Mercury
   B. Cadmium
   C. Lead
   D. Aluminium

7. **Cherry-red colouration of skin and mucous membrane is caused by poisoning of:**
   A. Carbon monoxide
   B. Lead paints in toys.
   C. Carbon dioxide
   D. Sulphur dioxide.

8. **Which of the following is associated with liver angiosarcoma?**
   A. Benzene
   B. Herbicide
   C. Alcohols
   D. Vinyl chloride

9. **Interstitial pulmonary fibrosis can occur due to all *except*:**
   A. Busulphan
   B. Nitrofurantoin
   C. Tetracycline
   D. Bleomycin

10. **All of the following are sedative hypnotics *except*:**
    A. Barbiturates
    B. Ethanol
    C. Methadone
    D. Mathaquilone

Answers

1. D	2. B	3. A	4. C	5. C	6. B	7. A	8. D
9. C	10. C						

Nutritional Disorders

PROTEIN ENERGY MALNUTRITION (PEM)

Protein energy malnutrition is one of the serious diseases affecting the children below 5 years of age and is a major cause of mortality and morbidity in developing countries like India. The main causes are poverty, economic fluctuations, famine because of draught or heavy rainfall with floods, etc.

Malnutrition is assessed by the body mass index (BMI). BMI is calculated by dividing weight (in kilograms) with square of height (in metres). The normal range is 18.5 to 25 kg/m². BMI <16 kg/m² is considered as malnutrition while >25 kg/m² is considered as obesity (Fig. 18.1).

$$\text{Body mass index} = \frac{\text{Weight (in kilograms)}}{\text{Height (in metres)}^2}$$

Fig. 18.1: Formula for BMI

In clinical setup, a child whose weight falls below 80% of normal (standard tables) is considered as malnourished. Additional clinical findings such as skin fold thickness, midarm circumference also help in assessing the nutritional status. Blood investigations such as serum total proteins and serum albumin are essential in diagnosis of PEM.

Marasmus and Kwashiorkar are the two ends of spectrum of protein energy malnutrition syndromes. This can be explained based on the differentially regulated protein compartments in the body. The central (visceral) compartment is represented by the protein in the liver while the peripheral (somatic) compartment represented by the protein in the skeletal muscle. The central (visceral) compartment is majorly affected in case of kwashiorkar while marasmus affects the peripheral (somatic) compartment. Hence, kwashiorkar can be diagnosed based on the liver

function test such as serum albumin, transferrrin levels, while marasmus can be analysed by skeletal muscle mass—midarm circumference and skin fold thickness.

MARASMUS

Definition

A child whose weight is below 60% of normal for age, sex and height is considered as marasmus.

Pathogenesis

The peripheral (somatic) compartment of proteins is mainly affected. The amino acids from skeletal muscles are the main source of energy. The central (visceral) compartment is not affected hence the serum albumin is nearly normal or slightly reduced. Along with skeletal muscle proteins, subcutaneous fat is also used up for production of energy. Leptins are reduced in these patients; hence this will activate the hypothalamic pituitary adrenal axis. This will increase the cortisol production which will further increase lipolysis (Fig. 18.2).

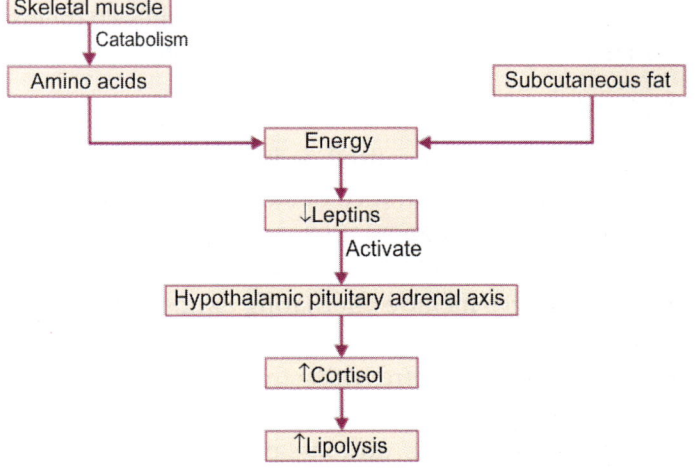

Fig. 18.2: Pathogenesis in marasmus

Clinical Features

- Growth retardation, loss of muscle mass, concurrent infections.
- Loss of skeletal muscle mass will make the head look larger than the extremities.
- Anaemia, multivitamin deficiency, immune deficiency (T cell-mediated immunity)
- Serum albumin is normal or slightly reduced.

Diagnosis

- Reduced midarm circumference.
- Reduced weight (<60%) as compared to standard for age, sex and height.
- Reduced subcutaneous fat.
- Normal or slightly reduced serum albumin.

KWASHIORKAR

Definition

It is a type of protein energy malnutrition wherein the protein deprivation is greater than the calorie deficiency. This is the most common type of malnutrition. It derives its name from the Ga language in Ghana describing "a disease of a baby due to the arrival of another child".

Pathogenesis

It is usually seen in children who are weaned off early from breastfeeding and started on pure carbohydrate diet. Less severe forms of the disease is seen worldwide secondary to chronic diarrhoeal states wherein proteins are not absorbed properly or protein loss due to protein-losing enteropathies, nephrotic syndrome and after extensive burns. Presently, kwashiorkor can also result from intake of fad diets.

In kwashiorkor, the central (visceral) compartment of proteins is affected. There will be severe hypo-albuminaemia leading to dependent or generalised oedema (anasarca). The loss of weight in these patients is masked by the increased fluid retention.

Clinical Features

- Dependent or generalised oedema
- 'Flaky paint' appearance of skin due to alternating zones of hyperpigmentation, areas of desquamation and hypopigmentation
- Hair changes include alternating bands of light and dark-coloured hair (flag sign).
- Enlarged fatty liver (resulting from reduced synthesis of the carrier protein component of lipoproteins)
- Apathy, listlessness, and loss of appetite
- Vitamin deficiencies

- Defects in immunity and secondary infections
- Relative sparing of subcutaneous fat and muscle mass

Morphology

The changes in PEM are:
- Growth failure
- Peripheral oedema in kwashiorkor
- Loss of body fat and atrophy of muscle more marked in marasmus.

Liver:
- In kwashiorkor, the liver is enlarged and shows fatty change.
- Cirrhosis is rare.

Gastrointestinal system: The small intestine shows:
- Mucosal atrophy
- Loss of villi and microvilli
- Decrease in the mitotic index in the crypts of the glands in kwashiorkor
- Disaccharidase deficiency
- The mucosal changes are reversible with treatment.

Bone marrow:
- The bone marrow is hypoplastic.
- Mainly erythroid hypoplasia.
- Mild to moderate anaemia (multifactorial in origin such as nutritional deficiencies of iron, folate, and protein, or anaemia of chronic disease secondary to infections).
- The RBC picture may be microcytic, normocytic, or macrocytic.

Central nervous system:
- Cerebral atrophy
- Reduced number of neurons
- Impaired myelinization of white matter

Other organs:
- Thymic and lymphoid atrophy
- Recurrent infections due to endemic worms and other parasites
- Deficiencies of other required nutrients such as iodine and vitamins.

Secondary PEM often develops in chronically ill, elderly and bedridden patients. They have an increased risk of developing infection, sepsis, impaired wound healing and death post-surgery.

The most evident signs of secondary PEM include:
1. Depletion of subcutaneous fat in the arms, chest wall, shoulders or metacarpal regions

2. Wasting of the quadriceps femoris and deltoid muscles
3. Ankle or sacral oedema.

VITAMIN DEFICIENCIES

Vitamins are very essential for healthy living. There are altogether 13 vitamins. Vitamins are classified as fat-soluble and water-soluble vitamins (Fig. 18.3). Vitamins A, D, E, and K are fat-soluble, while all others are water-soluble. The distinction between fat- and water-soluble vitamins is important. Fat-soluble vitamins are more readily stored in the body, but they may be poorly absorbed in fat malabsorption disorders. Certain vitamins can be synthesized endogenously and examples include: Vitamin D from precursor steroids, vitamin K and biotin by the intestinal microflora and niacin from tryptophan. However, just endogenous synthesis of vitamins is not sufficient hence a dietary supply of all vitamins is essential for health.

Vitamin deficiency can be classified as: (a) Primary or (b) Secondary. Primary is usually due to dietary deficiencies while secondary is because of disturbances in intestinal absorption, transport in the blood, tissue storage or metabolic conversion. However, it should be emphasized that deficiency of a single vitamin is uncommon, and that single or multiple vitamin deficiencies may be associated with PEM.

VITAMIN A

Vitamin A is the name given to a group of related compounds that include retinol, retinal, and retinoic acid, which have similar biologic activities. Retinol is the chemical name given to vitamin A. It is the transport form and, as retinol ester, also the storage form.

Sources

- **Animal-derived foods:** Liver, fatty fish, egg yolk, whole milk, and butter [preformed vitamins].
- **Plant-derived foods:** Yellow and leafy green vegetables such as carrots, squash and spinach.

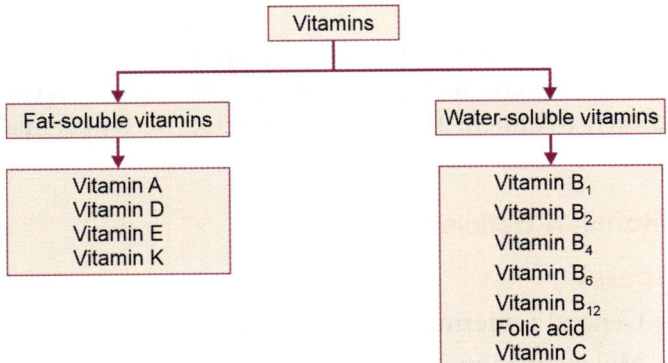

Fig. 18.3: Fat-soluble and water-soluble vitamins

[Provitamins which have to be metabolised to active vitamin A in the body.]

- Carotenoids contribute approximately 30% of the vitamin A in human diets; the most important of these is β-carotene, which is efficiently converted to vitamin A.

Daily requirement:
- Adults (above 6 years): 600 µg (retinol)
- Children (up to 6 years): 300 µg (retinol)

Metabolism (Fig. 18.4)

- Vitamin A is a fat-soluble vitamin.
- Retinol (retinol ester) and β-carotene are absorbed in the intestine. Absorption of vitamin A requires bile and pancreatic enzymes.
- Retinol is then transported by chylomicrons to the liver for esterification and storage.
- Liver cell uptake takes place through the apolipo-protein E receptor.
- Liver is the main site of vitamin A storage (>90%) mainly in perisinusoidal stellate (Ito) cells.
- In healthy persons, the body reserves of vitamin A are available for 6 months.
- Retinol esters stored in the liver can be mobilized. The retinol binds to a specific retinol-binding protein (RBP) in blood, which is synthesized in the liver.
- The uptake of retinol/RBP in peripheral tissues is by receptors present on the surface of the tissue.
- After uptake of retinol by the tissue receptors, the RBP is released back into the blood.
- Retinol may be stored in peripheral tissues as retinol ester or be oxidized to form retinoic acid.
- This retinoic acid is required for normal vision, epithelial development and differentiation.

Functions

1. **Normal vision** (Fig. 18.5): Vitamin A-containing pigments are required for the normal visual process. The most important and sensitive pigment is rhodopsin, which is present in the rods and other pigments are three iodopsins which are seen in cone cells, the rhodopsin pigment is mainly for dim light while the iodopsins are for bright light.
2. **Epithelial growth and maintenance of function:** Vitamin A and retinoids are required for the normal maturation and differentiation of the epithelial cells mainly the mucus-secreting epithelium
   - For example, mucous membrane of eyes
   - Mucous membrane of respiratory tract
   - Mucous membrane of genitourinary tract
   - Mucous membrane of gastrointestinal tract
   - Mucuos membrane of glands and ducts

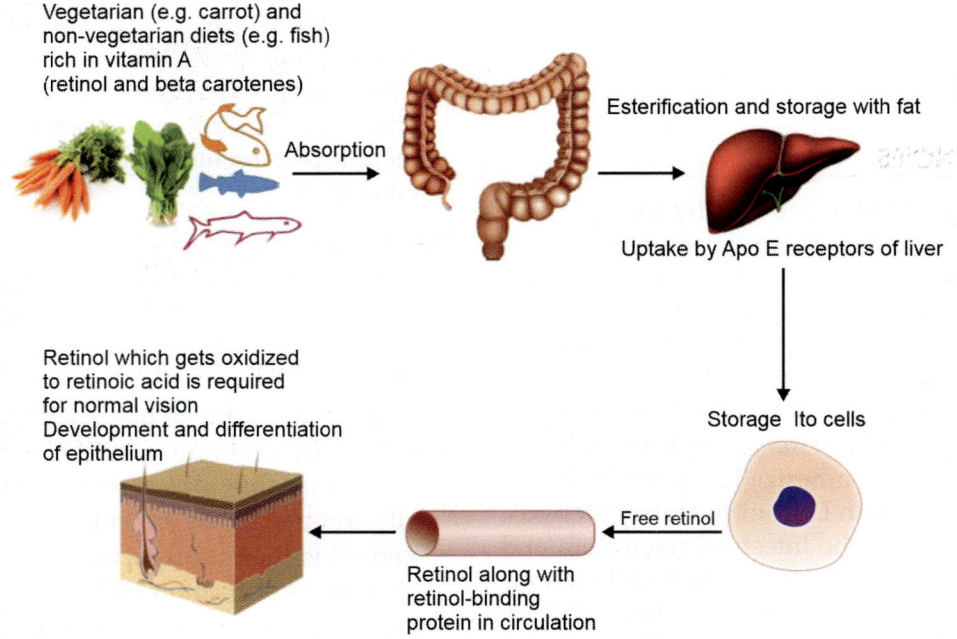

Fig. 18.4: Metabolism and functions of vitamin A

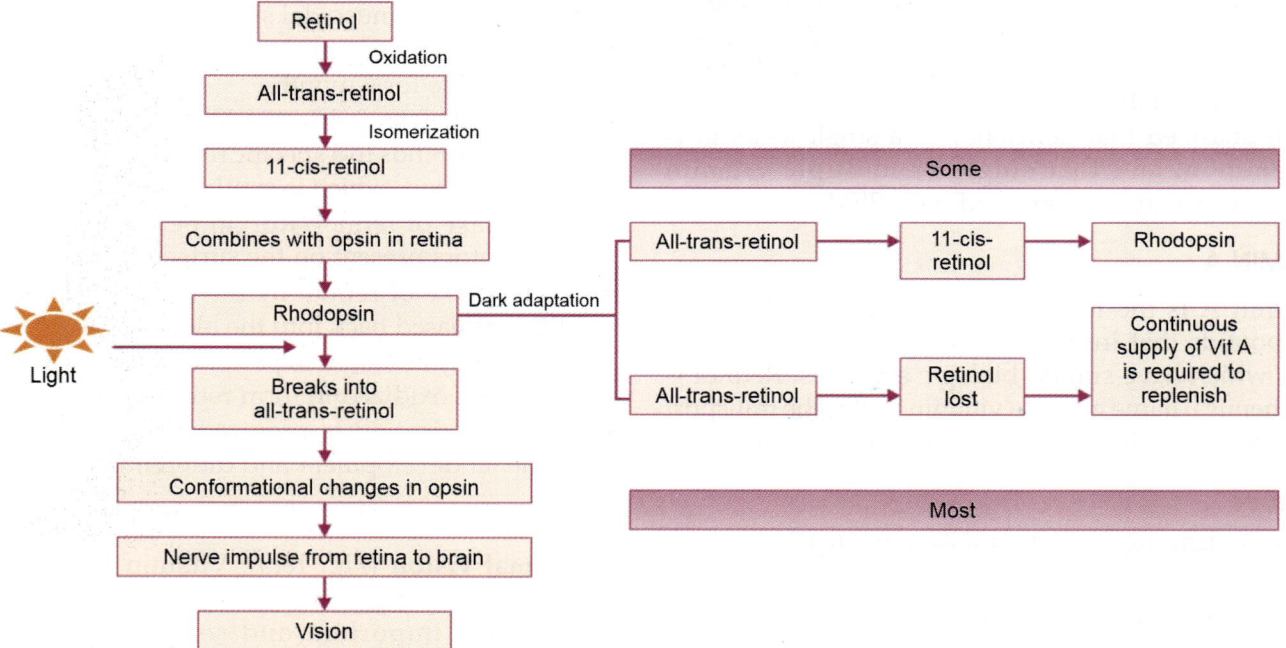

Fig. 18.5: Role of vitamin A in normal vision

- In case of vitamin A deficiency, the mucus-secreting epithelium will undergo squamous metaplasia and forms keratinizing squamous epithelium.
3. **Host resistance to infections:** Vitamin A supplementation is known to reduce morbidity and mortality from diarrhoea and measles in children. Vitamin A has an ability to stimulate the immune system.
4. **Antioxidant effect:** The retinoids, β-carotene, and some related carotenoids can function as photoprotective and antioxidant agents. Hence, it prevents the development of cancers.

Retinoids are used for the treatment of skin disorders such as severe acne and psoriasis. It is also a well-known treatment for acute promyelocytic leukaemia (APML).

Vitamin A Deficiency

Causes

- General undernutrition
- Malabsorption syndromes, such as celiac disease, Crohn's disease and colitis

- Infections (in infants)
- Poor absorption of the vitamins (newborn infants)
- Bariatric surgery
- Continuous use of mineral oil as a laxative (elderly persons)

Clinical Features

Eye (Fig. 18.6)
- The earliest manifestation of vitamin A deficiency is impaired vision in reduced light (**night blindness**).
- **Xerophthalmia (dry eye).** Firstly, there will be dryness of the conjunctiva (**xerosis conjunctivae**) due to keratinization of normal lacrimal and mucus-secreting epithelium, followed by buildup of keratin debris in small opaque plaques (**Bitot spots**) and eventually, erosion of the roughened corneal surface with softening and destruction of the cornea (**keratomalacia**) and total blindness.

Respiratory tract
- Epithelial metaplasia and keratinization.
- The epithelium lining is replaced by keratinizing squamous cells.
- Loss of the mucociliary epithelium of the airways predisposes to secondary pulmonary infections.

Genitourinary tract
- Epithelial metaplasia and keratinization.
- The epithelium lining is replaced by keratinizing squamous cells.
- Desquamation of keratin debris in the urinary tract predisposes to renal and urinary bladder stones.

Skin: Hyperplasia and hyperkeratinization of the epidermis with plugging of the ducts of the adnexal glands may produce follicular or papular dermatosis.

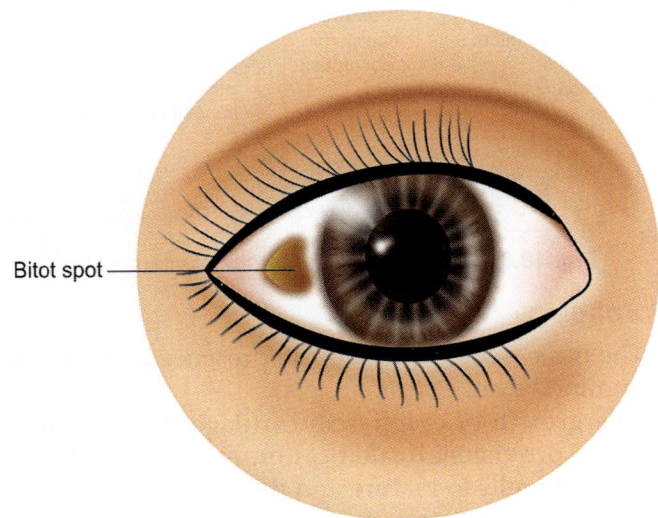

Fig. 18.6: Eye changes in vitamin A deficiency

Bitot spot

General:
- Immune deficiency can lead to common infections such as measles, pneumonia, and infectious diarrhoea.
- Dietary supplements of vitamin A reduce mortality by 20 to 30%.
- Increased risk of cancers due to reduction in antioxidants.

Vitamin A Toxicity

History

Acute hypervitaminosis A was first described by Gerrit de Veer in 1597. He was a ship's carpenter stranded in the Arctic. He noted the serious symptoms of vitamin A toxicity in the crew members after eating the liver of polar bear in his published diary.

Causes

Acute vitamin A toxicity has also been described in individuals who ingested the livers of whales, sharks, and tuna fish. Both short- and long-term excess consumption of vitamin A may produce toxic manifestations.

Clinical Features

- **Acute vitamin A toxicity** causes headache, dizziness, vomiting, stupor, blurred vision and papilloedema. These symptoms may be confused with those of a brain tumour, hence it is called pseudotumour cerebri.
- **Chronic vitamin A toxicity** is associated with weight loss, anorexia, nausea, vomiting, and bone and joint pain.
- High risk of fractures as retinoic acid stimulates osteoclast production and activity, which lead to increased bone resorption.
- They are teratogenic and hence contraindicated in in pregnancy.

VITAMIN D

- Vitamin D is a fat-soluble vitamin,
- The major function of vitamin D is to maintain the normal serum levels of calcium and phosphorus.
- It is required to support metabolic functions, bone mineralization, and neuromuscular transmission.
- Deficiency of vitamin D causes:
  - Rickets (in children)
  - Osteomalacia (in adults)
  - Tetany
- Tetany is a medical state with involuntary contraction of muscles caused by an insufficient extracellular concentration of ionized calcium, which is required for normal neural excitation and the relaxation of muscles.

Sources

- Endogenous synthesis of vitamin D in the skin by photochemical conversion of a precursor, 7-dehydrocholesterol by sunlight or artificial UV radiation in the range of 290 to 315 nm. 7-dehydrocholesterol forms cholecalciferol, known as vitamin D_3. This is subjected to 25-hydroxylation in the liver and converted to active 1,25 dihydroxycholecalciferol in the kidney (Fig. 18.7).
- Ninety per cent of vitamin D requirement of the body is done endogenously by the skin under the sunlight.
- Ten per cent of the remaining vitamin D comes from dietary sources.
- It mainly depends on adequate intestinal fat absorption.

Metabolism

Regulatory mechanism for production of vitamin D:

a. *Hypocalcaemia:* Stimulates secretion of parathyroid hormone (PTH), which helps the conversion of 25 hydroxycholecalciferol into 1,25 dihydroxycholecalciferol by activating 1α-hydroxylase.

b. *Hypophosphataemia:* Directly activates 1α-hydroxylase, increasing the production of 1,25 dihydroxycholecalciferol.

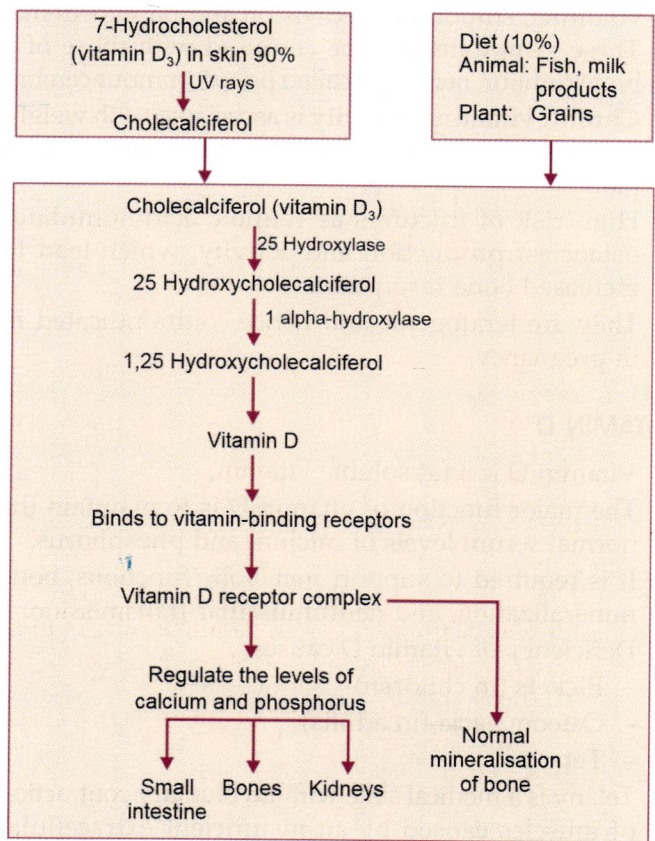

Fig. 18.7: Role of vitamin D regulating calcium, phosphorus and normal mineralization of bone

c. *Feedback mechanism:* Increased levels of 1,25 dihydroxycholecalciferol downregulate its own synthesis through inhibition of 1α-hydroxylase activity.

Deficiency of Vitamin D

Requirement

- Normal reference range of vitamin D: 20–100 ng/ml.
- Vitamin D deficiency: Value <20 ng/ml indicates vitamin D deficiency.

Deficiency of vitamin D in growing children is known as **rickets** and in adults as **osteomalacia**.

Causes

- Diets deficient in calcium and vitamin D
- Limited exposure to sunlight
- Renal disorders causing decreased synthesis of 1,25 dihydroxyvitamin D
- Phosphate depletion
- Malabsorption disorders such as celiac sprue, steatorrhoea
- Pancreatic insufficiency and biliary disorders
- Renal osteodystrophy and chronic renal disease
- Rare inherited disorders such as Fanconi's syndrome, X linked hypophosphataemia

Pathogenesis of Vitamin D Deficiency

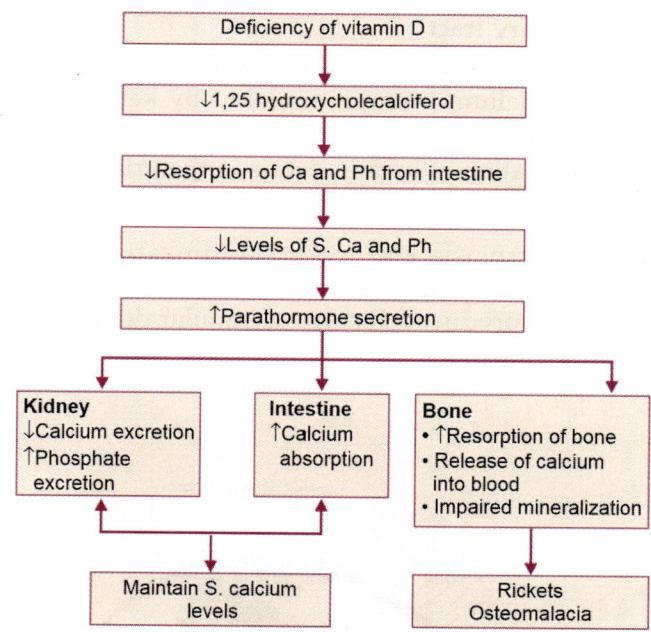

Fig. 18.8: Effects due to deficiency of vitamin D

Morphology

- The basic derangement is the presence of excess of unmineralized matrix.
- Overgrowth of epiphyseal cartilage due to inadequate provisional calcification and failure of the cartilage cells to mature and disintegrate.
- Persistence of distorted, irregular masses of cartilage, which project into the marrow cavity.

- Deposition of osteoid matrix on inadequately mineralized cartilaginous remnants.
- Disruption of the orderly replacement of cartilage by osteoid matrix, with enlargement and lateral expansion of the osteochondral junction.
- Abnormal overgrowth of capillaries and fibroblasts in the disorganized zone resulting from micro-fractures and stresses on the inadequately mineralized, weak, poorly formed bone.
- Deformation of the skeleton due to the loss of structural rigidity of the developing bones.

Clinical Features

- **Rickets:** Most common during the first year of life.
- The skeletal changes depend on the site of stress on individual bones, severity and duration of the process.
- **Non-ambulatory stage of infancy:**
  - Head and chest sustain the greatest stress.
  - Occipital bones become flattened.
  - **Craniotabes:** It is the earliest manifestation. Parietal bones can be bent inward due to pressure, however, once the pressure is released, there will be recoil phenomenon causing the bone to snap back into original position.
  - **Frontal bossing due to** excess of osteoid production.
  - **Squared appearance to the head.**
  - **Rachitic rosary:** Overgrowth of cartilage or osteoid tissue at the costochondral junction gives a beaded appearance of costochondral junctions.
  - **Pigeon breast deformity:** The weakened meta-physeal areas of the ribs are subject to the pull of the respiratory muscles and thus bend inward, creating anterior protrusion of the sternum.
  - **Harrison groove:** Due to the inward pull of the diaphragm during respiration, a horizontal depression is noted in the lower border of the rib cage.
- **Ambulatory stage:**
  - Lumbar lordosis and scoliosis
  - Bowing of the legs and knock knee
- **Adults (osteomalacia):**
  - **Deranges the normal bone remodelling**
  - The newly formed osteoid matrix laid down by osteoblasts is inadequately mineralized, thus producing the excess of persistent osteoid.
  - Gross fractures or microfractures
- **Microscopy:**
  - The presence of unmineralized osteoid.
  - Thickened layer of eosinophilic matrix arranged about the more basophilic, normally mineralized trabeculae.

- X-ray shows decreased bone density and saucerization of the radius and ulna.

Vitamin D Toxicity

Cause

Excess dose of orally administered vitamin D.

Clinical Features

- **Children:** Metastatic calcifications in soft tissue and kidney.
- **Adults:** Bone pain and hypercalcaemia.

VITAMIN K

Vitamin K is a fat-soluble vitamin necessary for synthesis of coagulation factors. The factors involved in pathways of coagulation are factors II, VII, IX, and X as well as protein C and protein S. Vitamin 'K', the word is derived from the original word 'koagulation factor' as it plays a major role in coagulation process.

- Vitamin K_1 (phylloquinone)—present in most edible fresh green vegetables.
- Vitamin K_2 (menaquinone)—present in fish and produced by intestinal bacteria.
- Vitamin K_3 (menadione)—all compounds are structurally related to this simple compound.

Sources

- Vitamin K_1—green leafy vegetables, alfalfa (*Medicago sativa*), spinach, cauliflower, cabbage, soybeans and tomatoes.
- Vitamin K_2—fish, egg yolk, meat, liver and product of normal intestinal flora.
- Cow's milk contains good amount of vitamin K as compared to breast milk.

Requirement

- Recommended dietary allowance: 1 µg/kg body weight.
- Males 120 µg and females 90 µg.

Functions

- It promotes coagulation of blood by helping in post-translational modification of clotting factors such as factors II (prothrombin), VII (SPCA), IX (Christmas factor) and X (Stuart-Prower factor).
- Formation of other calcium binding proteins such as c-reactive protein, osteocalcin of bone and structural proteins of kidney, spleen, lungs and placenta.
- Cofactor in oxidative phosphorylation.

Deficiency of Vitamin K

Causes

- Poor diet
- Malabsorption of fats due to bile salt deficiency in the intestines.
- Liver failure
- Gastrointestinal infections like tropical sprue and chronic diarrhoea.
- Use of antimicrobial drugs which temporarily eliminates intestinal flora.
- Anticoagulant agents such as dicumoral and warfarin
- Newborn infants, especially preterm infants.

Vitamin K deficiency produces:

- Impaired coagulation function and excessive bleeding and haemorrhage (internal bleeding, often severe).
- Haemorrhagic disease of the newborne
- Newborn infants are susceptible to vitamin K deficiency.

Clinical Features

- Easy bruising, echymotic patches, mucosal haemorrhage, profuse post-traumatic bleeding and gastrointestinal bleeding.
- Prolonged prothrombin time and delayed clotting time.
- All newborn infants should receive vitamin K prophylactically.
- A single dose of 0.5–1.0 mg of water miscible form of vitamin K_1 is given intramuscularly at birth.

VITAMIN B (Water-Soluble Vitamins)

VITAMIN B_1 (Thiamine)

Deficiency of thiamine causes beriberi.

Sources

- Whole grain cereals such as wheat, rice, pulses groundnuts, etc.
- Pork

Requirement

- Male: 1.2 mg, Female: 1.1 mg.
- 0.5 mg per 1000 kcal of energy intake.

Functions

- Thiamine acts as a cofactor in citric acid cycle (Krebs cycle) for the oxidative decarboxylation of alpha ketoglutaric acid to succinyl coenzyme.
- It plays a role in oxidative decarboxylation of alpha-ketoacids.

- Transketolase thiamine diphosphate plays a role in pentose monophosphate shunt.
- It helps to maintain the normal nerve conduction.

Thiamine Deficiency

Causes

- Chronic alcoholics
- Consumption of polished rice
- Excessive diarrhoea
- Chronic debilitating illness

Clinical Manifestations of Thiamine Deficiency

Deficiency of vitamin B_1 causes beriberi. There are three types of beriberi.
1. Dry beriberi (polyneuropathy)
2. Wet beriberi (cardiac failure)
3. Wernicke-Korsakoff syndrome

Dry beriberi:

- It is non-specific polyneuropathy with involvement of both motor and sensory nerves.
- Mainly involves the lower limbs and later may progress to arms, trunk and even vagus nerve.
- It is characterized by weakness, paraesthesia, decreased reflexes and muscle atrophy.

Wet beriberi:

- Dilated cardiomyopathy is known as wet beriberi.
- There is uncontrolled vasodilation which leads to peripheral arteriovenous shunting. Hence, there is reduction in the cardiac output. The ventricular wall is thinned out due to massive dilation of the heart which later leads to congestive heart failure.

Wernicke-Korsakoff syndrome: It is characterised by combination of two disorders namely Wernicke's encephalopathy and Korsakoff's psychosis. They usually present with a triad of confusion, ataxia and nystagmus.

Symptoms:

- Ocular disturbances such as ophthalmoplegia, nystagmus
- Unsteady gait and ataxia
- Confusion and changes in mental status
- Coma and death
- Amnesia

VITAMIN B_2 (Riboflavin)

Sources

- Animal products such as milk, meat, egg, fish, etc.
- Plant products such as green leafy vegetables.

Requirement

- Male: 1.3 mg, female: 1.1 mg
- 0.6 mg per 1000 kcal of energy

Functions

- Plays an important role in oxidation–reduction reactions.
- Required in formation of many mitochondrial enzymes such as monoamine oxidase, succinyl dehydrogenase.
- Cofactor of enzymes involved in energy metabolism.

Causes of Riboflavin Deficiency

- Rice is deficient in riboflavin. Hence, the places where rice is a staple diet, vitamin B_2 deficiency may be seen.
- Malabsorption syndromes

Deficiency of Riboflavin

- Angular cheilitis
- Oral ulcers
- Sore throat
- Dry scaly skin
- Eyes become itchy, watery and sensitive to light (photophobia)

VITAMIN B_4 (Niacin)

- It is formed by combination of two compounds, namely nicotinic acid and nicotinamide.
- Deficiency of vitamin B_4 causes pellagra.
- Tryptophan is a precursor of niacin.

Sources

- Animal products such as milk, meat, fish and eggs.
- Plant products such as legumes, groundnut, cereals.

Requirement

- Male: 16 mg/day and female: 14 mg/day
- 6.6 mg/1000 kcal

Functions

- Metabolism of carbohydrates, fat and proteins.
- Required in the formation of nicotinamide adenine dinucleotide (NAD) and nicotinamide adenine dinucleotide phosphate (NADP).
- NAD and NADP are essential for oxidation–reduction reactions.
- NADP is required for glucose metabolism.
- NAD acts as a coenzyme in the metabolism of carbohydrates, proteins and fat.

Causes of Deficiency

- Alcohol consumption
- HIV patients
- Maize diet: Maize has excess amounts of leucine which interferes with the conversion of tryptophan to niacin
- Poor protein diet
- Tryphophan malabsorption
- Deficiency of pyridoxine and riboflavin

Deficiency of Niacin

It is characterised by 3Ds:
  - Diarrhoea
  - Dermatitis
  - Dementia

- **Diarrhoea:**
  - Watery in nature
  - Colon is main site of involvement
  - Mucosal ulceration and atrophy
- **Dermatitis:**
  - Exposed areas such as face, hand, foot, knee, elbow later mouth and vagina
  - Significant glossitis and stomatitis are seen.
  - Skin becomes scaly and can form fissures.
  - Glove dermatitis
  - Bilaterally symmetrical involvement
- **Dementia:** Degeneration of myelin and ganglion cells.

VITAMIN B_6 (Pyridoxine)

- Vitamin B_6 occurs in three forms:
  - Pyridoxine
  - Pyridoxal
  - Pyridoxamine
- They get converted to pyridoxal 5 phosphate in the tissue which is a coenzyme.

Sources

- Animal products such as milk, meat, fish, pork and yolk egg.
- Plant products such as legumes, vegetables.

Requirement

- Adults 2 mg/day
- Pregnancy and lactation: 2.5 mg/day

Functions

- Cofactor for enzymes in lipid and protein metabolism.
- Coenzyme for enzymes such as transaminases and carboxylase.

Causes of Deficiency

- Increased demand: Pregnancy and lactation
- Alcohol intake
- Drugs: Antitubercular drugs—isoniazid and estrogens act as antagonist and cause deficiency of pyridoxine.
- Riboflavin deficiency: Impairs pyridoxine utilization

Clinical Features with Deficiency of Pyridoxine

- Peripheral neuritis
- Similar to vitamin B_{12} deficiency

Note: Details about vitamin B_{12} can be found in topic of megaloblastic anaemia.

VITAMIN C (Ascorbic Acid)

Deficiency of vitamin C causes **scurvy**. Scurvy is a bone disease characterised by haemorrhages and healing defects in both children and adults.

History

At the end of the eighteenth century, sailors of the British Royal Navy were provided with lime and lime juices to prevent the sailors from getting scurvy during their long sojourn at sea. They were given the nickname as "limeys," because of this.

Sources

- Vitamin C is not synthesized endogenously in human beings. Therefore, we are completely dependent on the diet.
- Animal products: Liver and fish.
- Plant products: Citrus fruits such as oranges and lemons, amla, bell peppers, guava, kiwi, papaya and strawberries. Vegetables such as brussels, cabbages, spinach and potatoes.

Requirement

- Males: 90 mg and females: 75 mg.

Functions

- **Collagen synthesis:** Hydroxylation of procollagen by the activation of prolyl and lysyl hydroxylases from inactive precursors is an essential step in formation of collagen. Vitamin C deficiency will lead to inadequate hydroxylation of procollagen which will lead to unstable helical configuration and inadequate cross-linked collagen. Hence, the collagen will lack tensile strength and easily degraded by enzymatic action.
- **Antioxidant properties:** Vitamin C can scavenge free radicals directly and can act indirectly by regenerating the antioxidant form of vitamin E.

- **Prevention of atheroma:** Decreases oxidation of low density lipoproteins and hence prevents formation of atheromatous plaques.
- **Iron absorption:** Helps in absorption of iron as ascorbic acid helps in reducing ferric to ferrous form.

Causes

- Deficiency is rare.
- Elderly individuals who live alone.
- Chronic alcoholics.
- Groups of people with erratic and inadequate eating patterns.
- Patients undergoing peritoneal dialysis and haemodialysis.
- Food faddists.
- Infants who are formula fed without supplementation of vitamin C.
- Heating of food destroys vitamin C.

Clinical Features

- Bleeding manifestations due to poor tensile strength of the collagen present in the blood vessels, e.g. gum bleeding, petechiae, purpura, subperiosteal haemorrhages, conjunctival haemorrhages, rarely intracerebral bleeds.
- Wound healing is poor and delayed.
- Skeletal changes in growing children such as generalized osteopaenia, cortical thinning: "pencil-point" cortex, periosteal reaction due to repeated subperiosteal haemorrhage.
- Scorbutic rosary due to expansion of the costochondral junctions secondary to fracture occurring at costochondral junction during normal respiration.
- Wimberger's ring sign: Circular, opaque radiologic shadow surrounding epiphyseal centres of ossification as a result of bleeding.
- Frankel's line: Dense zone of provisional calcification
- Haemarthrosis
- Adults show osteopaenia and pathologic fractures.
- Infections

OBESITY

Obesity is abnormal or excessive accumulation of body fat that threatens health and results with interaction of environment/lifestyle and genetic susceptibility factors.

Body Mass Index (BMI) Criteria

1. BMI of less than 25 kg/m^2 is normal.
2. 25 to 30 kg/m^2: Overweight
3. 30–35 kg/m^2: Moderate obesity
4. 35–40 kg/m^2: Severe obesity
5. More than 40 kg/m^2: Extremely high

Causes

1. Heredity
2. Sedentary lifestyle
3. Psychological problems
4. Fat and sugar rich diet

Pathogenesis

Obesity develops from imbalance in energy production and expenditure in the body. Mutation of leptin, disorders of adiponectin and ghrelin play role in pathogenesis of obesity. Leptin is a hormone produced from adipose tissue which acts on hypothalamus and suppresses food intake. Mutation of lectin cannot do this function. Adiponectin is another hormone produced from adipocytes which has anti-inflammatory, antidiabetic, antiatherogenic and cardioprotective properties. The secretion of adiponectin is reduced in obesity. Ghrelin is produced by stomach which increases appetite and stimulates release of growth hormones. Increased amounts of ghrelin can be observed in obesity.

Consequences of Obesity

1. Diabetes mellitus type 2
2. Atherosclerosis
3. Cardiovascular and lung diseases with premature death
4. Gallbladder diseases
5. Arthritis
6. Some cancers: Breast, colon, endometrial, esophageal, hepatocellular, renal, prostate, etc.

SELF-ASSESSMENT EXERCISE

1. **Features of marasmus are:**
   A. Flaky paint dermatosis
   B. Fatty liver
   C. Normal to slightly reduced albumin
   D. Hair change

2. **Amenorrhoea is classically seen in:**
   A. Anorexia nervosa   B. Bulimia
   C. Obesity   D. Vitamin D deficiency

3. **Fat-soluble vitamins are all** *except*:
   A. Vitamin A   B. Vitamin B
   C. Vitamin D   D. Vitamin K

4. **Vitamin A deficiency may lead to all** *except*:
   A. Bitot's spot
   B. Renal and urinary bladder stones
   C. Papular dermatoses
   D. Azoospermia

5. **Vitamin D deficiency causes:**
   A. Craniotabes
   B. Pigeon breast deformity
   C. Harrison's groove
   D. All of the above

6. **Vitamin C deficiency leads to all of the following** *except*:
   A. Bleeding tendency
   B. Inadequate osteoid synthesis
   C. Impaired wound healing
   D. Rachitic rosary

7. **Keshan's disease is due to deficiency of:**
   A. Zinc   B. Selenium
   C. Copper   D. Iron

8. **False statement among the following is:**
   A. Leptin decreases food craving
   B. Ghrelin secreted from stomach activates catabolic circuits
   C. Generalised obesity poses higher risk for certain diseases than central obesity
   D. Cholelithiasis is more common in obese individual than in lean individuals

9. **Clinical features of niacin deficiency are all** *except*:
   A. Dermatitis   B. Diarrhoea
   C. Dementia   D. Dental caries

Answers

1. C   2. A   3. B   4. D   5. D   6. D   7. B   8. C
9. D

Hypersensitivity Reactions

The immune response which can cause tissue injury is called hypersensitivity. The sensitized individual is one who can mount an immune response against an antigen.

These reactions are of four types (Coombs and Gell classification). They are as below:

Type I. Immediate/IgE-mediated/anaphylactic

Type II. Antibody-dependent cell-mediated cytotoxicity

Type III. Immune complex-mediated

Type IV. T cell-mediated, delayed hypersensitivity (antibody independent)

TYPE I. IMMEDIATE/IgE MEDIATED

Type I hypersensitivity is an allergic reaction which occurs in a previously sensitized individual. The reaction is triggered by binding of an antigen to the IgE antibody on the surface of mast cells. Allergens can be introduced by ingestion, inhalation, injection or direct contact.

Mechanism (Fig. 19.1)

Type I hypersensitivity is also known as **immediate** or anaphylactic hypersensitivity. Allergen when enters for the first time, the Th2 subtype of CD4 cells are activated which secrete cytokines and stimulate B cells and plasma cells. These produce IgE antibodies.

A subsequent exposure to the same allergen, the allergen binds to the IgE antibodies and crosslinks the cell-bound IgE and triggers the release of various pharmacologically active substances. Crosslinking of IgE antibodies to the Fc-receptor of mast cells activates signals with tyrosine phosphorylation, Ca^{++} influx, degranulation and release of mediators.

The reactions have two phases. The immediate reaction causes vasodilatation, vascular leakage, angio-edema, hypotension and bronchospasm due to smooth

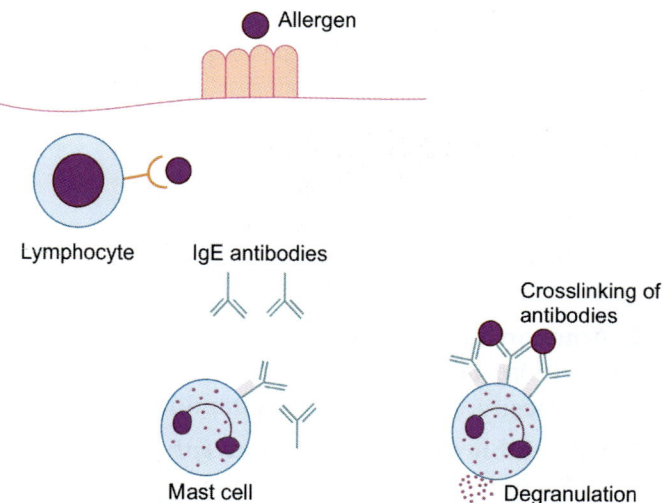

Fig. 19.1: Mechanism of type I hypersensitivity reaction (schematic)

muscle contraction or increased glandular secretions and urticaria. This reaction usually occurs within a few minutes from the time of re-exposure to the antigen or allergen. The late phase reaction may have a delayed onset (2–24 hours) after re-exposure.

Immediate effects are due to release of following chemical mediators (Table 19.1):

1. Histamine
2. Leukotrienes
3. Prostaglandins

Histamine is responsible for constriction of smooth muscles and constriction bronchioles which causes wheezing, intestinal wall contraction responsible for cramps and diarrhoea, vasodilatation which leads to oedema formation.

Late phase effects are due to eosinophils, neutrophils, basophils, monocytes and CD4 T cells present in the tissues. Eosinophils play a major role releasing

Table 19.1	Mediators in type I hypersensitivity
Mediator	**Effects**
Histamine	Increased vascular permeability and smooth muscle contraction
Bradykinin	Increased vascular permeability and smooth muscle contraction
Prostaglandin	Vasodilatation, smooth muscle contraction, platelet aggregation
Leukotrienes	Increased vascular permeability and contraction of smooth muscle cells
Cytokines (IL-1,TNFα)	Systemic anaphylaxis
Inflammatory cells (neutrophils, basophils)	Release proteases and tissue destruction
Eosinophils	Releases proteases, major basic protein and eosinophil cationic protein and tissue destruction

proteolytic agents, major basic protein and eosinophil cationic protein which damage the tissues.

The reaction may be either local or systemic. Symptoms vary from mild irritation to sudden death from anaphylactic shock. In systemic anaphylaxis, the allergen is introduced into bloodstream. Within minutes of exposure, in a sensitized host, there is systemic vasodilatation and fall of blood pressure with anaphylactic shock leading to collapse and death. Treatment usually involves epinephrine, antihistamines and corticosteroids.

Note: Hypersensitivity due to drugs, like pencillin, can be acute or subacute which may be mediated by IgE (Type I) or due to IgG antibodies (Type III), respectively. Acute reactions in the form of sudden anaphylaxis occur within a few minutes to hours due to preformed IgE antibodies and may take less dramatic picture due to preformed IgG antibody formation of 7–10 days.

Some examples of localised type I reactions are:
1. Familial predisposition to localized reaction—atopy skin
2. Eczema
3. Allergic asthma
4. Allergic conjunctivitis
5. Allergic rhinitis (hay fever)
6. Angioedema
7. Urticaria (hives)

Some examples of systemic anaphylaxis are:
1. Reaction to pencillin, sulfonamides, local anaesthetics, salicylates, etc.
2. Certain venoms, vaccines
3. Insect bites
4. Antigen from foods like nuts, eggs, peas, beans, milk sea food, etc.

TYPE II. ANTIBODY-MEDIATED CELL DESTRUCTION

The type II hypersensitivity is caused due to the antibodies which are directed against the antigens on the patient's own cell surfaces or tissue components.

The antigens recognized in this way may be either of intrinsic or extrinsic origin. The cytotoxic, cell damaging response occurs when IgG and/or IgM antibodies bind to these antigens or some drugs adsorbed on the surface of cells (RBCs).

Mechanism (Fig. 19.2)

1. **Opsonisation and phagocytosis of antigen and antibody bound cells:** The cells like RBCs, platelets, which are bound with autoantibodies with or without complement, they are phagocytosed by neutrophils and macrophages. NK cells (CD16 Fc receptor of NK cells) recognize and bind to cell bound antibody and release cytolytic enzymes—perforins and proteases. These are also called granzymes. The cells die by lysis. Phagocytosis by NK cells plays a crucial role in antibody dependent cell-mediated cytotoxicity (ADCC). Macrophages, neutrophils and eosinophils also can mediate ADCC.

2. **Complement-mediated lysis:** Can be mediated by antibodies of the IgM or IgG classes and complement, most often the antibodies are of IgG class. Cells bound with antigen and antibody form complexes activate the classical pathway of complement for eliminating cells presenting foreign antigens with formation of membrane attack complex (e.g. blood transfusion reactions). As a result, mediators of acute inflammation are generated at the site and membrane attack complex causes cell lysis and death. The reaction takes a few minutes to hours.

3. **Endogenous/exogenous antigens or haptens** can attach to cell membranes also lead to type II hypersensitivity.
   Examples:
   a. Drug-induced haemolytic anaemia
   b. Granulocytopenia
   c. Thrombocytopenia

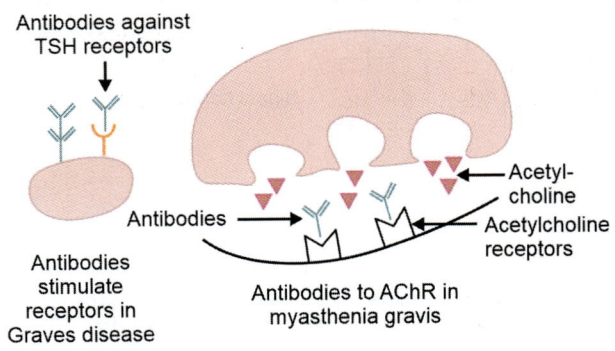

Fig. 19.2: Mechanism of type II reaction (schematic)

4. Antibodies bound to cell surface cause functional derangement (e.g. Graves disease and myasthenia gravis). Diagnostic tests include detection of circulating antibody against the tissues involved and the presence of antibody and complement in the lesion (biopsy) by immunofluorescence.

Type II hypersensitivity reactions are:
    i. Autoimmune haemolytic anaemia
    ii. Drug-induced haemolytic anaemia
    iii. Pernicious anaemia
    iv. Immune thrombocytopenia
    v. Transfusion reactions
    vi. Haemolytic disease of newborn
    vii. Hashimoto's thyroiditis
    viii. Graves' disease
    ix. Myasthenia gravis
    x. Farmer's lung
    xi. Pemphigus vulgaris
    xii. Rheumatic heart disease
    xiii. Malaria (reaction to parasite-derived antigen)
    xiv. Goodpasture disease
    xv. Hyperacute graft rejection

MYASTHENIA GRAVIS

This is acquired autoimmune disease characterised by muscle fatigue and is caused by circulating antibodies to acetylcholine (ACh) receptors at the myoneural junction. It affects all races, F:M ratio 2:1. Begins in young adults, can occur at any ages. Thymic hyperplasia is found in 65% and thymoma in 15% of the cases.

Pathogenesis (Fig. 19.3)

There are antibodies to ACh receptors of motor end plate and there is loss of function of receptors.

These patients may be associated with other autoimmune diseases.

The loss of functional receptors can be:
1. Increasing the internalization and degradation of the receptors, and/or
2. Blocking the binding of ACh to its receptors
   - The antibodies impair the transmission of ACh across the junction. Hence, weakness and fatigue is seen in the disease.
   - With the antigen antibody formation at the receptor site, complement is activated and disrupts the muscle cell membrane. Thymus is believed to be site of acetylcholine antibody development.
   - This is type II hypersensitivity reaction.

Pathology

Muscle biopsy may reveal atrophy of type II muscle fibres and focal collections of lymphocytes in muscle fascicles.

Clinical Features

Following are the clinical features:
1. There can be profound muscle weakness and fatiguability. Characteristically weakness begins in ocular and cranial muscles and then to limb muscles.
2. Respiratory muscles and respiratory functions are affected maximally.
3. Weakness of extraocular muscles, drooping of eyelids (ptosis), and double vision are the common features.
4. There can be generalized muscle weakness over the course of disease period and muscles of extremities may get affected.

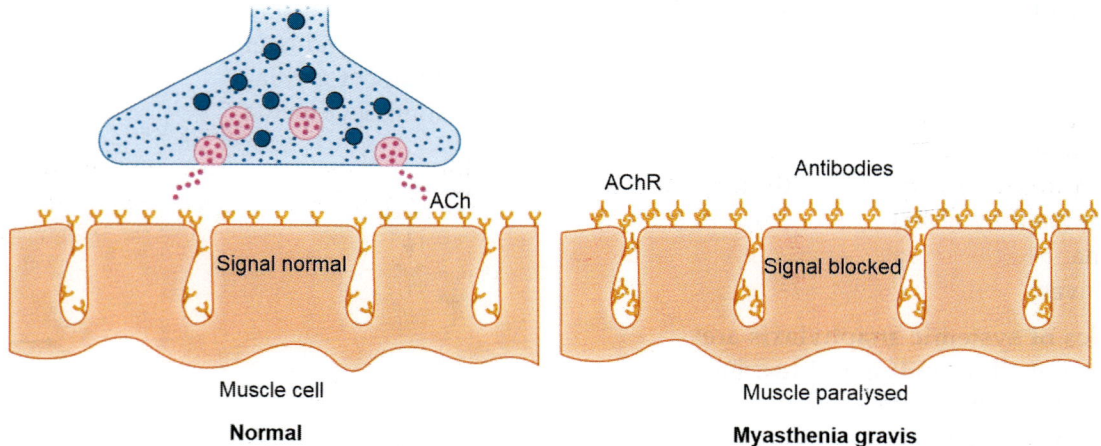

Note: Antibodies to post-synaptic receptor at NMJ. It is type II hypersensitivity and reduce AChR over the time. Muscle signal is blocked. This is complement-mediated destruction of receptor. The receptors are internalised and degraded. Thus AChR are reduced

Fig. 19.3: Pathogenesis in myasthenia gravis

5. There will be reduced muscle strength of electro-physiological stimulation.
6. Patients improve with anticholinesterase agents causing increased levels of ACh at neuromuscular synapse.
7. Sensory and autonomic functions are not affected.

Treatment

1. 95% patients show 5-year survival rate with acetyl-cholinesterase inhibitors, e.g. neostigmine, pyrido-stigmine, IV immunoglobulins, plasmapheresis, and thymic resection along with ventilatory support.
2. Thymectomy usually recommended when patients fail to respond to medication and particularly when less than 45 years old age.

Investigations

1. Repetitive stimulation during nerve conduction shows decremental response, if the muscle is cinically affected.
2. Muscle-specific kinase antibodies may be positive when AChR antibodies are negative.
3. CT scan for thymoma.
4. Screen for associated autoimmune disorders.

Management

- Action of acetylcholine is prolonged by inhibiting AChE (pyridostigmine, neostigmine).
- Short-term IV immunoglobulins can reduce anti-bodies.
- Plasma exchange removes antibodies.

Long-term therapy: Corticosteroids, immuno-suppression and thymectomy.

TYPE III. IMMUNE COMPLEX MEDIATED

In this hypersensitivity reaction, immune complexes (aggregations of antigens and IgG/IgM/IgA anti-bodies) formed in the blood and are deposited in various tissues (typically skin, kidneys, lung and joints). The antigen may be exogenous (microbial protein/animal origin) or endogenous (e.g. nucleoprotein). This may trigger an immune response with activation of classical pathway of complement. The reaction takes hours to days to develop. This is also known as **immune complex disease** which occurs when immune complexes (Ag-Ab complexes) are not removed from circulation.

Mechanism (Fig. 19.4)

Type III hypersensitivity reaction involve IgG and IgM antibodies with antigens to form immune complexes. These are intermediate sized and are difficult to be

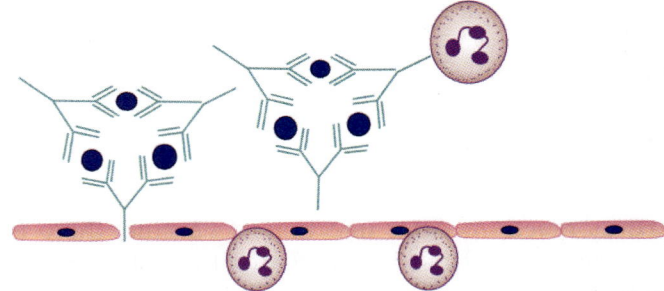

Fig. 19.4: Mechanism of type III hypersensitivity (schematic)

removed from the circulation by the process of phagocytosis.

These antigen–antibody complexes lodge in the capillaries between the endothelial cells and the base-ment membrane. These antigen–antibody complexes activate the classical complement pathway leading to vasodilatation. The complement proteins and antigen–antibody complexes attract leucocytes to the area. The leucocytes degranulate and release various pro-inflammatory chemical mediators and promote massive inflammation. This can lead to tissue death and haemorrhage.

The examples of type III immune complex-mediated diseases are:

1. Autoimmune diseases: SLE (lupus nephritis), rheumatoid arthritis
2. Drug reactions: Allergy to penicillin and sulfonamides
3. Infectious diseases: Post-streptococcal glomerulo-nephritis, hepatitis, infectious mononucleosis, malaria, trypanosomiasis
4. Vasculitis: Polyarteritis nodosa, necrotizing vasculitis
5. Serum sickness (arthritis, vasculitis, nephritis)
6. Arthus reaction (cutaneous vasculitis)

Serum sickness: This develops from injection of large amounts of heterologous or foreign proteins from other species, hapten or serum (e.g. anti-snake venom, anti-rabies vaccine and some medications). It takes 1–2 weeks for the development of antibodies. The simulta-neous presence of antigen and antibodies leads to formation of immune complexes which are deposited in various tissues giving rise to systemic effects. It is Type III hypersensitivity reaction with formation of immune complex deposits. The following are the features in these patients:

1. Systemic manifestations with fever and malaise
2. Diffuse erythema
3. Urticaria and itching
4. Subcutaneous oedema
5. Oedema and spasm of larynx
6. Athralgia
7. Features related to vasculits

8. Features related to nephritis
9. Wheezing
10. Tachycardia
11. CVS: Pericarditis, myocarditis
12. GI complaints
13. Hypotension and hypovolemic shock

Arthus reaction: After injection of vaccine, there is localized vasculitis due to deposition of immune complexes containing IgG antibodies and complement. There can be severe pain, swelling, induration, oedema, haemorrhage and occasionally necrosis after 4–12 hours of injection. It is type III hypersensitivity reaction.

Following are the treatment options:
1. Steroids
2. Immunosuppressive therapy

TYPE IV. HYPERSENSITIVITY (T Cell-mediated/ Delayed Hypersensitivity)

This is a cell-mediated response or also called delayed type of hypersensitivity. This takes several days to develop. CD4 Th1 helper T cells recognize the antigen in association with MHC class II histocompatibilty complex on the surface of antigen presenting cells (macrophages). The antigen presenting cells release IL-12 which stimulates further recruitment of Th1 CD4 T cells. The activated lymphocytes release interferon gamma which causes cell destruction by CD8 cells and macrophage activation. The activated macrophages release TNF and other mediators which convert macrophages to epithelioid cells and Langhans type of giant cell formation (Fig. 19.5). Examples include:
1. Lesions in tuberculosis
2. Lesions in tuberculoid leprosy

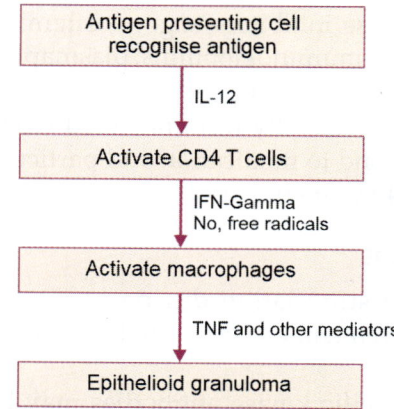

Fig. 19.5: Mechanism of type IV hypersensitivity reaction (schematic)

Note: Also refer to granulomatous inflammation.

SELF-ASSESSMENT EXERCISE

1. **Which of the following reactions is responsible for myasthenia gravis?**
   A. Type I HS reaction   B. Type II HS reaction
   C. Type III HS reaction   D. Type IV HS reaction

2. **Which of the following reactions is responsible for acute post-streptococcal glomerulonephritis?**
   A. Type I HS reaction   B. Type II HS reaction
   C. Type III HS reaction   D. Type IV HS reaction

3. **Which of the following reactions is responsible for blood transfusion reaction?**
   A. Type I HS reaction   B. Type II HS reaction
   C. Type III HS reaction   D. Type IV HS reaction

4. **Previously sensitized cell, binding of antigen with IgE antibody is:**
   A. Type I HS reaction   B. Type II HS reaction
   C. Type III HS reaction   D. Type IV HS reaction

5. **Which is antibody-mediated HS?**
   A. Type I HS reaction   B. Type II HS reaction
   C. Type III HS reaction   D. All of the above

6. **Which is cell-mediated HS?**
   A. Type I HS reaction   B. Type II HS reaction
   C. Type III HS reaction   D. Type IV HS reaction

7. **Stevens-Johnson syndrome:**
   A. Type I HS reaction   B. Type II HS reaction
   C. Type III HS reaction   D. Type IV HS reaction

8. **Acute haemolytic transfusion reaction is:**
   A. Type I HS reaction   B. Type II HS reaction
   C. Type III HS reaction   D. Type IV HS reaction

9. **In Type I HS, following are true *except*:**
   A. Allergen crosslinks the sensitized mast cell and release of various pharmacologically active substances in second exposure
   B. First exposure to allergen
   C. IgE binds FCR on mast cells
   D. First exposure mast cell are sensitized and cross-links with allergen

10. **Omalizumab can produce which of the following?**
   A. Type I HS reaction   B. Type II HS reaction
   C. Type III HS reaction   D. Type IV HS reaction

Answers

1. B	2. C	3. B	4. A	5. D	6. D	7. C	8. B
9. D	10. A						

Diseases of Immune System

AUTOIMMUNE DISEASES: MECHANISM

Definition

Developing an immune reaction to self-antigen is auto-immunity.

In normal health, an individual does not mount an immune response to a specific self-antigens. This unresponsiveness is called immunological tolerance. The breakdown of self-tolerance leads to development of autoimmunity.

Several mechanisms exist to prevent immune reaction against one's own antigens. These are broadly divided into (Table 20.1):

1. Central tolerance (clonal elimination or deletion)
2. Peripheral tolerance.

Central Tolerance

1. Central tolerance (Fig. 20.1) refers to deletion of self-reactive T and B cells during their maturation. This occurs during lymphocyte development in thymus

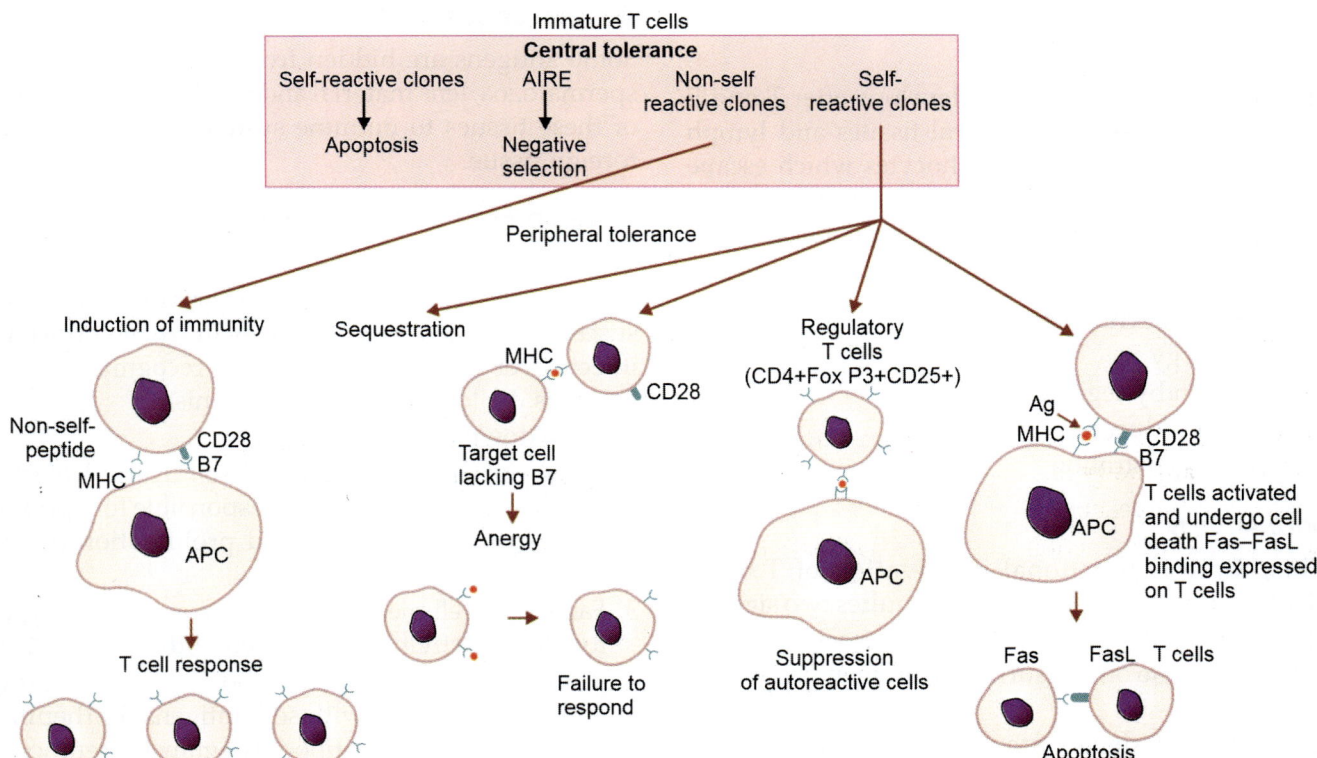

Fig. 20.1: Central and peripheral tolerance

Table 20.1	Differences between central and peripheral tolerance	
	Central tolerance	**Peripheral tolerance**
Origin	Thymus and bone marrow	Peripheral tissue
Mechanism	Clonal deletion of self-reacting cells AIRE	Clonal anergy Activation induced cell death Regulatory T cells + Antigen sequestration

(T cells) and bone marrow (B cells). The T and B cells which recognize self-antigens (MHC molecules bound to peptides of self-origin) are selected thus preventing autoimmunity.

Autoreactive (self) protein antigens are processed and presented by thymic antigen presenting cells (APC) in association with self-MHC. Any developing T cells that express a receptor are negatively selected and peripheral T cell pool is depleted of self-reactive T cells by apoptosis.

2. Another mechanism exists in central tolerance, i.e. autoimmune regulator (AIRE), a transcription factor prevents the immune system from attacking self-antigen and self-antigen recognizing T cells are negatively selected. AIRE gene mutations can lead to autoimmune, polyendocrinopathy, candidiasis and ectodermal dystrophy (APECED). These patients have autoimmune destruction of endocrine organs, fungal infection and dental abnormalities.

3. B cell receptors editing: With this mechanism, reactive B cells become less immunogenic.

Peripheral Tolerance

Peripheral tolerance (Fig. 20.1) develops after T and B cells mature and enter peripheral tissues and lymph nodes. Those self-reactive lymphocytes which escape negative selection in thymus, several mechanisms in the peripheral tissue exist to silence such autoreactive T cells.

The different mechanisms are:
a. Clonal anergy
b. Suppression by regulatory T cells
c. Activation-induced cell death
d. Antigen sequestration

Clonal Anergy

In this, there is functional inactivation of T cells. Activation of antigen specific T cell requires two signals.

1. Recognition of peptide antigen in association with MHC molecule on the surface of antigen presenting cell.

2. Costimulation signals provided by the APC.

T cell-associated molecules such as CD 28 must bind to their ligands B7 on APC. If the APC does not bear CD28 ligand, i.e. B7, negative signal is generated to induce anergy.

Suppression by Regulatory T Cells

Populations of lymphocytes, called regulatory T cells, have an ability to downregulate function of autoreactive T cells. This is mediated by secretion of cytokines. These T cells express CD 25 and FOX P3 CD4 +ve. T cells of Th2 type are the regulatory cells to mediate their action by cytokines like IL-4 and IL-10.

Activation-Induced Cell Death

T cells that are repeatedly stimulated by antigens undergo apoptosis. Death receptor Fas (CD 95), a member of TNF receptor family, is expressed on CD4 +ve T cells. The activated T cells express Fas ligand (Fas L).

Binding of Fas by Fas L induces apoptosis of activated T cells and thus the autoreactive T cells are deleted at the periphery. Self-reactive B cells are also deleted by Fas L expressed on helper T cells.

Antigen Sequestration

Some antigens are hidden from immune system, e.g. spermatozoa, lens material and myelin tissue. Exposure of these tissues to immune system will be treated as foreign tissue.

Development of Autoimmunity

The breakdown of self-tolerance and development of autoimmunity is related to inheritance of various susceptibility genes and changes in tissue induced by infection or injury that makes the recognition of self-antigens. Following are the mechanisms:

1. Breakdown of T cell anergy.

2. Failure of activation induced cell death: Defects in Fas-FasL system which are responsible for apoptosis may lead to persistence and proliferation of autoreactive T cells.

3. Failure of T cell-mediated suppression: Reduced regulatory T cell activity is associated with autoimmunity.

4. Molecular mimicry: Antibodies against foreign antigens crossreact with self-antigens. In rheumatic heart disease, the antibodies against streptococcal bacterial antigens crossreact with antigens of cardiac muscle which is known as molecular mimicry.

5. Polyclonal lymphocyte activation: B cells directly get activated by complex substances that contain many antigenic sites.
6. Release of sequestered antigens.
7. Exposure of cryptic antigens.

Classification of Autoimmune Diseases

Systemic:
a. Systemic lupus erythematosus
b. Rheumatoid arthritis
c. Sjögren's syndrome
d. Systemic sclerosis (scleroderma)
e. Inflammatory myopathies
f. Polyarteritis nodosa

Organ-specific:
a. AIHA
b. Autoimmune thrombocytopenia
c. Atrophic gastritis
d. Goodpasture syndrome
e. Insulin deficiency DM
f. Graves disease
g. Myasthenia gravis
h. Hashimoto's thyroiditis
i. Inflammatory bowel diseases
j. Vitiligo
k. Primary biliary cirrhosis
l. Autoimmune hepatitis

SYSTEMIC LUPUS ERYTHEMATOSUS

Systemic lupus erythematosus (SLE) is a multisystem disease of autoimmune origin with protean manifestations. It may involve many organs of the body. It principally affects skin, kidneys, serosal membranes, joints and heart. Clinically, it has unpredictable, remitting and relapsing disease of acute or insidious onset.

Prevalence

1:2500 persons, F : M ratio is 10:1.

Etiology

The exact etiology is unknown. But has several predisposing factors.
1. Heredity: Inherited susceptibility genes, higher concordance in monozygotic twins
2. Genetics: Mutations of C1q, C2 and C4
3. HLA-DQ locus has been linked.
4. Sex hormone status: Estrogen excess with reduced androgens
5. Drugs like hydralazine, isoniazid, procainamide, pencillamine

6. Environmental triggers: Ultraviolet rays
7. Epstein-Barr virus
8. Overproduction of cytokine IFN-α
9. Failure of T and B cells tolerance to self-antigens
10. Defective clearance of nuclear antigens released by apoptotic cells

Mechanism of Tissue Injury

The potential etiological factors are either to initiate acquired sensitization to self-antigens or there is defect in failure to maintain self-tolerance. The helper T and B cells specific for self-antigens are activated. There is production of autoantibodies which can damage tissues directly or in the form of immune complex deposits.
1. The injury is mainly due to deposition of immune complexes (Type III hypersensitivity).
   DNA—anti-DNA complexes are detected in glomeruli. Low levels of complement and granular complement deposits support the role of immune complexes.
2. Auto-Abs to RBCs, white blood cells and platelets promote phagocytosis and destruction by type II hypersensitivity.

Spectrum of Antibodies

Spectrum of antibodies include: Antibodies to nuclear and cytoplasm components, cell membrane of RBCs and to proteins with phospholipids. There will be antinuclear antibodies directed against nuclear antigens and these can be grouped into:
1. Antibodies to DNA (double or single stranded)
2. Antibodies to histones
3. Antibodies to non-histone proteins bound to RNA
4. Antibodies to nucleolar antigens.

Indirect immunofluorescence is the technique used to detect these antibodies, the patterns being:
a. Homogenous/diffuse staining: Antibodies to histones and dsDNA
b. Rim or peripheral staining pattern supports antibodies to dsDNA
c. Speckled pattern: Antibodies to non-DNA nuclear material such as histones and ribonucleoproteins (RNPs).

If the damaged nuclei are exposed to ANAs, DNA can bind to ANAs and this is called **positive LE cell phenomenon.** After binding to ANAs, nuclear material becomes homogenous and loose chromatin pattern. These are **LE bodies or haematoxylin bodies**. The LE cell is any phagocytic leucocyte that has engulfed the denatured nucleus of an injured cell.

Other autoantibodies:

1. Anti-Ro
2. Anti-La
3. Anti-Sm
4. Antiphospholipid antibody: This is present in 40–50% of the SLE patients. This can give false positive test for syphilis, thrombotic tendency and recurrent abortions possibly due to placental thrombosis or poor implantation. These have prolonged APTT test.
5. Red cell antibodies: Cause autoimmune haemolytic anaemia.
6. Antibodies to WBCs and pletelets: Neutropenia, thrombocytopenia.
7. Rheumatoid factor may be positive in Class IV and Class V kidney involvement.
8. Cell or organ specific antibodies: Antibodies to mitochondria, smooth muscle, gastric parietal cells (pernicious anaemia) can be present.

The most diagnostic amongst these investigations are anti-dsDNA antibodies and anti-Smith antibody. Serum complement levels will be low.

Clinical presentation of SLE is variable and symptoms may overlap with rheumatoid arthritis, polymyositis and other autoimmune diseases. Hence, diagnosis has to be established using criteria given in Table 20.2.

Clinical Features

SLE affects predominantly the young females, in 2nd and 4th decade of life, i.e. during child-bearing age. They may present with:

1. Butterfly rash over cheeks: Painful, itchy, erythema-tous rashes occur on cheeks sparing nasolabial folds.

Table 20.2	Criteria for diagnosis of SLE (1997 revised criteria for SLE)[14]
1. Malar rash: Flat or raised erythematous lesions over the malar eminences
2. Discoid rash: Erythematous raised patches with keratotic scaling and follicular plugging
3. Photosensitivity
4. Oral ulcers
5. Arthritis
6. Serositis
7. Renal disorder: Persistent proteinuria and cellular casts
8. Neurological disorder: Seizures and psychosis
9. Haematological disorder: Haemolytic anaemia, leukopenia, lymphopenia, thrombocytopenia
10. Immunological disorder: Anti-DNA antibody, anti-Sm, anti-phospholipid antibody
11. Antinuclear antibody: IF and assay positive

Note: Four or more of the 11 criteria to be present to diagnose SLE

2. Arthritis: Occurs in 90% of the cases, morning stiffness.
3. Pleuritic chest pain
4. Photosensitivity
5. Raynaud's phenomenon
6. May present as PUO
7. Renal involvement: Abnormal urinary findings—haematuria, proteinuria, casts
   Renal failure and may present as nephrotic syndrome.
8. Neuropsychiatric manifestations including psychosis
9. Cardiovascular manifestations
10. Haematological disorders

Pathology of Systemic Lupus Erythematosus

The morphological changes in SLE are variable. The most characteristic morphological changes in SLE are due to deposition of immune complexes. The following are the changes.

Acute necrotizing vasculitis: The small arteries and arterioles are commonly affected. There is arteritis, wall has necrosis, fibrinoid deposits containing antibodies, DNA, complement components and fibrinogen. Transmural and perivascular leucocytic infiltrate is also present. In chronic stages, vessels show fibrous thickening with narrowing of lumina.

Skin changes: Erythematous rash may be annular or psoriasiform, or discoid form with hyperkeratosis, hydropic degeneration of basal layer and periadnexal lymphocytic infiltrate. These patients may have scarring or non-scarring with alopecia. Direct IF shows irregular band of coalescing clumps of IgG or IgM and complements (C5b, C6, C7, C8 and C9) in 90% of the cases.

Kidney involvement is common and most important finding in SLE. Renal failure is the common cause of death in these patients.

According to WHO classification, six patterns are recognized and these are:[15]

- Class I: Minimal mesangial lupus nephritis (normal by light microscopy)
- Class II (A and B): Mesangial lupus glomerulo-nephritis
- Class III: Focal proliferative glomerulonephritis
- Class IV: Diffuse proliferative glomerulonephritis
- Class V: Membranous glomerulonephritis
- Class VI: Advanced-stage lupus nephritis

The details of the different types of renal involvement in SLE (lupus nephritis) are given below.

1. Minimal mesangial lupus nephritis (Class I): This is normal by light microscopy, but has mesangial immune deposits (Fig. 20.2).

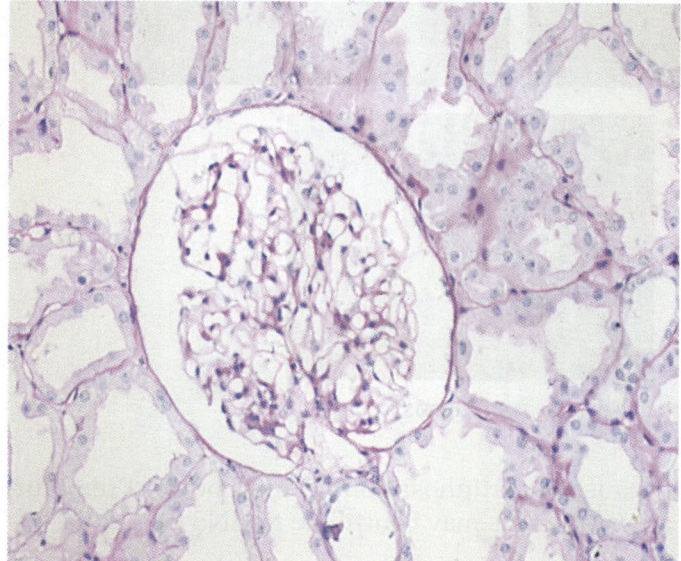

Fig. 20.2: Class I lupus nephritis. The glomerulus appears mildly enlarged unremarkable morphology resembling minimal change disease (PAS, 200×)

2. Mesangial lupus glomerulonephritis (Class II): This is seen in 10–25% of SLE cases and associated with mild symptoms. Class IIA has minimal changes on light microscopy and IF has immune complexes. Class IIB shows slight increase in the cellularity of mesangial cells and increase in matrix. The immune complex deposits are seen in the mesangium (Fig. 20.3).

3. Focal proliferative glomerulonephritis (Class III): This accounts for 20–35% of the cases. This is associated with mild haematuria and proteinuria. A few glomeruli and segments of glomeruli show necrosis, fibrinoid necrosis and neutrophilic infiltrate. Fragmented nuclei may be visible as haematoxylin bodies. May show focal interstitial inflammation and oedema. Immune complexes and complement are evident with IF in mesangium and subendothelial region.

4. Diffuse proliferative glomerulonephritis (Class IV): This is the most serious form and accounts for 35–60% of the cases.

These patients have haematuria, moderate to severe proteinuria, hypertension and renal insufficiency. Most glomeruli show hypercellularity with mesangial and endothelial cell proliferation. Epithelial crescents may fill the Bowmans space. With extensive disease, the capillary wall is thickened giving wire loop on light microscopy (Fig. 20.4).

Electron microscopy shows electron dense subendothelial deposits. Granular IF staining is seen with immunoglobulins (IgG) and complement (C3 and C1q are frequently found). When C3, C1q, IgM and IgA are present along with IgG it is termed as "Full House" (Figs 20.5A to E). These may be subendothelial/mesangial and sometimes subepithelial or membranous deposits. Fibrin is found in cresentic and necrotising lesions.

5. Membranous glomerulonephritis (Class V): These accounts for 10–15% of the SLE cases, patients have severe proteinuria and overt nephrotic syndrome. The capillary wall is thickened spike and dome patternon silver stain. There is deposition of basement membrane like material and immune complexes.

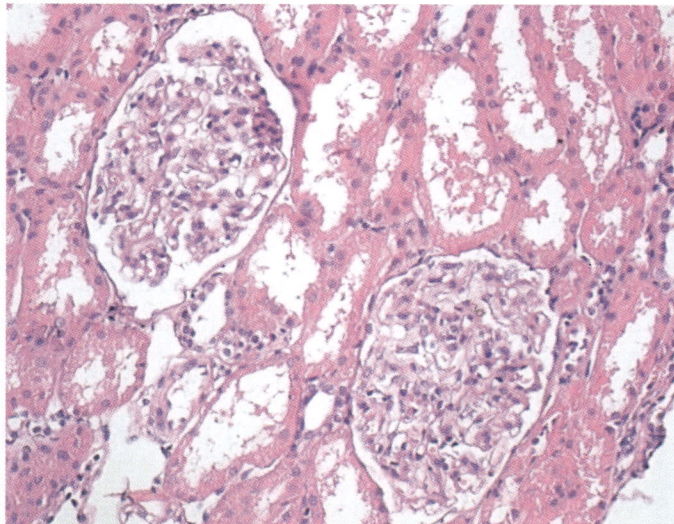

Fig. 20.3: Class II lupus nephritis. The glomerulus appears mildly enlarged with mild mesangial expansion and mild hypercellularity (HE, 200×)

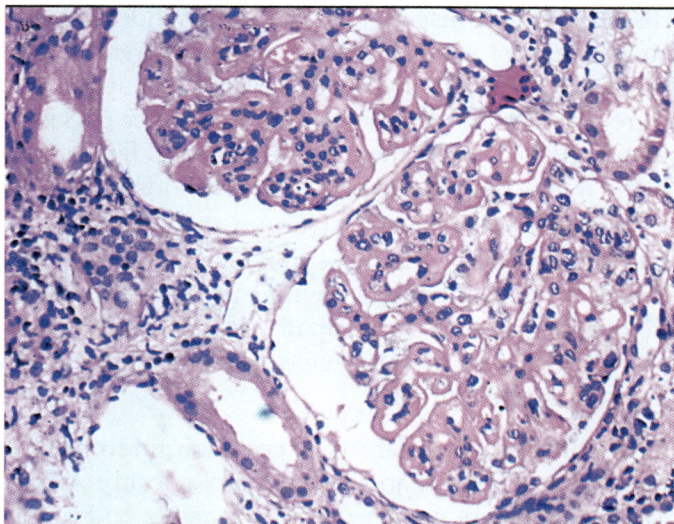

Fig. 20.4: Class IV lupus nephritis, the glomeruli have lobular accentuation with capillary lumina lined by thickened membranes (wire loop lesion) (PAS, 200×)

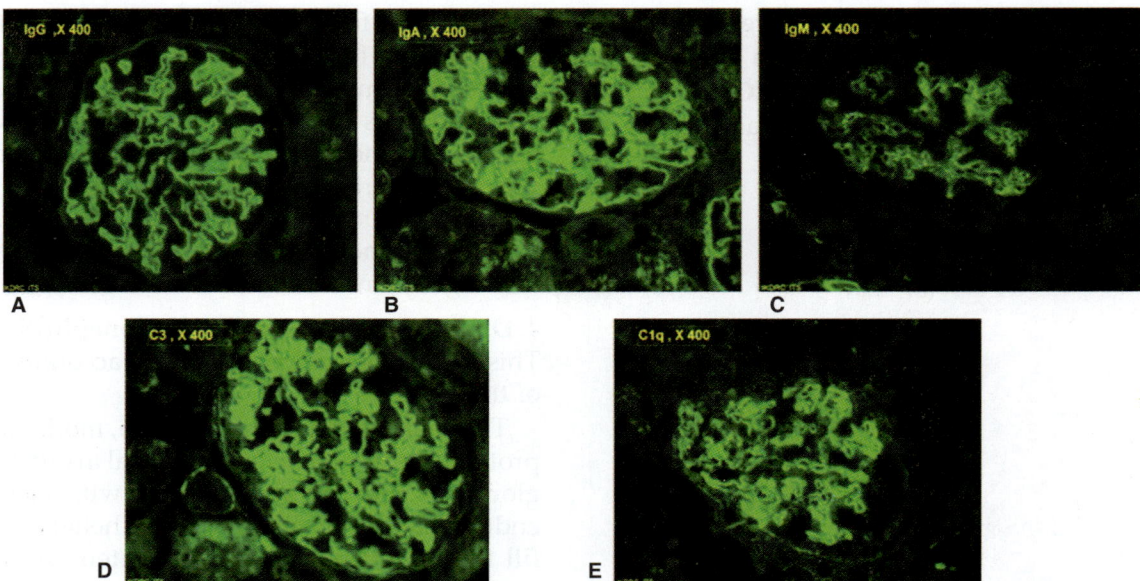

Figs 20.5A to E: IF with 'Full House' positivity in Class IV lupus nephritis

6. Advanced-stage lupus nephritis (Class VI): In this, more than 90% of the glomeruli will show (global glomerulosclerosis). There is absence of active glomerular disease. There is interstitial fibrosis, inflammation and tubular atrophy. There is small amounts of immune complexes in mesangium and capillary walls. These patients have proteinuria and renal insufficiency.

Class VI may represent the advanced stage of chronic class III, class IV, or class V lupus nephritis. Without the use of sequential renal biopsies, it may not be possible to comment on which class of renal disease has advanced to sclerotic glomerular lesions.

With clinical findings of mild haematuria and/or proteinuria, the renal lesions may be in class I or II disease; when presents like nephritic syndrome with some degree of acute or rapidly progressive renal failure the lesions may be of class III or IV; when appears as pure nephrotic syndrome the disease may be of class V histology; and when there is chronic renal failure probably it may be sclerosing advanced lesions of class VI.

Joint involvement is frequent. There is early morning stiffness with tenosynovitis. Swelling of joint is rare and non-specific synovitis may be present. Joint deformity (Jaccoud's arthropathy) may occur. Erosion and destruction of cartilage as seen in rheumatoid arthritis is uncommon.

CNS changes: These are very common findings with neurological deficits and neuropsycological problems. These lesions are mainly due to ischaemia and micro-infarcts. Small vessel angiopathy with intimal proliferation is the most frequent lesion. Frank vasculitis is less common. Angiopathy is mainly due to thrombosis because of antiphospholipid antibodies. Premature atherosclerosis may contribute to CNS ischaemia.

Other Findings in SLE

1. **Spleen** may be moderately enlarged.
2. **Heart** shows endocarditis, myocarditis and pericarditis. There is infiltration mainly by mononuclear cells. The valvular lesions are called **Libman-Sacks endocarditis.** These are 1–3 mm warty deposits on either surface of the leaflets.
3. **Serositis:** There is pericarditis and pleuritis with effusion.
4. **Lung:** Pneumonitis, atelectasis, pulmonary fibrosis may occur.
5. **Haematological changes:** There can be neutropenia, lymphopenia, thrombocytopenia and autoimmune haemolytic anaemia.
6. Many other organs and tissue may be involved.

Clinical Course of the Disease

Following is the course of the disease:

1. The clinical course is variable. Even without therapy, some patients will have indolent course with skin manifestations and/or with mild haematuria.
2. Some progress rapidly and die within a few months.
3. The disease may have remissions and relapses for years and decades.
4. Acute flare-ups are controlled by steroids and immunosuppressive drugs.
5. With therapy, 90% 5-year survival and 80% 10-year survival can be expected.
6. Renal failure, recurrent infections and CNS involvement are the causes of death in SLE patients.

Criteria for classification of SLE (2012 SLICC SLE criteria):[16]

SLICC: Systemic Lupus International Collaborating Clinics.

Requirements: More than 4 criteria (at least 1 clinical and 1 laboratory criteria) or biopsy proven lupus nephritis with positive ANA or anti-DNA.

Clinical Criteria

1. Acute cutaneous lupus
2. Chronic cutaneous lupus
3. Oral or nasal ulcers
4. Non-scarring alopecia
5. Arthritis
6. Serositis
7. Renal disorder
8. Neurological disorder
9. Haemolytic anaemia
10. Leukopenia or lymphopenia
11. Thrombocytopenia (<1,00,000/cmm)

Immunological Criteria

1. ANA
2. Anti-DNA
3. Anti-Sm
4. Antiphospholipid Abs
5. Low complement (C3, C4, CH50) levels
6. Direct Coombs' test (in absence of haemolytic anaemia)

RHEUMATOID ARTHRITIS

Rheumatoid arthritis (RA) is a systemic, chronic inflammatory disease, affecting many tissues, principally affecting the joints to produce non-suppurative proliferative synovitis which progress and destroys articular cartilage and underlying bone causing deformities. When extra-articular organs are involved like skin, heart, blood vessels, muscles and lungs, RA may resemble SLE or scleroderma.

Pathogenesis

The disease is initiated by CD4 T helper cells, possibly to microbial and self-antigen.

The activated T cells produce cytokines (IL-1, TNF) which are responsible for the following:

i. The cytokines activate macrophage and other cells in the joint space, releasing degenerative enzyme and other factor for inflammation.
ii. Activated B cells—release antibodies which may be directed against self-antigen in joint.
iii. Cytokines promote macrophage activation and proliferation of synovial cells and fibroblasts. Cytokines also stimulate synovium and chondrocytes to release matrix degradative and proteolytic enzymes.

- T cells in RA express RANK ligand which induces osteoclast differentiation and activation which plays role in bone resorption.
- RA factor (IgM/IgG) is an autoantibody. This may lead to immune reactions of joints and other tissue leading to inflammation and tissue damage.
- The patients have family history with disease affecting first degree relatives and high concordance rate in monozygotic twins. HLA-DR4 and polymorphism in PTPN22 gene is common in RA.
- Infectious agents like EBV, *Borrelia*, *Mycoplasma* and parvovirus have role in RA which may activate T and B cells.

Pathology

RA presents as symmetrical arthritis, principally involving the small joints of hands and feet, ankles, knees, wrists, elbows, and shoulders. Proximal interphalangeal and metacarpophalangeal joints are involved, but distal interphalangeal joints are spared. Upper cervical spine may be involved. Hip joint is rarely involved.

Microscopy shows following features:

i. Synovial cell hyperplasia
ii. The synovium is infiltrated by CD4+ T cells, plasma cells, and macrophages.
iii. There is increased vascularity.
iv. Dense perivascular inflammatory cell infiltrate (frequently forming lymphoid follicles)
v. There is granulation tissue.
vi. Organizing fibrin and neutrophils on the synovial surface and in the joint space.
vii. There is increased osteoclast activity in the underlying bone, leading to synovial penetration and bone erosion.

The proliferating synovial lining cells admixed with inflammatory cells, granulation tissue, and fibrous connective tissue is called "**pannus**".

The synovium is oedematous and has villous projections. There is fibrinoid necrosis with palisade of macrophages and rimmed by granulation tissue and lymphocytes. In severe cases, periarticular soft tissue oedema develops with fusiform swelling of involved joints. The articular cartilage is eroded and destroyed. The subarticular bone also destroyed. Eventually, the pannus fills the joint space.

There is effusion in the joints and juxta-articular osteopenia with erosions and narrowing of the joint space and loss of articular cartilage. There is destruction of tendons, ligaments, and joint capsules forming deformity with radial deviation of the wrist, ulnar deviation of the fingers, and flexion-hyperextension abnormalities of the fingers (swan-neck deformity, boutonnière deformity).

Patients with severe erosive disease, rheumatoid nodules and high titers of rheumatoid factor may develop vasculitic syndromes of small and large arteries. One-fourth of patients present with rheumatoid subcutaneous nodules occurring along the extensor surface of the forearm and areas of pressure. These can be rarely in organs like lungs, spleen, heart, aorta, and other viscera. These are firm, non-tender, oval or rounded masses, 2 cm in diameter.

There can be fibrinous pleuritis or pericarditis or both. Lung parenchyma may show progressive interstitial fibrosis. Ocular changes like uveitis and keratoconjunctivitis can occur.

Clinical Features

RA may present with weakness, malaise, and low-grade fever along with symmetric polyarticular arthritis. There is morning stiffness with pain. The joints become enlarged, movements limited and later ankylosis develops. Vasculitis can present as Raynaud's phenomenon and chronic leg ulcer. RA has to be distinguished from lupus, scleroderma, polymyositis, dermatomyositis and lyme disease.

Clinical Course of the Disease

The clinical course of RA is highly variable. The disease has remitting and relapsing course. There is progressive joint destruction with disability in 10 to 15 years. There can be secondary amyloidosis in 5 to 10% of cases. Cytokine IL-1 and TNF cause the damage and therapy to antagonize this has improved the outcome of the disease.

Characteristic findings for diagnosis are:
i. X-ray findings
ii. Sterile synovial fluid with inflammatory cells
iii. Poor mucin clot formation
iv. Rheumatoid factor (in 80% of the cases)
v. CRP: Raised
vi. Anti-CCP: Positive

Juvenile rheumatoid arthritis: RA occurs in children which is associated with HLA-B27. Juvenile rheumatoid arthritis is destructive in nature. RF is typically absent. Rheumatoid nodules are absent.

Spondyloarthopathies: These are RF negative. It is associated with HLA-B27. The ligaments rather than synovium are predominantly affected. Sacroiliac joints are affected. Ankylosing spondylitis, Reiter syndrome, psoriatic arthritis, spondylitis associated with inflammatory bowel diseases and arthropathies after infections (e.g. *Yersinia, Shigella, Salmonella, Campylobacter*) may be encountered.

SJÖGREN SYNDROME

Sjögren syndrome is an entity characterised by:
i. Dry eyes (keratoconjunctivitis sicca)
ii. Dry mouth (xerostomia)
iii. Immune-mediated destruction of the lacrimal and salivary glands.

Pathology

Lacrimal and salivary glands are the targets, but other secretory glands, including nasopharynx, upper airway, and vagina, also may be involved. Tissues are inflamed with activated CD4+ T cells and plasma cell infiltrate, occasionally forming lymphoid follicles with germinal centres. There is lack of tears, leading to drying of the corneal epithelium, with subsequent inflammation, erosion, and ulceration (keratoconjunctivitis). Xerostomia is present since salivary glands are involved, giving rise to mucosal atrophy, inflammation, fissuring and ulceration. Dryness and crusting of the nose may lead to ulceration and even perforation of the nasal septum. Laryngitis, bronchitis and pneumonitis may occur. Anti-SS-A antibodies are present in 25% of the cases. CNS, skin, kidneys, and muscles may be involved. Kidney shows mild interstitial nephritis with tubular transport defects.

Clinical Course

Females between the ages of 35 and 45 years are commonly affected. Dry mouth, lack of tears are common symptoms. Salivary glands are enlarged with lymphocytic infiltrate. Synovitis, pulmonary fibrosis and peripheral neuropathy may occur. 60% of the Sjögren patients have another accompanying autoimmune disorder such as RA. There is a 40-fold increased risk for developing a non-Hodgkin's lymphoma.

SYSTEMIC SCLEROSIS (Scleroderma)

Systemic sclerosis (SS) is characterised by extensive fibrosis throughout the body including skin. Cutaneous involvement is the commonest presenting symptom and is present in 95% of the cases.

The involvement of organs like GIT, lungs, kidneys, heart and skeletal muscle causes major morbidity and mortality.

It can be grouped as:
- **Diffuse:** Includes widespread skin lesions with rapid progression and visceral involvement.
- **Localised:** This has mild skin involvement limited to fingers and face. Visceral involvement is late in the disease process.

CREST syndrome is described in systemic sclerosis because of:
  i. Calcinosis
  ii. Raynaud's phenomenon
  iii. Esophageal dysmotility
  iv. Sclerodactyly
  v. Telangiectasia

Etiology and Pathogenesis

Fibroblast stimulation and microvascular injury are the important findings in SS. CD 4 T cells release cytokines that activate mast cells and macrophages. In turn these cells release fibrogenic cytokines like IL-1, PDGF, TGF-α, and FGF. B cell activation occurs, these patients have hypergammaglobulinaemia and ANAs. Antibodies directed to DNA topoisomerase I (Anti-Scl70) is specific. The anti-centromere antibody is found in 90% of the cases with limited scleroderma.

Endothelial damage is present with platelet aggregation, release of PDGF with periadventitial fibrosis and narrowing.

Pathology

All the organs may be affected prominent being skin, skeletal muscle, bones, GIT, lungs, kidneys and heart.

Skin: Shows diffuse sclerotic atrophy of skin beginning in the fingers and extending proximally.

Initially skin is oedematous.

Microscopy: There is oedema, perivascular lymphocytic infiltration, capillaries and small arterioles show thickening of basal lamina, endothelial damage and occlusion of vessels. Later progresses to fibrosis. The dermal collagen is increased with atrophy of skin appendages and hyaline thickening of wall of the vessels (arterioles and capillaries). Focal and diffuse subcutaneous nodules may develop. Fingers become claw-like due to limitation of joint movements, with loss of blood supply cutaneous ulceration, atrophic changes in terminal phalanges may progress to auto-amputation.

GIT: In gastrointestinal tract, there is progressive increase in collagen tissue, which subsequently replaces muscularis mucosae and submucosa. It is severe in esophagus, with loss of flexibility and there is dysfunction of lower esophageal sphincter giving rise to GE reflux and its complications, including Barrett's metaplasia and strictures. Mucosa is thin and may be ulcerated. There is loss villi which may lead to malabsorption syndrome.

Musculoskeletal system: Synovial hyperplasia and inflammation are common findings. There is erosive osteoarthritis and later fibrosis occurs. There may be myositis.

Lungs: The changes manifest as pulmonary hypertension, and/or interstitial fibrosis. Endothelial dysfunction is the cause of pulmonary hypertension.

Kidneys: The interlobular vessels show endothelial cell proliferation and in the wall deposition of glycoproteins and mucopolysaccharides. In hypertensive patients, there is fibrinoid necrosis of the vessel walls. Thrombosis and infarction are common. Such patients die of renal failure.

Heart: There has patchy myocardial fibrosis with thickening of walls of the arteries. The changes in lung may lead to right ventricular hypertrophy and failure (cor pulmonale).

INFLAMMATORY MYOPATHIES

Inflammatory myopathies are characterised by immune-mediated muscle injury and inflammation.

These can be:
  i. Polymyositis
  ii. Dermatomyositis
  iii. Inclusion body myositis
  These can occur alone, or along with other autoimmune diseases such as systemic sclerosis.

Females with dermatomyositis have high risk of developing visceral carcinomas of ovary, lung, and stomach.

Pathogenesis

In dermatomyositis, immunological evidence supports the antibody-mediated tissue injury.

In polymyositis and inclusion body myositis, there is cytotoxic T cell-mediated cell injury. ANAs are present in most patients. Jo-1 antibodies are directed against tRNA synthetase.

Pathology

Microscopically, there is lymphocytic infiltration with regeneration and degeneration of muscle fibres. Perifascicular atrophy and microangiopathy strongly support dermatomyositis.

Diagnosis

The diagnosis depends on:
  i. Clinical features, and
  ii. Laboratory evidence of immune antibodies, elevated creatinine kinase and biopsy.

Clinical Features

There is systemic weakness, initially affecting larger muscles of trunk, neck, and limbs. Dermatomyositis is associated with rash having lilac or heliotrope (reddish-purple) discolouration, affects upper eyelids and causes periorbital oedema.

SELF-ASSESSMENT EXERCISE

1. Which of the following is associated with auto-antibodies to thyroglobulin and thyroid peroxidase?
   A. Hashimoto's thyroiditis
   B. Graves
   C. Both of the above
   D. None of the above

2. In autoimmune reactions, all are true *except*:
   A. High tire of antibodies found
   B. Autoreactive T cells found
   C. NK cells found
   D. Antibodies to self-antigens present

3. Butterfly rash is found in:
   A. SLE
   B. Sjogren's disease
   C. Serum sickness
   D. Lambert-Eaton myasthenic syndrome

4. Autoimmune disease is found in:
   A. Reproductive females
   B. Children
   C. Men older than 60
   D. Females more than 50

5. Hashimoto's thyroiditis has all *except*:
   A. Has destruction of follicles
   B. Can be associated with papillary carcinoma
   C. Can have lymphoma
   D. Proliferation of follicles

6. Hashimoto's thyroiditis leads to:
   A. Hypothyroidism   B. Hyperthyroidism
   C. Normal thyroid   D. All of the above

7. Which sex has preference for autoimmune disease?
   A. Male affected   B. Female affected
   C. Males not affected   D. Both affected

8. Which of the following is AI disease?
   A. Type I DM   B. Rheumatoid arthritis
   C. Psoriasis   D. All of the above

9. In AI disease:
   A. Mistakenly antibodies attack tissue antigens
   B. Immune cells proliferate
   C. Immune cells die
   D. None

10. In ability to differentiate self and non-self leads to:
    A. HS   B. AI disease
    C. Immunodeficiency   D. Tolerance

11. HIV attacks:
    A. B cells   B. T helper cells
    C. T cytotoxic cells   D. Null cells

12. Severe combined immunodeficiency has absence of adenosine deaminase are deficient in or have defects of:
    A. T cells   B. B cells
    C. Both of the above   D. None of the above

Answers

1. A	2. C	3. A	4. A	5. D	6. A	7. B	8. D
9. A	10. B	11. B	12. C				

Genetic Disorders

The genetic disease can involve numerical and structural defects of chromosomes. The numerical defects can affect autosomes or sex chromosomes. The structural proteins can involve proteins, receptors or enzymes. There can be mutation which is a permanent damage to DNA. Mutation can be of following ways.

1. *Point mutations:* There is substitution of single nucleotide base by different bases, e.g. sickle cell anaemia. This is also referred to as missenrre mutation.

2. *Stop codons (nonsense mutation):* Cause termination of production of proteins, e.g. thalassaemia.

3. *Frame shift:* Deletion or insertion of one or two basepairs alters the reading frame of DNA.

Some of the genetic diseases are listed below.

1. **Cytogenetic disorders: Autosomal and X chromosomal disorders:**
   - Trisomy 21
   - Trisomy 18
   - Trisomy 13
   - Chromosome 22q11.2 deletion syndrome
   - Klinefelter syndrome
   - Turner syndrome

2. **Single gene disorders with atypical pattern of inheritance:**
   - Fragile X syndrome

3. **Genomic imprinting:**
   - Prader-Willi syndrome
   - Angelmann syndrome

4. **Mandelian disorders:**
   - Autosomal dominant
   - Autosomal recessive
   - X-linked

5. **Diseases with mutations in structural proteins:**
   - Marfan syndrome
   - Ehlers-Danlos syndrome

6. **Diseases with mutation in receptor proteins:**
   - Familial hypercholesterolaemia

7. **Diseases with mutation in enzymes:**
   - Phenylketonuria
   - Galactosaemia

8. **Lysosomal storage diseases:**
   - Tay-Sachs syndrome
   - Niemann-Pick syndrome
   - Gaucher syndrome
   - Mucopolysaccharidosis

9. **Glycogen storage disease**

10. **Maple syrup urine disease**

11. **Aplha-1-antitrypsin deficiency**

12. **Cystic fibrosis**

TRISOMY 21 (Down Syndrome)

This is the most common chromosomal disorder. About 95% of the people affected have trisomy 21. The chromosome count is 47. Incidence is 1:700 live births.

Risk factors: Advancing maternal age has a strong influence on incidence. Women older than 45 years have higher risk (1:25 live births). At the age of 35, the risk is 1:400 live births.

This occurs from meiotic non-disjunction of chromosome 21 in meiosis I or meiosis II (95%), Robertsonian translocation between 21 and 14 (4%) or non-disjunction in mitosis (mosaicism) in 1% of the cases. Mosaicism is not-inherited.

These patients have following features (Fig. 21.1):
- Epicanthal folds
- Simian crease
- Abundant neck skin
- Flat facial profile
- Hypotonia of muscles
- Mental retardation (IQ 25 to 50)
- Congenital heart defects: Atrioventricular septal defect is most common. Other defects include ventricular septal defect, atrial septal defect, tetralogy of Fallot and patent ductus arteriosus.
- Serious infections
- Gap between 1st and 2nd toes
- Umbilical hernia
- Intestinal stenosis

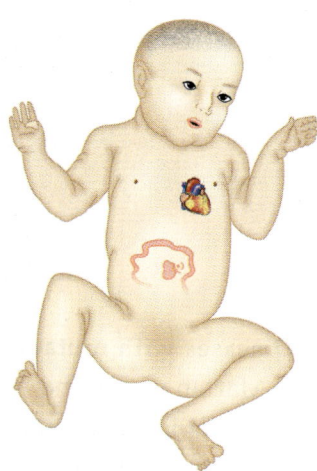

Fig. 21.1: Features of trisomy 21

Prognosis: Most of the patients survive till adult life. The overall prognosis of Down syndrome cases improved due to better control of infections. These patients have higher risk of developing acute leukaemias.

TRISOMY 13 (Patau Syndrome)

Incidence is 1:5000.

Risk factors: Advanced maternal age.

Cause: Non-disjunction in meiosis or non-disjunction in mitosis.

Most affected infants die during first few days or weeks of life.

These patients have the following features (Fig. 21.2):
- Microphthalmia
- Microcephaly
- Cleft lip and palate
- Polydactyly
- Cardiac defects
- Umbilical hernia
- Renal defects
- Rocker bottom feet

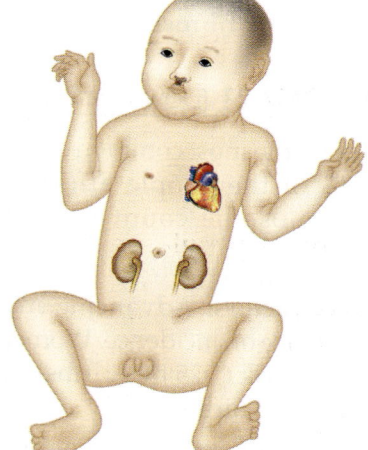

Fig. 21.2: Features of trisomy 13

Prognosis: There are multiple defects and develop life-threatening complications.

TRISOMY 18 (Edward Syndrome)

Incidence is 1:800.

Risk factors: Advanced maternal age.

Cause: Non-disjunction in meiosis or mosaicism due to non-disjunction in mitosis.

These patients have the following features (Fig. 21.3):
- Mental retardation
- Prominent occiput
- Micrognathia
- Low set ears
- Short neck
- Overlapping fingers
- Congenital heart diseases
- Renal anomalies
- Limited hip abduction

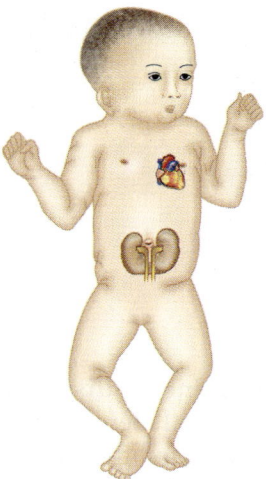

Prognosis: The disease is usually associated with life threatening complications.

Fig. 21.3: Features of trisomy 18

DELETION OF CHROMOSOME 22q11.2 (DiGeorge's Syndrome)

There is interstitial deletion of band 11 on long arm of chromosome 22. This has heart diseases, palate abnormalities, facial dysmorphism, developmental delay, thymic hypoplasia, parathyroid associated features like hypocalcaemia, dominant features of T cell immunodeficiency, hypocalcaemia and thymic hypofunction. This is called DiGeorge's syndrome.

SEX CHROMOSOMAL DISORDERS

Under X chromosome disorders, the following are encountered:
1. Klinefelter's syndrome
2. Turner's syndrome

Klinefelter Syndrome

Risk factors: Advanced maternal age, history of irradiation to either of the patients. Following are the features:
1. Most are 47XXY, there is non-disjunction during meiosis.
2. Male with hypogonadism.

Findings (Fig. 21.4):
a. Tall, narrow shoulders, wide hip and gynaecomastia.
b. Reduced facial and pubic hair.
c. Mental retardation is mild. The reduction of intelligence depends upon number of extra X chromosomes.

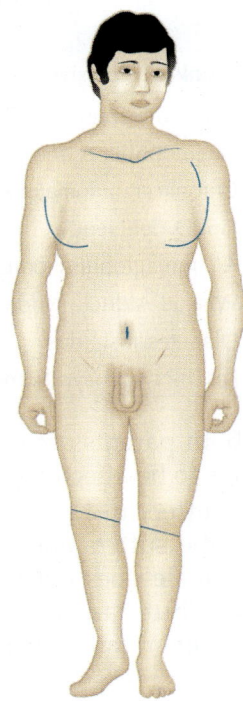

47 XXY
Mosaic (47 XXY, 46XY)

Features
Tall
Hypogonadism with
small testes
No sperms
Infertility
Gynaecomastia
Lower IQ
Poor muscle tone
Reduced secondary
sexual characters:
Sparse facial and
chest hair, poor beard
growth
Narrow shoulders
Wide hips

Fig. 21.4: Features of Klinefelter syndrome

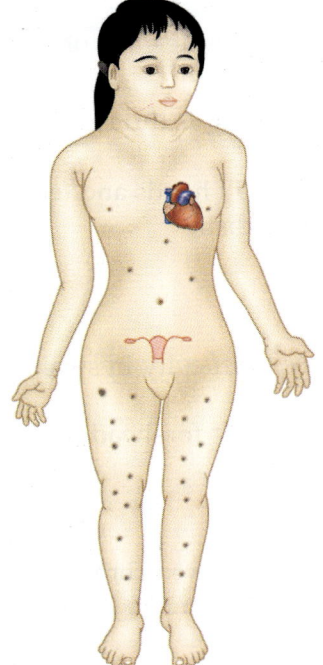

Phenotypic female
45XO
Short stature
Webbing of neck
Cubitus valgus
Broad chest
Widely spaced nipples
Coarctation of aorta
Amenorrhoea
Infertility
Streak ovaries
Pigmented nevi

Fig. 21.5: Features of Turner syndrome

d. Testis reduced in size, may be atrophied.

e. These patients have azoospermia. Sterility is due to impaired spermatogenesis.

f. Serum testosterone is low.

g. Urinary gonadotropins increased.

h. Histopathology of testes shows:
   • Leydig cell hyperplasia
   • Hyalinisation of tubules

i. Klinefelter syndrome may be associated with increased risk of breast cancer (20 times more than normal males), extragonadal germ cell tumours and systemic lupus erythematosus.

Turner Syndrome

• The incidence of Turner syndrome in live born females is: 1 in 5000 to 1 in 10,000.

• These are of 45X (45XO). These patients have hypogonadism in phenotypic females. One X chromosome is missing during paternal meiosis.

Following are the features found in these patients (Fig. 21.5):

• The diagnosis is made at birth or early in childhood.

• Intalligence is normal.

• There is significant growth retardation. They are of short stature. They have:
   a. Webbing of neck
   b. Cubitus valgus (increase in the carrying angle of arms)

c. Shield-like chest with widely spaced nipples

d. Low posterior hair line

• Patients may have lymphoedema of hands and feet.

• Patients have lack of secondary sexual characteristics, primary amenorrhoea; genitalia are infantile, ovarian failure, no follicle formation and have streak ovaries. Patients are infertile.

• Breast poorly developed.

• Have osteoporosis.

• Tiny brown spots of naevi.

• Cardiovascular malformations are common: Most common is coarctation of aorta. These attribute to common cause of death in these patients.

• Short stature and primary amenorrhoea are the important findings.

SINGLE GENE DISORDERS WITH ATYPICAL PATTERN OF INHERITANCE: FRAGILE X SYNDROME

In normal population, the number of CGG repeats are small (around 29), but the affected individuals have these repeats ranging to 50 to 200. These repeats are located in the 5' untranslated region of the FMR1 gene. These have familial mental retardation. Patients have macro-orchidism, and abnormal facial features.

GENOMIC IMPRINTING

1. Prader-Willi syndrome
2. Angelman syndrome

Prader-Willi Syndrome

In Prader-Willi syndrome, there is deletion of chromosome 15q11–13 of paternal origin.

The syndrome has the following features:
- Mentle retardation
- Short stature along with small hands and feet
- Hypogonadism/cryptorchidism
- Obese with central obesity
- Hypotonia
- Hyperphagia
- Newborns have weak cry, difficulty in swallowing and sucking
- Almond shaped eyes, narrow forehead and nasal bridge.

Angelman Syndrome

In this syndrome, the maternal derived chromosome 15 is affected with deletion of chromosome 15q11–13 region.

These patients have:
- Mentle retardation
- Ataxic gait
- Inappropriate laughter (happy puppet syndrome)
- Seizures
- Speech delay

MANDELIAN DISORDERS

Mandelian disorders are mutant genes involving single large gene and are hereditary and familial. These are (Tables 21.1 and 21.2):
- Autosomal dominant (AD),
- Autosomal recessive (AR), and
- X-linked.

AD diseases manifest in heterozygote state. Both males and females are affected. One parent is affected. If parents are not affected, can be attributed to new mutation.

Table 21.1	Autosomal dominant and recessive disorders
Autosomal dominant	**Autosomal recessive**
Hereditary spherocytosis and elliptocytosis	Phenylketonuria
Marfan's syndrome	Galactosaemia
Ehlers-Danlos syndrome	Homocystinuria
Osteogenesis imperfecta	Alkaptonuria
Achondroplasia	Lysosomal storage disorder (Gaucher disease, Niemann-Pick disease, etc.)
Familial hypercholesterolaemia	α-1 antitrypsin deficiencies
Acute intermittent porphyria	Wilson disease
Tuberous sclerosis	Haemochromatosis
Huntington disease	Cystic fibrosis
Myotonic dystrophy	Sickle cell disease
von Willebrand disease	Thalassaemia
Adult polycystic kidney disease	Congenital adrenal hyperplasia
Wilms tumour	Criggler-Najjar syndrome type I

Table 21.2	X-linked disorders
X-linked dominant	**X-linked recessive**
Vitamin D resistant rickets	Duchenne muscular dystrophy
Rett syndrome	Haemophilia A and B
Alport's incontinentia pigmenti	Chronic granulomatous disease
	G6PD deficiency
	Agammaglobulinaemia
	Wiskott-Aldrich syndrome
	Diabetes insipidus
	Lesch-Nyhan syndrome

AR disease occurs when both parents are affected. There is 25% chance of siblings to be affected.

The X-linked diseases can affect in heterozygous form. The affected males are the suffers and females are the carriers. The diseased male does not transmit the disease to male children but can transmit to daughters who are carries. Mother can transmit the disease to son.

DISEASES WITH MUTATIONS IN STRUCTURAL PROTEINS

The common ones are:
1. Marfan syndrome
2. Ehlers-Danlos syndrome

Marfan Syndrome

The patients of Marfan syndrome have skeletal disorders, defect with eyes, high arched palate and cardiovascular defects. They are tall, have long fingers, bilateral subluxation of lens, osteogenesis imperfecta, floppy mitral valve, aortic aneurysm and aortic dissection.

Gene defect: There is mutation in gene encoding fibrillin 1 (FBN 1) which is on chromosome 15 (15q21.1). This fibrillin is required for structural integrity of connective tissue. There are 500 varieties of Marfan syndromes. Important test done is echocardiogram.

Ehlers-Danlos Syndrome

There is defect in collagen synthesis and assembly. This has more than 10 variants. Affects mainly skin, joints, and blood vessels. Patients have fragile, hyperextendable and hypermobile joints and are vulnerable to trauma. There can be rupture of internal organs like colon, cornea, and large arteries. Healing is poor.

DISEASES WITH MUTATION IN RECEPTOR PROTEINS

These include familial hypercholesterolaemia and mutations with G-protein-coupled receptors.

Familial Hypercholesterolaemia

This is due to mutations of genes of LDL receptors (LDLR) which binds LDL and delivers to the hepatic cells. It is an AD disorder. The prevalence is 1:500 in the general population. The LDLR is encoded by gene on chromosome 19. Mutation of this gene causes the functional defects of LDLR.

Cholesterol in the body comes from diet and endogenous synthesis. Dietary triglycerides and cholesterol are incorporated into chylomicrons in the intestinal mucosa, hydrolysed in the vessels by an endothelial lipoprotein lipase, the cholesterol-rich chylomicrons are taken to liver.

Pathophysiology

- Cholesterol will be transported in blood with LDL, VLDL, HDL or IDL. About 70% of the cholesterol is transported with LDL (Fig. 21.6).
- In familial hypercholesterolaemia, cholesterol or fat bound lipoproteins cannot be taken inside the liver as receptors are abnormal in function.
- Also there is increased synthesis of LDL and VLDL by the liver cells as cholesterol is not available to the liver cells.
- When VLDL particles reach the capillaries of adipose tissue or muscle, it is cleaved by lipoprotein lipase, a process that extracts most of the triglycerides. The resulting molecule is intermediate-density lipoprotein (IDL), is enriched in cholesterol esters, has two of the three apoproteins (B-100 and E) present in the parent VLDL particle. VLDL and IDL are sources for LDL formation. These carry more amount of cholesterol. Hence, these are termed as bad lipoproteins. HDL liproteins carry less cholesterol and are called good lipoproteins.
- As LDL receptors are mutated, the lipoproteins LDL, VLDL, IDL, cholesterol and triglycerides are increased in the blood.

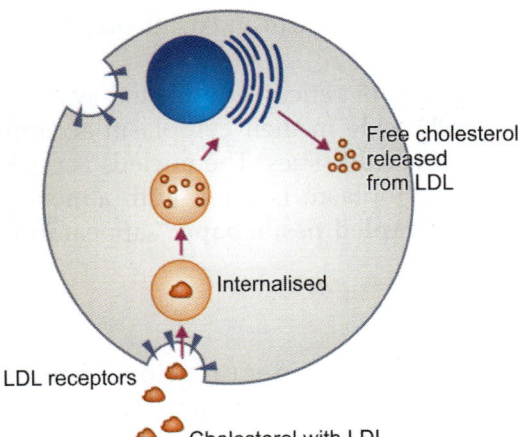

Fig. 21.6: Normal function of LDL receptors (diagrammatic)

Cholesterol is used for cell membrane synthesis and also maintains intracellular cholesterol homeostasis by:
1. Suppressing endogenous synthesis of cholesterol by HMG-CoA.
2. Activates enzyme acyl-CoA which helps in esterification and stoge of cholesterol.
3. Reduced synthesis of LDLR and thus reducing incoming excess LDL and cholesterol to liver.

Familial hypercholesterolaemia is characterised by high levels of LDL, VLDL, IDL, cholesterol and triglycerides in the blood with deposition of cholesterol in the wall of arteries, tendons and skin. The LDL receptors are:
1. Synthesized in endoplasmic reticulum
2. Get transferred to the golgi complex
3. Transported to the cell surface
4. Internalized by receptor-mediated endocytosis after binding to LDL.

Thus, there are four types of functional defects of LDLR:
1. Reduced or defective biosynthesis of receptors
2. Reduced or defective transportation
3. Abnormal binding
4. Abnormal internalization.

Clinical features and laboratory findings: Xanthelasma, cardiovascular diseases and atherosclerosis with obesity and high serum cholesterol are the findings.

Effects: With defective LDLR function, risk of atherosclerosis and heart diseases is common in males of 20–40 years.

DISEASES WITH MUTATION IN ENZYMES

These include phenylketonuria and galactosaemia.

Phenylketonuria (PKU)

This is due to absence of an enzyme phenylalanine (PA) hydroxylase produced by liver which converts PA to tyrosine which is required for synthesis of melanin, thyroxine, dopamine, epinephrine and nor-epinephine. Substantia nigra lacks this pigment. It is an essential amino acid and has to come from protein-rich diet. Phenyl hydroxylase is located on chromosome 12q24.1.

Pattern of inheritance: AR

Incidence: 1:10000 to 15000

Clinical features:
- Eczematous rash
- Blond hair
- Blue eyes
- Fair skin
- Mental retardation, irritability, scizures, brain damage

Investigations: Soon after birth, test blood sample for PA in blood and urine. PA in blood is 1 mg/dl in normal individuals and more than 20 mg/dl is seen in classical PKU. Urine has mousy odour.

Treatment: Diet free of phenylalanine should be given. Meat, fish, eggs, cheese, milk products, legumes, and bread which have high protein content to be avoided. Substitute with tyrosine.

Galactosaemia

- This is an AR disease of galactose metabolism.
- Incidence: Affects 1 in 30,000 live born infants.
- Normally lactose splits milk into glucose and galactose in the intestinal villi. Galactose later gets converted to glucose, and this requires an enzyme galactose-1-phosphate uridyltransferase (GALT). Lack of this enzyme results in accumulation of galactose-1-phosphate and its metabolites.
- Children have failure to thrive, hepatomegaly, vomiting and diarrhoea. Older children have jaundice, liver damage, cataract, speech defects, abnormal neurodevelopment and premature ovarian failure. Renal function affected with aminoaciduria and hence *E. coli* sepsis. Diagnosis is done by assay of transferase enzyme in leucocytes and red cells. Antenatal diagnosis is possible with DNA-based testing of amniocytes and chorionic villi.
- Treatment is to restrict the diet free of milk.

LYSOSOMAL STORAGE DISEASES

Most common ones are: Tay-Sachs disease, Niemann-Pick disease, Gaucher disease and mucopolysaccharidosis.

Tay-Sachs Disease (GM2 Gangliosidosis)

- This occurs in 1:3600 newborns.
- Common in Ashkenazi Jewish ancestry.
- Mutant hexosaminidase A leads to fatal neuro-degenerative lysosomal disease. There is accumulation of GM2 gangliosides, which cannot be broken down due to deficiency of the enzyme hexosaminidase A. GM2 gangliosides accumulate in neurons, axon cylinders of nerves, and glial cells. The cells appear swollen and foamy. EM of these lysosomes appears as whorled configuration.
- Affected children are normal until 3 to 6 months of age, but deteriorate to death by 2 to 4 years.

Niemann-Pick Disease

- AR disease.
- This belongs to a group of lipid storage disorder. There is dysfunction in metabolizing sphingolipid and sphingomyelin in lysosomes.

- Monocytes and macrophages are converted into **foam cells** in the bone marrow, spleen, liver, lungs, brain and other tissues with sphingomyelin accumulation.
- There is enzyme deficiency of sphingomyelinase.
- Jewish Ashkenazi, Eastern European ancestry are commonly affected.
- Infants of Niemann-Pick disease present with:
  1. Failure to thrive, abdominal distension
  2. Hepatosplenomegaly
  3. Jaundice
  4. Anaemia
  5. Thrombocytopenia
  6. Neurological disorders
  7. Cherry red spot on macula
- Type A, B and C1 and C2 forms exist.
- Type A has developmental regression by one year, rapidly progressive neurodegenerative course and death by 4 years.

Gaucher's Disease

- AR disease
- This is the common sphingolipidosis. There is deficiency of an enzyme beta-glucocerebrosidase. Gaucher cells store sphingolipid in spleen, liver, bone marrow, skeletal tissue, brain and other tissues.
- Type I occurs in children and adults, affects spleen and liver, there is mild anaemia, thrombocytopenia and bony pains, however, CNS spared.
- Type II occurs in children (infantile form). The disease presents by 3 to 6 months of life. There is neurological involvement. Child presents with:
  1. Failure to thrive
  2. There is hepatosplenomegaly
  3. Neurological deterioration present with spasticity, recurrent pulmonary infections
  4. Death occurs by 2 years
- Type III is juvenile or subacute neuropathic form, slowly progressive form and death occurs by 15 years of age.
- Macrophages of reticuloendothelial system having glucocerebroside in their cytoplasm accumulate in various affected tissues. The nucleus is pushed to a side and cytoplasm is filled with abnormal lipid giving **"crumpled tissue paper"** appearance.

Mucopolysaccharidosis

- AR disease
- There is defective degradation of mucopolysaccharides and thus accumulation of heparan sulphate, dermatan sulphate, and keratan sulphate. They are of different types.

– Type I: This is called Hurler syndrome and this is caused due to deficiency of lysosomal enzymes needed to degrade glycosaminoglycan (GAG).

– Type II: This is called Hunter syndrome due to deficiency of iduronate 2-sulfatase.

– Type III: Sanfilippo syndrome, is due to deficiency or absence of 4 different enzymes, those are necessary to degrade the GAG heparan sulphate.

– Type IV: Morquio syndrome, deficiency of lysosomal enzymes required for the degradation of muco-polysaccharides or glycosaminoglycans (GAGs).

– Type V: Scheie syndrome, mild form of Type I.

– Type VI: Maroteaux-Lamy syndrome, is due to deficiency of N-acetylgalactosamine 4-sulfatase. (arylsulfatase B) activity and the lysosomal accumulation of dermatan sulphate.

– Type VII: This is due to deficiency of specific lysosomal enzymes required for the degradation of glycosaminoglycans (GAGs).

• Mucopolysaccharides accumulate in liver, spleen, blood vessels, heart, brain, cornea, and joints. Affected patients have coarse facial features.

• In Hurler syndrome, there is corneal clouding, coronary arterial and valvular deposition and death in childhood. Hunter syndrome has milder course.

GLYCOGEN STORAGE DISEASE

Glycogen storage disease (GSD) or glycogenosis is due to inherited deficiency of enzymes involved in glycogen synthesis or breakdown. The disease affects most often cytoplasm or nucleus except Pompe's disease wherein lysosomes are affected. Most glycogen storage diseases are inherited as AR disease and they are of various types as mentioned below:

• GSD type I: von Gierke disease. There is deficiency of glucose-6-phosphatase.

• Type Ia: G-6-phosphatase deficiency, patients experience weakness of muscles and cramps, hypo-glycaemia, seizures and cardiomegaly.
Type Ib: Defect in G-6-P transportor protein.
Type Ia GSD is commoner than than Type Ib GSD.

• GSD type II: Lysosomal acid maltase deficiency or Pompe's disease, there is deficiency of alpha-1, 4-glucosidase, manifests in childhood, patients have muscle weakness, seizures and cardiomegaly.

• GSD type III: Forbes–Cori disease has deficiency of debranching enzyme, liver and skeletal muscle are involved.

• GSD type IV: Amylopectinosis or Anderson disease has deficiency of transglucosidase and patients have hepatosplenomegaly.

• GSD type V: McArdle disease has muscle phosphory-lase deficiency, develops in adolescents and adults.

• GSD type VI : Liver phosphorylase is deficient (Her's disease). This is similar to Type I, but has milder course.

• GSD type VII: Tarui disease has deficiency of phosphofructokinase. Symptoms begin in early childhood. Skeletal muscle is affected.

Depending upon organ/tissue involvement, GSDs can be grouped into three categories:

1. **Hepatic type:** Deficiency of hepatic enzyme G-6-P, causing von Gierke disease, these patients have hepatomegaly and hypoglycaemia.

2. **Myopathic type:** McArdle disease due to deficiency of muscle phosphorylase, marked muscle cramps after exercise, myoglobinuria, and failure of exercise to induce an elevation of blood lactate levels because of block in glycolysis.

3. **Pompe's disease** does not fit into any of the above categories. There is deficiency of enzyme from lysosomal origin, i.e. lysosomal acid maltase.

MAPLE SYRUP URINE DISEASE

This disease was described by Dr Menkes for the first time in 1954 and has following features:

1. This is due to deficiency of branched chain ketoacid hydroxylase which is required for metabolism of branched chain AA (valine, leucine and isoleucine).

2. Pattern of inheritance: AR

3. Presents during first week of life with vomiting, muscle tone changes, seizures, coma and death in a few weeks, if not treated. Urine smells of maple syrup (sweet odour).

Alpha-1 Antitrypsin Deficiency

• Alpha-1 antitrypsin (A-1-AT) is an enzyme inhibitor. It inhibits proteases particularly elastase released by the neutrophils.

• AR disease.

• It is associated with emphysema and cirrhosis of liver.

Note: Please refer to Emphysema in Respiratory System.

CYSTIC FIBROSIS

Cystic fibrosis transmembrane conductance regulator (CFTR) which is present on the cell membrane is a cAMP regulated chloride channel that regulates Cl^- and has a critical role in hydration of secretions. Genetics and clinical feture are given below.

• It is located on chromosome 7.

• It is an AR disease.

• The hydration of secretions in airways and ducts is mainly affected. The chloride ions cannot reach the cell surface. The dehydrated secretions damage the mucociliary function of airway lining epithelium and also block the ducts in pancreas, skin and other organs and allow growth of organisms.

SELF-ASSESSMENT EXERCISE

1. **Trisomy 21 is due to all** *except*:
   A. Meiotic non-dysjunction
   B. Mosaicism
   C. Robertsonian translocation
   D. Mitosis

2. **Fragile X syndrome has all** *except*:
   A. CGG triplet repeats
   B. CGG repeats in FRM1 gene
   C. Mental retardation
   D. X-linked recessive disease

3. **Angelman syndrome has all** *except*:
   A. Named after Harry Angelman
   B. Happy puppets
   C. Normal gait
   D. Maternal gene deletion

4. **Prader-Willi syndrome has all** *except*:
   A. Paternal gene deletion
   B. Short stature
   C. Tall stature
   D. Hypotonia

5. **In X-linked disorders, all are true** *except*:
   A. Males are sufferers
   B. Females are carriers
   C. Male does not transmit the disease to daughters
   D. Female can transmit to sons

6. **Turner syndrome patient has all** *except*:
   A. Osteoporosis   B. Brown spots of naevi
   C. Intelligence poor   D. CVS anomalies

7. **Turner syndrome has all** *except*:
   A. One X chromosome missing
   B. Heart murmur
   C. Ovarian function normal
   D. Naevi

8. **Familial hypercholesterolaemia has all** *except*:
   A. AD disease
   B. Chromosome 12 with mutation of LDLR
   C. Risk of atherosclerosis
   D. Prone for MI

9. **Phenylketonuria has:**
   A. Deficiency of enzyme involved in melanin synthesis
   B. Musty odour in breath
   C. Blond hair
   D. Urine confirmation

10. **A child with splenomegaly, failure to thrive, wrinkled tissue paper macrophages in marrow can be:**
    A. Gaucher's disease
    B. Mucopolysaccharidosis
    C. Niemann-Pick disease
    D. Glycogen storage disease

Answers

1. D	2. D	3. C	4. C	5. C	6. C	7. C	8. B
9. B	10. A						

Neoplasia

Neoplasia literally means **'new growth'**, i.e. 'Neo' meaning new and 'plasia' is proliferation. Willis defines neoplasm as, **"an abnormal mass of tissue, the growth of which exceeds and is uncoordinated with that of the normal tissues and persists in the same excessive manner after the cessation of the stimuli which evoked the change".**

Fundamental to the origin of all neoplasms are the genetic **changes** that allow excessive and unregulated proliferation that is independent of physiologic growth-regulatory stimuli.

A tumour is said to be **benign** when its microscopic and gross characteristics are considered to be:

*   Relatively innocent.
*   Localized to its site of origin.
*   Cannot spread to other sites.
*   It can be surgically excised.
*   Not harmful to the patient generally.
*   However, benign tumours on occasions are responsible for serious problems, e.g. benign tumours of pancreas arising from beta cells can produce marked hypoglycaemia.

Malignant tumours, referred to as cancers, are derived from the Latin word for **crab** that is, they adhere to any part that they seize in an obstinate manner, similar to a crab's behaviour.

Malignant tumours can:

*   **Invade and destroy** adjacent structures and spread to distant sites **(metastasis).**
*   Histologically they may resemble the cell of origin or may not.
*   Their progression depends on the surgical stage and histological grade of the tumour. In early stages, they can be treated successfully. Thus detection of malignant tumours in early stages and proper treatment at right time gives long life to the patients.

Difference between benign and malignant tumours and nomenclature of tumours are given in Tables 22.1 and 22.2.

EPIDEMIOLOGY OF CANCER

According to national cancer registry programme, more than 1300 Indians die of cancer every day. The most common tumours in Indian males are: oral and lung cancer. In Indian women, breast and cervical cancers are common. In Western population, lung and colon cancers and malignant melanoma are prevalent. In a few geographical areas, some malignancies are common like carcinoma stomach in Japan due to food habits and carcinoma bladder is frequent in Africa and Middle East countries (e.g. Egypt), where Schistosomiasis is endemic.

ETIOLOGY OF CANCER

The following are implicated in causation of cancer, and can be classified as:

1. Physical agents: Radiation such as UV rays, ionizing radiation like electromagnetic: X-rays, γ-rays, particles like α and β.
2. Biological carcinogens
    a. Oncogenic viruses
    b. Bacteria and cancer: *H. pylori*: Gastric carcinoma and gastric lymphoma
    c. Fungi and cancer: Aflatoxin B1 from *Aspergillus flavus*
3. Chemical carcinogens
4. Others: Metals and asbestos

Table 22.1   Differences between benign and malignant tumours

Characteristics	Benign	Malignant
Rate of growth	Slow growing	Fast growing
Capsule	Usually present	Absent/lacking
Localisation	Localised to site of origin, may compress underlying tissue	Not localised
Differentiation and anaplasia	Well differentiated, resemble cell of origin	Well/ moderate/poorly differentiated, may or may not resemble cell of origin
Microscopic findings:		
Cell cohesiveness	Cohesive clusters and sheets	Non-cohesive or dis-cohesive with loss of polarity, seen singly and small groups
Pleomorphism	Absent, uniform in size and shape	May show variation in size and shape Hyperchromatic
Nuclear features: N:C ratio	1:4 to 1:6	1:1
Bizarre cells	Absent	Present
Tumour giant cells	Absent	Present
Increased mitosis	Absent	Present
Abnormal mitoses	Absent	Present
Local invasion	Absent	Present, invade surrounding tissues
Metastasis	Absent	Present, spread by lymphatic/haematogenous or body cavities

Table 22.2   Nomenclature of tumours

Tissue of origin	Benign	Malignant
Tumours arising from one parenchymal cell type		
Connective tissue origin	Fibroma	Fibrosarcoma
	Lipoma	Liposarcoma
	Chondroma	Chondrosarcoma
	Osteoma	Osteosarcoma
Endothelial and related tissues		
Blood vessels	Haemangioma	Angiosarcoma
Lymph vessels	Lymphangioma	Lymphangiosarcoma
Mesothelium		Mesothelioma
Meninges	Meningioma	Invasive meningioma
Muscle		
Smooth muscle	Leiomyoma	Leiomyosarcoma
Striated	Rhabdomyoma	Rhabdomyosarcoma
Blood cells and related tissues		Leukaemia, lymphoma
		Multiple myeloma
Epithelia		
Stratified squamous epithelium	Squamous cell papilloma	Squamous cell carcinoma
Basal cells of skin and adenexa		Basal cell carcinoma
Glandular/ductal epithelia	Adenoma	Adenocarcinoma
Renal	Renal cell adenoma	Renal cell carcinoma
Urinary tract	Transitional cell papilloma	Transitional cell carcinoma
Respiratory Tract	Adenoma/papilloma	Bronchogenic carcinoma
		Carcinoid
Melanocytes	Naevus	Malignant melanoma
Liver cells	Liver cell adenoma	HCC
		Cholangiocarcinoma

(Contd.)

Table 22.2	Nomenclature of tumours (*contd.*)	
Tissue of origin	**Benign**	**Malignant**
Placental tissue	Hydatidiform mole	Choriocarcinoma
Germ cells:		
• Ovary		Dysgerminoma
• Testis		Seminoma
Ovary surface epithelium	Adenoma/cystadenoma	Adenocarcinoma
Tumours arising from more than one parenchymal cell type: Mixed tumours derived from one germ layer		
Salivary glands	Pleomorphic adenoma	Malignant mixed tumour
Breast	Fibroadenoma	Malignant cystosarcoma
Renal		Phyllodes, Wilms
Tumours arising from more than one parenchymal cell type: Mixed tumours derived from more than one germ layer		
Totipotential cells of ovary, testis, midline germ cell tumours	Mature teratoma	Immature teratoma
		Teratocarcinoma

Radiation Effects

UV rays and cancer: Have high risk for **basal cell carcinoma, squamous cell carcinoma and malignant melanoma.** For details of radiation effects, please refer to topic on Environmental Diseases.

Biological Carcinogens: Viruses, Bacteria and Fungi

Oncogenic Viruses

The most common oncogenic DNA viruses causing cancer are:

1. Human papillomavirus (HPV): HPV commonly produces warts, and squamous cell carcinoma of cervix and skin.
2. Epstein-Barr virus (EBV): EBV is implicated in Burkitt's lymphoma, patients of organ transplantation, Hodgkin's lymphoma, nasopharyngeal carcinoma.
3. Hepatitis B virus (HBV): Hepatocellular carcinoma.
4. Kaposi sarcoma herpes virus (KSHV, human herpes virus 8).

The oncogenic RNA viruses are:

1. **HTLV-1 (human T cell leukaemia virus):** It causes T cell leukaemia and lymphoma in Japan and the Caribbean region.
2. **HCV:** Hepatocellular carcinoma.

Pathogenesis: In DNA viruses, the viral DNA enters the cell after uncoating of its envelop proteins. The viral DNA gets integrated into the host DNA and proliferates in host cells using its enzymes.

In RNA viruses, using reverse transcriptase makes DNA and then DNA gets integrated into host DNA as provirus and virus proliferates. The oncoproteins released act through signal transduction pathways or activating transcription factors.

The HPV produces two viral proteins—E6 and E7.
- The E7 binds to RB gene and displaces E2F transcription factor, thus neutralizing RB gene's function.
- E6 binds to P53 and degrades it with loss of its tumour suppressor activity. Also activates cyclin A and E, inducing cell proliferation and inhibits apoptosis thus increasing the cell survival or immortalizing the cells.

HBV and HCV oncoproteins activate variety of signal transduction pathways which contributes to carcinogenesis.

Bacteria and Cancer Association

H. pylori is known to cause gastric carcinoma.

Fungi And Cancer Association

Aflatoxin B1, a natural product of **fungus *Aspergillus flavus*,** is metabolized to epoxide **which can bind to DNA** is known to produce **hepatocellular carcinoma.**

Chemical Carcinogens

Chemical carcinogens (Table 22.3) causing cancer can be divided into:

1. Initiators
2. Promoters

Initiators

Application of initiator may cause mutational activation of genes such as RAS. Subsequent application of promoter leads to clonal expansion of initiated cell.

After initiation, there should be sustained exposure to promoter which stimulates proliferation of initiated cell (example of initiator—alkylating agents).

Promoters

These do not cause mutations, however, act on a mutated cell. These are: Pharbol esters, hormones, phenols and benzopyrines, azo dyes and aflatoxins.

Table 22.3   List of chemical carcinogens

Chemical carcinogens

Direct-acting carcinogens
- *Alkylating agents*
  - β-propiolactone
  - Dimethyl sulphate
  - Diepoxybutane
  - Anticancer drugs (cyclophosphamide, chlorambucil, nitrosoureas, and others)
- *Acylating agents*
  - 1-Acetyl-imidazole
  - Dimethylcarbamyl chloride

Procarcinogens that require metabolic activation
- Polycyclic and heterocyclic aromatic hydrocarbons
  - Benz(a)anthracene
  - Benzo(a)pyrene
  - Dibenz(a,h)anthracene
  - 3-methylcholanthrene
  - 7,12-dimethylbenz(a)anthracene
- Aromatic amines, amides, azo dyes
  - 2-Naphthylamine (β-naphthylamine)
  - Benzidine
  - 2-Acetylaminofluorene
  - Dimethylaminoazobenzene (butter yellow)
- Natural plant and microbial products
  - Aflatoxin B_1
  - Griseofulvin
  - Cycasin
  - Safrole
  - Betel nuts
- Others
  - Nitrosamine and amides
  - Vinyl chloride, nickel, chromium
  - Insecticides, fungicides
  - Polychlorinated biphenyls

Mechanism of carcinogenesis: Chemical carcinogens produce mutations and the chemical carcinogenesis is a multistep process which includes the following steps (Fig. 22.1):
1. Initiation
2. Promotion
3. Progression
4. Cancer

Directly acting chemical carcinogens have:
1. Highly reactive electrophilic groups which damage the DNA and leads to mutations.
2. These do not require metabolic conversion to become carcinogen.

Note: Indirectly acting chemical carcinogens need metabolic activation by enzyme like P450.

Alkylating agents: Mainly the chemotherapeutic drugs like cyclophosphamide, cisplatin, busulphan and these have significant risk for solid and haematological malignancies.

Polycyclic hydrocarbons derived from **coal tar** are Benzo(a)pyrene, Dibenz(a,h)anthracene and 3-methylcholanthrene. These need metabolic activation by cytochrome P450-dependent oxidase to electrophilic epoxides which inturn react with proteins and nucleic acids.

Aromatic amines and azo dyes: Produce **bladder and liver tumours.**

Nitrosamines: Nitrites commonly added as preservatives along with other dietary compounds are conveted to **nitrosamines, and these can produce carcinoma stomach.**

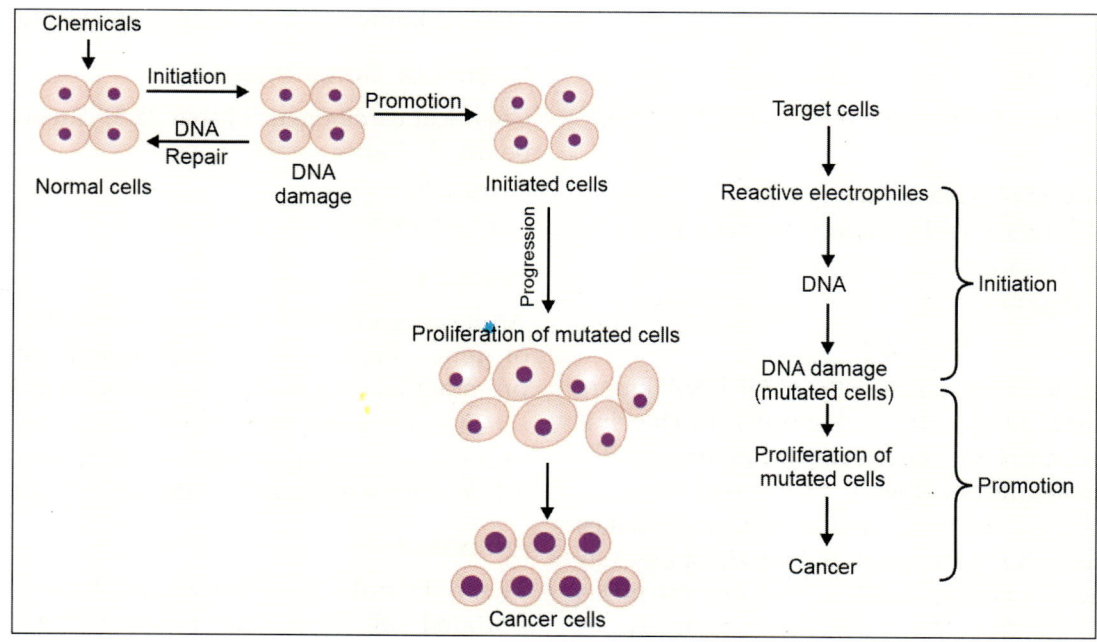

Fig. 22.1: Multistep process of chemical carcinogenesis (schematic)

Vinyl chloride: This is used in production of plastics and can produce **hepatic angiosarcomas.**

Others

Metals and Cancer

Nickel, lead, cadmium, cobalt, beryllium are electrophilic and can cause cancers.

Asbestos and Cancer

Produce malignant **mesothelioma** and **lung carcinoma.** Crocidolite fibres have greater risk than shorter and thicker amosite and flexible chrysolite fibres for mesothelioma and lung cancer.

PRENEOPLASTIC LESIONS

Preneoplastic conditions include disorders that are associated with a significantly increased risk of cancer. They are:

1. Chronic atrophic gastritis of pernicious anaemia
2. Solar keratosis
3. Oral lichen planus
4. Oral submucous fibrosis
5. Endometrial hyperplasia
6. Chronic gastritis
7. Ulcerative colitis
8. Adenomatous polyps of colon
9. Xeroderma pigmentosum
10. Epidermolysis bullosa hereditaria

The WHO specifies the following diseases with increased risk of oral squamous cell carcinoma:

1. Sideropenic dysphagia (in case of chronic iron deficiency: Plummer-Vinson syndrome, or Paterson-Kelly syndrome)
2. Oral lichen planus
3. Oral submucous fibrosis
4. Discoid lupus erythematosus
5. Xeroderma pigmentosum
6. Epidermolysis bullosa hereditaria

Table 22.4	AD and AR diseases associated with cancer
AD diseases associated with cancer	**AR diseases associated with cancer**
1. Inherited retinoblastoma	1. Xeroderma pigmentosum
2. Neurofibromatosis	2. Friedreich's ataxia
3. Breast carcinoma	3. Bloom's syndrome
4. Ovarian cancer	4. Fanconi's anaemia
5. Familial polyposis coli	5. Ataxia telengiectasia
6. MEN1 and 2	
7. NHPCC	
8. Li-Fraumeni syndrome	

Xeroderma pigmentosum: AR disease with inability to repair DNA after UV radiation has greater risk of cancers.

PATHOGENESIS OF CANCER (Molecular Basis)

The cancer causing agents set in a non-lethal genetic damage in a host nucleus which is the basis for carcinogenesis.

In normal health, the cell proliferation is under control by different mechanisms.

1. Proto-oncogenes (with normal cellular genes)
2. Tumour suppressor genes
3. Programmed cell death
4. Genes involved in DNA repair

Carcinogenesis is multistep process at both the phenotypic as well as genotypic levels with accumulation of multiple mutations.

Properties of Malignant Cells

1. **Self-sufficiency in growth signals:** Cancer cells control their proliferation by producing growth signals themselves. There can be:
   a. Over stimulation to growth factors, e.g. PDGF; this has self-stimulatory loop.
   b. Over expression of normal or mutated growth factor receptors, e.g. EGRF in small cell carcinoma of lung, HER2/NEU in breast cancers.
   c. Over production of signal transducing proteins, e.g. PI3K I which initiate gene transcription, e.g. RAS and ABL. **Activation of these signaling molecules** can be by:
      i. Mutation of proto-oncogenes, e.g. RAS
      ii. Chromosome re-arrangements, e.g. ABL (tyrosine kinase)
      iii. Gene amplification
   d. Over production of nuclear transcription factors, e.g. transcription factor Myc promotes cyclin production for cell cycle.
   e. Cyclins and cyclin dependent kinases: Cyclins along with their CDKs are responsible for controlling the progression of cell cycle.
2. **Insensitivity to growth inhibitory signals:** Cancer cells ignore or escape the growth inhibitory signals, e.g. loss of tumour suppressor genes, e.g. RB and P53.
3. Evasion of apoptosis
4. Limitless replicative potential (telomerase activity)
5. Sustained angiogenesis
6. Ability to invade
7. Micro-RNAs
8. Genomic instability

Oncogenes and Proto-oncogenes

The mutations of proto-oncogenes are oncogenes. The products of these mutated genes bring about:

a. Autonomous proliferation of cells
b. Uncontrolled proliferation
c. The proliferation does not require normal growth promoting signals.

Proto-oncogenes become oncogenes by one of the following mechanisms:

i. Point mutation
ii. Reduplication
iii. Chromosomal translocations

Philadelphia Chromosome

This has tyrosine kinase activity. The ABL gene when translocated from its normal position on chromosome 9 to 22 where it fuses with part of break point cluster region (BCR) gene. The BCR-ABL hybrid protein has upregulated tyrosine kinase activity and proliferation of cells as in chronic myeloid leukaemia (Fig. 22.2).

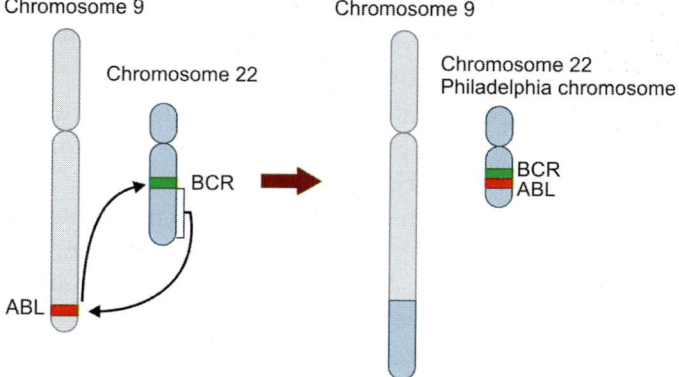

Fig. 22.2: Philadelphia chromosome, t (9;22) (q34;q11)—reciprocal translocation between chromosome 9 and 22 (schematic)

Cancer Suppressor Genes

RB gene and P53 are good examples of cancer suppressor genes.

SPREAD OF MALIGNANT TUMOURS

The important properties of malignant tumour can spread by following ways:

1. Direct invasion
2. Metastasis
   a. Body cavities
   b. Lymphatic spread
   c. Haematogenous spread

Direct Invasion

Most malignant tumours grow as localized masses but later spread by progressive infiltration and invasion of neighbouring structures. These do not have a well-developed capsule or may have a pseudocapsule from host tissue. This requires wide excision of the mass and careful examination of the resected mass for invasion of the borders.

The epithelial tumours initially develop within the epithelium. The dysplastic features are confined only to the epithelium without breach of the basement membrane. This is called carcinoma *in situ*. Diagnosing the cancers early in the stage can cure the cancer. However, in this stage, the patients are asymptomatic and may not consult their physicians.

The organs which are easily approachable can be detected in this stage by regular screening programs. This is true with breast and cervical cancers for early detection of cancer.

With direct invasion, the squamous cell carcinoma of cervix can spread to ureters and cause obstruction or may cause vesicovaginal fistulas. The broncho-pleural fistulas can be encountered in lung carcinomas and pancreatic carcinoma can cause severe pain due to direct invasion of the celiac nerve plexus.

The breast cancer can invade the overlying skin by direct invasion causing ulceration and eczematous change (pagetoid change).

Metastasis

This is spread of the tumour away from its primary origin. Thus from site of origin, the tumour can spread to distant sites. The neoplastic cells penetrate the coelomic cavities, wall of the lymphatic vessels and blood vessels and thus spread to distant sites. The secondary deposits usually resemble the primary tumour histologically, but occasionally may show poor differentiation.

The aggressive primary tumours of larger or smaller size, poorly differentiated or anaplastic tumours would have been metastasized at the time of diagnosis.

Spread through Body Cavities

- The CNS tumours may spread through CSF pathway: CNS tumours may penetrate the ventricles and carried through CSF to other parts of brain and spinal cord.
- Lung tumours through pleural cavity.
- GIT, ovarian and breast tumours may spread through peritoneal cavity. Peritoneal implants and peritoneal effusions with presence of malignant cells are very common with ovarian cancers especially serous and mucinous carcinomas. Invasive and non-invasive implants are looked for the prognosis of the tumours. The invasive implants have bad prognosis compared to the non-invasive ones.

Spread through Lymphatics

This type of metastasis is characteristic of carcinomas, while the sarcomas usually spread by haematogenous route. The enlargement of draining lymph nodes, size of the lymph nodes, presence of invasion and number of lymph nodes are factors taken into account in staging of some carcinomas (e.g. breast carcinoma). The sentinal lymph node is the first lymph node to receive malignant cells amongst the draining lymph nodes. Blue dye or radiolabelled materials are injected to find out the presence of tumour cells in sentinal node.

Haematogenous Spread

This is the most common mode of spread in sarcomas but carcinomas too can use this mode of spread. Amongst the blood vessels, venous route is more often used by the tumour cells than the arterial route. The cancer cells easily invade capillaries and venules. The vessels are observed for tumour emboli in the histopathological sections of the resected specimen. The liver and lungs are the most common organs of secondary deposits in haematogenous spread followed by brain and bone.

MECHANISM OF METASTASIS (Fig. 22.3)

The malignant cells have the capacity to invade the surrounding tissue and metastasize to distant site.

Following are the mechanisms:

1. Normally E-cadherin keeps the cells together. Because of mutations or activation of beta-catenin or SNAIL and TWIST transcription factors which suppress E-cadherin or its function is lost. Thus, the cells are loosened.

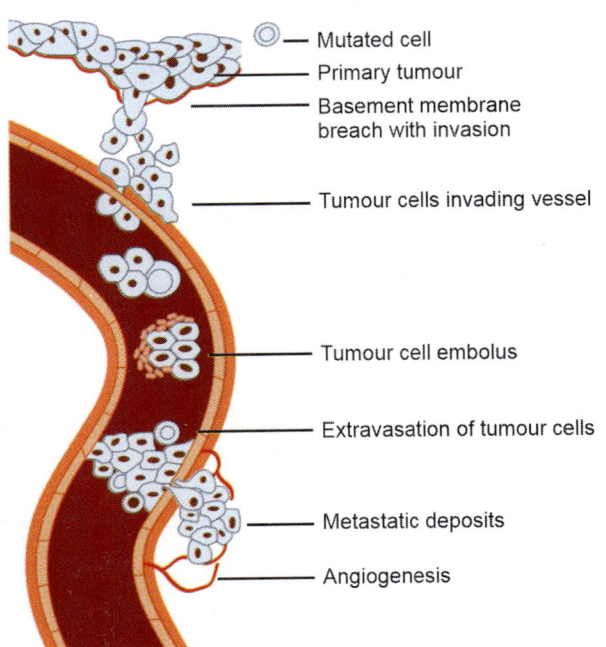

Fig. 22.3: Invasion and metastasis of tumour cells (schematic)

Mutated cell
Primary tumour
Basement membrane breach with invasion
Tumour cells invading vessel
Tumour cell embolus
Extravasation of tumour cells
Metastatic deposits
Angiogenesis

2. The next step is degradation of BM and ECM. The tumour cells secrete proteolytic enzymes like matrix metalloproteinases, cathepsin, urokinase plasminogen activator are implicated in tumour invasion. Matrix metalloproteinases, cleaves collagen and vascular BM.

3. The tumour cells get attached to ECM proteins (fibronectin, laminin and collagen) through the receptors present on the basal surface of the cells.

4. Locolisation and migration is the next step. The tumour cells move to other places through degrading the basement membrane.

5. Vascular dissemination and homing of malignant cells: The tumour cells enter vessels and can lodge in distant site after coming out of the vessel. Receptors for adhesion molecules on the tumour cells are expressed in high levels, e.g. CXCR4, CCR7.

DIAGNOSIS OF MALIGNANCY (Cancer)

1. Proper clinical history
2. Relevant examination findings
3. Relevant tumour markers/tumour antigens, e.g.
   PSA—prostatic carcinoma
   CEA—colorectal cancers and other cancers
   Alpha-fetoprotein—hepatocellular carcinoma, yolk sac tumour
4. USG/X-ray
5. FNAC/core biopsy for palpable or deep seated masses
6. Exfoliative cytology—pap smears for cervical cancer
7. Cytology for malignant cells—sputum and body fluids and bronchoalveolar lavage (BAL) samples, etc.
8. Biopsy
9. Frozen section—for rapid diagnosis of cancers when the patient is on the operation table
10. Excision of tumour
11. Suitable molecular diagnostic modality like:
    - PCR
    - FISH
    - For prognosis and behaviour: HER2/neu, N–myc
    - For treatment purposes: ER, PR, HER2/neu
    - Hereditary predisposition: BRCA 1 and 2 as in breast and ovarian cancers
12. Immunohistochemistry (suitable markers)
13. Immunofluorescence
14. Cytogenetics
15. Recognition of paraneoplastic syndromes: These may be early symptoms in some cancers.

PARANEOPLASTIC SYNDROMES

These are symptom complexes that occur in patients with cancer and these symptoms occur at sites distant to tumour or its metastasis. The symptoms cannot be readily explained by local or distant spread of tumour or by elaboration of hormones indigenous to the tissue of origin of tumour (Table 22.5).

These may be:
1. Earliest manifestation of cancer.
2. May have significant clinical problems and even be fatal.
3. May mimic metastatic disease.

Mucin-secreting adenocarcinomas of pancreas, lung and GIT can have:
1. Non-bacterial thrombotic endocarditis (marantic endocarditis)
2. Hypercoagulability leading to venous thrombosis
3. Trousseau's syndrome (migratory thrombosis in superficial veins and uncommon site)

Syndromes which can occur in lung carcinoma are:
1. Hypercalcaemia (non-small cell carcinoma/sqamous cell carcinoma)

Table 22.5 Paraneoplastic syndromes with clinical symptoms, underlying malignancy and mechanism

Clinical syndromes	Major forms of underlying cancer	Causal mechanism
Endocrinopathies Cushing syndrome	Small-cell carcinoma of lung Pancreatic carcinoma Neural tumours	ACTH or ACTH-like substance
Syndrome of inappropriate antidiuretic hormone secretion	Small-cell carcinoma of lung; intracranial neoplasms	Antidiuretic hormone or atrial natriuretic hormones
Hypercalcaemia	Squamous cell carcinoma of lung Breast carcinoma Renal carcinoma Adult T cell leukaemia/lymphoma Ovarian carcinoma	Parathyroid hormone-related protein (PTHRP), TGF-α, TNF, IL-1
Hypoglycaemia	Hepatocellular carcinoma Fibrosarcoma Lung cancer Other mesenchymal sarcomas	Insulin or insulin-like substance
Carcinoid syndrome	Gastric carcinoma Bronchial adenoma (carcinoid) Atypical carcinoid of lung Small cell carcinoma of lung Pancreatic carcinoma	Serotonin, bradykinin
Polycythemia	Renal carcinoma Cerebellar haemangioma Hepatocellular carcinoma	Erythropoietin
Nerve and muscle syndromes Myasthenia	Bronchogenic carcinoma	Immunological
Disorders of the central and peripheral nervous system	Breast carcinoma	
Dermatologic disorders Acanthosis nigricans	Gastric carcinoma Lung carcinoma Uterine carcinoma	Immunological; secretion of epidermal growth factor
Dermatomyositis	Bronchogenic, breast carcinoma	Immunological
Osseous, articular, and soft-tissue changes Hypertrophic osteoarthropathy and clubbing of the fingers	Bronchogenic carcinoma	Unknown
Vascular and haematologic changes Venous thrombosis (Trousseau phenomenon)	Pancreatic carcinoma Bronchogenic carcinoma Other cancers	Tumour products
Nonbacterial thrombotic endocarditis	Advanced cancers	Hypercoagulability
Red cell aplasia	Thymic neoplasms	Unknown
Others Nephrotic syndrome	Various cancers	Tumour antigens, immune complexes

2. Syndrome of inappropriate antidiuretic hormone secretion (SIADH) (non-small cell carcinoma/ sqamous cell carcinoma)
3. Carcinoid (small cell carcinoma)
4. Venous thrombosis (Trousseau phenomenon)
5. Hypertrophic osteoarthropathy and clubbing of the fingers
6. Dermatomyositis
7. Myasthenia gravis
8. Acanthosis nigricans
9. Hypoglycaemia

Paraneoplastic syndromes which can occur in breast carcinoma are:
1. Hypercalcaemia
2. CNS and nerve disorders

Paraneoplastic syndromes which can occur in renal cell carcinoma are:
1. Polycythaemia
2. Hypercalcaemia

SOME COMMON TUMOURS

Haemangiomas

Haemangiomas lie in a grey zone between hamartomatous lesions and true neoplasms.

Some syndromes associated with haemangiomas:
1. *Kasabach–Merritt syndrome* has giant haemangioma with thrombocytopenic purpura and coagulopathy.
2. *Maffucci's syndrome* is rare non-hereditary syndrome characterised by multiple haemangioma and enchondroma, less commonly with lymphangiomas.
3. *Von Hippel-Lindau syndrome* consists of cavernous haemangiomas or haemangioblastoma which occurs in cerebellum or brainstem and retina. It is a inherited multisystem disorder. The gene is on chromosome 3 and inherited dominantly.
4. *Sturge-Weber syndrome* occurs in brain and skin with haemangiomas and neurological abnormalities.

Capillary Haemangioma

These commonly involve the skin, subcutaneous tissue, mucous membranes of oral cavity and lips; and they also occur in the internal viscera such as liver, spleen and kidneys. They frequently occur on the skin of newborn children and fade away, when the child is of 1 to 3 years of age.

The strawberry type or **juvenile haemangioma** is very common in newborn.

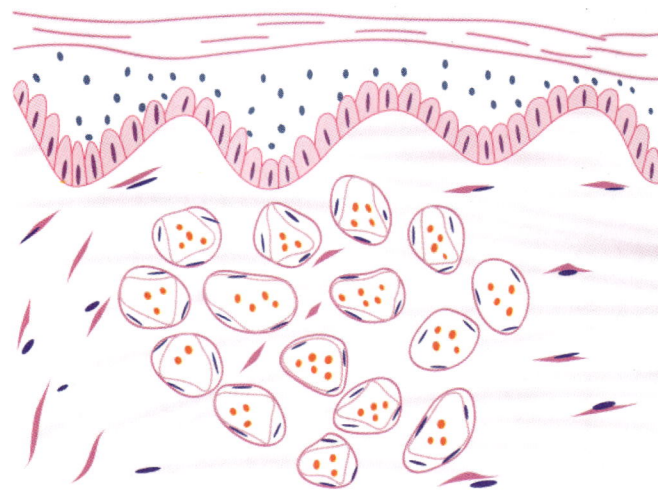

Fig. 22.4: Microscopy of capillary haemangioma (schematic)

Gross: These are a few mm to several cm, bright red to blue-coloured, slightly elevated or strawberry shaped.

Microscopy: These show blood-filled capillary-sized vascular channels lined by endothelial cells separated by scant connective tissue. The lumen of these vascular channels may be partially or completely thrombosed (Fig. 22.4).

Cavernous Haemangioma

These are less commom than capillary haemangiomas. They are larger and less circumscribed.

Grossly, cavernous haemangioma can occur in skin, mucosal surfaces, and visceral organs including spleen, liver and pancreas. May occur in brain, when enlarges produce neurological symptoms (Fig. 22.5).

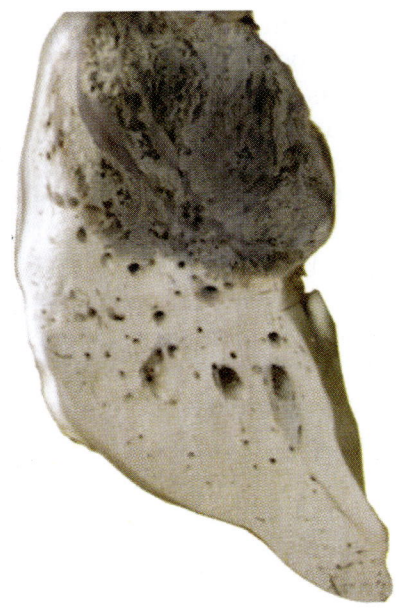

Fig. 22.5: Cavernous haemangioma liver (gross picture)

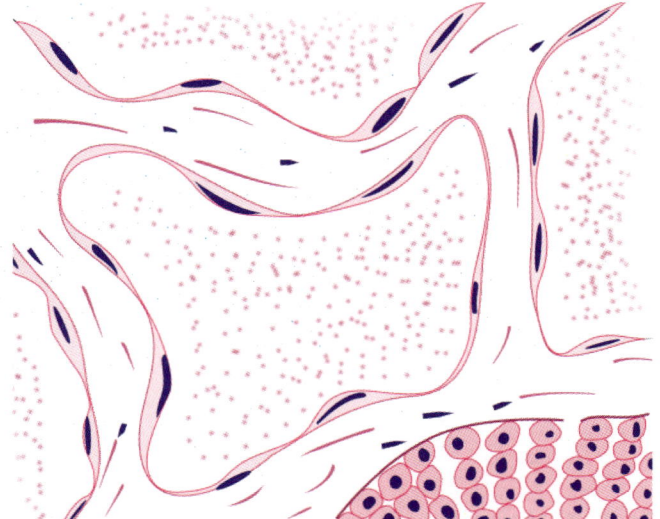

Fig. 22.6: Microscopy of cavernous haemangioma (schematic)

Cavernous haemangioma of skin has portwine stains. In organs, cavernous haemangioma may be red blue, soft spongy mass with diameter of several centimetres. These are not encapsulated; usually do not regress as that of capillary haemangioma. They may undergo thrombosis, fibrosis, cystic cavitation or haemorrhage. Rarely giant forms occur as in Kasabach–Merritt syndrome.

Microscopy: The lesion is sharply defined and not well encapsulated. It has cavernous vascular spaces filled with blood and separated by connective tissue stroma. Intravascular thrombosis with associated dystrophic calcification is common (Fig. 22.6).

Lipoma

It is a benign tumour of fat cells. The subcutaneous lipomas are common and occur in regions like arms, shoulder and buttocks.

Deep lipomas may be detected late and have larger size and are found in the omentum, mesentery, retroperitoneum, intramuscular location, juxta-articular regions, periosteum, thorax, mediastinum, paratesticular region and so on.

Apart from subcutaneous plane, they can occur in planes like intramuscular, intermuscular, myelolipoma (in bone marrow), tendon sheath, joints, intraneural, perineural, etc.

They are most common in 5th or 6th decade.

They are single or multiple.

These are soft, mobile, painless and well circumscribed masses and slip under the palpating fingers.

Angiomyolipoma is common in kidney.

Histological variants like pleomorphic lipoma, spindle cell lipoma, fibrolipoma, chondroid lipoma, myolipoma, angiolipoma, etc. are rare.

Areas of infarct, necrosis and calcification may be present.

Malignant form is called **liposarcoma** and these are usually deep seated.

Gross: These tumours are well circumscribed, thinly capsulated and measure several cm in dimension. They are rounded yellow-coloured masses (Fig. 22.7).

Microscopy: The neoplasm shows lobules of mature adipocytes separated by thin fibrous septae.

The amount of connective tissue and blood vessels may vary (Figs 22.8 and 22.9).

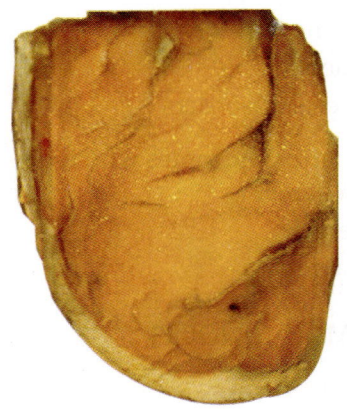

Fig. 22.7: Lipoma (gross picture)

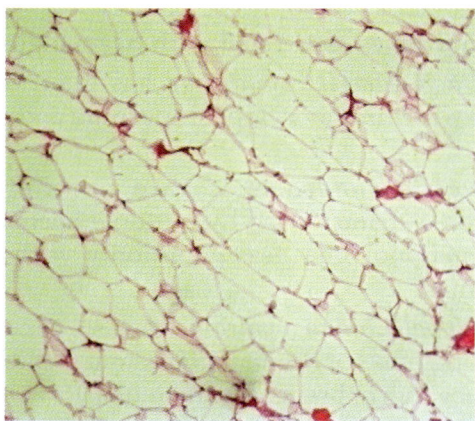

Fig. 22.8: Microphotograph of lipoma

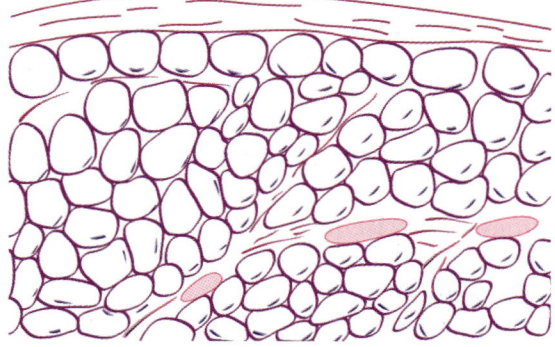

Fig. 22.9: Microscopy of lipoma (schematic)

Schwannoma

These tumours arise from the neural crest-derived Schwann cells. These are usually solitary. Most common locations are flexor aspects of extremities, neck, mediastinum, retroperitoneum, posterior spinal roots, and cerebellopontine angle. The commonest location is cerebellopontine angle; the vestibular branch of 8th cranial nerve is affected. Cranial nerves III, IV, or VI may be affected.

Other cranial and sensory nerves also can be affected. Schwannoma usually involves sensory rather than motor nerves.

Local recurrence with incomplete resection is known. Malignant change is extremely rare in contrast to neurofibroma.

Schwannomas can have 'Antoni A' with cellular areas and in 'Antoni B' schwannomas areas of degenerative changes and cystic spaces are found. Occasionally isolated cells with bizarre hyperchromatic nuclei are seen. They are common in long-standing or ancient schwannoma. Mitoses are usually absent. Blood vessels are prominent with large vascular spaces which may be confused with vascular neoplasm. Hemosiderin-laden macrophages may be present.

The tumour is positive for S-100, Leu-7 and myelin basic protein.

Schwannomas are composed of proliferated Schwann cells in a background of collagenous tissue.

Initially, the tumour is fusiform, but later the nerve bundle is compressed and displaces it eccentrically. While excision, the nerve can be restored.

Gross: The tumour is well circumscribed and encapsulated. It is attached to the nerve and can be separated from it. It is firm, grey to yellow and areas of cystic degeneration are present.

Microscopy: The elongated spindle-shaped Schwann cells are arranged in fascicles with high cellularity. There is palisading of nuclei of these cells and these cells at places form Verocay bodies (Antoni A pattern). The less cellular areas may show myxoid and cystic degeneration (Fig. 22.10). Areas of haemorrhage are sometimes encountered (Antoni B pattern).

Neurofibroma

Neurofibromas are different from schwannomas. They are softer than schwannomas. They are superficial, small, soft and pedunculated. They are not capsulated. Sometimes these tumours, especially deeper ones grow into larger masses and may produce tortuous enlargement of peripheral nerves and are designated as plexiform neurofibromas.

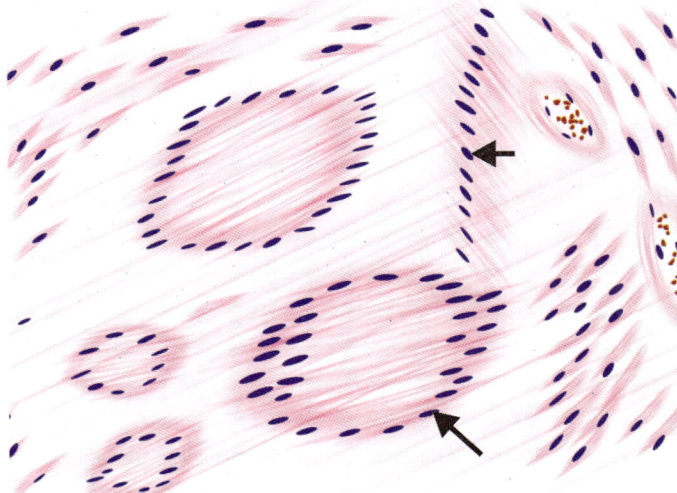

Fig. 22.10: Microscopy of neurilemmoma. Note densely cellular areas (Antoni A pattern) with nuclear palisading (thick arrow—verocay body, thin arrow—palisading of nuclei) (schematic)

Multiple neurofibromas represent important component of genetically determined disorder known as **neurofibromatosis or Recklinghausen's disease type 1** which is **autosomal dominant** disease. **The NF gene is at chromosome 17.** This is also associated with **café au lait spots. Type 2 Recklinghausen's disease** is genetically different and the gene is located at chromosome 22.

Gross: Fusiform, grey white, soft tissue mass, solitary or multiple.

Microscopy: Composed of nerve cells which are spindle shaped with varying amounts of reticulin and collagen. No areas of myxoid or cystic degeneration seen (Figs 22.11 and 22.12).

Table 22.6 describes differences between schwannom and neurofibroma.

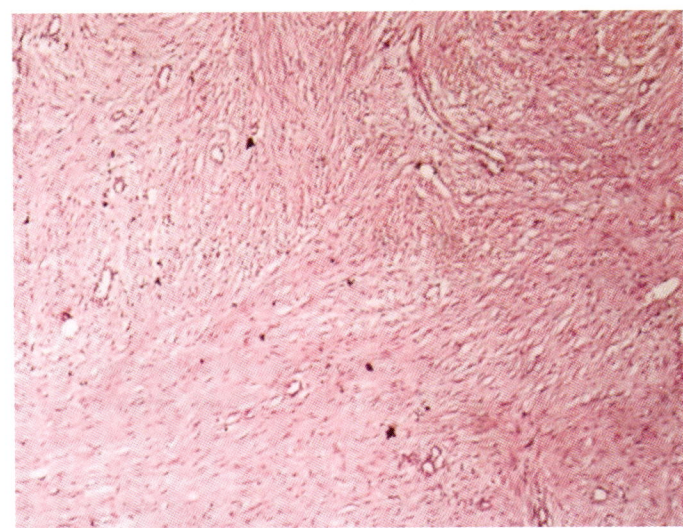

Fig. 22.11: Microphotograph of neurofibroma

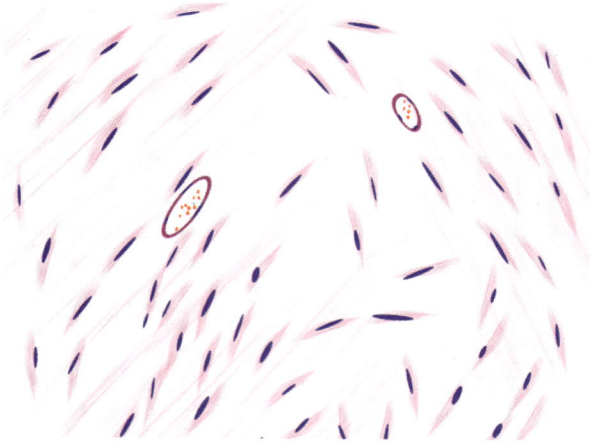

Fig. 22.12: Microscopy of neurofibroma (schematic)

Table 22.6	Differences between schwannoma and neurofibroma
Schwannoma	**Neurofibroma**
Arises from Schwann cells	Arises from nerve cells
Initially fusiform, but later nerve is compressed and is displaced eccentrically	Fusiform, involves/infiltrates nerve
Well circumscribed, capsulated	Soft-well circumscribed, non-encapsulated
Nerve can be restored during surgery	As nerve is involved needs to be cut
Cystic degeneration, hemorrhage, xanthomatous changes are common	Not seen

NICE TO KNOW

RAS PROTEIN

Normal RAS protein belongs to low molecular weight G proteins family, becomes inactive when bound to GDP. Stimulation of cells by growth factors leads to exchange of GDP for GTP and subsequently generates active RAS protein. Mutant RAS has uncontrolled proliferation.

Most commonly, point mutations of RAS are seen in colon and pancreatic cancers.

CANCER SUPPRESSOR GENES

The tumour suppressor genes are of two types.
1. **Gatekeeper genes (promoter genes):** These act as guards for passing through cell cycle. These directly or indirectly interact with Cyclin-CDK complexes. Mutations of the promoter genes (p53 gene, RB gene, APC gene) lead to cancer transformation by releasing brakes on cellular proliferation.
2. **Caretaker genes:** These maintain and protect the integrity of genes. These are involved in DNA repair, mismatch repair (schematic) etc. The caretaker genes (P53, BRCA1 gene, MLH1 gene, MSH2 gene) repair the non-lethally damaged DNA and suppress mutations.

BRCA1: These resolve DNA crosslinks and mutations. Commonly, the mutations are associated with familial breast and ovarian cancers.

Mismatch repair genes: MSH2 and MLH genes. These are not directly involved with cell proliferation.

RB Gene

The gene product binds to DNA. The active form is hypophosphorylated. The hyperphosphorylated form is inactive form. The RB gene exerts antiproliferative effects in G1-S transition of cell cycle. RB gene with less of phosphates binds to E2F transcription factor. With this cyclin E is not formed which is required for DNA replication and thus cells are arrested in G1 phase of cell cycle. RB gene is located on chromosome 13q14. RB gene mutations cause retinoblastoma. In inherited form, one allele has loss of RB gene. The second copy is lost by somatic mutation. In sporadic form, both are lost by somatic mutations. Oncogenic DNA viruses like HPV, EBV and HBV may render RB gene non-functional.

P53 Gene (Guardian of Genomes)

It acts as both promoter and caretaker genes. The following are the important findings as regards to P53 gene:
1. P53 genome senses the DNA damage, assists in DNA repair, by arresting cell division in G_1 phase of cell cycle.
2. It also induces DNA repair genes.
3. MDM2 acts as a negative regulator; P53 gets detached from MDM2 and gets activated.
4. Any DNA damage or chromosomal abnormalities, P53 gene causes cell cycle arrest followed repair and cell cycle restart or induces apoptosis causing death of damaged cells.
5. P53 gene is located on 17p13.1. It has AD inheritance pattern.
6. Li-Fraumeni syndrome is associated with mutations of P53 gene. It is known to be associated with many of the cancers such as osteosarcoma, soft tissue sarcomas, acute leukaemias, breast, brain and adrenal gland.
7. Similar to RB gene, DNA viruses may render P53 gene non-functional.

CYCLINS AND CYCLIN-DEPENDENT KINASES

The cyclin-CDK complexes phosphorylate target proteins which drive the cell through cell cycle.

1. Cyclin D/CDK4 is overexpressed in many cancers (breast, esophagus, liver and glioblastomas).
2. Amplication of CDK4 occurs in melanomas and sarcomas.
3. Mutations of cyclin B, cyclin E and CDKs occur in some cancers.
4. There can be downregulations of CDK inhibitors by mutations, thus promoting cell cycle, e.g. mitogenic p27 relieving inhibition of cyclin E-CDK2 complexes.

TGF BETA PATHWAY

The TGF beta belongs to a family of growth factors. It has inhibitory effects. It binds to TGFR I and II. This binding leads to transcriptional activation of CDKIs with growth suppressive activity as well as repression of growth promoting genes such as MYC and CDKs.

TGF beta binds to type II receptors, this in turn phosphorylates type I receptors. Type I receptors in turn phosphorylates receptor regulated SMADs which can bind to SMAD4. RSMAD/SMAD4 complex accumulates in the nucleus and acts as transcription factor.

APC BETA-CATENIN IN WNT SIGNALING PATHWAY

APC is a tumour suppressor gene and it is an intracellular protein which regulates intracellular levels of beta-catenin. It has anti-proliferative effects. Beta-catenin binds to E-cadherin which mediates intercellular interactions; on the other hand it can translocate to nucleus and activate cell proliferation binding to transcription factor (TF).

Beta-catenin is an important component of Wnt signaling pathway which regulate cell proliferation. Wnt binds to its receptors and sends signals to prevent degradation of beta-catenin, allowing it to translocate to nucleus. Those cells which are not exposed to Wnt, cytoplasmic beta-catenin is degraded by a destruction complex of which APC is a component.

With mutation of APC, beta-catenin is prevented from destruction and individuals develop hundreds of colonic polyps by teen age and later can have loss of one more allele which can have malignant transformation of some of the polyps in early age (Fig. 22.13).

DETAILS ABOUT CANCER CELLS

1. **Evasion of apoptosis:** The DNA damaged cells may escape death by apoptosis. The cancer cells produce excess of anti-apoptotic or less of pro-apoptotic factors. Bcl-2 is upregulated in many of the cancers. In 85% of the follicular B cell lymphomas and other types of NHLs, the anti-apoptotic gene Bcl-2 is activated by t(14;18)(q32:q21). This translocation results in juxtaposition of Bcl-2 on 18q21, and JH locus immunoglobulin Ig heavy chain on 14q32 gene. This leads to activation and overexpression of Bcl-2.

2. **Limitless replicative potential:** There is progressive shortening of telomerase at the ends of chromosomes, during cell division.

The short telomeres are recognized by DNA repair genes and arrest cells entering cell cycle which is mediated by P53 and RB genes. With mutations of P53 and RB gene, the check points are disabled. And also, the tumour cells develop ways to avoid cellular senescence and mitotic catastrophes. The cancer cells

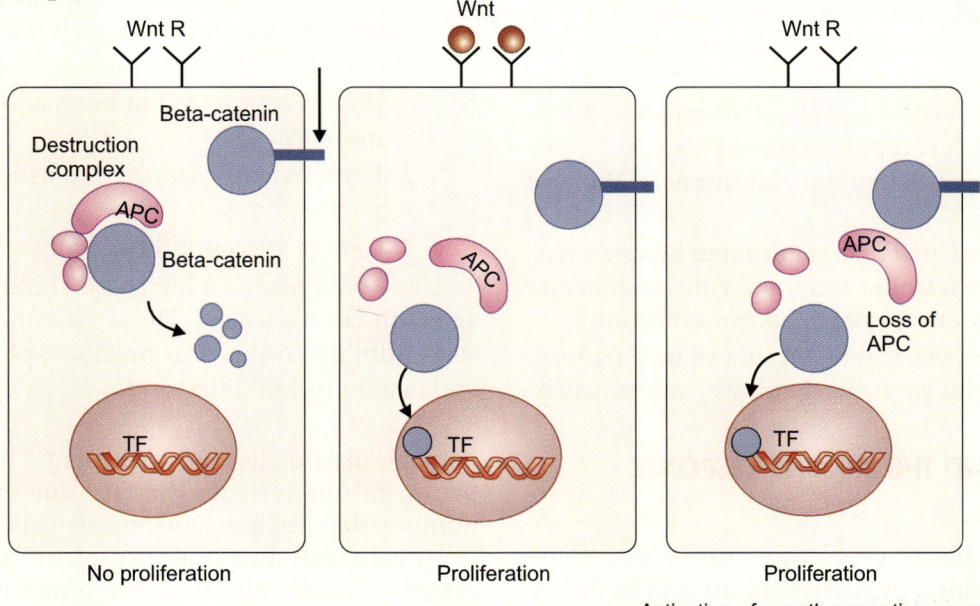

Fig. 22.13: Functioning of APC beta-catenin in Wnt signaling pathway (schematic)

upregulate the enzyme telomerase and with telomerase maintenance, the cancer cells become immortal.

3. **Development of sustained angiogenesis:** The tumour tissue requires oxygen and nutrients. Hence, cancer tissues need to be vascularised. Sustained angiogenesis is essential for invasive tumour growth. Hypoxia triggers angiogenesis by HIF-1-alpha. Von Hippel-Lindau (VHL) gene degrades HIF-1-alpha and thus acts as tumour suppressor gene. Hypoxia also triggers VGEF through hypoxia-inducible factor 1-alpha which is a transcription factor.

Mutations of VHL gene are associated with VHL syndrome which has renal cell carcinoma, pheochromocytoma, haemangiomas of CNS, retinal angiomas and renal cysts.

In normal health, the development of new blood vessels is highly regulated by both positive and negative controls.

4. **Ability to invade and metastasize:** This is already described in spread of tumours.

5. **Genetic instability:** Persons born with high frequency of mutations are at high risk of developing cancer. Following are some of the examples:
   a. Hereditary non-polyposis colon cancer (HNPCC)
   b. Xeroderma pigmentosum
   c. Chromosomal breakage syndromes

   • *Hereditary non-polyposis colon cancer (HNPCC):* This is also called **Lynch syndrome.** It has autosomal dominant inheritance with high risk of colon cancer as well as other cancers. There is defect in the DNA repair genes.

   • *Xeroderma pigmentosum:* These patients are at increased risk of cancers of skin exposed to UV light/sunlight and can develop multiple malignancies. This has AR pattern of inheritance. There is defect in DNA repair in these patients.
   Note: Refer pre-malignant conditions of the oral cavity.

   • *Chromosomal breakage syndromes:* Bloom's syndrome, ataxia telangiectasia, and Fanconi anaemia fall under chromosomal breakage syndromes.
   Bloom's syndrome: It has AR inheritance pattern. These patients have short stature, sun sensitive

skin changes, immunodeficiency, reduced fertility and are prone for many cancers. Dr David Bloom (German, 1969) first described this. There is tendency for chromosomal breakage and rearrangements.

Central and Eastern European (Ashkanazi) Jewish people are frequently affected. 1;50,000 population are affected.

Ataxia telangiectsia (Louis-Bar syndrome): It is an AR disorder and is characterised by chromosomal breakages. It is an ataxic dyskinetic syndrome beginning early in childhood. There is neuronal degeneration predominantly affecting cerebellum. There is loss of Purkinge cells and and granular cells. There is loss of dorsal columns, spinocerebellar tracts, anterior horn cells and has peripheral neuropathy. There is primary immunodeficiency. These patients are hypersensitive to ionizing radiation. The disease progresses to death early in second decade. There is mutation of ATM gene encoding repair enzyme.

The four "As" to remember are:
1. **ATM** gene
2. **A**taxia (cerebellar defects)
3. Spider **A**ngioma (telangiectasia)
4. Ig**A** deficiency

The ataxia telangiectasia syndrome has ataxia and telangiectasia in early childhood and recurrent sinopulmonary (ear, sinuses and lungs) infections.

Fanconi anaemia: Fanconi anaemia is an inherited chromosomal instability syndrome with variable clinical manifestations which include:
1. Congenital anomalies: Short stature, skin pigmentation, radial bone and thumb abnormalities.
2. Bone marrow failure: Aplastic anaemia with pancytopenia.
3. Cancer susceptibility.

These patients have increased chromosomal breakage with DNA damage. These patients have increased susceptibility to develop myelodysplastic syndrome and acute myeloid leukaemia.

IMMUNOLOGY AND THE IMMUNE RESPONSE TO CANCER

Cancer is a major health problem worldwide and one of the most important causes of morbidity and mortality to the humans. The lethality in cancer is due to their uncontrolled growth within normal tissues, causing damage and functional impairment. The malignant cell proliferation reflects the tumour evasion of host immune defence mechanisms, defects in regulation of cell proliferation, resistance of the tumour cells to apoptotic death, ability of the tumour cells to invade the basement of the host tissues and metastasize to distant sites.

Tumour development can be controlled by innate and adaptive immune cells:

1. **Innate immunity:** It is the body's first line of defence. These immune cells are programmed to attack cells they sense as a threat to the host. Among the cells in the innate immune system are **natural killer (NK) cells.** These can attack and kill cancerous and pre-cancerous cells.

2. **The acquired immune system:** It is also called adaptive immunity. The tumour cells can be recognized and destroyed by CD8+ T lymphocytes. These are also called cytotoxic T cells. Tumour antigens are presented to cytotoxic T cells as small peptides via major histocompatibility complex class I molecules (MHC-I, or HLA-I in humans). It is likely that T cell-mediated immune surveillance is, in fact, destroying the tumour cells without any noticeable signs of the rejection process. Spontaneous regression, regression of metastasis after removal of primary tumour, infiltration of lymphocytes around the tumour cells, etc., higher incidence cancer after immunosuppression and immunodeficiency, children and old people prone for cancers suggests the role of immunity in normal health.

As the clinically detectable tumours develop, cancer cells evolve different mechanisms that mimic peripheral immune tolerance in order to avoid tumouricidal attack. Following are some of the ways of survival of cancer cells:

1. **Tumour immune escape** is associated with the loss of tumour HLA class I (HLA-I) expression commonly found in malignant cells. They may acquire new antigens.

2. **Insensitivity to growth inhibitory signals:** Cancer cells ignore or escape the growth inhibitory signals, e.g. loss of tumour suppressor genes, e.g. RB and P53.

3. **Evasion of apoptosis**

SELF-ASSESSMENT EXERCISE

1. **Not true about tumour marker:**
   A. Tumour marker is used to diagnose residual tumour or recurrence of the tumour.
   B. PSA for diagnosis of carcinoma prostate.
   C. To diagnose cancer
   D. CEA is used for colon cancer

2. **The immune response against tumour cells is:**
   A. CD8 T cells
   B. CD4 T cells
   C. Null cells
   D. Null cells and CD4 T cells

3. **The tumour antigens are displayed by:**
   A. MHC II   B. Toll molecules
   C. Adhesion molecules D. MHC I molecules

4. **DNA repair defect is seen in all *except*:**
   A. Xeroderma pigmentosum
   B. Bloom's syndrome
   C. Ataxia telangiectasia
   D. Li-Fraumani syndrome

5. **All are true about hybridoma cells *except*:**
   A. Immortal
   B. Monoclonal
   C. Involves fusion of myeloma cells and B cells
   D. Involves separation of cells

6. **Kohler and Milstein are known for:**
   A. PCR technique
   B. Sothern blot technique
   C. Hybridoma technique
   D. Western blot technique

7. **Pap smear, a screening method is used for early detection of:**
   A. Breast cancer   B. Lung cancer
   C. Oral cancer   D. Cervical cancer

8. **Self-examination, a screening method, is detection of:**
   A. Cervical cancer   B. Oral cancer
   C. Breast cancer   D. Liver cancer

9. **Marjolin's ulcer can have following *except*:**
   A. Squamous cell carcinoma
   B. Chronic venous insufficiency
   C. Chronic non-healing ulcer
   D. Adenocarcinoma

10. **CA125 is elevated in:**
    A. Surface epithelial ovarian tumours
    B. Stromal tumours of ovary
    C. Germ cell tumours of ovary
    D. All of the above

Answers

1. C   2. A   3. D   4. D   5. D   6. C   7. D   8. C
9. D   10. A

Systemic Pathology I

Lymph Node Lesions

NORMAL STRUCTURE

The lymph node has cortex, paracortex and medulla. The cortex is situated just beneath the capsule and the medulla is close to the hilum. The cortex represents the B cell zone. The paracortex is situated between the cortex and the medulla and represents T cell zone. The medulla deep to cortex and paracortex has medullary cords and medullary sinuses (Fig. 23.1).

REACTIVE LYMPHADENITIS

Infectious and non-microbial stimuli may cause lymphadenopathy. This may be acute or chronic. In most instances, the histologic changes are non-specific.

ACUTE NON-SPECIFIC LYMPHADENITIS

In acute non-specific lymphadenitis, lymph nodes are swollen, confined to local infections or generalized as in bacterial and viral infections. They are tender; fluctuant with abscess formation, overlying skin is red and can have draining sinuses. With control of infection, lymph node reverts back to its normal size or may undergo scarring, if damaged by infection.

Microscopy shows large germinal centres and numerous mitoses of the cells. When infection is caused

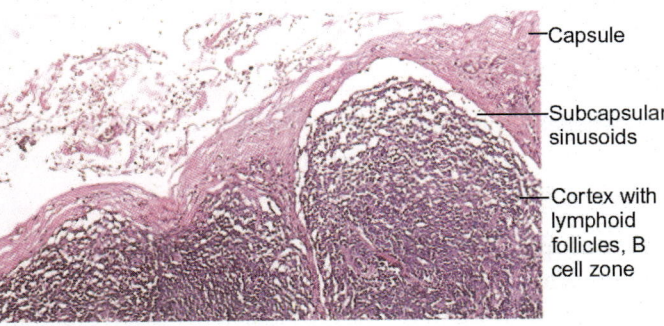

— Capsule

— Subcapsular sinusoids

— Cortex with lymphoid follicles, B cell zone

Fig. 23.1: Microphotograph of normal structure of lymph node

by pyogenic organisms, neutrophilic infiltrate is seen in the follicles and sinuses with severe infection. Necrosis with abscess formation can be present.

CHRONIC NON-SPECIFIC LYMPHADENITIS

This can have follicular hyperplasia, paracortical hyperplasia or sinus histiocytosis.

FOLLICULAR HYPERPLASIA

This is seen in infectious and non-infectious conditions. When reactive follicles are large following should be considered.
1. Infection by Epstein-Barr virus should be suspected.
2. Rheumatoid arthritis
3. Toxoplasmosis
4. Early stage of HIV infection

In reactive hyperplasia, following are the important features:
1. The follicles vary in size and shape.
2. Their margins are sharply defined.
3. The germinal centres have crisp or sharp edge.
4. Follicle is surrounded by mantle of small lymphocytes, often arranged circumferentially (onion skin pattern) or at one pole of the follicle (at the point of antigenic stimulation).
5. The follicles are composed of two distinct areas: A darker peripheral zone has proliferating blast like B cells termed as centroblasts, and central pale area having admixture of small and large lymphoid cells with cleaved nuclei.
6. Mitoses are numerous.
7. Phagocytosis of nuclear debris with Tingible body macrophages.

Table 23.1 highlights the differences between follicular lymphoma and follicular hyperplasia.

Table 23.1	Differences between follicular lymphoma and follicular hyperplasia	
Follicular lymphoma	**Follicular hyperplasia**
Architectural features	
Complete effacement of architecture	Nodal architecture preserved
Follicles evenly spread in cortex and medulla	Follicles only in cortex
Slight variation in size and shape of follicles	Follicles with marked variation in size and shape
Fading of follicles	Sharp or crisp-edged germinal centres
Follicles extend beyond capsule	No
Reticulin fibres condensed around the follicles	No change in the reticulin network
Cytological features	
Follicles with monomorphic or polymorphic cells with nuclear irregularities	Centre of follicles with lymphoid cells, histiocytes, reticulum cells, no nuclear irregularities
Similarity of cells inside and outside the follicles	Infiltration of inflammatory cells between the reaction centres
No phagocytosis	Active phagocytosis in reactive centres, tangible body macrophages present
No apoptosis, Bcl-2 positive	Apoptosis present, Bcl-2 negative
Paucity of mitoses inside the follicles, no much difference with mitoses outside the follicles, atypical mitoses present	Centre with increased mitoses, rare mitoses outside, no atypical mitoses

PARACORTICAL HYPERPLASIA

In this, reactive changes are seen in T cell regions. The T cells transform into immunoblasts, proliferate and efface upon B cell regions (follicles). Paracortical hyperplasia is observed in viral infection (e.g. EBV), following certain vaccination and reaction to certain drugs.

SINUS HISTIOCYTOSIS

In this pattern, there is distension and prominence of lymphoid sinusoids. The endothelial cells are hypertrophied. Histiocytes/macrophages are seen in the distended sinuses. This is usually encountered in lymph nodes draining cancer and may represent an immune response.

CAT-SCRATCH DISEASE

This is a self-limited lymphadenitis, caused by bacteria *Bartonella henselae*. It is a disease of childhood. It presents with axillary and cervical lymphadenopathy. The enlargement is usually after a feline scratch (scratch of cat) or uncommonly after a thorn injury. The lymph nodes regress after 2–4 months, rarely encephalitis occurs.

Microscopy: Shows partial distortion of architecture, capsulitis, sarcoid-like granulomas; these may surround **central necrosis which has plenty of neutrophils.** Similar lesion can be seen in lymphogranuloma venereum. Diagnosis can be made by silver stain, EM, serology, IHC, PCR or the positive skin test to the microbial antigen.

KIKUCHI-FUJIMOTO DISEASE
(Histiocytic Necrotising Lymphadenitis)

The etiology of this Kikuchi-Fujimoto disease is unknown. Viruses like EBV, Hepatitis B, HSV6 and 8 and parvovirus B19 are linked with this pathology. Patients have fever and painless cervical lymphadenopathy often accompanied by leucopenia.

Microscopy: Lymph node shows partially effaced architecture with large discrete areas of **necrosis with abundant nuclear debris surrounded by transformed lymphocytes, histiocytes, dendritic cells and plasmacytoid cells.** These plasmacytoid cells are 2–3 times the size of small lymphocytes with round nuclei, open chromatin small nucleoli and variable amount of cytoplasm. Transformed lymphocytes are cytotoxic CD8+ T cells. Neutrophils are absent, follicular centres are not hyperplastic. Absence of neutrophils and lack of follicular hyperplasia can differentiate **Kikuchi-Fujimoto disease** from cat-scratch disease. Overt necrosis and partial effacement of lymph node architecture, dendritic cells, bland cytologic features differentiate this lesion from malignant lymphoma.

KIMURA DISEASE

This disease commonly affects young Asian men. There is subcutaneous cervical mass with lymph node involvement.

Microscopy: The soft tissue lesion shows proliferation of thin-walled vessels with tissue eosinophilia. Lymph node shows follicular hyperplasia with interfollicular increased eosinophils and proliferation of thin-walled vessels. Late lesions may show sclerosis with Charcot-Leyden crystals. This lesion needs to be differentiated from angiolymphoid hyperplasia with eosinophilia which affects only the skin and lymph nodes are spared.

HODGKIN DISEASE (Hodgkin Lymphoma)

Hodgkin disease (HD) or Hodgkin lymphoma (HL) is a malignant neoplasm of the lymphoid system with potential to spread to many sites and produce large tumour masses containing dysplastic cells (Reed-Sternberg cells).

Etiology: Viral infections like EBV, HIV, etc. are known to cause the disease. Patients having EBV related diseases such as infectious mononucleosis have two- to threefold higher risk of Hodgkin's disease. Family history and genetic mutations involving lymphocyte function have higher incidence of HD.

Classification of Hodgkin's lymphoma (WHO)

1. Classical Hodgkin lymphoma
   • Nodular sclerosis
   • Lymphocyte-rich
   • Mixed cellularity
   • Lymphocyte depleted
2. Nodular lymphocyte predominant Hodgkin lymphoma

HL shares the following characteristics:

1. Usually arise in the lymph nodes preferably cervical lymph nodes. These are painless, single or contiguous lymph nodes involved.
2. Constitutional symptoms like fever, night sweats, weight loss may be present.
3. Majority of them manifest clinically in young adults.
4. Liver, spleen, bone marrow involvement may be present.
5. It is characterized by Reed-Sternberg cells.

6. The tumour cells are usually ringed by T lymphocytes in a rosette-like manner.

The important finding in Hodgkin lymphoma is the Reed-Sternberg (RS) cell. This is a large cell (15–45 μm in diameter) with mirror image nuclei, exceptionally prominent nucleoli, distinct nuclear membrane and abundant, basophilic to amphophilic cytoplasm. The nucleus has inclusion-like acidophilic nucleolus surrounded by a distinctive clear zone (halo); together they impart an **owl-eye appearance**.

In general, in Hodgkin disease, following are the gross and microscopic features.

Gross: The lymph nodes are enlarged, grey white, and are of rubbery consistency.

Microscopy: This varies depending upon the type of Hodgkin's disease. In **mixed cellularity,** there is diffuse effacement of the lymph node architecture with polymorphic cellular infiltrate which includes small lymphocytes, eosinophils, plasma cells and macrophages admixed with plenty of Reed-Sternberg (RS) cells (classical and mononuclear varieties). The nodular sclerosis Hodgkin disease may show abundant fibrosis; the classical RS cells are less frequent and show lacunar variety of RS cells. Lymphocyte-rich Hodgkin disease shows lymphocyte predominance with mononuclear and classical RS cells. In lymphocyte depletion Hodgkin's disease, RS cells with bizarre configuration and atypical mononuclear variants are present.

In nodular lymphocyte predominance Hodgkin disease, there is effacement of lymph node architecture which shows nodular infiltrate of small lymphocytes admixed with histiocytes. In this histological type, the classical RS cells are difficult to find and, however, they have L and H variants (popcorn cells).

Various types of RS cells and microscopy in Hodgkin disease are shown in Figs 23.2 to 23.4.

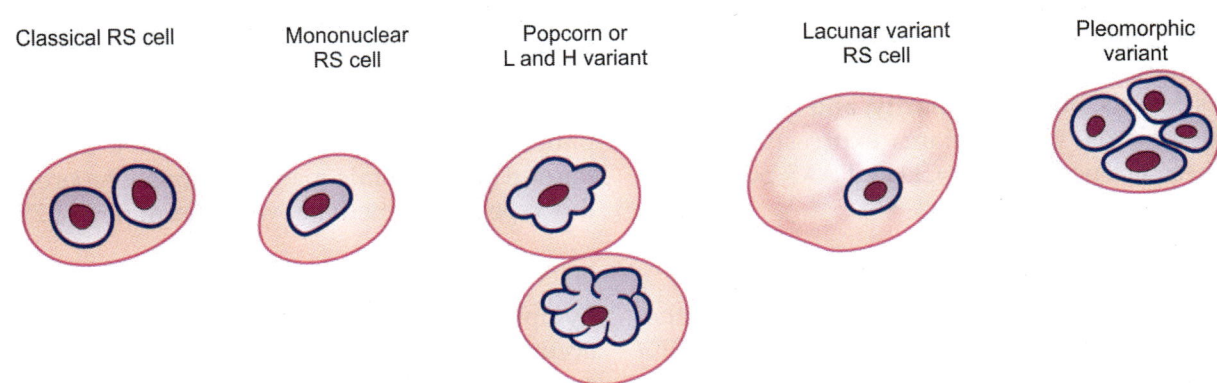

| Classical RS cell | Mononuclear RS cell | Popcorn or L and H variant | Lacunar variant RS cell | Pleomorphic variant |

Fig. 23.2: Various types of RS cells

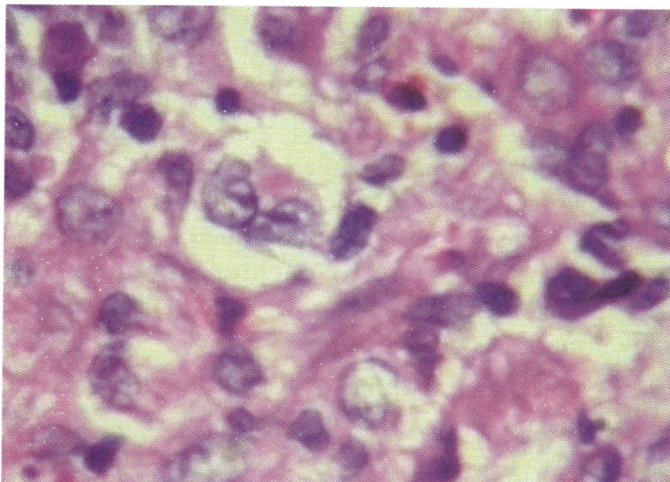

Fig. 23.3: Microphotograph of Hodgkin disease, note RS cell

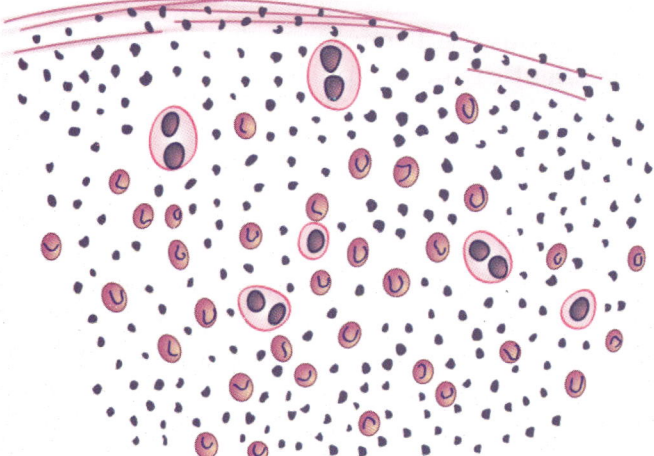

Fig. 23.4: Microscopy of Hodgkin disease (mixed cellularity) (schematic)

CLASSICAL HODGKIN LYMPHOMA

Classical Hodgkin lymphoma (CHL) is characterised by clonal proliferation of typical mononuclear Hodgkin cells and multinucleated Reed-Sternberg cells. A variable inflammatory background of lymphocytes, eosinophils, macrophages, neutrophils, plasma cells, fibroblasts, and collagenous tissue determines the morphologic appearance.

Four different types of CHL are **lymphocyte-rich, nodular sclerosis, mixed cellularity, and lymphocyte-depleted variants.** CHL variants express CD15 and CD30. These are negative for CD45. PAX5 positive in RS cells.

Nodular Sclerosis Hodgkin Lymphoma

Nodular sclerosis Hodgkin lymphoma (NSHL) is the most common form of HL and accounts for 70% of CHL. Commonly affects adolescent girls and young women in the age range of 15 to 35 years and manifests as lower

cervical, supraclavicular and mediastinal adenopathy (stage II). Symptoms occur in up to 40% of patients.

Microscopy: NSHL features nodular architecture in which lymphoid tissue is surrounded by broad bands of collagen tissue. The fibrous bands show birefringence under polarized light. In NSHL, there is presence of a particular variant of the RS cells called **lacunar cells, in addition to classical RS cells**. The lacunar cells are large and have a single multilobate nucleus with multiple small nucleoli and an abundant, pale-staining cytoplasm. In formalin-fixed tissue, the cytoplasm often retracts, giving rise to the appearance of cells lying in empty spaces, or lacunae. The fibrosis may be scant or abundant, and the cellular infiltrate may show varying proportions of lymphocytes, eosinophils, histiocytes, and lacunar cells. Classical RS cells are infrequent.

Prognosis: The prognosis is good, with a cure rate of 80 to 85%. Untreated, NSHL is fatal, with a 10-year survival rate of only 1%. With irradiation and chemotherapy, a 70% cure rate can be achieved.

Mixed Cellularity Hodgkin Lymphoma

The mixed cellularity Hodgkin lymphoma has following features:
1. Most common form of **Hodgkin lymphoma** in older patients (>50 yrs).
2. Most frequent HL subtype in HIV1-infected patients and shows the highest association with EBV.
3. Accounts for 25% of cases of Hodgkin disease.
4. Has male predominance.
5. Cervical lymph nodes are commonly affected. However, after staging, most patients are found to have stage II or III disease. A minority have visceral involvement (stage IV).
6. Mediastinal involvement is uncommon.

Microscopy: Classic RS cells are plentiful within a distinctive heterogeneous cellular infiltrate, which includes small lymphocytes, eosinophils, plasma cells, histiocytes and atypical mononuclear RS cells. Focal necrosis may be present but fibrosis is absent or minimal.

Prognosis: Compared with the other common subtypes, patients with mixed cellularity have disseminated disease and systemic manifestations. The prognosis of this type is intermediate, with a cure rate of 75%.

Lymphocyte-Rich Hodgkin Lymphoma

Lymphocyte-rich Hodgkin lymphoma (LRHL) variant occurs in **older population and mediastinal involvement** is common. It is characterised by classical and mononuclear RS cells in an abundant background of small lymphocytes. Mixed inflammatory cells and collagen bands are missing.

Prognosis: Prognosis is favourable and similar to NLPHL.

Lymphocyte-Depleted Hodgkin Lymphoma

Lymphocyte-depleted Hodgkin lymphoma (LDHL) has the following features:

1. Least common type of CHL.
2. Frequently **associated with HIV** infection and most are positive for EBV too.
3. Advanced stage and symptoms are seen in more than 70% of patients.
4. Affects middle-aged to elderly men.
5. Advanced clinical stage (III and IV) and signs and symptoms are present in two-thirds of patients.
6. Those with the diffuse fibrosis subtype of LDHL commonly present with fever of undetermined origin, pancytopenia, and wasting.
7. There is usually **no peripheral or mediastinal lymphadenopathy**. However, retroperitoneal lymphadenopathy and involvement of the spleen, liver, and bone marrow are common.

Microscopy: Shows marked absence of background lymphocytes and has bizarre RS cells.

Prognosis: LDHL is the most clinically aggressive type. The overall cure rate of LDHL is 40 to 50%. Without treatment, this type of HL has the worst prognosis. Profound immunodeficiency develops and death commonly results from secondary infections.

NODULAR LYMPHOCYTE PREDOMINANT HODGKIN LYMPHOMA

Nodular lymphocyte predominant Hodgkin lymphoma (NLPHL) has following features:

1. Accounts for 5% of HL cases.
2. Presents in young adult men.
3. Presents with isolated cervical or axillary lymphadenopathy.
4. Usually in stage I or II, stage IV rare.
5. Uncommonly involves bone, liver and spleen unless when changes to aggressive pattern.

Microscopy: It is characterised by a large number of small resting lymphocytes admixed with a variable number of histiocytes, often within large, poorly defined nodules. Eosinophils, neutrophils, and plasma cells are scanty or absent, and classic RS cells are extremely difficult to find. Scattered among the reactive cells are **lymphohistiocytic (L and H) variant** RS cells that have a delicate multilobed, puffy nucleus that has been likened in appearance to popcorn (**popcorn cell**).

L and H variants have rearranged and somatically hypermutated IgH genes, strongly supporting a follicular B cell origin.

Nodular lymphocyte predominant HD express B markers (CD19, 20, LCA), PAX5, MUM1 and CD15 and 30 negative.

Prognosis: The disease has excellent prognosis.

NICE TO KNOW

STAGING OF HODGKIN DISEASE

Ann Arbor staging of Hodgkin disease

Stage IA or B	I or	Single lymph node group
	I E	Single extranodal organ or site
Stage IIA or B	II or	Two or more lymph node groups on same side of diaphragm
	II E	With localized contiguous involvement of extralymphatic organ or site
Stage IIIA or B	III	Two or more lymph node groups on both sides of diaphragm
	III E	With localized contiguous involvement of extralymphatic organ or site
	IIIS	With spleen involvement
	IIIES	With extralymphatic organ or site and spleen
Stage IVA or B	IV	Diffuse or disseminated with one or more extralymphatic organs with or without lymph node involvement

A: Asymptomatic, B: Symptomatic

Cotswolds modification of Ann Arbor staging system for Hodgkin lymphoma

Stage	Area of involvement
I	Single lymph node group
II	Multiple lymph node groups on same side of diaphragm
III	Multiple lymph node groups on both sides of diaphragm
IV	Multiple extranodal sites or lymph nodes and extranodal disease
X	Bulk >10 cm
E	Extranodal extension or single, isolated site of extranodal disease
A/B	A: Asymptomatic B: Symptoms: Weight loss >10%, fever, drenching night sweats

The Cotswolds modification maintains the original 4-stage clinical and pathologic staging framework of the Ann Arbor staging system but also adds information regarding the prognostic significance of bulky disease (denoted by an X designation) and regions of lymph node involvement (denoted by an E designation).

Table 23.2   Differences between Hodgkin lymphoma and non-Hodgkin lymphoma

Hodgkin lymphoma	Non-Hodgkin lymphoma
More often localized to single group of lymph nodes (either cervical, mediastinal or para-aortic)	Multiple groups of lymph nodes are involved
Spread by contiguity	Non-contiguous spread
Mesenteric lymph nodes and Waldeyar ring rarely involved	Mesenteric lymph nodes and Waldeyar ring commonly involved
Extranodal involvement less common	Extranodal involvement more common
Leukaemic phase absent	Leukaemic phase present
Has association with virus EBV	Has association with virus HIV and immunosuppression
Low grade fever, night sweats and weight loss are common constitutional symptoms	Fewer symptoms
Responsive to treatment	Depends upon type of NHL
Curable with 5-year survival 90%	Prognosis varies with type of NHL and overall survival lesser compared to HD

Hodgkin lymphoma has to be differentiated from non-Hodgkin lymphoma for treatment purposes and Table 23.2 shows the differences between the two.

NON-HODGKIN LYMPHOMA
(Malignant Lymphoma)

Non-Hodgkin lymphoma (NHL) or malignant lymphomas (ML) are neoplastic disorders which originate from the lymphoid tissue similar to Hodgkin's disease but do not have the RS cells. NHLs are common in men than women. It is common malignancy occurring in developed countries accounting for 4.3% of all malignancies in USA.[17]

Risk Factors and Etiology

The risk factors for development of lymphoma are not fully understood. However, following factors are implicated and association is seen in the causation of the disease.

1. Environmental association with pesticides, chemicals, hair dyes, radiation and chemotherapy are known.
2. Viruses: HIV infection, EBV in Burkitt lymphoma, Human T cell leukaemia Virus-1(HTLV-1) in T cell lymphomas and leukaemias.
3. Immune-suppression with inherited disorders like severe combined immunodeficiency disease, Wiskott-Aldrich syndrome.
4. Infection with *H. pylori* with ongoing antigenic stimulation is known to cause NHLs and especially MALT lymphomas.
5. Patients with chronic diseases.
6. Patients with autoimmune diseases: Hashimoto's thyroiditis is known to cause primary NHL in thyroid gland.

7. Chromosomal translocations play an important role in the causation of NHLs. Chromosomal translocations like t(14:18) in follicular lymphoma, t(11:14) in mantal cell lymphoma, etc. are known in non-Hodgkin's lymphomas.

Classification of NHL

There have been different classifications proposed from time to time for non-Hodgkin lymphomas or malignant lymphomas. Initial classifications were based on histomorphology. The REAL/WHO 2001, WHO 2008 and revision of WHO 2016 classification of lymphoid neoplasms are based on immunophenotype, karyotype and molecular features (Table 23.3).

The 2016 revision clarifies the diagnosis, management at very early stages of lymphoid neoplasms, refines the diagnostic criteria of some of the entities, expands genetic and molecular markers, their clinical correlation and targeted therapeutic strategies.

SMALL LYMPHOCYTIC LEUKAEMIA/CHRONIC LYMPHOCYTIC LYMPHOMA (SLL/CLL)

These two disorders are morphologically, phenotypically and genotypically identical, differing only in peripheral blood involvement. Arbitrarily, if the absolute lymphocyte count exceeds 4000 cells/cmm, the diagnosis of CLL is made, otherwise labelled as SLL. Most often SLL/CLL is preferred.

Epidemiology

Small lymphocytic lymphoma/chronic lymphocytic leukaemia is the malignant lymphoma accounting for 11.3% of the cases.

Table 23.3	2016 WHO classification of mature lymphoid, histiocytic and dendritc neoplasms[18]

Non-Hodgkin lymphoma

Mature B neoplasms

- Chronic lymphocytic leukaemia/small lymphocytic lymphoma (CLL/SLL)
- Monoclonal B cell lymphocytosis
- B-prolymphocytic leukaemia
- Splenic marginal zone lymphoma
- Hairy cell leukaemia (HCL)
- Splenic B cell lymphoma/leukaemia
- Lymphoplasmacytic lymphoma (Waldenstrom's macro-globulinaemia)
- MUGS-IgM/IgG/IgA
- Heavy chain diseases (Mue, gamma and alpha)
- Plasma cell myeloma
- Solitary plasmacytoma of bone
- Extra osseous plasmacytoma
- MALT lymphoma
- Nodal marginal zone lymphoma
- Follicular lymphoma
- Large B cell lymphoma
- Mantle cell lymphoma
- Diffuse large B cell lymphoma (DLBCL)
- T cell rich large B cell lymphoma
- CNS large B cell lymphoma
- Thymic/mediastinal large B cell lymphoma
- ALK positive large B cell lymphoma
- Plasmablastic lymphoma
- Burkitt lymphoma
- High Grade B cell lymphoma

Mature T and NK cell neoplasms

- T cell prolymphocytic leukaemia
- T cell large cell lymphoma
- Aggressive NK cell leukaemia
- Adult T cell lymphoma/leukaemia
- Extranodal T/K cell lymphoma, nasal type
- Enteropathy associated T cell lymphoma
- Mycosis fungoides
- Sezary syndrome
- Primary cutaneous CD30 positive T cell lymphoproliferative disease
- Peripheral T cell lymphoma
- Angioimmunoblastic lymphoma
- Anaplastic large cell lymphoma (ALK+ /ALK–)

Hodgkin's lymphoma

Post-transplant lymphoproliferative disorder

Histiocytic and dendritic cell neoplasms

Histiocytic and dendritic neoplasms

Morphology

In SLL/CLL, lymph nodes are enlarged and the architecture is effaced. There is diffuse proliferation of small round lymphocytes with regular nuclear contours, inconspicuous nucleoli, scanty cytoplasm, mitoses are minimal and scattered larger cells (prolymphocytes and paraimmunoblasts) with vesicular nuclei and prominent nucleoli.

Bone marrow, spleen and liver are also infiltrated with such cells. There is absolute lymphocytosis and these cells are fragile and gets disrupted during preparation of smears. These are called smudge cells. Smear also shows variable number of larger activated lymphocytes.

Immunophenotype, karyotype and molecular features: The cells of small lymphocytic lymphoma are always of B cell type. They express pan B cell markers (CD19, CD20, CD23 and surface Ig heavy and light chains). The cells express CD5 similar to cells of mantle cell lymphoma. These are negative for CD10. Trisomy 21, deletions of chromosomes 11 and 12 are frequent karyotypic anomalies. ZAP-70 positivity has unfavourable prognosis.

Clinical Features

The patients are elderly or middle aged; often have fewer or no symptoms. The symptoms are non-specific and these include easy fatigability, weight loss and anorexia. Generalised lymphadenopathy and hepato-megaly are present in 50–60% of the cases. The total count is increased and may exceed 2 lac cells/cmm. Hypogammaglobulinaemia is present in 50% of the cases late in the disease process and this is the reason for increased susceptibility to bacterial infections. This may be associated with monoclonal gammopathy (50% of the cases involve bone marrow) with plasmacytoid differentiation. Less commonly, these patients may present with autoimmune haemolytic anaemia and thrombocytopenia.

Prognosis

The prognosis is good. These patients survive for more than 10 yrs after diagnosis. The lesion may transform into prolymphoctic lymphoma or large B cell lymphoma (Richter's syndrome) with median survival of less than one year.

FOLLICULAR LYMPHOMA

Follicular lymphoma (FL) is relatively common and accounts for 40% of the adult NHLs. They are unusual before 20 years of age.

Pathology

The lymph nodes are enlarged. The architecture is effaced and cortex and medulla show nodular pattern of growth of lymphoid follicles. The tumour cells resemble normal follicular centre B cells, most of these are centrocytes. These are slightly larger than resting B cells, angular cleaved nuclei, nuclear chromatin is coarse and condensed and nucleoli are indistinct. These cells are mixed with larger centroblasts having vesicular chromatin, several nucleoli with moderate amount of cytoplasm. Mitoses are infrequent; apoptotic cells are not seen. Uniform follicles and indistinct/fading of lymphoid follicles are common. Condensation of reticulin fibres around the follicles helps to distinguish follicular lymphoma from follicular hyperplasia.

Immunophenotype, karyotype and molecular features: The cells express pan B markers CD19, CD10 and CD20. CD5 and CD43 are negative. t(14:18)(q32;q21) is found in 85% of FL. The chromosomal translocation juxtaposes IgH with Bcl-2 gene and over expresses Bcl-2 protein, an anti-apoptotic protein. Hence, there is no apoptosis. Bcl-6 translocation, P53 and Bcl-2 mutations can be seen. Bcl-6 and CD10, the follicular centre cell markers are helpful in diagnosis.

Depending upon number of centroblasts, follicular lymphoma is graded as below:

Grade 1. Follicular lymphoma with 0–5 centroblasts/hpf

Grade 2. Follicular lymphoma with 6–15 centroblasts/hpf

Grade 3. Follicular lymphoma with >15 centroblasts/hpf

Clinical Features

Follicular lymphoma predominantly occurs in adults or elderly persons, males and females are equally affected. It presents with painless generalized lymphadenopathy, extranodal involvement is common. Bone marrow is almost always involved at the time of diagnosis. It has median survival of 7–9 yrs, but not easily curable. About 40% of the cases progress to diffuse large B cell lymphoma with or without treatment.

Prognosis

Grade 1 follicular lymphoma has good prognosis with indolent clinical course, whereas Grade 3 has aggressive course, while Grade 2 follicular lymphoma has intermediate clinical course.

MANTLE CELL LYMPHOMA

These contribute 4% of NHLs and occur mainly in elderly males. It is of low grade nature. It is also called by names of intermediate lymphocytic mantle zone, centrocytic and diffuse small cleaved cell lymphoma.

Pathology

There is diffuse proliferation with occasional presence of small germinal centre like structures (naked germinal centres). The cells are slightly larger than small lymphocytes, irregular and cleaved nucleoli and indistinct nucleoli. These cells may be admixed with some larger cells resembling lymphoblasts. Bone marrow is involved in majority of the cases and 20% of the cases have peripheral spillage. These may have gastrointestinal tract involvement in the form of multifocal submucosal nodule which resemble as polyps (lymphomatoid polyps).

Immunophenotype, karyotype and molecular features of mantle cell lymphoma:

1. The cells express surface IgM and IgD
2. Pan B cell antigens CD19, CD20 positive
3. CD5 positive (similar to CLL/SLL). CD23 negative. It is to be differentiated from CLL/SLL by the presence of Cyclin D1 and absence of CD23. There is t(11:14) (q13:q32) that fuses Cyclin D1 gene on chromosome 11 to IgH on chromosome 14. Thus, there is overexpression of Cyclin D1.

Clinical Features

Most patients have fatigue and lymphadenopathy. Bone marrow, spleen, liver and often GIT are involved. These tumours are aggressive and incurable and median survival is 3 to 5 years.

MARGINAL ZONE LYMPHOMA

Marginal zone lymphoma (MZL) cells have the capacity to develop into B cells or plasma cells. These account for 8% of NHLs.

Pathology

The tumour cells are small to medium sized. The nodal MZL is usually sinusoidal and interfollicular or sometimes with follicular colonization.

The extranodal MZL of mucosa associated lymphoid tissue (MALT lymphoma) has small round lymphocytes, monocytoid B cells, plasmacytoid cells and plasma cells. Splenic MZL also can occur.

Prognosis

MALT lymphoma has good prognosis. Nodal MZL and splenic MZL have indolent course.

DIFFUSE LARGE B CELL LYMPHOMA

Diffuse large B cell lymphomas (DLBCL) have diffuse growth pattern, aggressive clinical history, can occur in children and adults and accounts for 50% of adult NHLs.

Pathology

The B cells are four times the size of small lymphocytes, nucleus may be round, irregular or with cleaved nuclear contours. The chromatin is dispersed, nucleoli are several and distinct. They have moderate amount of pale cytoplasm. These cells are centroblasts. A few large cells resembling immunoblasts are present. These are large cells, have multilobated vesicular nuclei, 1–2 centrally placed nucleoli, pale or deeply staining amphophilic and pyroninophilic cytoplasm with nuclear hof.

Immunophenotype, karyotype and molecular features: These cells are of mature B cell type, express pan-B-cell antigens CD19 and CD20. Cells may express IgM and/or IgG. CD10 usually expressed. Diffuse large B cell lymphomas may be associated with t(14:18) involving Bcl-2. Minority express CD30.

Anaplastic lymphoma kinase (ALK) DLBCLs expressing ALK have poor prognosis. This is an uncommon form of DLBCL with plasmacytic differentiation. It is CD30 negative and there is t (2;17) (p23;p23) which fuses ALK gene with CLTC gene.

DLBCL with CD 30+ expression have favourable outcome. However, CD30+ EBV+ DLBCL has aggressive clinical course. T cell/histiocyte-rich DLBCL has aggressive clinical course.

Clinical Features

These can arise at any age. Most commonly occur around the age of 60 years. They constitute about 15% of childhood lymphomas. Patients of DLBCL have rapidly enlarging, symptomatic mass/ masses at one or several sites. Extranodal involvement of GIT and brain is common.

Prognosis

These are of aggressive nature and rapidly fatal, if untreated. With intense combination chemotherapy, complete remission can be achieved in 60 to 80% of the cases.

BURKITT LYMPHOMA

Burkitt lymphoma (BL) is a high grade NHL, has germinal centre B cells and presents in three clinical forms.

1. Endemic
2. Sporadic
3. Immunodeficiency associated

Endemic BL: Most often this occurs in equatorial parts of Africa. Most common in childhood, characteristically involve jaw and orbit. GIT, ovaries, breast and kidneys may be involved with this type of ML. There is 100% association of EBV with BL.

Sporadic form of BL: This occurs throughout the world, mainly children and adolescents are affected. Abdominal cavity is often affected. Only 20–30% are associated with EBV.

Immunodeficiency associated BL: This is seen primarily in HIV infection (25–40% association).

Morphology

There is diffuse proliferation of neoplastic cells. The cells are uniform, of intermediate size, have round or oval nuclei containing 2–5 prominent nucleoli. The cells have basophilic or amphophilic cytoplasm, has fat containing vacuoles, a high mitotic index is characteristic of this tumour. The necrotic debris is ingested by the macrophages which are numerous giving the appearance of "starry sky" (Fig. 23.5).

Immunophenotype, karyotype and molecular markers:

1. BLs are of B cell lineage. They express immuno-globulins (predominantly IgM).
2. B cell markers CD19, CD20, CD22, germinal centre markers like CD10 and Bcl-6 are positive.
3. They do not express TdT.
4. Helpful markers: CD20 positive, CD10 positive and Bcl-2 negative and Ki-67 index over 95%.
5. t(8:14), t(2:8) or t(8:22) fuses Myc gene with Ig heavy chain, kappa light chain or lambda light chain genes. The Myc gene is on chromosome 8 and IgH gene on chromosome 14. Kappa and lambda light chain loci are on chromosome 2 and 22, respectively.

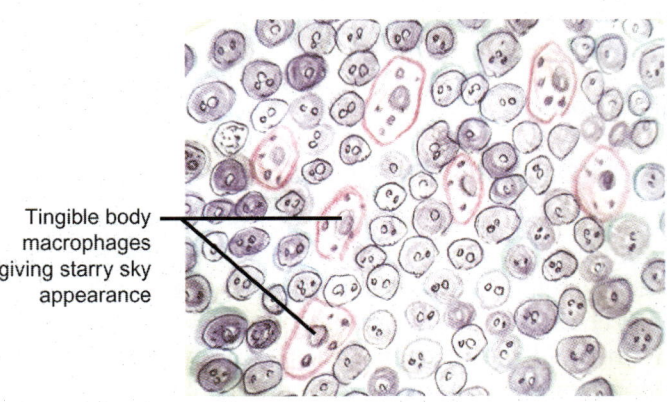

Tingible body macrophages giving starry sky appearance

Fig. 23.5: Microphotograph of Burkitt's lymphoma

Clinical Features

Both endemic and non-endemic forms affect children and young adults. BL accounts for 30% NHL. In both forms, extranodal origin is common. Maxilla and mandible usually are affected, bowel retroperitoneum and ovaries also can be affected. Peripheral blood spillage is less common especially in endemic form. BL is a high grade tumour, however, responds to aggressive chemotherapy and majority of the patients can be cured.

Prognosis

Fatal, if left untreated. Early diagnosis and chemotherapy has long survival in children (60–90%) compared to adults.

ANAPLASTIC LARGE CELL LYMPHOMA/KI-1 LYMPHOMA (ALK Positive)

Anaplastic large cell lymphoma (ALCL) is also called Ki-1 lymphoma, this is of T cell origin, clinically has systemic and cutaneous forms. This can involve extranodal sites. It can be seen in children and adults. These may be associated with HIV and mycosis fungoides. These can be ALK positive or negative. ALK positive are commonly seen in young adults while negative are in old age. The prognosis of ALK negative ALCL has worse than ALK positive lymphomas.[19]

Pathology

The infiltrate is polymorphic with variable admixture of neutrophils, lymphocytes, histiocytes and highly atypical large lymphoma cells showing kidney-shaped nuclei with pleomorphism.

Immunophenotype, karyotype and molecular markers: ALCL is CD30 and Ki-1 positive. CD3 and CD4 are positive. They are also EMA+, positive for IL-2R, clusterin, cadherins and galectin-3. B cell markers are absent. PAX5 absent and ALK can be +/−. There is variable expression of T cell markers. The T cell receptor genes are clonally rearranged in 90% of ALK+ ALCL. These are negative for EBV.

Prognosis: ALCL has an aggressive course.

LYMPHOBLASTIC LYMPHOMA

Lymphoblastic lymphoma (LL) is primarily seen in children and adolescents, but also in adults. In 50% of the cases, there is mediastinal mass in the thymic region. The clinical course of untreated cases is extremely poor with rapid multisystem dissemination and leukaemic blood picture (acute lymphoblastic lymphoma) and death occurs in a few months.

Pathology

Grossly, lymph nodes are whitish and soft, foci of haemorrhage and necrosis are present.

Microscopy: It shows diffuse and monomorphic population of cell proliferation with focal starry sky appearance. The tumour extends outside the thymus/node and invades adipose tissue. Permeation of blood vessels in targetoid fashion is another feature. Neoplastic cells have scanty cytoplasm, nucleus has round contours, shows delicate convolutions in small percentage of cells. Chromatin is finally stippled, nucleoli inconspiculous, mitosis are extremely high. The convoluted cells are similar to cerebroid cells of mycosis fungoides—Sezary syndrome. The nuclear membrane is thin and chromatin is dispersed.

Immunophenotype, karyotype and molecular markers:

1. Acid phosphatase positive (focally strong in paranuclear location).
2. Beta glucuronidase, alpha-naphthyl acetate esterase and TdT are positive.
3. 85% of the LL neoplasms express T cell markers. Pan T antigens CD1, CD2, CD7, CD3 and CD43 are positive.
4. 15–20% of these lesions express B cell markers CD19, 20, 21 and 24 (Precursor B LL).
5. Differential diagnosis for these lesions is thymoma, Ewings/PNET, Burkitt's lymphoma and blastoid variants of mantle cell lymphoma.

ADULT T CELL LYMPHOMA/LEUKAEMIA

This involves CD4 T cells and occurs in regions where HTLV virus is endemic. Skin lesions, generalised lymphadenopathy, enlarged liver and spleen, peripheral spillage of lymphocytosis and hypercalcaemia are common features.

Microscopy shows T cells having multilobated nuclei (clover leaf or flower like). The tumour cells contain HTLV-1 provirus.

Prognosis: Fatal and progresses fast within a year.

MYCOSIS FUNGOIDES/SEZARY SYNDROME

Mycosis fungoides involves CD4 helper T cells which infiltrate skin lesions. The disease has three phases:
1. Premycotic phase
2. Plaque phase
3. Tumour phase

In Sezary syndrome, there is skin involvement with exfoliative erythroderma. Tumour phase is less common and peripheral spillage with leukaemic phase is common.

Microscopy: The cells are cerebriform and infiltrate epidermis and upper dermis.

METASTASIS TO LYMPH NODES

The primary malignant tumours can metastasize to regional lymph nodes. The common groups of lymph nodes involved are:

1. **Cervical (high jugular, posterior cervical) lymph nodes:** Head and neck malignancies (nasopharynx, tonsils, tongue, floor of mouth, thyroid, extrinsic larynx, facial skin, scalp).

2. **Low cervical group lymph nodes:** Intrathoracic (lungs) and intra-abdominal malignancies.

3. **Supraclavicular (left supraclavicular) lymph nodes:** Gastric malignancy.

4. **Axillary lymph nodes:** Breast and upper extremities malignancies.

5. **Inguinal lymph nodes:** Malignancies of lower extremities, vulva, cervix, endometrium, ovary, penis, prostate, rectum, anus.

6. **Pelvic lymph nodes:** Prostate, testes, female genital tract, lower extremities.

Sometimes lymph node metastasis can be the earliest manifestation as in occult malignancies of head and neck and papillary carcinoma thyroid. The tumour cells in nests, islands, and cords are seen in the sinusoids of

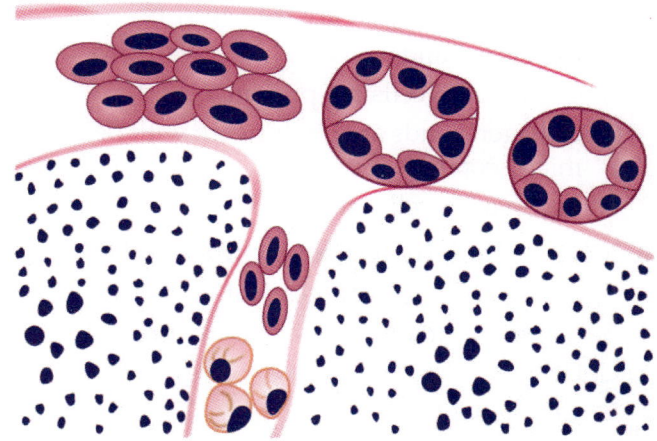

Fig. 23.6: Microscopy of metastatic adenocarcinoma lymph node (schematic)

the lymph node with preservation of the integrity of the capsule (Fig. 23.6).

The sites of origin of other metastatic tumours may be indicated by the following:

- Papillary structures with psammoma bodies in adenocarcinomas of the thyroid and ovary
- Keratin pearls in squamous cell carcinomas
- Melanin pigment in melanomas
- Neurofibrils in neuroblastomas
- Neurosecretory granules in neuroendocrine tumours
- Argyrophil granules in carcinoid tumours

SELF-ASSESSMENT EXERCISE

1. **B cells are located in:**
   A. Cortex B. Interfollicular region
   C. Subcortical sinuses D. Medullary sinuses

2. **Small lymphocytic lymphoma has:**
   A. Indolent course
   B. High mitotic rate
   C. Conspicuous nucleoli
   D. All of the above

3. **RS cells are:**
   A. CD15 positive B. CD 30 positive
   C. EBV positive D. All of the above

4. **Peripheral T cell lymphomas, all are true** *except*:
   A. Extranodal
   B. High stage at presentation
   C. Aggressive
   D. CD19 positive

5. **Non-caseating granulomas are seen in all** *except*:
   A. Sarcoidosis
   B. Tuberculoid leprosy

   C. Advanced tuberculosis
   D. Berylliosis

6. **t(14: 18) is known in:**
   A. Follicular lymphoma
   B. Mantle zone lymphoma
   C. Burkitt's lymphoma
   D. Diffuse large B cell lymphoma

7. **t(11:14) is known in:**
   A. Mantle cell lymphoma
   B. Burkitt's lymphoma
   C. Diffuse large B cell lymphoma
   D. Follicular lymphoma

8. **t(8:14) is seen in:**
   A. Burkitt's lymphoma
   B. Diffuse large B cell lymphoma
   C. Follicular lymphoma
   D. Mantle cell lymphoma

9. **Nodular sclerosis, all are true** *except*:
   A. Collagen bands+
   B. Classical RS cells are present
   C. Collagen bands are birefringent with polarising microscope
   D. Lacunar RS cells are present

10. **Mixed cellularity HD, all are true** *except*:
    A. Classical RS cells are present
    B. Different inflammatory cells are present
    C. CD20 +
    D. CD15+, CD30+

11. **Lymphocyte rich HD, all are true** *except*:
    A. Small lymphocytes plenty
    B. Admixed with eosinophils and neutrophils

C. RS cells present
D. CD20+

12. **Mediastinal involvement is seen in:**
    A. Nodular sclerosis   B. Mixed cellularity HD
    C. LDHD   D. LRHD

13. **Hodgkin disease is:**
    A. EBV positive   B. HPV positive
    C. HSV positive   D. All of the above

14. **Nodular lymphocyte predominant HD has all** *except*:
    A. Classical RS cells
    B. L and H variants of RS cells
    C. CD15+ and CD30+
    D. CD20 +

Answers

1. A	2. A	3. D	4. D	5. C	6. A	7. A	8. A
9. B	10. C	11. D	12. A	13. A	14. C		

Respiratory Pathology

NORMAL ANATOMY AND HISTOLOGY

The upper respiratory tract comprises nasal cavity, paranasal sinuses, and nasopharynx which is lined by pseudostratified columnar epithelium with numerous goblet cells.

The lower respiratory tract begins with larynx, and continues with trachea. The trachea divides into primary, secondary and tertiary (segmental) bronchi. The tertiary bronchi ramifies into smaller airways called bronchioles, the smallest is terminal bronchiole, which continues as respiratory bronchiole and alveolar duct. This terminates into alveolar sacs. The terminal bronchiole with respiratory bronchiole and alveoli is called acinus (Fig. 24.1).

The respiratory bronchiole contains small number of alveoli. The wall of respiratory bronchi has ciliated cuboidal cells, and a few cells with short villi/non-ciliated cells called Clara cells. The distal part of respiratory bronchiole is predominantly lined by Clara cells. These Clara cells produce surfactant, act as reserve cells and contain enzymes which can detoxify noxious substances.

The respiratory bronchiole divides into alveolar duct and end into alveolar sacs. The alveolar sac has many alveoli. The alveolar wall has lining epithelium. There are blood vessels in the septum. The epithelium has two types of cells. The type I pneumocytes are squamous cells with dense nucleus and are infrequently seen in the tissue sections. These help in gas exchange. Type II pneumocytes are a few in number and have large nucleus with prominent nucleoli and vacuolated cytoplasm. These secrete surfactant and prevent collapse during expiration. Alveolar septa contain macrophages which have engulfed particulate matter.

ATELECTASIS (Collapse)

Atelectasis is loss of lung volume caused due to inadequate expansion of air spaces.

There are different types of atelectasis and they are briefed below.

Resorption Atelectasis

Obstruction prevents air from reaching distal airways. The air which is already present gradually gets absorbed and collapse follows. Depending upon the level of obstruction, an entire lung, whole lobe or one or more segments of lobe may be involved. The causes of obstruction are:

1. Mucus or mucopurulent plug in bronchial asthma, bronchiectasis and chronic bronchitis
2. Postoperatively
3. Aspiration of foreign bodies

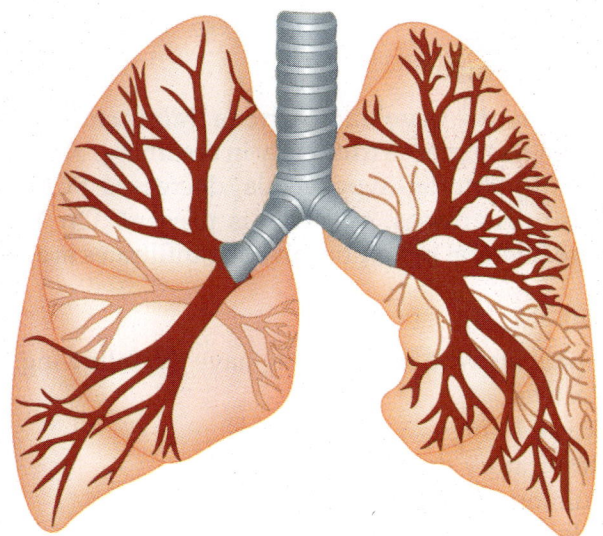

Fig. 24.1: Normal anatomy of bronchial tree (schematic)

Compression Atelectasis

This is also referred to as passive or relaxation atelectasis and is associated with fluid, blood, air within the pleural cavity. This is frequent with congestive heart failure.

Basal atelectasis occurs in patients who are bed-ridden, ascites and in patients during or after surgery due to elevated position of the diaphragm.

Contraction Atelectasis

Generalized fibrotic changes in the lung or pleura hamper expansion and elastic recoil of lung.

Atelectasis except for contraction induced, the others need to be promptly treated to prevent hypoxaemia and superimposed infection of the collapsed lung.

ACUTE LUNG INJURY

Acute lung injury (ALI) clinically manifests as:
1. Acute onset of dyspnoea
2. Decreased arterial oxygen pressure—hypoxaemia/cyanosis
3. Development of bilateral pulmonary oedema—non-cardiogenic pulmonary oedema
   Acute lung injury can progress to acute respiratory distress syndrome.
4. Absence of left-sided heart failure.

ACUTE RESPIRATORY DISTRESS SYNDROME (ARDS)

ARDS is a clinical syndrome with diffuse alveolar capillary and epithelial damage. There is rapid onset of:
1. Respiratory insufficiency
2. Cyanosis
3. Severe hypoxaemia refractory to oxygen
4. Multiorgan failure

According to the 2012 Berlin definition, ARDS characterises the following:
1. Lung injury of acute onset with a week of clinical condition with respiratory symptoms
2. Bilateral lung opacities (X-ray/CT) not explained by other lung pathology
3. Respiratory failure not explained by heart failure or volume overload
4. Decreased PaO_2/FiO_2 ratio

The histological manifestations are known as **diffuse alveolar damage.** This occurs in many clinical settings and is associated with lung injury (Table 24.1)

Pathology

In ARDS, there can be injury to the endothelium or epithelium or injury to both. There is imbalance in pro- and anti-inflammatory mediators causing injury to the

Table 24.1	Clinical conditions associated with ARDS
1. Pneumonia	2. Sepsis
3. Trauma	4. TRALI
5. Drug injuries	6. Inhalation injuries
7. Severe burns	8. Severe inflammation
9. Panceatitis	10. Drowning
11. Other aspirations	

epithelium and endothelium. Neutrophils have crucial role to play in the pathogenesis of ARDS.

The characteristic findings are:
1. Oedema
2. Epithelial necrosis
3. Accumulation of neutrophils and
4. Hyaline membrane lining the alveoli

ARDS can be divided into:
1. Exudative phase
2. Organising phase

In early phase, i.e. exudative phase, there is injury to the epithelium which allows leakage of protein-rich fluid from alveolar capillary into interstitium with destruction of type I pneumocytes. There is exudation of fluid into alveolar space. Intra-alveolar oedema develops. There is formation of eosinophilic hyaline membrane composed of proteinaceous exudate and cell debri. This starts on second day and conspicuous on 4th to 5th day. The basement membrane is intact and there is proliferation of type II pneumocytes at the end of first week and line the lung surface. Grossly, lungs are heavy, oedematous, and airless.

In organising phase, that is a week after initial injury, there is proliferation of fibroblasts in the alveolar walls. There is interstitial inflammation, and proliferation of type II pneumocytes persists. Hyaline membrane is no longer formed. The alveolar macrophages digest the hyaline membrane and debris. The alveolar septa are thickened.

Clinical Features

The patients have tachypnoea (abnormal rapid breathing), dyspnoea (difficulty in breathing/shortness of breath), arterial hypoxaemia, decreased PCO_2. As disease progresses, cyanosis is present. On X-ray, diffuse bilateral interstitial alveolar infiltrates are seen.

Prognosis

The patients who survive may have the following:
1. Recover
2. Scarred lungs
3. Respiratory dysfunction
4. Pulmonary hypertension
5. Infection
6. Pneumothorax

PNEUMONIA

Pneumonia is a bacterial infection of lung parenchyma.

LOBAR PNEUMONIA

Classical lobar pneumonia now is infrequent. In 90–95% of the cases, *Streptococcus pneumoniae* types 1, 3, 7 and 2 cause the infection. Occasionally, *Klebsiella pneumoniae, Streptococcus, Staphylococcus, H. influenzae, Pseudomonas* and *Proteus* may also cause pneumonia.

The organisms reach the lungs by four ways:

a. Inhalation

b. Aspiration

c. Hematogenous

d. Direct spread from contiguous infection

   Normally, lung has defence mechanisms. When defence mechanisms (mucociliary function, alveolar macrophages, phagocytosis, humoral and cellular immunity) fail, infection spreads. Infection spreads through pores of Kohn.

Clinical Features

Sudden onset of fever, chills, and rigors. There is cough, breathlessness, hemoptysis (rusty sputum), and chest pain due to pleuritis. Loss of appetite, body ache and headache are present. Patient is dyspnoeic, has trachy-cardia, high grade fever.

Investigations

1. Total count increased
2. Pulmonary opacities on X-ray/CT establishes diagnosis
3. Pleural tap for microscopy and culture
4. Blood gas analysis impaired

Gross (Fig. 24.2)

- **Stage of congestion:** Lung is heavy, boggy and red.
- **Stage of red hepatisation:** Lung is dry, solid, granular and reddish coloured.
- **Stage of grey hepatisation:** Affected lobe is solid, dry and grey white. Pleural surface is covered with exudate.
- **Stage of resolution:** Exudate undergoes progressive enzymatic digestion to produce granular debris that is reabsorbed.

Microscopy (Fig. 24.3)

- **Stage of congestion:** The lung parenchyma shows vascular engorgement, intra-alveolar fluid with a few neutrophils and numerous bacteria.
- **Stage of red hepatisation:** Alveoli show marked fibrinous exudate with polymorphs and RBCs.

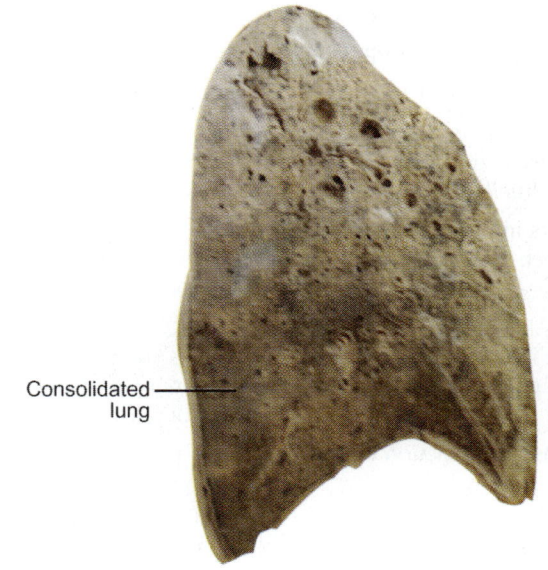

Fig. 24.2: Lung in lobar pneumonia (gross picture)

Consolidated lung

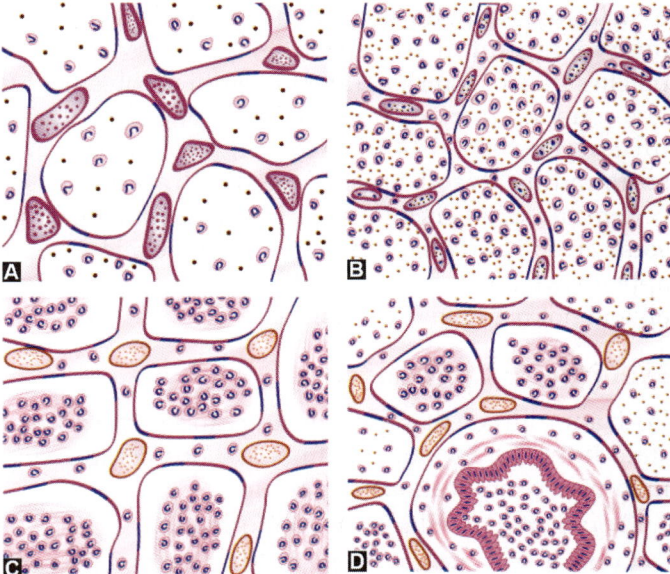

Fig. 24.3: Microscopy in lobar pneumonia—congestion stage (A), red hepatisation stage (B), grey hepatisation stage (C), broncho-pneumonia (D) (schematic)

- **Stage of grey hepatisation:** Alveoli show exudate with contracted fibrin; the RBCs are lysed. The septal capillaries are congested.

Differences between lobar pneumonia and broncho-pneumonia are described in Table 24.2.

BRONCHOPNEUMONIA

This occurs during extremes of age groups (children and old age people), debilitating illness, pre-existing lung diseases and local obstruction to the upward flow of mucus. The organisms which can cause broncho-pneumonia are: *Staph. aureus,* streptococci, *Klebsiella. E.coli, Proteus, Pseudomonas.*

Table 24.2	Differences between lobar pneumonia and bronchopneumonia
Lobar pneumonia	**Bronchopneumonia**
Caused by pneumococci in 90% of cases, a few cases are caused by *Klebsiella, Staph aureus*	Caused by staphylococci, streptococci, *H. influenzae, Proteus* and *Pseudomonas*
Occurs in healthy individuals between 30 and 50 years of age	Occurs in infants, old age people and those suffering from chronic debilitating illness or immunosuppression
Onset is sudden with high grade fever, chills and rusty sputum	Onset is insidious with low grade fever and productive cough of purulent sputum
Causes consolidation of whole lobe	Causes patchy consolidation
Complications: Bacteremia, meningitis, endocarditis, septic arthritis	Complications: Fibrosis, bronchiectasis, lung abscess

Unlike in lobar pneumonia, the inflammation is **distributed in patches** around the bronchioles with intervening uninvolved normal lung tissue. These patches may become confluent. Pleural involvement is less common than lobar pneumonia. The suppurative inflammation fills the **bronchi, bronchiole and surrounding alveoli**. Some of the alveoli are filled with oedema fluid, others may show fibrinous exudate while some alveoli are collapsed, thus giving the microscopic appearance different from that of lobar pneumonia, all alveoli not being in one stage.

Sequelae or Complications

With appropriate therapy, the lung can resume normal state in both types of pneumonias, but occasionally following complications can occur:
1. **Organisation**—fibrous tissue formation
2. **Lung abscess** due to tissue destruction and necrosis
3. **Empyema**—accumulation of exudate in the pleural cavity
4. Meningitis
5. Septic arthritis
6. Infective endocarditis

PULMONARY TUBERCULOSIS

Tuberculosis is a chronic granulomatous inflammation. The causative organism is *Mycobacterium tuberculosis/* Koch's bacillus. The organism is a strict aerobe and thrives in tissues with high oxygen tension. Organisms can be demonstrated by the following methods.
1. Ziehl-Neelson/acid-fast staining
2. Fluorescent dye methods
3. Culture of the organism in LJ medium for 6 weeks
4. Guinea pig inoculation method

Occasionally, human tuberculosis may be caused by atypical mycobacteria which are non-pathogenic to guinea pigs and resistant to the usual anti-tubercular drugs. There are 4 groups of atypical mycobacteria: Photochromogens (group 1), scotochromogens (group 2), non-chromogens (group 3), rapid growers (group 4).

Mode of Transmission of Tuberculosis
1. Inhalation
2. Ingestion
3. Inoculation
4. Transplacental route

Spread of Tuberculosis in the Body
1. Local spread
2. Lymphatic spread
3. Haematogenous spread
4. By natural passages to pleura (tuberculous pleurisy)
5. Transbronchial spread into adjacent lung segments
6. Tuberculous salpingitis into peritoneal cavity
7. Infected sputum into larynx
8. Swallowing of infected sputum
9. Renal lesions

PRIMARY TUBERCULOSIS

It is the infection of an individual who has not been previously infected or immunised. It is also called **'Ghon's complex or childhood tuberculosis'**.

Primary complex or Ghon's complex: It is the lesion produced at the portal of entry with foci in the draining lymphatic vessels and lymph nodes. It has three components:
1. *Ghon's focus* (Fig. 24.4): Lesion in the lung is the primary focus or Ghon's focus. It is 1–2 cm, solitary, located peripherally near the fissure, in any part of the lung but more often in the subpleural focus in the upper part of lower lobe or lower part of upper lobe. Microscopically, the lung lesion consists of tuberculous granulomas with caseation necrosis.
2. *Lymphatic vessels:* The lymphatics draining the lung lesion may develop tuberculous lymphangitis.
3. *Lymph nodes:* Hilar and tracheobronchial lymph nodes in the area drained are enlarged. The affected lymph nodes are matted and show caseation necrosis.

Fate of Primary Tuberculosis
1. Healing by fibrosis and further may undergo **calcification and even ossification**.
2. **Progressive primary tuberculosis** where infection is disseminated through bronchi to other parts of the same lung or to the other lung.

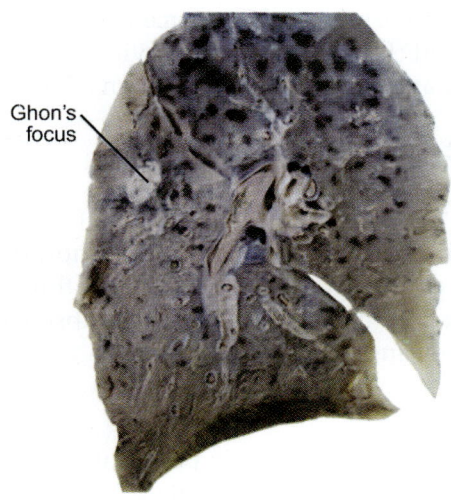

Fig. 24.4: Tuberculosis lung—Ghon's focus (gross picture)

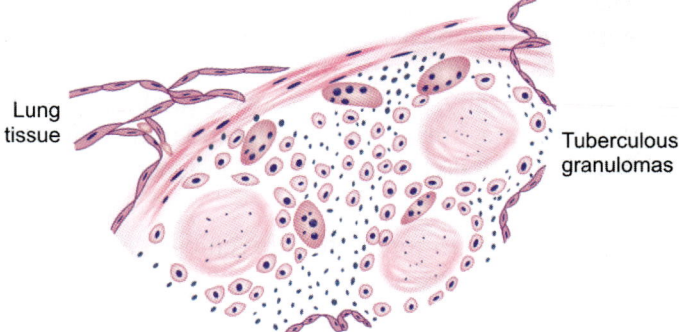

Fig. 24.5: Microscopy of tuberculosis lung (schematic)

3. **Primary miliary tuberculosis** where bacilli enter circulation and spread to various tissues and organs.
4. **Progressive secondary tuberculosis** where healed lesions get reactivated. This is seen with lowered host resistance.

SECONDARY TUBERCULOSIS

It is the infection of an individual who has been previously infected or sensitised. It is also called '**secondary or post-primary or reinfection tuberculosis'.**

The infection may be acquired from:
- **Endogenous source:** Reactivation of dormant primary complex
- **Exogenous source:** Fresh dose of reinfection by tubercle bacilli.

Fate of Secondary Pulmonary Tuberculosis

The lesions may heal with fibrous scarring and calcification. The lesions may extend to progressive secondary pulmonary tuberculosis with the following pulmonary and extrapulmonary organ or tissue involvement.

1. **Fibrocaseous tuberculosis:** Grossly, tuberculous cavity is spherical with thick fibrous wall, lined by yellowish, caseous, necrotic material and the lumen is traversed by thrombosed blood vessels. The overlying pleura may also be thickened and shows adhesions. **Microscopically** widespread coalesced tuberculous granulomas composed of epithelioid cells, Langhans giant cells and peripheral mantle of lymphocytes and having central caseation necrosis are seen (Fig. 24.5). The outer wall of cavity shows fibrosis.
2. Fibrocaseous cavitatory tuberculosis (Fig. 24.6).
3. **Miliary tuberculosis** (Fig. 24.7): There is lympho-haematogenous spread of tuberculous infection. The spread may occur to systemic organs or isolated organ. The spread through pulmonary vein produces

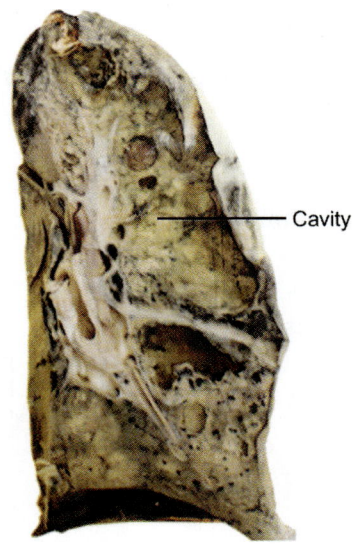

Fig. 24.6: Fibrocaseous cavitatory tuberculosis (gross picture)

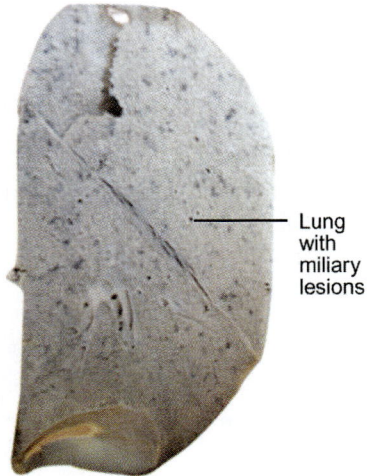

Fig. 24.7: Miliary tuberculosis (gross picture)

disseminated or isolated organ lesion in different **extrapulmonary sites** (e.g. liver, spleen, kidney, brain and bone marrow). Spread into the pulmonary artery restricts the development of miliary lesions within the lung. The miliary lesions are millet seed-sized (1 mm diameter), yellowish, firm areas. Microscopically, the lesions show the structure of tubercles with minute areas of caseation necrosis.

4. **Tuberculous pneumonia:** Individuals with high degree of hypersensitivity, tuberculosis may spread to the rest of the lung producing caseous pneumonia. Microscopically, the lesions show exudative reaction with oedema, fibrin, polymorphs and monocytes but numerous tubercle bacilli can be demonstrated in the exudate.

Note: Also refer to topic on Tuberculosis, in Chapter on Infectious Diseases.

OBSTRUCTIVE PULMONARY DISEASES

These are associated with airflow obstruction. They are listed below:

I. Chronic obstructive lung/pulmonary disease (COPD)
  i. Chronic bronchitis
  ii. Emphysema
II. Bronchial asthma
III. Bronchiectasis
IV. Small airways disease
V. Cystic fibrosis

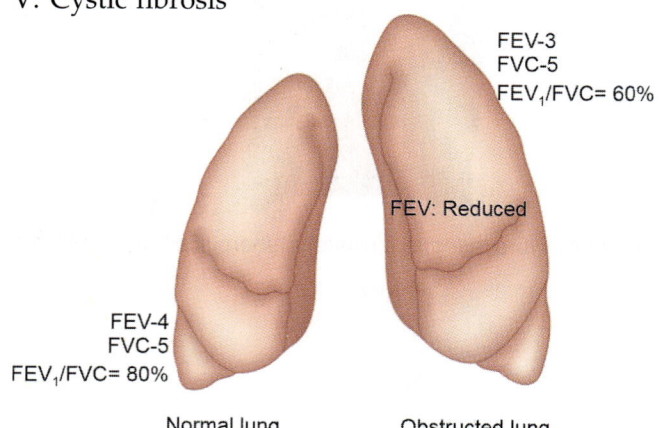

FEV-3
FVC-5
$FEV_1/FVC = 60\%$

FEV: Reduced

FEV-4
FVC-5
$FEV_1/FVC = 80\%$

Normal lung   Obstructed lung

Fig. 24.8: Lung functions in obstructive lung diseases (comparision to normal)

In obstructive lung diseases, forced expiratory volume in 1st second (FEV_1) is less, forced vital capacity (FVC) is reduced and FEV_1/FVC is less than 0.7 (Fig. 24.8).

CHRONIC BRONCHITIS

Definition

The diagnosis on clinical grounds should include persistent productive cough for at least three months, in at least two consecutive years in absence of any identifiable cause.

Pathogenesis

Cigarette smoking, other air pollutants such as SO_2, NO_2 may contribute. These irritate leading to hypertrophy and hyperplasia of mucus glands of surface epithelium of smaller bronchi and bronchioles. The irritants cause inflammation with infiltration of CD8+ T cells, macrophages and neutrophils. No eosinophils are present.

Pathology

In large airways, the mucosa is hyperaemic and oedematous. It is covered by mucopurulent secretion. Small bronchi and bronchioles also contain similar secretion. Normally, the Reid index is 0.4. Reid index is ratio of the thickness of the submucous glands to the thickness between the epithelium and the cartilage. In chronic bronchitis, there is hyperplasia and hypertrophy of submucosal glands with Reid index more than 0.4. The small airways (small bronchi and bronchioles) show increase in goblet cells and mucous plugging with inflammation and fibrosis. The bronchial epithelium may show increase in goblet cells, squamous metaplasia, basal cell hyperplasia, mucus plugging, inflammation and fibrosis. There is narrowing of lumen and airway obstruction (Fig. 24.9).

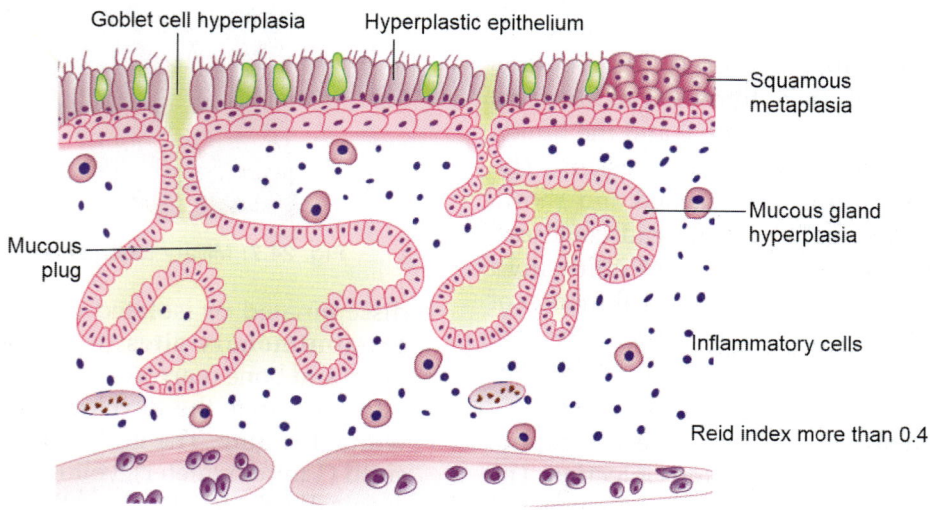

Goblet cell hyperplasia   Hyperplastic epithelium

Squamous metaplasia

Mucous plug

Mucous gland hyperplasia

Inflammatory cells

Reid index more than 0.4

Fig. 24.9: Changes in chronic bronchitis (schematic)

In severe form, complete obstruction of the lumen due to fibrosis can occur. Peribronchiolar fibrosis and luminal narrowing result in airway obstruction.

Clinical Features

Patients have cough with copious purulent sputum without ventilatory dysfunction. Some develop outflow obstruction with hypercapnia, hypoxaemia, cyanosis (blue bloaters), peripheral oedema and polycythemia. In pink puffers, chronic bronchitis leads to pulmonary hypertension and cardiac failure.

EMPHYSEMA

Emphysema is defined as permanent dilatation of air spaces distal to the terminal bronchioles with destruction of the walls without obvious fibrosis.

The elastic recoil of lung is lost. There is low FCV1 with normal or near normal FCV and the ratio of FEV1 to FVC is reduced.

Emphysema can be classified according to its anatomic distribution within the lobule as below:
- Centriacinar
- Panacinar (panlobular)
- Paraseptal (distal acinar)
- Irregular (paracicatricial)

A number of other conditions to which the term 'emphysema' is loosely applied to over inflation, are given below:
- Compensatory over inflation (compensatory emphysema)
- Senile hyperinflation (aging lung, senile emphysema)
- Obstructive over inflation (infantile lobar emphysema)
- Unilateral translucent lung (unilateral emphysema)
- Interstitial emphysema (surgical emphysema)

Etiopathogenesis

The most important etiologic factors are tobacco smoke and air pollutants. Other less significant contributory factors are occupational exposure, infection and somewhat poorly understood familial and genetic influences.

However, the pathogenesis of the most significant event in emphysema, the destruction of alveolar walls, is closely related to the deficiency of serum alpha-1 antitrypsin commonly termed as protease–antiprotease theory/hypothesis.

Protease–Antiprotease Theory

Alpha-1 antitrypsin (alpha-1-AT) is a glycoprotein that is normally synthesized in the liver and is distributed in the circulating blood, tissues, body fluids and inflammatory cells. The normal function of alpha-1-AT is to inhibit proteases and hence its name alpha-1-protease inhibitor.

In lung, the proteases are derived from neutrophils. Neutrophil elastase has the capability of digesting lung parenchyma but is inhibited from doing so by anti-elastase effect of alpha-1-AT.

There are several known alleles of alpha-1-AT which have an autosomal codominant inheritance pattern and are classified as normal, deficient, null type having no detectable level, and dysfunctional type having about half the normal level.

The normal alpha-1-AT phenotype called PiMM is present in 90% of the population. The most abnormal phenotype homozygous state PiZZ has alpha-1-AT deficiency and emphysema occurs in early age and has greater severity in smokers.

The mechanism of alveolar wall destruction in emphysema by **elastolytic action** is based on the imbalance between proteases and anti-proteases:
- By decreased anti-elastase activity, i.e. deficiency of alpha-1-AT.
- By increased activity of elastase, i.e. increased neutrophilic infiltration in the lungs causing excessive elaboration of neutrophil elastase.

Smoking promotes emphysema. Oxidants in cigarette smoke have inhibitory influence on alpha-1-AT, thus lowering the level of anti-elastase activity. Smokers have up to ten times more phagocytes and neutrophils in their lungs than non-smokers. Thus, they have very high elastase activity.

Pathologic Changes

Emphysema can be diagnosed with certainty only by gross and histologic examination of sections of whole lung. The lungs should be perfused with formalin under pressure in inflated state to grade the severity of emphysema with naked eye.

Grossly, the lungs are voluminous, pale with little blood. The edges of the lungs are rounded. Mild cases show dilatation of the air spaces visible with hand lens. Advanced cases show subpleural bullae and blebs bulging outwards from the surface of the lungs with rib marking between them. The bullae are air-filled, cyst-like structures, larger than 1 cm in diameter. The rupture of bullae directly into the subpleural interstitial tissue is the common cause of spontaneous pneumothorax.

Microscopy reveals **destruction of alveolar walls, leading to enlarged air spaces**. In addition to alveolar loss, the number of alveolar capillaries is diminished. Terminal and respiratory bronchioles may be deformed because of the loss of septa. With **loss of elastic tissue** in the surrounding alveolar septa, radial traction on the small airways is reduced. As a result, they tend to collapse during expiration, this is an important cause of chronic airflow obstruction in severe emphysema. Bronchiolar inflammation and submucosal fibrosis are consistently present in advanced disease (Figs 24.10 to 24.12).

Clinical Features

- There is a long history of slowly increasing severe exertional dyspnoea.
- Patient is quite distressed with obvious use of accessory muscles of respiration.

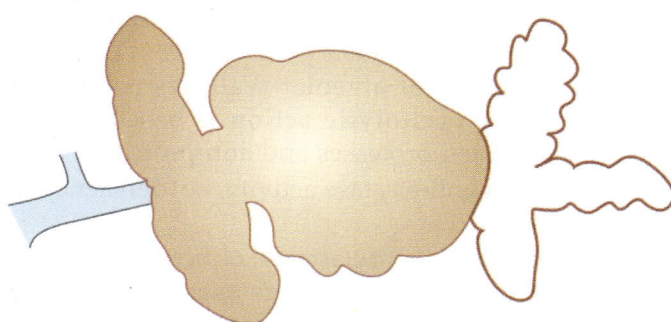

Fig. 24.10: Emphysema—centriacinar (diagrammatic)

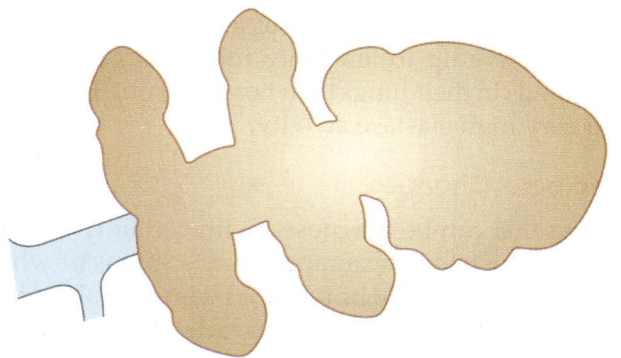

Fig. 24.11: Panacinar emphysema (schematic)

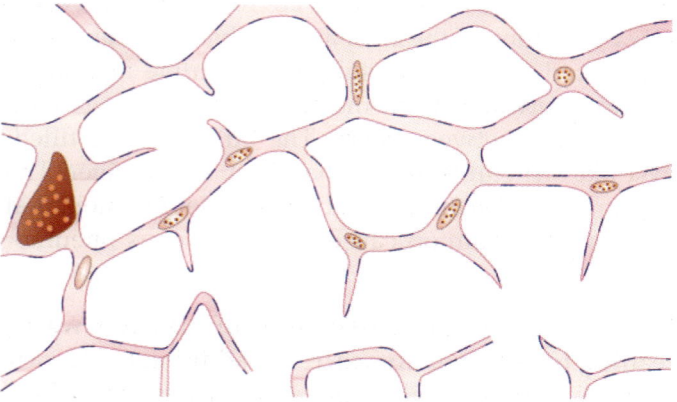

Fig. 24.12: Microscopy, emphysema lung

- Chest is barrel shaped and hyper-resonant.
- Cough occurs after dyspnoea starts and is associated with scanty mucoid sputum.
- Recurrent respiratory infections are frequent.
- Patients are called "pink puffers" as they remain well oxygenated but have tachypnoea.
- Weight loss
- Chest X-ray shows small heart with hyperinflated lungs.
- Features of right heart failure and hypercapneic respiratory failure are the usual terminal events. Cor pulmonale and congestive cardiac failure are secondary to pulmonary hypertension. Death in these patients is due to coronary artery disease, respiratory failure, right-sided heart failure or collapse of the lungs secondary to pneumothorax.

Different types of emphysema are described below.

Centriacinar (Centrilobular) Emphysema

In this type of emphysema, the central or proximal parts of the acini are affected while the distal parts are spared. Grossly, lesions are more common and more severe in the upper lobes of the lungs. Large amount of black pigment is often present in the walls of emphysematous areas. In more severe cases, distal parts of acini are also involved and the appearance may closely resemble panacinar emphysema. This type of emphysema is common in chronic smokers.

Microscopically, there is distension and destruction of the respiratory bronchiole in the centre of the lobules, surrounded peripherally by normal uninvolved alveoli. The terminal bronchioles supplying the acini show chronic inflammation and are narrowed.

Panacinar (Panlobular) Emphysema

Pan meaning entire acinus, this type of emphysema is seen in alpha-1-AT deficiency.

Grossly, this condition involves the lower zone of lungs more frequently and more severely than the upper zone. The involvement may be confined to a few lobules or may be more widespread affecting a lobe or part of lobe of the lung. The lungs are enlarged and over-inflated.

Microscopically, all the alveoli within a lobule are affected to the same degree. All portions of acini are distended. The respiratory bronchioles, alveolar ducts and alveoli are all dilated and their walls are stretched and thin. Ruptured alveolar walls and spurs of broken septa are seen between the adjacent alveoli. The capillaries are stretched and thinned. Special stains show loss of elastic tissue. Inflammatory changes are usually absent.

Paraseptal (Distal Acinar) Emphysema

This type involves the distal part of acinus while the proximal part is normal. It is localized adjacent to the pleura, at the margins of the lobules and along the perilobular septa. It occurs adjacent to areas of fibrosis, scarring or atelectasis and severe in the upper half of the lungs. Grossly, the subpleual portion of the lung shows air-filled cysts, 0.5 to 2 cm in diameter. Rupture of these bullae can cause pneumothorax in young adults.

Irregular (Paracicatricial) Emphysema

This type is seen surrounding scars from any cause. The involvement is irregular as regards to the portion of the acinus involved as well as within the lung as a whole.

BRONCHIAL ASTHMA

Asthma is a chronic inflammatory disorder of airways which causes repeated episode of wheezing, breathlessness, chest tightness and cough. There is hyper-responsiveness to various stimuli leading to bronchospasm and mucus hypersecretion. This may be with:

1. Intermittent and reversible airway obstruction
2. Chronic bronchiolar inflammation with eosinophils
3. Bronchial smooth muscle cell hypertrophy and hyperactivity

Asthma may be classically divided into:
1. Extrinsic (atopic)
2. Intrinsic (non-atopic)

Extrinsic/atopy/allergic asthma: About 70% of the cases, the etiological agent is extrinsic or atopic due to IgE and Th2 cells mediated immune response. The bronchospasm is induced by inhaled antigens, can occur at any age, but usually begins in childhood with family history of allergic diseases.

Risk factors and triggers: Environmental antigens such as dust, pollen, animal dander, foods or any antigen may be implicated.

Intrinsic/non-atopic asthma: In other 30% of patients, it is intrinsic (non-atopic) triggered by non-immune causes. No family history is available in these patients. These can be:
1. Infectious asthma
2. Exercise-induced asthma
3. Occupational asthma
4. Drug-induced asthma
5. Air pollution
6. Emotional factors
7. Obesity
8. Diet
9. Allergens

Pathogenesis

The etiological factors cause **type I IgE-mediated hypersensitivity (atopy)**, acute on chronic airway inflammation and bronchial hyper-responsiveness to stimuli to Th2 cells to release cytokines (IL-4, IL-5, IL-13). IL-4 stimulates IgE production. IL-5 activates eosinophils and IL-13 is responsible for mucus production. Epithelial cells are activated to produce chemokines which promote Th2 cells and eosinophils accumulate (Table 24.3).

In sensitized person, type I IgE-mediated hypersensitivity occurs with acute and late phase response. IgE-coated mast cells, when exposed to same antigen, there occurs cross-linking of IgE and release of cytokines and cause accumulation of neutrophils, mononuclear cells, mast cells and eosinophils. These release chemical mediators. Eosinophils are important in late phase reaction. Major basic protein and eosinophil cationic protein of eosinophils cause injury to airway epithelial cells.

The mechanism of bronchial inflammation and hyper-responsiveness is less clear for intrinsic (non-atopic) asthma. These patients have normal serum concentrations of IgE and some negative for skin tests.

Pathology

The changes are seen in prolonged and severe attack (status asthmaticus).

Gross: Lungs are over distended due to overinflation. Small areas of atelectasis, occlusion of the bronchi and bronchioles by viscid mucus plugs are present.

Microscopy: Lumen has mucus plugs having normal or degenerated respiratory epithelium forming twisted strips called Curschmann's spirals and Charcot-Leyden

Table 24.3	Action of chemical mediators in asthma
Leukotrienes (LC4, D4, E4)	Vasoconstriction, increased VP, increased mucus secretion
Thromboxane A2	Platelet activation and vasoconstriction
Acetylcholine from motor nerves	Smooth muscle contraction
Histamine	Bronchospasm, increased VP
Bradykinin	Increased vascular permeability, vasodilatation and smooth muscle contraction
Prostaglandin D2	Bronchoconstriction, vasodilation
Platelet activating factor (PAF)	Aggregation of platelets and release of histamine

crystals (crystals of eosinophilic proteins). The bronchial wall shows thickened basement membrane of the bronchial epithelium, submucosal oedema and inflammatory infiltrate consisting of mast cells, eosinophils and other inflammatory cells. There is hypertrophy of submucosal glands as well as of the bronchial smooth muscle.

Clinical Features

Characteristic symptoms of asthma are:
1. Wheezing
2. Dyspnoea
3. Coughing

Symptoms are worse at night and patients awake in the morning hours. Some patients may have increased sputum production which is tenacious and difficult to expectorate.

BRONCHIECTASIS

It is defined as permanent dilatation of the bronchi and bronchioles, developing secondary to inflammation with weakening of the bronchial walls. The most characteristic manifestation of bronchiectasis is persistent cough with production of copious amounts of foul smelling and purulent sputum.

Etiopathogenesis

The origin of **inflammatory destructive process** of bronchial walls nearly always is a result of two basic mechanisms:
1. Obstructive cause
2. Non-obstructive cause: Infection or defects in the defence mechanism.

Obstructive Causes

The obstructive causes are generally localised to a segment of the lung distal to the site of mechanical obstruction.

The causes of endobronchial obstruction include:
- Foreign bodies
- Endobronchial tumours
- Compression by enlarged hilar lymph nodes and post-inflammatory scarring (e.g. in healed tuberculosis), all of which favour the development of post-obstructive bronchiectasis.
- Mucus plugs as in asthma

Acquired disorders causing obstruction:

1. Neuropathic disorders that impair consciousness, swallowing, cough
2. Incompetence of the lower esophageal sphincter
3. Nasogastric intubation
4. Chronic bronchitis

Hereditary and congenital factors (obstructive or non-obstructive): Several hereditary and congenital factors may result in diffuse bronchiectasis. These include:
1. *Congenital bronchiectasis:* This is caused by developmental defects of the bronchial system.
2. *Cystic fibrosis:* It is a generalised defect of exocrine gland secretions, resulting in obstruction, infection and bronchiectasis.
3. *Hereditary immune deficiency diseases:* They are often associated with high incidence of bronchiectasis.
4. *Immotile cilia syndrome:* It includes Kartagener's syndrome (bronchiectasis, situs inversus and sinusitis) which is characterised by ultrastructural changes in the microtubules causing immotility of cilia of the respiratory tract epithelium, sperms and other cells. Males in this syndrome are often infertile.
5. *Atopic bronchial asthma:* These patients often have positive family history of allergic diseases and may rarely develop diffuse bronchiectasis.

Non-Obstructive Causes

The causes for non-obstructive localised bronchiectasis include childhood bronchopulmonary infections such as measles, pertussis and other bacterial infections. **As a secondary complication,** necrotizing pneumonias such as in staphylococcal suppurative pneumonia and tuberculosis may develop bronchiectasis as a complication.

Pathologic Changes

The disease characteristically affects distal bronchi and bronchioles beyond the segmental bronchi.

Grossly, the lungs may be involved diffusely or segmentally. Bilateral involvement of lower lobes occurs most frequently. More vertical air passages of left lower lobe are more often involved than the right. The pleura is usually fibrotic and thickened with adhesions to the chest wall. The dilated airways, depending upon their gross or bronchographic appearance, have been subclassified into the following different types (Fig. 24.13):

- **Cylindrical:** The most common type characterised by uniform and moderate tube-like bronchial dilatation.
- **Fusiform:** Having spindle-shaped bronchial dilatation.
- **Saccular:** Having rounded sac-like bronchial distension, affects the proximal 3rd to 4th branches of the bronchi. The bronchi are severely dilated and end blindly in dilated sacs with collapse and fibrosis of the distal lung parenchyma.
- **Varicose:** Having irregular bronchial enlargements.

Cut surface of the affected lobes, generally the lower zones, shows characteristic honey-combed appearance.

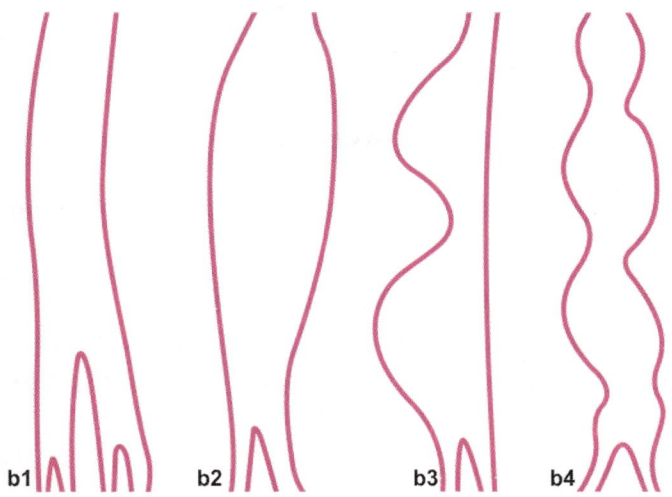

Fig. 24.13: Types of air passages in bronchiectasis: Cylindrical (b1)—note dilated and prominent bronchioles, fusiform (b2), saccular (b3), and vericose (b4)

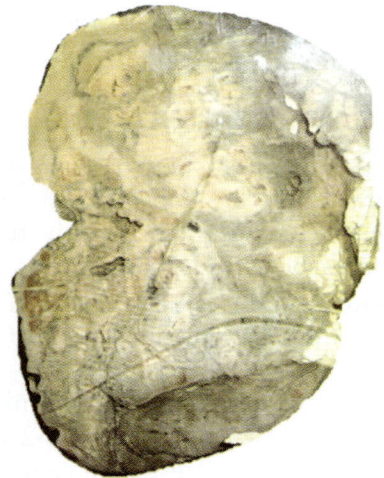

Fig. 24.14: Bronchiectasis (gross picture)

The bronchi and bronchioles are extensively dilated nearly up to the pleura, their walls are thickened and the lumina are filled with mucus or mucopus. The intervening lung parenchyma is reduced and fibrotic (Fig. 24.14).

Microscopically, the bronchial epithelium may be normal, ulcerated or may show squamous metaplasia. The bronchial wall shows infiltration by acute and chronic inflammatory cells and destruction of normal muscle and elastic tissue with replacement by fibrosis. The intervening lung parenchyma shows fibrosis, while the surrounding lung tissue shows changes of interstitial pneumonia.

Clinical Features

- Chronic cough with foul-smelling sputum
- Haemoptysis
- Recurrent pneumonia

- Sinusitis in diffuse bronchiectasis
- Clubbing of fingers
- Amyloidosis
- Cor pulmonale

RESTRICTIVE LUNG DISEASES

These are also called diffuse interstitial or infiltrative lung diseases. These are heterogeneous group of disorders predominantly involving pulmonary interstitium and also have intra-alveolar components. It is of diffuse and chronic nature. In these diseases, the lungs are restricted from fully expanding. The lungs are not able to expand and fill with air. There is decreased total lung capacity (Fig. 24.15).

In restrictive lung diseases, FEV_1 is reduced and FVC is much more reduced and FEV_1/FVC more than 0.8. These are classified as given in Table 24.4.

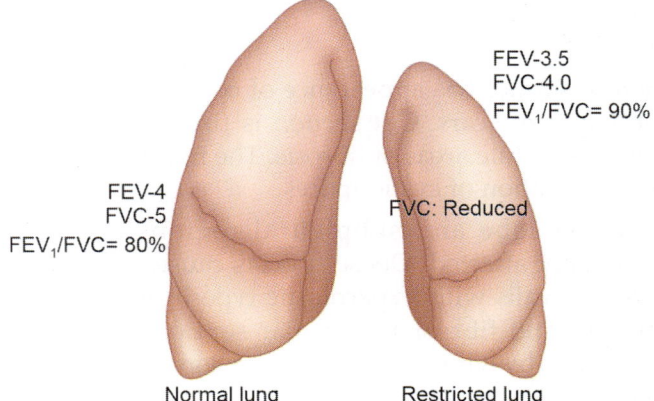

FEV-3.5
FVC-4.0
$FEV_1/FVC= 90\%$

FEV-4
FVC-5
$FEV_1/FVC= 80\%$

FVC: Reduced

Normal lung   Restricted lung

Fig. 24.15: Lung size and functions in restrictive lung diseases (comparision to normal)

Table 24.4	Restrictive lung diseases

- Fibrosing
  - Interstitial pneumonia
  - Non-specific interstitial pneumonia
  - Cryptogenic organizing pneumonia
  - Collagen vascular disease associated
  - Pneumoconiosis
  - Therapy related
- Granulomatous
  - Sarcoidosis and other causes
- Hypersensitivity pneumonitis
- Pulmonary eosinophilia
- Smoking related
  - Desquamative interstitial pneumonia
  - Respiratory bronchiolitis
- Neuromuscular diseases, e.g. amyotrophic lateral sclerosis

Pathogenesis

The initial common manifestation is alveolitis. The septa and alveoli show inflammatory cells.

Injury is usually mild, self-limited and resolution occurs. With the persistence of injurious agent, there is parenchymal injury, and progressive fibrosis. The activated macrophages secrete IL-8 and LB4 which recruit and activate neutrophils. The oxidants and proteases released by these inflammatory cells injure alveolar epithelium and degrade connective tissue. Fibrogenic growth factors like FGR, TFG beta and PDGF attract fibroblasts with proliferation of connective tissue.

IDIOPATHIC PULMONARY FIBROSIS/CRYPTOGENIC FIBROSING ALVEOLITIS

This is of unknown etiology. There is diffuse interstitial fibrosis. There is severe hypoxaemia and cyanosis.

Pathology

Pleural surface has appearance of cobble stone due to retraction of scars. Cut section is firm and rubbery. There are white areas of fibrosis. The fibrosis is patchy with formation of cystic spaces.

Lower lobe and subpleural regions are more commonly affected. Dense fibrosis causes collapse of alveolar walls with hyperplastic type II pneumocytes (honeycomb fibrosis). Alveolar septa show patchy infiltration by lymphocytes and occasional plasma cells, mast cells and eosinophils.

Secondary pulmonary hypertension changes, like thickening of artery with intimal fibrosis, are present. The histology of idiopathic pulmonary fibrosis is referred to as usual interstitial pneumonitis (UIP).

Clinical features include non-productive cough and progressive dyspnoea.

On examination, there are dry/velcro-like crackles during inspiration. Cyanosis, peripheral oedema and cor pulmonale develops in later stages.

NON-SPECIFIC INTERSTITIAL FIBROSIS

This has diffuse interstitial lung disease. This has two patterns. These are: (1) Cellular, and (2) fibrosing patterns.

There will be interstitial fibrosis with mild to moderate lymphocytes and plasma cells. The fibrosis is diffuse or patchy.

Prognosis: Patients with cellular pattern have better prognosis than the fibrosing pattern.

CRYPTOGENIC ORGANIZING PNEUMONITIS

This is also called bronchiolitis obliterans organizing pneumonitis. Patients have cough and dyspnoea. X-ray shows subpleural and peribronchial patchy consolidation.

Microscopy shows loose organising connective tissue within the ducts, alveoli and bronchioles.

LUNG IN COLLAGEN VASCULAR DISEASES

Systemic lupus erythematosus, systemic sclerosis, rheumatoid arthritis, dermatomyositis and polymyositis are associated with lung manifestations.

PNEUMOCONIOSIS

These encompass a group of chronic fibrosing diseases of lung due to exposure to organic and inorganic particulates.

Coal workers, pneumoconiosis, silicosis, asbestosis, etc. cause lung injury followed by fibrosis. For details refer to topic on Occupational Lung Diseases.

GRANULOMATOUS DISEASES OF LUNG

Sarcoidosis is a multisystem disease of unknown etiology characterized by non-caseating granulomas. Other causes of granulomas include tuberculosis, fungal infections, berylliosis, etc.

Multisystem involvement and bilateral hilar lymphadenopathy are the major manifestation of the disease sarcoidosis. Etiology of sarcoidosis is unknown. However, may be it is a disease of immune dysregulation. CD4 T helper cells release IL-2 and IFN-γ. Epithelioid cells, lymphocytes, giant cells, Schaumann bodies and asteroid bodies are present. Schaumann bodies are laminated concretions and asteroid bodies are stellate inclusions within the giant cells.

The granulomas are present in the interstitium and some localise around the bronchiole, venules and pleura. Bronchioalveolar lavage shows CD4 T cells. Granulomas are later replaced by fibrosis with honeycomb lung.

DISEASES OF VASCULAR ORIGIN

These include:
1. Pulmonary embolism, haemorrhage and infarction
2. Pulmonary hypertension
3. Diffuse alveolar haemorrhage syndrome: Goodpasture syndrome, idiopathic pulmonary haemosiderosis and Wegener's granulomatosis.

GOODPASTURE SYNDROME

There is presence of autoantibodies to the antigenic targets within the glomerulus and pulmonary basement membrane. Around 40 to 60% patients of the glomerular diseases develop lung haemorrhage. There is destruction of lung alveoli giving rise to necrotizing hemorrhagic interstitial pneumonitis in addition to RPGN.

Clinical Features

Patients have haemoptysis. There is uraemia due to rapidly progressive renal failure because of RPGN.

Pathology

The lungs are heavy with red brown consolidation. Microscopy shows focal fibrinoid necrosis, hemosiderin-laden macrophages, and late stage fibrosis of septa, hyperplasia and hypertrophy of type II pneumocytes.

Note: For details refer to the topic on Kidney Diseases.

LUNGS IN WEGENER'S GRANULOMATOSIS

Wegener's granulomatosis causes necrotizing vasculitis and granulomatous vasculitis of small and medium-sized vessels. Wegener's granulomatosis involves mainly lungs and kidneys, however, sometimes it may be limited to lungs only.

Patients of Wegener's granulomatosis develop upper respiratory and pulmonary manifestations during the course of the disease like sinusitis, epistaxis, nasal perforation, cough, haemoptysis and chest pain. There is necrotizing vasculitis, parenchymal necrotizing granuloma, inflammation and haemorrhage. Pulmonary vessels show fibrinoid necrosis with acute on chronic inflammation. The granulomas coalesce to form visible nodules which may cavitate.

Patients with Wegener's granulomatosis have the following clinical features:
- Fever with night sweats
- Fatigue
- Palpitation
- Lethargy
- Weight loss

Other clinical features include:
- *Eyes:* The clinical features are related to the vascular pathology.
- *CNS:* Manifestations include cranial nerve palsies; small and medium sized vessels of brain and spinal cord are affected.
- *Kidney:* Crescentic necrotizing glomerulonephritis. (may lead to renal failure).

LUNG CARCINOMA

It is the most common primary tumour of the lung. Most common in men and people from industrialized nations are affected.

Etiology

1. Smoking
2. Atmospheric pollution
3. Occupational causes include workers exposed to asbestos, nickel, beryllium, arsenic and metallic iron
4. Dietary factors: Vitamin A deficiency
5. Genetic factors
6. Chronic scarring

Smoking: More than 90% of the lung cancer is associated with smoking. Two packs of cigarettes/day increase the risk by 6–7-fold while cessation of smoking reduces the risk. Passive smoking and radon gas produced from radioactive decay of uranium found in soil and rocks increases the risk twofold. Polycyclic hydrocarbons and 3,4 benzopyrines present in the tobacco smoke has the highest risk of malignancy. Squamous cell carcinoma is common with smoking while adenocarcinoma can be encountered in non-smokers.

Exposure to industrial pollutants: This has been associated with lung cancer.

Genetic factors: Mutations of K-ras, enzyme aryl hydrocarbon hydroxylase (metabolises benzopyrines and hydrocarbons), P53 and RB genes, Myc gene over-expression (small cell carcinoma), 3p deletions, Bcl-2 overexpression (inhibits apoptosis) can be associated in lung cancer.

Classification of Lung Tumours[20]

Epithelial tumours
- Benign: Papilloma, adenoma
- Pre-invasive: Adenocarcinoma *in situ*, squamous carcinoma *in situ*
- Adenocarcinoma: Lepidic, acinar, papillary, micropapillary, solid, mucinous, non-mucinous, minimally invasive
- Squamous cell carcinoma: Keratinising, non-keratinising, basaloid
- Adenosquamous carcinoma
- Neuroendocrine: Small cell carcinoma, large cell neuroendocrine carcinoma, carcinoid tumours (typical, atypical), preinvasive (neuroendocrine cell hyperplasia)
- Large cell carcinoma
- Sarcomatoid carcinoma
- Lymphoepithelioma-like carcinoma
- NUT carcinoma
- Salivary gland type carcinoma

Mesenchymal tumours: Hamartoma, PEComa, pleuropulmonary blastoma, inflammatory myofibroblastic tumour.

Lymphohistiocytic tumours: Lymphomas and other related tumours

Tumours of ectopic origin: Germ cell tumour, intrapulmonary thymoma, melanoma and others

Pleural tumours: Benign mesothelioma, Malignant mesothelioma

Metastatic tumours

Note: Modified from 2015 WHO classification of tumours of lung, pleura, thymus and heart.

Pathologic Changes

Gross

Squamous cell carcinoma (Fig. 24.16): Most commonly, the lung cancer arises in the main bronchus or one of its segmental branches in the hilar parts of the lung, more often on the right side. The tumour begins as a small roughened area on the bronchial mucosa at the bifurcation. As the tumour enlarges, it thickens, the bronchial mucosa has nodular or ulcerated surface. As the nodules coalesce, the carcinoma grows into a friable mass, 1 to 5 cm in diameter, narrowing and occluding the lumen.

The cut surface of the tumour is yellowish-white with foci of necrosis and haemorrhage which may produce cavitary lesions. It is common to find secondary changes in bronchogenic carcinoma of lung such as broncho-pneumonia, abscess formation and bronchiectasis as a result of obstruction and intercurrent infections. The tumour soon spreads within the lungs by direct extension or by lymphatics, and to distant sites by lymphatic or hematogenous routes.

Adenocarcinoma (Fig. 24.17): A small proportion of lung cancers chiefly adenocarcinomas, originate from a small peripheral bronchioles. The tumour may be a

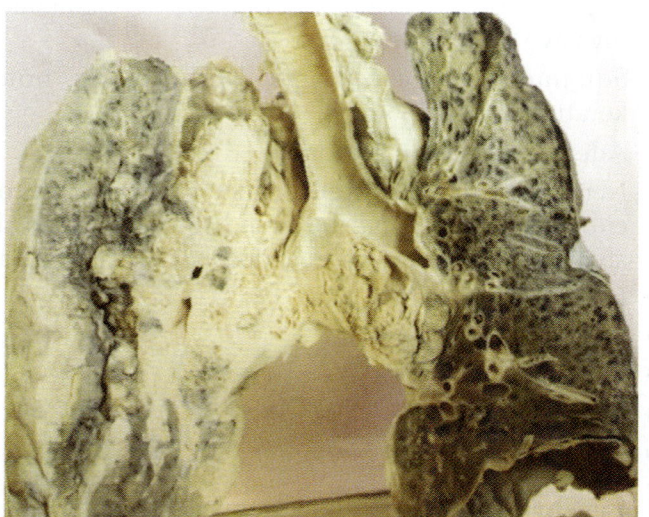

Fig. 24.16: Carcinoma lung, squmaous cell carcinoma (gross picture)

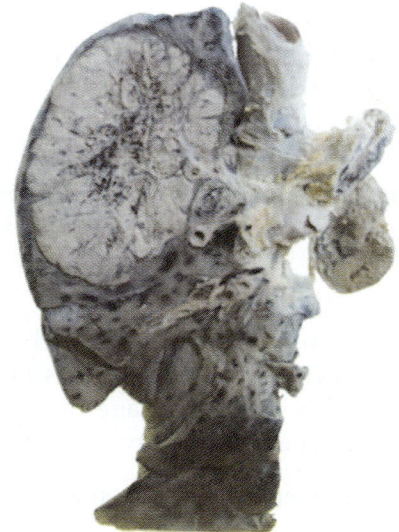

Fig. 24.17: Carcinoma lung, adenocarcinoma (gross picture)

single nodule or multiple nodules in the periphery of the lung producing pneumonia-like consolidation of a large part of the lung. The cut surface of the tumour is grayish and mucoid.

Microscopy

Squamous cell carcinoma: It is the most common type of lung carcinoma. It arises in a large bronchus and is prone to massive necrosis and cavitation. It is diagnosed microscopically by intercellular bridges, keratinisation and can be well-differentiated, moderately differentiated or poorly differentiated. Frequently, the edge of the growth and the adjoining uninvolved bronchi show squamous metaplasia, epithelial dysplasia and carcinoma *in situ* changes.

Adenocarcinoma: The predominant patterns include:
1. *Acinar type:* This type has predominance of closely packed glandular or tubular structures separated by fibrous stroma.
2. *Lepidic pattern:* There is recognisible alveolar septum and alveolar architecture and malignant cells line the inner surface.
3. *Papillary adenocarcinoma:* It has pronounced papillary configuration with fibrovascular core lined by columnar to cuboidal cells.
4. *Micropapillary adenocarcinoma:* Papillae lack fibrovascular core.
5. *Solid variant:* Poorly differentiated adenocarcinoma lacking acini, tubules or papillae but having mucus-containing vacuoles in many tumour cells.

Adenocarcinomas are positive for TTF-1 and Napsin-A.

Adenosquamous carcinoma: There is clear evidence of both keratinisation and glandular differentiation.

Small cell carcinoma: The cells of small cell carcinoma of lung are derived from neuroendocrine cells and express variety of neuroendocrine markers. It is also accompanied by many paraneoplastic syndromes. The lesion appears as pale gray centrally located mass with early involvement of hilar and mediastinal nodes. These are most aggressive tumours with poor prognosis. These have strong association with smoking. Mutation of P53 and RB genes is common. The cells may express chromogranin A, synaptophysin, CD56, TTF1, CD117, etc. Ki-67 is a proliferative marker. Non-small cell lung tumours (squamous cell carcinoma and adeno-carcinoma) have better prognosis than this tumour.

Grossly the tumour is tan, homogenous, soft, and rubbery and has necrosis. **Microscopy** shows round, oval or fusiform-shaped, scant cytoplasm, nuclei two to three times of small lymphocyte, nuclear molding present, inconspicuous nucleoli, nuclear chromatin appears salt and pepper pattern. Cells are fragile and show fragmentation and crush artifacts. Mitoses are high. There is basophilic staining of the vascular wall due to deposition of nuclear debris from necrotic tumour cells.

Clinical Features in Patients with Carcinoma Lung

Following are the clinical features in patients with carcinoma lung:

- Cough, haemoptysis, anorexia, weight loss, wheeze, stridor, and dyspnoea are common symptoms in these patients.
- Dry cough and haemoptysis may be the earliest signs.
- Fever and productive cough may be seen in carcinoma lung with postobstructive pneumonitis.
- Obstructive emphysema, segmental collapse followed by infection and abscess distal to the obstruction.
- **Extension to pleura:** There can be pain/pleurisy/pleural effusion.
- May involve ribs.
- **Hilar lymph node metastasis:** Progressive dyspnoea and collapse of part or whole lung.
- **Secondaries in mediastinum:**
  - Tracheal obstruction: Strider
  - Recurrent laryngeal nerve compression: Hoarseness of voice
  - Phrenic nerve compression: Elevation of hemi-diaphragm with paralysis
- **Cervical sympathetic nerve palsy:** Invasion of the sympathetic chain by the lung cancer produces Horner's syndrome (pneumonic: SAMPLE: sympathetic nerve compression, anhidrosis, miosis, ptosis, loss of ciliospinal reflex, and enophthalmos).

Pancoast syndrome: Lung cancer in the superior sulcus (apex) of the lung invades lower part of brachial plexus and sympathetic trunk with pain in the arm and wasting of muscles of hands.

Syndromes which can occur in lung carcinoma are:
1. Hypercalcaemia (non-small cell carcinoma/sqamous cell carcinoma)
2. SIADH (non-small cell carcinoma/squamous cell carcinoma): ADH secretion causing hyponatraemia and hypo-osmolarity
3. Cushing syndrome (ACTH)
4. Hypoglycaemia **due to insulin-like growth factors**
5. Carcinoid syndrome (neuroendocrine tumours)
6. Venous thrombosis (Trousseau phenomenon)
7. DIC with haemorrhage and anaemia
8. Hypertrophic osteoarthropathy and clubbing of the fingers
9. Cutaneous manifestations: Dermatomysitis, acanthosis nigricans
10. Neurological syndromes
11. Non-bacterial thrombotic endocarditis with emboli

Spread
1. Lung cancer spreads by lymphatic route: Supra-clavicular, axillary and groin lymph nodes can be enlarged.
2. Liver: May show metastatic deposits.
3. Bone: May show metastatic deposits.
4. Brain: May show metastatic deposits with convulsions and neurological deficits.

Investigations

Following investigations are useful in diagnosis of lung cancer:
1. CT/USG/X-ray
2. Bronchoscopy and washings: To visualize and to take biopsy of study washings for malignant cells
3. Fine needle aspiration cytology (FNAC)
4. Cytology of pleural effusion for malignant cells
5. Liver biopsy: For staging
6. Bone marrow: Trephine biopsy for staging

OCCUPATIONAL LUNG DISEASES

It is the term used for lung diseases caused by inhalation of dust, mostly at work, also called **'dust diseases'** or **'occupational diseases'**.

The type of lung disease varies according to the nature of dust inhaled. Some of the dusts are inert and cause no reaction and no damage, while others cause immunologic damage and predispose to tuberculosis or neoplasia (Table 24.5).

Table 24.5	A comprehensive list of various types of occupational lung diseases caused by inorganic (mineral) dusts and organic dusts
Agent	**Diseases**
Inorganic (mineral) dusts	
Coal dust	Simple coal workers' pneumoconiosis, progressive massive fibrosis, Caplan's syndrome
Silica	Silicosis, Caplan's syndrome
Asbestos	Asbestosis, pleural diseases, tumours
Beryllium	Acute berylliosis, chronic berylliosis
Iron oxide	Pulmonary siderosis
Organic (biologic) dust	
Mouldy hay	Farmer's lungs
Bagasse	Bagassosis
Cotton, flax, hemp dust	Byssinosis
Bird droppings	Bird breeder's lung
Mushroom compost dust	Mushroom workers' lung
Mouldy barley, malt dust	Malt workers' lung
Mouldy maple bark	Maple-bark disease
Silage fermentation	Silo-filler's disease

The factors which determine the extent of damage caused by inhaled dust are:
1. Size and shape of the particles
2. Their solubility and physicochemical composition
3. The amount of dust retained in the lungs
4. The additional effects of other irritants such as tobacco smoke
5. Host factors such as efficiency of clearance mechanism and immune status of the host.

In general, most of the inhaled dust particles larger than 5 μ reach the terminal airways where they are ingested by alveolar macrophages. Most of these too are eliminated by expectoration but the remaining accumulate in alveolar tissue. Of particular interest are the particles smaller than 1μ which are deposited in the alveoli most efficiently.

Most of the dust-laden macrophages accumulated in the alveoli die, leaving the dust, around which fibrous tissue is formed. Some macrophages enter the lymphatics and reach regional lymph nodes. The tissue response to inhaled dust may be one of the following 3 types:
1. **Fibrous nodules,** e.g. coal workers' pneumoconiosis and silicosis
2. **Interstitial fibrosis,** e.g. asbestosis
3. **Hypersensitivity,** e.g. berylliosis.

COAL WORKERS' PNEUMOCONIOSIS

This is the commonest form of pneumoconiosis and is defined as the lung disease resulting from inhalation of coal dust particles especially in coal miners engaged in handling soft bituminous coal for a number of years often 20 to 30 years.

It exists in two forms:
1. Simple coal workers' pneumoconiosis—a milder form
2. Progressive massive fibrosis—an advanced form

Anthracosis, on the other hand, is not a lung disease in true sense but is the common, accumulation of carbon dust in the lungs of most urban dwellers due to atmospheric pollution and cigarette smoke. **Anthracotic pigment** is deposited in the macrophages, in the alveoli and around the respiratory bronchioles and into the draining lymph nodes but does not produce any respiratory difficulty or radiologic changes.

Pathogenesis

It appears that anthracosis, simple coal workers pneumoconiosis and progressive massive fibrosis are different stages in the evolution of fully developed coal workers' pneumoconiosis. However, progressive massive fibrosis develops in a small proportion of cases of simple coal workers' pneumoconiosis. A number of predisposing factors have been implicated in this transformation. These are:
1. Older age of the miners
2. Coal dust burden
3. Duration of exposure (20–30 years)
4. Concomitant tuberculosis
5. Additional role of silica dust

Activation of alveolar macrophages plays the most significant role in the pathogenesis of progressive massive fibrosis by release of various mediators:
1. Free radicals
2. Chemotactic factors like leukotrienes, TNF, IL-8 and IL-6
3. Fibrogenic cytokines such as IL-1, TNF and platelet-derived growth factors.

Pathologic Changes

The pathologic changes in lung in coal workers' pneumoconiosis is graded by radiologic appearance according to the size and extent of opacities.

Simple Coal Workers' Pneumoconiosis

Gross: The lung parenchyma shows small, black focal lesions, measuring less than 5 mm in diameter and evenly distributed throughout the lung but have a tendency to be more numerous in the upper lobes. These are termed as **coal macules** and if palpable, are called **nodules**. The air spaces around coal macules are dilated with destruction of alveolar walls. Similar blackish pigmentations are found on the pleural surface and in the regional lymph nodes.

Microscopy:

1. Coal macules are composed of aggregates of dust-laden macrophages. These are present in the alveoli and bronchiolar walls.
2. There is some increase in the network of reticulin and collagen in the coal macules.
3. Respiratory bronchioles and alveoli surrounding the macules are distended without significant destruction of the alveolar walls.

Progressive Massive Fibrosis

Gross: Besides the coal macules and nodules of simple pneumoconiosis, there are larger, hard, black scattered areas measuring more than 2 cm in diameter and sometimes massive. They are usually bilateral and located more often in the upper parts of the lungs posteriorly. Sometimes, these masses breakdown centrally due to ischaemic necrosis or due to tuberculosis forming cavities filled with black semifluid resembling India ink. The pleura and the regional lymph nodes are also blackened and fibrotic.

Microscopy:

1. The fibrous lesions are composed almost entirely of dense collagen and carbon pigment.
2. The wall of respiratory bronchioles and pulmonary vessels included in the massive scars are thickened and their lumina obliterated.
3. There is scanty inflammatory infiltrate of lymphocytes and plasma cells around the areas of massive scars.
4. The alveoli surrounding the scars are markedly dilated.

Rheumatoid Pneumoconiosis (Caplan's Syndrome)

The development or rheumatoid arthritis in a few cases of coal workers' pneumoconiosis, silicosis or asbestosis is **termed rheumatoid pneumoconiosis or Caplan's syndrome.**

Gross: The lungs have rounded, firm nodules with central necrosis, cavitation or calcification.

Microscopy: The lung lesions have rheumatoid nodules with central zone of dust-laden fibrinoid necrosis enclosed by palisading of fibroblasts and mononuclear cells.

SILICOSIS

Silicosis is caused by the prolonged inhalation of silicon dioxide commonly called silica. Silica constitutes about one-fourth of the earth's crust. Therefore, a number of people engaged working with siliceous rocks or sand and products manufactured from them are at increased risk. These include miners (e.g. granite, sandstone, slate, coal, gold, tin and copper), quarry workers involved in the manufacture of abrasives containing silica.

Pathogenesis

Silicosis appears after prolonged exposure to silica dust, often after a few decades. Besides it depends upon a number of other factors such as total dose, duration of exposure, type of silica inhaled and individual host factors.

Mechanism

1. Silica particles of 0.5 to 5 μ size on reaching the alveoli are taken by the macrophages which undergo necrosis. New macrophages engulf the debris and thus a repetitive cycle of phagocytosis and necrosis is set in.
2. Some silica-laden macrophages are carried to the respiratory bronchioles, alveoli and in the interstitial tissue. Some of the silica dust is transported to the subpleural and interlobar lymphatics and into the regional lymph nodes. The cellular aggregates containing silica are associated with lymphocytes, plasma cells, mast cells and fibroblasts.
3. Silica dust is fibrogenic. Crystalline form, particularly quartz, is more fibrogenic than non-crystalline form of silica.
4. Silica is cytotoxic and kills the macrophages which engulf it. The released silica dust activates viable macrophages leading to secretion of macrophage-derived growth factors such as interleukin-1 that favors fibroblast proliferation and collagen synthesis.
5. Simultaneously, there is activation of T and B lymphocytes. This results in increased serum levels of immunoglobulins (IgG and IgM), antinuclear antibodies, rheumatoid factor and circulating immune complexes as well as proliferation of T cells.

Pathologic Changes

Gross: The chronic silicotic lung is studded with well-circumscribed, hard, fibrotic nodules, 1–5 mm in diameters. They are scattered throughout the lung parenchyma but are initially more often located in the upper zones of the lungs. These nodular lesions frequently have simultaneous deposition of coal-dust and may develop calcification

The pleura is grossly thickened and adherent to the chest wall. There may be similar fibrotic nodules on the pleura and within the regional lymph nodes.

The nodular lesions are detectable as egg-shell shadows in chest X-rays. The lesions may undergo ischaemic necrosis and develop cavitation, or be complicated by tuberculosis and rheumatoid pneumoconiosis.

Microscopy: The silicotic nodules are located in the region of respiratory bronchioles, adjacent alveoli, pulmonary arteries, in the pleura and the regional lymph nodes. The silicotic nodules consist of central hyalinised material with scanty cellularity and some amount of dust. The hyalinised centre is surrounded by concentric laminations of collagen which is further enclosed by more cellular connective tissue, dust-filled macrophages and a few lymphocytes and plasma cells. Some of these nodules may have calcium deposits.

The collagenous nodules have cleft-like spaces between the lamellae of collagen which when examined polariscopically may demonstrate numerous birefringent particles of silica.

The severe and progressive form of the disease may result in coalescence of adjacent nodules and cause complicated silicosis similar to progressive massive fibrosis of coal workers' pneumoconiosis.

The intervening lung parenchyma may show hyperinflation or emphysema. Cavitation when present may be due to ischaemic necrosis in the nodules or may reveal changes of tuberculosis or rheumatoid pneumoconiosis (Caplan's syndrome).

ASBESTOSIS

Asbestos is a Greek word meaning 'unquenchable'. In general, if coal is with a lot of dust and little fibrosis, asbestos is with little dust and lot of fibrosis.

Prolonged exposure for a number of years to asbestos dust produces three types of severe diseases:
1. Asbestosis of lungs
2. Pleural disease
3. Tumours

In nature, asbestos exists as long thin fibrils which are fire-resistant and can be spun into yarns and fabrics suitable for thermal and electrical insulation and has many applications in industries.

Particularly at risk are workers engaged in mining, fabrication and manufacture of a number of products from asbestos such as asbestos pipes, tiles, roofs, textiles, insulating boards, water conduit systems, brake lining, clutch castings, etc.

There are two major forms of asbestos:
1. *Serpentine* consists of curly and flexible fibres. It includes the most common chemical form chrysotile (white asbestos) comprising more than 90% of commercially used asbestos.
2. *Amphibole* consists of straight, stiff and rigid fibres. It includes the less common chemical forms crocidolite, amosite, tremolite, anthophyllite and actinolyte. However, the group of amphibole, though less common, is more important since it is associated with induction of malignant lung and pleural tumours, particularly in association with crocidolite.

Asbestosis of Lungs

Pathogenesis

Over exposure to asbestos for more than a decade may produce asbestosis of the lung, pleural lesions and certain tumours.

Mechanism

The inhaled asbestos fibres are phagocytosed by alveolar macrophages from where they reach the interstitium. Some of the engulfed dust is transported via lymphatics to the pleura and regional lymph nodes.

The asbestos-laden macrophages release chemo-attractants for neutrophils and macrophages, thus inciting cellular reaction around them.

Asbestos fibres are coated with glycoprotein and endogenous haemosiderin to produce characteristic beaded or dumb-bell-shaped asbestos bodies.

All types of asbestos are fibrogenic and result in interstitial fibrosis. Fibroblastic proliferation may occur via macrophage-derived growth factor such as interleukin-1. Alternatively, fibrosis may occur as a reparative response to tissue injury by lysosomal enzymes released from macrophages and neutrophils or by toxic free radicals.

A few immunological abnormalities such as anti-nuclear antibodies and rheumatoid factor have been found in cases of asbestosis.

Asbestos fibres are carcinogenic, the most carcinogenic being crocidolite. There is high incidence of bronchogenic carcinoma in asbestosis which is explained on the basis of the role of asbestos fibres as tumour promoters or by causing cell death of the airways so that it is exposed to the carcinogenic effects of cigarette smoke. The development of pleural mesothelioma in these cases is probably by carrying of asbestos fibres via lymphatics to the pleura.

Pathologic Changes

Gross: The affected lungs are small and firm with cartilage-like thickening of the pleura. The sectioned surface shows variable degree of pulmonary fibrosis, especially in the subpleural areas and in the bases of lungs. The advanced cases may show cystic changes.

Microscopy: There is non-specific interstitial fibrosis. There is presence of characteristic asbestos bodies in the involved areas. These are asbestos fibres coated with glycoprotein and haemosiderin and appear beaded or dumb-bell-shaped and these are positive for Prussian blue stain (Ferruginous bodies).

There may be changes of emphysema in the pulmonary parenchyma between the areas of interstitial fibrosis.

Pleural Diseases and Asbestosis

- **Pleural effusion:** It develops in about 5% of asbestos workers.
- **Visceral pleural fibrosis:** Quite often, asbestosis is associated with dense fibrous thickening of the visceral pleura encasing the lung.
- **Pleural plaques:** Fibrocalcific pleural plaques are the most common lesions associated asbestosis exposure.

Gross: The lesions appear as circumscribed, flat, small (up to 1 cm in diameter), firm or hard, bilateral nodules. They are seen often on the posterolateral part of parietal pleura and on the pleural surface of the diaphragm.

Microscopy: They consist of hyalinised collagenous tissue which may be calcified so that they are visible on chest X-ray.

Lung Tumours and Asbestosis

Asbestos exposure predisposes to a number of cancers, most importantly bronchogenic carcinoma and malignant mesothelioma. A few others are: Carcinomas of esophagus, stomach, colon, kidneys, larynx and lymphoid malignancies.

Bronchogenic carcinoma: It is the most common malignancy in asbestos workers. Its incidence is 5 times higher in non-smoker asbestos workers than the non-smoker general population and 10 times higher in asbestos workers who smoke than the other smokers.

Malignant mesothelioma: It is an uncommon tumour but association with asbestos exposure is present in 30–80% of cases with mesothelioma.

SELF-ASSESSMENT EXERCISE

1. **Pulmonary TB is more common in following diseases, *except*:**
   A. AIDS
   B. Diabetes mellitus
   C. Chronic renal failure
   D. Mitral stenosis

2. **Grey hepatisation of lung is seen on the following day:**
   A. 1
   B. 2–3
   C. 3–4.
   D. 5–7

3. **ARDS syndrome has:**
   A. Diffuse alveolar damage
   B. Respiratory bronchiolitis
   C. Diffuse interstitial pneumonia
   D. Hypersensitivity pneumonitis

4. **Maximum smooth muscle mass relative to wall thickness is seen in:**
   A. Terminal bronchiole
   B. Trachea
   C. Bronchi
   D. Respiratory bronchioles

5. **Creola bodies are seen in:**
   A. Asthma
   B. Chronic bronchitis
   C. Emphysema
   D. Bronchiectasis

6. **Alpha-1-antitrypsin deficiency occurs in:**
   A. Emphysema
   B. Bronchiectasis
   C. Empyema
   D. Bronchogenic carcinoma

7. **Which of the following is characteristic feature of adult respiratory distress syndrome?**
   A. Diffuse alveolar damage
   B. Interstitial tissue inflammation
   C. Alveolar exudates
   D. Interstitial fibrosis

8. **Ferruginous bodies are seen with:**
   A. Silicosis
   B. Byssinosis
   C. Asbestosis
   D. Bagassosis

9. **Which of the following is characteristically not associated with development of interstitial lung disease?**
   A. Organic dusts
   B. Inorganic dusts
   C. Toxic gases, e.g. chlorine, sulphur dioxide
   D. None of the above

10. **Which of the following is associated with hypersensitive pneumonitis?**
    A. Silicosis
    B. Asbestosis
    C. Byssinosis
    D. Berylliosis

11. **End stage lung disease is usually not seen in:**
    A. Sarcoidosis
    B. Interstitial lung disease
    C. Langerhans cell histiocytosis
    D. Aspergillosis

12. **Which of the following occupational pollutant produces extensive nodular pulmonary fibrosis?**
    A. Silica
    B. Asbestos
    C. Wood dust
    D. Carbon

13. **Pleural calcification is seen in:**
    A. Pneumonia
    B. Tuberculous pleural effusion
    C. None of the above
    D. Both of the above

14. **Bronchopulmonary sequestration is seen in which lobe?**
    A. Left lower lobe
    B. Right upper lobe
    C. Left middle lobe
    D. Left upper lobe

15. **Inappropriate antidiuretic hormone (SIADH) secretion is seen in which lung carcinoma?**
    A. Adenocarcinoma
    B. Small cell carcinoma
    C. Large cell carcinoma
    D. Bronchoalveolar carcinoma

16. **Emphysema with jaundice possibility is:**
    A. Alph-1-antitrypsin deficiency
    B. Wegener's granulomatosis
    C. Microscopic angiitis
    D. Churg-Strauss disease

Answers

1. D	2. D	3. A	4. A	5. A	6. A	7. A	8. C
9. D	10. C	11. D	12. A	13. B	14. A	15. B	16. A

Cardiovascular Pathology: Vascular Lesions

ATHEROSCLEROSIS

Atherosclerosis has been derived from Greek words meaning gruel and hardening.

Definition

It is an intimal disorder of vessels with formation of atherosclerotic plaque that protrudes into the vascular lumina. This plaque consists of a soft, yellow grumous core which is covered by a fibrous cap.

These atherosclerotic plaques can:
1. Obstruct the blood flow
2. Weaken the underlying media
3. May rupture and bleed
4. Invite formation of thrombus

Epidemiology

Atherosclerosis is common among developed nations and less common in Southern America, Africa and Asia. The mortality rate for ischaemic heart disease (IHD) in US is highest in the world and 5 times higher than Japan. Population from low incidence countries who migrate to US and adopt American styles and dietary habits acquire atherosclerosis as that of US.

There are multiple risk factors as shown in Table 25.1.

Non-modifiable major risk factors:
1. *Family history* is an independent risk factor. Hypertension, diabetes mellitus run in families.
2. *Increasing age* has dominant influence, although atherosclerosis starts in early age and progresses to manifest with clinical features in later age. The effects are common between the age groups of 40 to 60 years.
3. Premenopausal females are protected because of estrogen, but postmenopausal females and other males have the risk.

Table 25.1	Risk factors for atherosclerosis	
Major	**Minor/lesser**
Non-modifiable	Obesity
Increasing age	Physical inactivity
Male gender	Stress (Type A personality)
Family history	High carbohydrate diet
Genetic abnormality	Post-menopausal estrogen deficiency
	Unsaturated fat intake
Potentially controllable/ modifiable	Higher levels or defects in apolipoprotein [Lp(a)]
Hyperlipidemia	
Hyperhomocysteinaemia	
Hypertension	
Cigarette smoking	
Diabetes mellitus	
C-reactive protein	

The modifiable risk factors can control atherosclerosis, if the levels or severity is less.
1. *Hypertension (HT)* is a major risk factor. Both systolic and diastolic levels are important. Chronic HT increases the risk of cardiovascular (CV) accidents.
2. *Smoking* is a well-established risk factor. Years of smoking and number of cigarettes has effect on vessel wall injury and atherosclerosis.
3. *Hypercholesterolaemia* is major risk factor. High levels of high density lipoproteins (HDL) and low levels of low density lipoproteins (LDL) and very low density lipoproteins (VLDL) are to be monitored. Omega 3 fatty acids and exercise will help to keep the HDL levels high whereas unsaturated fatty acids have adverse effects with with high levels of bad cholesterol (LDL).
4. *Uncontrolled diabetes mellitus* has direct correlation with atherosclerosis and its effects.

Pathogenesis

There are many hypotheses for atherosclerosis. They are as below.

1. Thrombogenic theory
2. Incorporation theory
3. Imbibation theory
4. Monoclonal theory
5. Reaction to injury hypothesis

The atherosclerosis is well explained by "reaction to injury hypothesis". Endothelial injury or loss of endothelial cells of any cause, e.g. denudation, haemodynamic forces, hypercholesterolaemia, immune complexes, irradiation, chemicals, toxins, smoking, homocysteine, infectious agents all can induce atherosclerosis.

The most important two factors which contribute to atherosclerosis are:

1. Haemodynamic disorders
2. Hypercholesterolaemia

The haemodynamic stress can injure endothelial cells and the effect is more at the region where vessels branch and also on the parts of the vessel which lie on the bony parts. This is the reason, atherosclerosis more prominent at the ostia and on the posterior surface of the abdominal aorta.

Lipids: Lipids play a pivotal role in atherogenesis. The lipids are transported in the blood, bound to specific apoproteins after forming lipoprotein complexes. The important lipids found in atherosclerosis are cholesterol and cholesterol esters. About 70% of the cholesterol found in blood is bound to LDL followed by VLDL and intermediate density lipoproteins (IDL). The cholesterol can be increased due to:

1. Homozygous familial hypercholesterolaemia (FH) due to defective LDLR and inadequate uptake of lipoproteins by hepatocytes.

2. There can be deficiency of LDLR and apolipoproteins which can lead to early onset of atherosclerosis.
3. Other causes include:
   - Diabetes mellitus
   - Hypothyroidism
   - Nephrotic syndrome
   - Alcoholism

In these patients, there is increased LDL, decreased HDL and increased levels of Lp (a).

Lowering of cholesterol either by diet or drugs that inhibit synthesis of cholesterol (HMG-CoA) can slow the process of atherosclerosis and reduce the risk of cardiovascular events.

Reaction to Injury Hypothesis: Mechanism of Atherosclerosis (Fig. 25.1)

1. Endothelial injury: Multiple factors and hyperlipidaemia cause endothelial injury and with this there is adhesion of platelets and monocytes to the endothelium. These release cytokines including platelet-derived growth factor. There is local production of reactive oxygen species. The injured endothelium allows lipids to enter into intima due to increased permeability.

2. There is inflammation of the wall which is responsible for initiation, progression and complications of atherosclerosis.

3. There is accumulation of lipoproteins mainly LDL and oxidised forms of LDL due to ROS in the intimal layer of the vessel wall. The endothelial cells express leucocyte adhesion molecules. T cells and monocytes gain entry into intima and these monocytes transform into macrophages and foam cells as they ingest LDL and thus become foamy macrophages. There is platelet adhesion and activation.

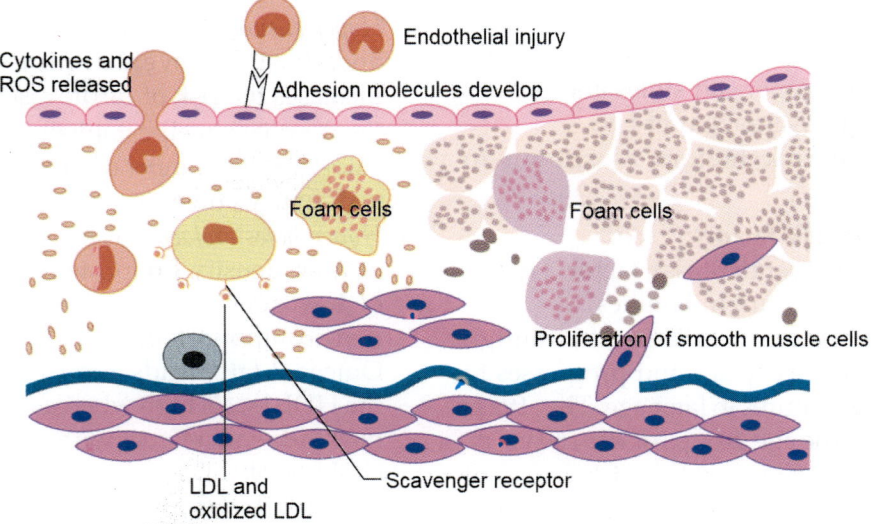

Fig. 25.1: Pathogenesis of atherosclerosis (diagrammatic)

4. Oxidised LDL stimulates release of cytokines by endothelial cells and macrophages and recruits more inflammatory cells. Oxidised LDL is also toxic to endothelial cells and smooth muscle cells (SMCs).
5. Growth factors, released from activated platelets, and macrophages (e.g. PGDF, FGDF, TGF-α), induce extracellular matrix deposition and SMCs recruitment from media. Thus there are smooth cells and deposition of collagen and proteoglycans.
6. Lipid accumulation: Lipid accumulates extracellularly and within the cells (macrophages and SMCs).
7. Thus, central core of lipids, necrotic debris, lipid-laden macrophages and smooth muscle cells and fibrous cap are components of atherosclerosis. Lipid and necrotic debris can get calcified in due course of time. Disruption of the fibrous cap with super-imposed thrombus leads to complications (Figs 25.2 and 25.3).

Classification

Morphologically, atherosclerotic lesions can be classified as below:

1. **Streaks:** Earliest lesions, followed by
2. **Plaque** which has:
   - *Fibrous cap* which has cells—SMCs, macrophages and T cells and extracellular matrix having dense collagen, elastic fibres and proteoglycans.
   - *Core* has intracellular and extracellular lipids mainly cholesterol and cholesterol esters.
3. **Complicated atherosclerotic plaque:**
   - Calcification
   - Rupture
   - Ulceration
   - Erosion
   - Thrombosis
   - Haemorrhage
   - Occlusion/stenosis
   - Atheroemboli
   - Aneurysmal dilatation

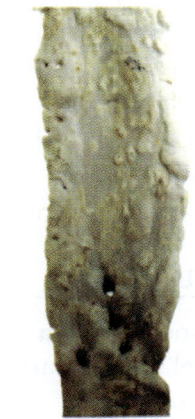

Fig. 25.2: Atherosclerosis (gross picture)

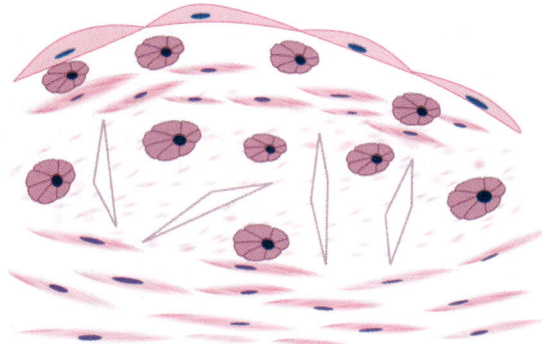

Fig. 25.3: Microscopy of atherosclerosis (schematic)

Table 25.2 shows AHA classifications of athero-sclerosis for histologic diagnosis.

Table 25.2	American Heart Association (AHA) classification of atherosclerotic plaques for histologic diagnosis[21]
Type	**Nature of histology**
Type I	Initial lesion; isolated macrophages and foam cells (fatty dot)
Type II	Fatty streaks; foam cells, intracellular lipid
Type III	Preatheroma; raised fatty streak, small extracellular lipid core, foam cells contain lipid droplets, increasing number of smooth muscle cells
Type IV	Atheroma; covered by a proteoglycan-rich layer infiltrated with foam cells and smooth muscle cells, extracellular lipid
Type V	Fibroatheroma; lipid core, fibrotic layer, or mainly calcific or mainly fibrotic
Type VI	Complications: Surface defect, haemorrhage, thrombus

HYPERTENSIVE VASCULAR DISEASE

Elevated blood pressure is called hypertension (HT). A systolic blood pressure of more than 140 mm Hg and diastolic blood pressure of more than 90 mm Hg is taken as hypertension. Hypertension is a common health problem with devastating outcomes. The causes are listed in Table 25.3.

Table 25.3	Causes of hypertension
Types and causes of HT	

Essential HT (90 to 95% cases)
Secondary causes
Renal
1. Acute glomerulonephritis
2. Cronic renal failure
3. Polycystic kidney
4. Renal artery stenosis
5. Renal vasculitis
6. Renin-producing tumours

Endocrine
1. Adrenocortical hyperfunction: Cushing syndrome, primary aldosteronism, congenital adrenal hyperplasia
2. Exogenous hormones: Glucocorticoids, estrogen, oral contra-ceptives
3. Pheochromocytoma
4. Acromegaly
5. Hypothyroidism
6. Hyperthyroidism

CVS
1. Coarctation of aorta
2. Polyarteritis nodosa
3. Raise of intra-arterial pressure
4. Raised cardiac output
5. Rigidity of aorta

Neurologic
1. Psychological
2. Raises intracranial pressure
3. Sleep apnoea
4. Acute illness and stress

Before going into details of essential and secondary hypertension, let us know in short about regulation of blood pressure.

Regulation of Blood Pressure

Cardiac output and vascular resistance are important in regulation of blood pressure. Cardiac output is dependent on sodium concentrations. Peripheral resistance is influenced by neural and hormonal inputs.

Kidney is the major organ influencing vascular resistance through renin. When blood pressure is reduced, juxtaglomerular cells of kidney produce renin. This converts angiotensin to angiotensin I and this further gets converted to angiotensin II by angiotensin-converting enzyme. Angiotensin II increases blood pressure by increasing peripheral resistance by inducing vasoconstriction and aldosterone secretion by the adrenal cortex which conserves sodium in distal convoluted tubules. Kidney also produces vasorelaxant substances like prostaglandins and NO to counter-balance the vasopressor effect of angiotensin II.

Essential hypertension (EHT): This type of EHT represents 90–95% of cases of HT. It is complex and multifactorial disorder. The etiology of essential hypertension is idiopathic and compatible with long life unless major cardiovascular or CNS problems occur. In EHT:

- Sodium homeostasis and vessel wall tone or structure contributes to the increased blood volume and peripheral resistance.
  Reduced renal sodium excretion will cause increase in fluid volume and thus increases cardiac output.
  Vascular changes cause functional vasoconstriction and changes in vascular wall structure which results in increased vascular resistance.
- Genetic component with family history is known in hypertension. Environmental factors modify the genetic determinants.
- Stress, obesity, smoking, physical inactivity, heavy salt consumption are associated with hypertension.
  There is increase of blood pressure, has long clinical course and has little clinical effects in early stages.

Secondary hypertension (malignant hypertension): About 5% of the HT cases have rapidly rising blood pressure. This is termed as accelerated HT or malignant HT. The diastolic blood pressure is more than 120 mm Hg. This has severe impact on renal, CVS and CNS system.

VASCULAR PATHOLOGY IN HYPERTENSION

Hypertension is associated with atherosclerosis and degenerative changes of the large- and medium-sized vessels. Small blood vessels in hypertension show hyaline arteriolosclerosis and hyperplastic arteriolosclerosis.

Hyaline Arteriolosclerosis

There is accumulation of homogenous pink hyaline material in the walls of arterioles with loss of underlying structures and narrowing of lumen. This type of hyaline arteriolosclerosis is commonly encountered in elderly people (normotensive and hypertensive patients). It is more generalized and severe in patients with hypertension. It is encountered in patients with diabetes mellitus and benign nephrosclerosis.

Hyperplastic Arteriolosclerosis

This type of vessel pathology is common with malignant hypertension, wherein the diastolic blood pressure is more than 120 mm Hg and associated with acute renal or cerebral injury.

Hyperplastic arteriolosclerosis is associated with onion skin concentric laminated thickening of the walls of the arterioles with luminal narrowing.

The laminations consist of smooth muscle cells and thickened and duplicated basement membrane. There is deposition of fibrinoid material and vessel wall necrosis (necrotizing arteriolitis). This is more pronounced in vessels of kidneys.

HT usually remains asymptomatic until late in its course. Hypertension can cause the following:
1. Cardiac hypertrophy
2. Heart failure
3. Aortic dissection
4. Renal failure
5. Cardiovascular accidents

ANEURYSMS

An aneurysm is a localized abnormal dilatation of blood vessel or the heart walls (Fig. 25.4). These can be:
1. True, or
2. False.

True aneurysm is the one with involvement of all the three layers (intima, media, and adventitia). Example: Atherosclerotic, syphilitic, congenital and ventricular aneurysms.

False aneurysm or pseudoaneurysm is a branch in the vascular wall leading to an extravascular haematoma that freely communicates with the intravascular space, e.g. ventricular wall rupture after MI, arterial wall dissection.

Depending upon shape, aneurysm can be classified as:
1. Saccular (Berry aneurysm)
2. Fusiform

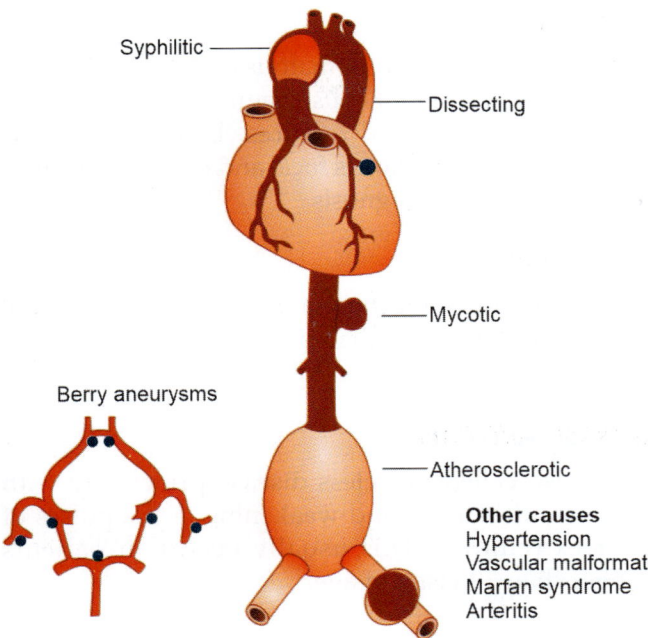

Syphilitic

Dissecting

Mycotic

Berry aneurysms

Atherosclerotic

Other causes
Hypertension
Vascular malformation
Marfan syndrome
Arteritis

Fig. 25.4: Different causes of aneurysms

SACCULAR ANEURYSMS

These are spherical outpouchings involving only a portion of a vessel. They are 5–20 cm in diameter. Saccular aneurysms are thin walled; round shaped and are outpouchings of an artery. At the neck of the artery, muscle layer and internal elastic lamina are absent.

Saccular/Berry aneurysms are the most common type of intracranial aneurysms. Rupture can occur at any time, and in one-third of the cases, it is associated with increased intracranial pressure. Rupture of saccular aneurysm causes subarachnoid haemorrhage.

Clinical Features

As there is increased arterial pressure, these patients have sudden headache, vomiting and unconsciousness with rupture and subarachnoid haemorrhage.

FUSIFORM ANEURYSMS

These involve a long segment of the vessel. The causes include:
1. Atherosclerosis and arterial medial degeneration—abdominal aorta commonly affected. Iliac, arch and descending part of thoracic aorta also can be involved. The media undergoes degeneration and necrosis.
2. Trauma
3. Congenital
4. Vasculitis
5. Infection (mycotic)

Mycotic Aneurysm

Infection weakens the arterial wall. Thrombosis and rupture are common complications in this type of aneurysms. These originate usually from bacteria or fungi:
1. Septic emboli as in infective endocarditis
2. Extension of suppurative process
3. Circulating organisms directly infect the vessel, e.g. salmonella gastroenteritis
4. Infection by *Aspergillus* and *Mucor* species

Syphilitic Aneurysm

T. pallidum causes obliterative endarteritis. The vessels show luminal narrowing, obliteration, scaring and dense rim of inflammatory cell infiltration, predominantly lymphocytes and plasma cells. The narrowing of vasa vasorum causes ischaemic injury of media with loss of medial elastic fibres and muscle cells followed by inflammation and scaring. Damage to media leads to aneurysm. Scarring leads to wrinkling of the intima (tree bark appearance).

AORTIC DISSECTION

There is dissection in the laminar plane of the media. Blood flows in the media and ruptures the adventitia and into various spaces. This causes massive haemorrhage or cardiac temponade.

It occurs most commonly in:
1. Men aged 40 to 60 years with hypertension.
2. Younger patients with systemic or localized abnormalities of connective tissue (Marfan syndrome, Ehlers-Danlos syndrome, vitamin C deficiency, copper metabolic defects).

Marfan syndrome is a disease with AD inheritance of fibrillin which is required for elastic tissue synthesis. These patients have elongated axial bones, lens subluxation and CVS manifestations. There is a trigger for intimal tear; blood flow dissects the media causing medial haematoma. These can be type A or type B. The type A involves ascending aorta or descending aorta. Type B lesions are distal to subclavian artery.

RAYNAUD'S PHENOMENON

Raynaud's phenomenon is exaggerated vasoconstriction of digital arteries and arterioles. The involved digits show red (rubor), white (pallor), and blue colour (cyanosis) changes from proximal to distal correlating with proximal vasodilatation, central vasoconstriction and distal cyanosis.

Primary Raynaud's phenomenon (Raynaud's disease), the cause of which is not known, shows exaggeration of vasomotor response to cold or emotion with predilection for young women. The course is benign. Long-standing Raynaud's disease has atrophy of skin, subcutaneous tissues and muscles. Ulceration and gangrene are rare.

Secondary Raynaud's phenomenon can be observed in:

1. Collagen vascular disease: SLE, scleroderma, rheumatoid arthritis, dermatomyositis and polymyositis
2. Occlusive arterial diseases: Buerger disease and atherosclerosis
3. Blood disorders: Waldenstrom's macroglobulinaemia, cryoglobulinaemia, cold agglutinins, myeloproliferative disorders
4. Neurological disorders: Carpel tunnel syndrome, syringomyelia, spinal cord tumours, intervertebral disc disease
5. Trauma
6. Drugs: Ergot alkaloids, beta blockers

VASCULITIS

Vasculitis is inflammation of the vessels. Vessels of any organs can be affected.

According to the pathologic mechanisms, it can be:
1. Immune-mediated vasculitis or
2. Direct injury to the vessels by the organisms

In immune-mediated vasculitis, large-sized, medium-sized or small-sized vessels can be affected and the classification is given in Table 25.4.

GIANT CELL ARTERITIS

It is chronic granulomatous inflammation of vessels and large- to small-sized arteries are usually involved. Most commonly temporal, vertebral and ophthalmic arteries are affected. This occurs after the age of 50 years.

Etiology

Exact etiology not known. However, it is linked to bacterial infection, vius, antibiotics and auto-immunity.

Pathology

Intimal thickening, granulomatous inflammation of the wall, mainly with giant cells, fragmentation of elastic lamina are the classical features. Late stages show fragmentation. The lesion is focal and negative findings do not rule out the diagnosis.

Clinical Features

Facial pain and headache mainly along the temporal artery are common. Ophthalmic artery involvement has diplopia to complete vision loss.

TAKAYASU ARTERITIS

This is also called pulseless disease principally with ocular manifestations and weakening of the pulses of upper extremities. This usually occurs in patients younger than 50 years of age.

Pathology

There is fibrous thickening of the aorta mainly aortic arch and affects other large- and medium-sized arteries. The microscopy of involved vessel shows dense mononuclear cells with granulomatous inflammation having giant cells in the media and perivascular cuffing of vasavasorum.

Clinical Features

Symptoms due to reduced blood pressure, weak pulse of carotids, ocular vessels, and upper extremities are common features. Visual defects, retinal haemorrhages, and blindness may occur. Neurological defects and claudication of legs with involvement of distal aorta, pulmonary hypertension, myocardial infarction, renal involvement leading to systemic hypertension may be present in these cases.

Table 25.4	Classification of vasculitis	
Vasculitis type	**Diseases**	**Description**
Mainly large vessel vasculitis along with medium and small vessel vasculitis	Giant cell arteritis	Granulomatous inflammation, patients older than 50 years affected
	Takayasu arteritis	Granulomatous inflammation, patients younger than 50 years affected
Mainly medium vessel vasculitis along with small vessel vasculitis	PAN	Necrotising vasculitis usually renal vessels affected
	Kawasaki disease	
	Buerger disease	Acute or chronic inflammation of arteries and veins with thrombus formation
Small vessel vasculitis, inflammation of capillaries	Wegener's disease	Granulomatous inflammation usually lung involved
	Churg-Strauss syndrome	Granulomatous inflammation with plenty of eosinophils
	Microscopic polyangiitis	Capillaries and venules also involved. Segmental necrotizing vasculitis and leukocytoclastic vasculitis

POLYARTERITIS NODOSA (PAN)

There is systemic vasculitis mainly affecting visceral and renal blood vessels. The pulmonary vessels are not involved. Exact etiology is not known, in about 30% of the cases associated with immune complex deposits in cases of hepatitis B infections.

Pathology

There is segmental transmural inflammation of small- and medium-sized vessels. There is weakening of vessel wall with aneurysm formation and sometimes rupture.

In acute phase, there is transmural necrotizing inflammation with mixed infiltrate of neutrophils, eosinophils and mononuclear cells along with fibrinoid necrosis.

Clinical Features

This is a disease of young age. But can occur in all age groups. Rapid onset of hypertension due to renal vessel involvement, abdominal pain, blood-tinged stools due to involvement of vessels of GIT, myalgias and neuritis can be the features.

KAWASAKI DISEASE

This is also known as mucocutaneous lymph node syndrome. Usually affects children; large-, medium-sized and even small-sized vessels are affected. The pathogenesis is not known; mostly viral etiology has been implicated.

Pathology

Microscopy is similar to polyarteritis nodosa. There can be scarring of old lesions. Aneurysms, thrombosis, rupture and infarction of the area supplied are seen. Fibrinoid necrosis is less common than PAN.

Clinical Features

Mucous membranes of conjunctiva and oral cavity with erythema and blisters along with desquamative rash on hands and feet, mainly palms and soles are seen. It is associated with lymphadenitis. Prognosis is good unless CVS is affected with coronary arteritis which can lead to rupture, thrombosis, and myocardial infarction.

WEGENER DISEASE (Granulomatosis)

This has acute necrotising granulomas of small and medium sized vessels. Granulomas with c-ANCA positivity represent disease activity.

CHURG-STRAUSS SYNDROME

This involves small vessels. This is also called allergic angiitis, as it is associated with asthma, allergic rhinitis and eosinophilia. The disease may be associated with antineutrophil cytoplasmic antibodies (ANCAs). This is a multisystem disease involving skin and many organs including renal and cardiovascular systems. Death can be because of heart involvement.

Pathology

Shows necrotizing granulomas along with eosinophils.

MICROSCOPIC ANGIITIS

In microscopic angiitis, all the systems are affected including skin and mucous membranes. These features may be seen in Henoch-Schonlein purpura and connective tissue disorders.

Pathology

This affects capillaries, venules and small arterioles. There is segmental necrotizing vasculitis with leukocytoclastic vasculitis.

THROMBOANGIITIS OBLITERANS (TAO)/ BUERGER'S DISEASE

It is a segmental, acute on chronic disease of medium- and small-sized vessels causing thrombosis. Arteries and veins of extremities are affected. It is common in young male smokers, before 35 to 40 years of age.

Pathology

It shows acute or chronic inflammation of vessel wall with thrombus formation.

Clinical Features

Claudication pain in legs and less commonly of hands, may lead to gangrene. Pain even on rest, digital ulcers and association with smoking are classical features.

SELF-ASSESSMENT EXERCISE

1. **c-ANCA is associated with:**
   A. Wegener's granulomatosis
   B. Kawasaki disease
   C. TAO
   D. PAN

2. **c-ANCA is characteristic of:**
   A. Sjogren's syndrome
   B. Giant cell arteritis
   C. Wegener's granulomatosis
   D. Kawasaki's disease

3. **An elderly with headache and visual disturbances point towards:**
   A. Organising thrombus
   B. Infarction brain
   C. Giant cell arteritis
   D. Aneurysm of vessel

4. **Hallmark feature of benign hypertension is:**
   A. Hyaline arteriolosclerosis
   B. Medial calcification
   C. Fibrinoid necrosis
   D. Hyperplastic arteriolosclerosis

5. **Feature of temporal arteritis?**
   A. Bacterial infection
   B. Bleeding
   C. Benign tumour
   D. Capillary haemangioma

6. **All are small vessel vasculitis *except*:**
   A. Kawasaki's disease
   B. Churg-Strauss syndrome
   C. Wegener's granulomatosis
   D. Microscopic polyangiitis

7. **Polyarteritis nodosa can occur in association with which of the following?**
   A. Hypertension   B. Trauma
   C. Drugs   D. Bronchial asthma

8. **In 60 years male, kidneys are smaller with hyalinised vessels. Possibility is:**
   A. PAN
   B. Kawasaki's vasculitis
   C. Systemic HT (benign)
   D. Malignant HT

9. **Child with IgA deposits in glomerulus with skin biopsy showing vasuculitis is possibly:**
   A. PAN
   B. Giant cell arteritis
   C. Takayasu arteritis
   D. Henoch-Schonlein purpura

10. **Claudication pain is characteristic of:**
    A. TAO
    B. GCA
    C. Takayasu arteritis
    D. Henoch-Schonlein purpura

11. **Atherosclerotic plaque has all *except*:**
    A. Fibrous cap
    B. Lipid core
    C. Migration of smooth muscle cells
    D. Seen in media

12. **Most common cause of secondary HT:**
    A. Renal disease
    B. Coarctation of aorta
    C. Stress
    D. Pheochromocytoma

Answers

| 1. A | 2. C | 3. C | 4. A | 5. A | 6. A | 7. A | 8. C |
| 9. D | 10. A | 11. D | 12. A | | | | |

Cardiovascular Pathology: Heart Lesions

CONGENITAL HEART DISEASES

Congenital heart diseases (CHDs) are abnormalities of the heart or great vessels that are present at birth.

Most such disorders arise from faulty embryogenesis during gestational weeks of 3 through 8, when major cardiovascular structures develop.

Pathogenesis

1. Cause is unknown in almost 90% of cases.
2. *Environmental factors,* such as congenital rubella infection.
3. *Genetic* with certain chromosomal abnormalities (e.g. trisomies 13, 15, 18, and 21 and Turner syndrome).

Congenital heart diseases subdivided into three groups (Table 26.1).

Table 26.1	Different types of congenital heart diseases
Right-to-left shunt	Tetralogy of Fallot, transposition of great arteries, tricuspid atresia, total anomalous pulmonary venous connection, persistent truncus arteriosus
Left-to-right shunt	VSD, ASD, PDA, atrioventricular septal defect
Malformations causing *obstruction*	Coarctation of aorta, aortic valvular stenosis, pulmonary stenosis

Some of the important congenital heart diseases (CHDs) are mentioned below.

CHDs CAUSING LEFT-TO-RIGHT SHUNT

Atrial Septal Defect (ASD)

An abnormal opening in the atrial septum that allows communication of blood between the left and right atria. ASDs are usually asymptomatic until adulthood (until the age of 30 years).

Three major types of ASDs are:
a. **Secundum ASDs (90%)**—single, multiple or fenestrated oval fossa near the centre of the atrial septum (mid-septum).
b. **Primum anomalies (5%)** adjacent to the AV valves associated with cleft in the anterior mitral leaflet.
c. **Sinus venosus defects (5%)** located near the entrance of the superior vena cava and may be associated with anomalous pulmonary venous return to the right atrium.

Effects of ASD
- Increased pulmonary flow (2 to 4 times than normal) with pulmonary hypertension
- Right ventricular hypertrophy

Ventricular Septal Defect (VSD)

There is incomplete closure of the ventricular septum, with free communication of blood between the left-to-right ventricles. This is the most common form of congenital cardiac anomaly.
- Most VSDs are associated with other congenital cardiac anomalies such as **tetralogy of Fallot.**
- **About 90% involve the region of the membranous interventricular septum (membranous VSD).** The remainder lies below the **pulmonary valve (infundibular VSD) or within the muscular septum.**
- Although most VSDs are **single, those in the muscular septum may be multiple (so-called "Swiss-cheese" septum).**
- 50% close spontaneously and remainder are tolerated.
- Large defects produce left-to-right shunts.

Effects of VSD
- Increased pulmonary flow with pulmonary hypertension.
- Right ventricle hypertrophy

Patent Ductus Arteriosus (PDA)

PDA results when the ductus arteriosus, an essential fetal structure that normally spontaneously closes, remains open after birth and shunts blood from the aorta to pulmonary artery. 90% occur as isolated anomalies. Remainder occurs with VSD and coarctation of aorta.

Coarctation with PDA presents early in life. Murmer is present. Initially no cyanosis as the shunt is left to right. When there is obstructive pulmonary vascular disease flow reverses.

Effects of PDA

- Increased volume on left side of ventricle, later with increased pulmonary flow.
- Left atrium and left ventricle hypertrophy.

CHDs CAUSING RIGHT-TO-LEFT SHUNTS

These patients have cynosis with dimished pulmonary flow and poorly oxygenated blood enters the systemic circulation.

More over bland or septic emboli arising from peripheral vein can bypass pulmonary circulation and can enter systemic circulation (paradoxical emboli).

Tetralogy of Fallot (TOF) (Fig. 26.1)

Four cardinal features of TOF are:
1. VSD
2. Obstruction of the right ventricular outflow tract (subpulmonary stenosis)
3. An aorta that overrides the VSD
4. Right ventricular hypertrophy

This results from anterosuperior displacement of the infundibular septum and has following features.

- Heart is often enlarged and "boot-shaped" due to marked right ventricular hypertrophy, particularly of the apical region.
- The VSD is usually large, aortic valve forms the superior border and override the defect (VSD).
- There is obstruction to the right ventricular outflow due to narrowing of infundibulum/complete atresia of pulmonary valve.
- If the subpulmonary stenosis is mild, the abnormality resembles an isolated VSD, and the shunt may be left-to-right, without cyanosis (so-called pink tetralogy).
- As the obstruction increases in severity, there is greater resistance to right ventricular outflow. *Right-sided pressure exceeds that of left-sided pressure and right-to-left shunt develops with cyanosis* (Classic TOF).
- Most infants with TOF are cyanotic from birth or soon thereafter.

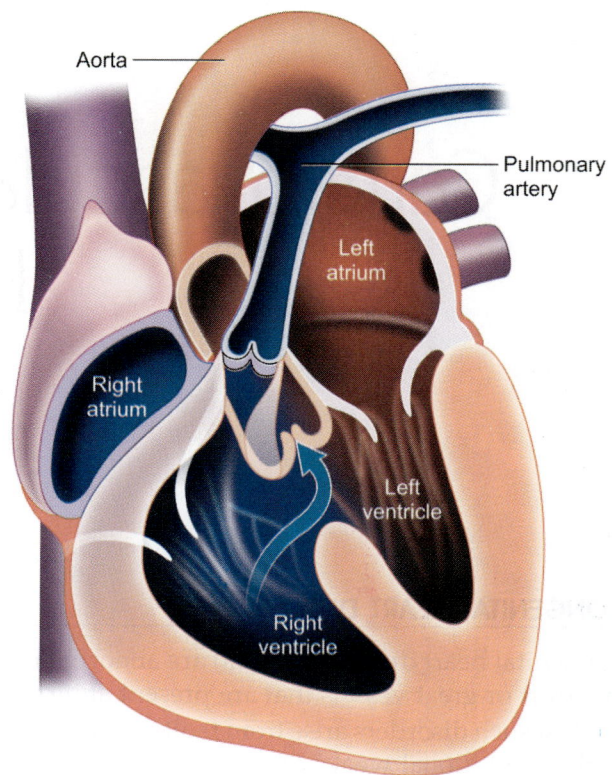

Fig. 26.1: Congenital heart diseases, Fallot's tetralogy

Transposition of the Great Arteries (TGA)

- TGA is a discordant connection of the ventricles to their vascular outflow.
- The embryologic defect is an abnormal formation of the truncal and aortopulmonary septa, so that the aorta arises from the right ventricle and the pulmonary artery from the left ventricle.
- The atrium-to-ventricle connections, however, are normal (concordant). The functional outcome is separation of the systemic and pulmonary circulations. Incompatible with life unless shunts exists.

OBSTRUCTIVE LESIONS

Coarctation of Aorta

- It is narrowing or constriction of aorta.
- M:F = 2:1, although females with Turner syndrome frequently have aortic coarctation.
- **Two classic forms:** Infantile (preductal) form, and adult (postductal) form.

Infantile (Preductal) Form (Fig. 26.2)

- Hypoplasia and tubular narrowing of the aortic arch between the left subclavian artery and the ductus arteriosus.
- Ductus arteriosus is usually patent.
- Right ventricle is hypertrophied and dilated.
- Manifests immediately after birth.

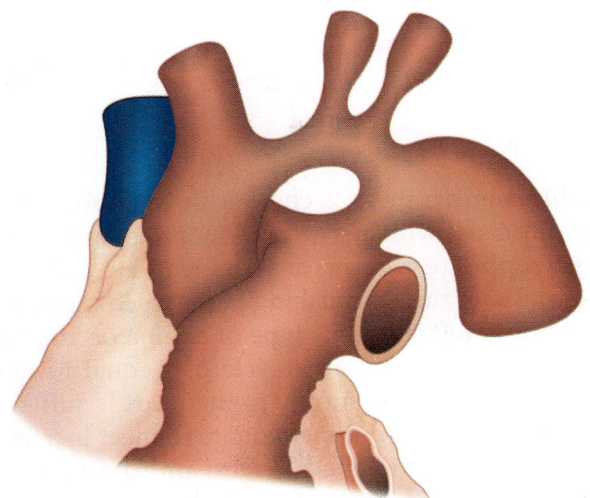

Fig. 26.2: Coarctation of aorta with PDA

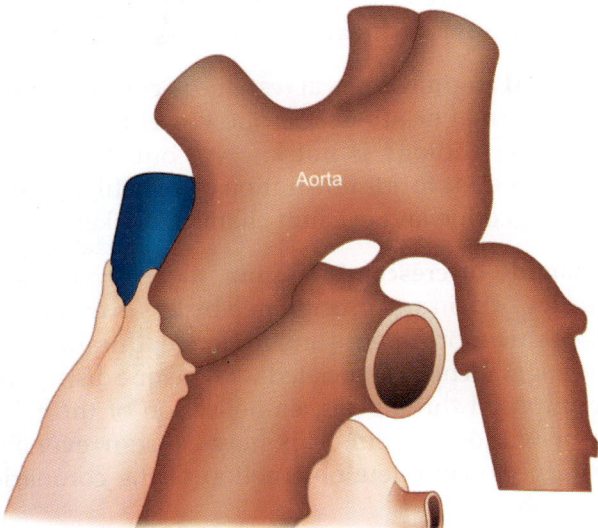

Fig. 26.3: Coarctation of aorta (Figs 26.1 to 26.3 *From* Burford TH. Symposium on clinical surgery. Coarctation of aorta and its treatment. Surg Clin North Am 1950, 30:1249–1258)

- Cyanosis localized to the lower half of the body.
- Femoral pulses are almost always weaker than those of the upper extremeties.

Adult (Postductal) Form (Fig. 26.3)

- Aorta is sharply constricted by a ridge of tissue at or just distal to the ligamentum arteriosum.
- The ductus arteriosus is closed.
- Proximal to the coarctation, the aortic arch and its branch vessels are dilated.
- Left ventricle is hypertrophic.
- Usually asymptomatic.
- Upper extremity hypertension, but weak pulse and lower blood pressure in the lower extremities. Claudication and coldness of the lower extremities.
- Adults show exuberant collateral circulation "around" the coarctation involving markedly enlarged inter-

costal and internal mammary arteries—radiographically visible "notching" of the ribs.

Aortic Stenosis and Atresia

Most common congenital anomaly of aorta is bicuspid aortic valve.

- Congenital aortic atresia—incompatible with life.
- Acquired aortic stenosis—rheumatic heart disease, calcified aortic stenosis.

Congential aortic stenosis—three types:

1. Valvular stenosis—aortic valve cusps are malformed and are irregularly thickened. The aortic valve may have one, two and three malformed cusps.
2. Subvalvular stenosis—thick fibrous ring under the aortic valve causing subaortic stenosis.
3. Supravalvular stenosis—there is fibrous constriction above sinuses of Valsalva.

Effects of aortic stenosis and atresia:

- Left atrium and left ventricle—volume hypertrophy
- Aortic root—dilated

CARCINOID HEART DISEASE

This represents cardiac manifestations of a carcinoid syndrome which includes flushing, diarrhoea, dermatitis and bronchoconstriction.

The effects are due to serotonine produced by these cells. About 70% tryptophan is converted to serotonin which further gets converted to 5-hydroxyindoleacetic acid (5-HIAA). Liver inactivates bioactive products. Cardiac lesions do not occur until there is hepatic metastatic burden and only occurs when vasoactive mediators are no longer catabolised by the liver.

Bronchial carcinoids have symptoms in 10% of the cases. Hindgut carcinoids are silent. Right side of heart is the first tissue to get exposed to the effect of bioactive substances. Left side of the heart gets affected with patent foramen ovale, right-to-left flow or with pulmonary carcinoids.

Pathology

The heart in carcinoid syndrome has glistening white plaque-like thickening of endocardial surface of chambers and valve leaflets. The lesion is composed of smooth muscle cells and sparse collagen fibres embedded in acid mucopolysaccharide-rich matrix.

HEART FAILURE

Heart failure or congestive cardiac/heart failure (CCF or CHF) is an end result of many conditions. The heart is unable to pump blood, to meet the requirements of the tissues.

In CHF, there is inadequate cardiac output, i.e. forward failure which is accompanied by backward failure (increased congestion of venous circulation).

Left-sided failure is due to:
1. Ischaemic heart disease
2. Systemic hypertension
3. Mitral/aortic valve diseases
4. Primary myocardial diseases

Right-sided failure is due to:
1. Left-sided failure with pulmonary congestion or increased arterial pressure
2. Cor pulmonale (occurs in intrinsic disease of lung parenchyma or due to chronic pulmonary hypertension)
3. Congenital heart diseases with left-to-right shunts

In left-sided failure, the following are seen:
1. Left ventricle is hypertrophied and dilated.
2. Left atrium may dilated.
3. There is pulmonary congestion and oedema.

Clinical features in left-sided failure include:
1. Dyspnoea
2. Orthopnoea
3. Paroxysmal nocturnal dyspnoea—night awakening with extreme dyspnoea

In right-sided failure, the following features are seen:
1. Liver is enlarged, shows chronic venous congestion features.
2. There is portal hypertension with centrilobular necrosis.
3. May develop cardiac cirrhosis and congestive splenomegaly.
4. Pericardial and pleural effusion may be present.
5. Peripheral oedema of dependent portions is present, e.g. pedal (ankle), pre-tibial, pre-sacral or may become generalized (anasarca).

ISCHAEMIC HEART DISEASES (IHD)

Ischaemic heart disease is due to lack of blood supply to the heart and this can lead to:
1. Angina pectoris
2. Myocardial infarction
3. Chronic ischaemic heart disease
4. Sudden cardiac death

ANGINA PECTORIS

Intermittent chest pain with reversible myocardial injury is called angina pectoris.

There are variants:
1. Stable
2. Prinzmetal
3. Unstable.

In stable angina, there is chest pain with exertion or due to any cause with increased demands of myocardial oxygen supply (e.g. fever, anxiety, fear, etc.). There is substernal sqeezing or crushing pain which radiates to left arm or to left jaw. This type of angina occurs with blockage of vessels by atherosclerosis equal to more than 75%. The oxygen supply to the heart is sufficient for basal conditions, but inadequate to meet increased demands. Pain is relieved by rest or administering nitroglycerine or peripheral vasodilator drugs which increases blood supply to the myocardium by dilatation of the coronaries and also reduces venous blood coming to the heart, thus reducing workload on heart.

Prinzmetal angina occurs at rest due to coronary artery spasm. Normal or atherosclerotic vessel can undergo spasm. The etiology is not known, but this type of angina responds to administration of vasodilators such as nitroglycerine and calcium channel blockers.

In unstable or crescendo angina, there is increasing frequency of pain and precipitated by less exertion. The episodes are more intense and for longer duration than stable angina. This is associated with plaque disruption, superimposed thrombosis, embolisation of thrombus with or without spasm. This may cause irreversible injury due to complete obstruction of the coronaries by thrombus.

MYOCARDIAL INFARCTION (MI)

Myocardial infarction is death of the cardiac muscle due to blockage of the coronary vessel supplying or prolonged severe ischaemia.

Incidence and Epidemiology

Myocardial infarction is common with increased age. It can occur in younger age with genetic (familial hypercholesterolaemia) and type A personality people. Females are protected in reproductive age. However, postmenopausal period has increased incidence of myocardial infarction due to reduced estrogen levels.

Causes

1. In 90 to 95% of the cases, the cause is occlusion of the coronary artery with atherosclerosis having complications (haemorrhage, rupture, fissure, erosion or ulceration) and thrombus formation.
2. In another 5 to 10% of the cases: Vasospasm.

3. Emboli: Embolisation in atrial fibrillation, mitral valve disease, vegetations bacterial endocarditis, rheumatic heart disease with prosthetic valves, mural thrombus, and paradoxical emboli can occlude the coronaries.

Types or Patterns of Myocardial Infarction (Classification)

1. **Depending on involvement of thickness of myocardium:** Transmural or subendocardial. In transmural infarcts, necrosis involves full thickness of the ventricle in the area supplied by the blocked coronary vessel. Subendocardial infarcts usually occur in the inner one-third portion of the myocardium as it is less perfused tissue. This is more common with chronic ischaemia and prolonged shock; infarct is circumferential and is not according to the distribution of the coronary vessel. Circumferential infarcts can occur due to severe reduction of blood flow, involves ventricles in circumferential manner.

2. **Area of myocardium involved:** This depends upon supply of blood by different coronaries. LAD branch supplies apex and anterior wall of left ventricle and anterior two-thirds of interventricular septum. Left coronary artery (LCA) supplies remaining part of the left ventricle including lateral free wall. Right coronary artery (RCA) perfuses entire right ventricular free wall.

   In a right dominant circulation, RCA in 80% of the cases supplies posterior one-third of the septum and posterobasal portion of the left ventricle. In rest 20%, left circulation may be dominant and LCA supplies posterior one-third of the interventricular septum. Thus, depending upon area involved, the infarcts are named, e.g. apical, septal, anterolateral, posterior, etc.

3. **On ECG findings:**
   - Transmural infarcts are ST elevation infarcts (STEMI).
   - Subendocardial infarcts are non-ST elevation (NSTEMI).

   For gross, microscopy and laboratory findings refer to topic on infarction.

CHRONIC ISCHAEMIC HEART DISEASE

There is progressive heart failure and most commonly this is consequence of myocardial infarction with following gross and microscopic changes.

Gross: Heart is enlarged, with left ventricular dilatation and hypertrophy. Aorta has varying degrees of atherosclerosis. Foci of old healed MI can be present. The endocardium shows patchy thickening and can show mural thrombi.

Microscopy: Shows myocardial hypertrophy, diffuse subendocardial myocyte vacuolization and fibrosis due to old infarcts.

SUDDEN CARDIAC DEATH (SCD)

Unexpected death from cardiac causes without symptoms or death occurring within 1 to 24 hours of onset of symptoms.

Causes

Coronary artery disease is the commonest cause in adults. In younger patients, non-atherosclerotic causes are common and these include:

1. Congenital coronary artery anomalies
2. Aortic valve stenosis
3. Mitral valve prolapse
4. Myocarditis
5. Sarcoidosis
6. Dilated cardiomyopathy
7. Pulmonary hypertension

   These patients usually have arrhythmias and ventricular fibrillation.

Pathology

Coronaries show severe atherosclerosis with stenosis of more than 75%. Plaque disruption is seen in some patients. Old MI or in resuscitated individuals recent MI may be found. Subendothelial myocyte vacuolations are common which are indicative of ischaemia. In minority of the cases non-atherogenic cause may be encountered.

HYPERTENSIVE HEART DISEASE

Chronic hypertension affects many organs, including heart, brain, and kidneys. There is cardiac myocardial hypertrophy. The myocardial fibres cannot divide, but they undergo hypertrophy. This is mainly due to increased workload from increased pressure, volume or from trophic signals. Hypertension can affect left or right side of heart.

The average weight of normal heart is given below:
- Indian males: 250–300 g
- Indian females: 200–250 g
- Western population: 300–350 g

   Heart may weigh 2–3 times of the normal in systemic hypertension (HT), aortic stenosis (AS), miltral incompetence/mitral regurgitation (MI/MR), dilated CMP and hypertrophic cardiomyopathy (CMP). Average heart weight in these patients is 500 g.

   Pressure overload (HT or AS) shows **concentric hypertrophy** of left ventricle with increased wall

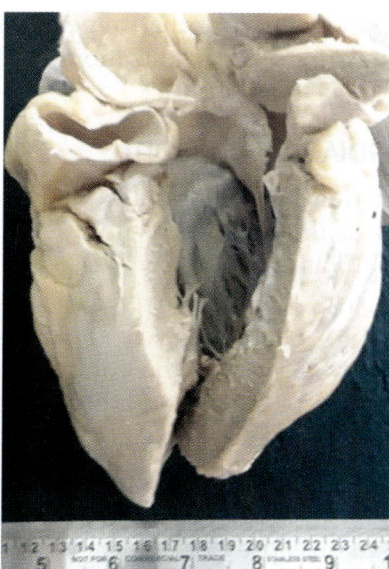

Fig. 26.4: Concentric hypertrophy of heart (gross picture) (*Courtesy:* HOD and staff of Pathology, SDM College, Dharwad)

thickness. The wall may show thickness of 2 cm or more (Fig. 26.4).

Volume overload as in AI or MR has hypertrophy and ventricular dilatation. This is called **eccentric hypertrophy.** The myocytes are hypertrophic, with prominent, irregular nuclear enlargement and hyperchromasia and interstitial fibrosis.

Cor pulmonale is associated with right-sided hypertrophy and dilatation due to pulmonary hypertension caused by lung parenchymal or vascular diseases. Cor pulmonale can be acute or chronic. Acute cor pulmonale occurs due to massive embolism and chronic cor pulmonale occurs because of pulmonary vascular pathology or compression or obliteration of capillary vessels resulting from emphysema, interstitial fibrosis or primary pulmonary hypertension.

VALVULAR HEART DISEASES

Valvular heart diseases cause stenosis or insufficiency or both. With stenosis, there is obstruction to the forward flow. Insufficiency results from failure of valve to close completely and results in backflow. Valve diseases can be congenital or caused due to variety of acquired causes. They can be categorised as below:

1. Rheumatic heart disease
2. Non-rheumatic heart disease
   a. Infective endocarditis
   b. Non-infected vegetations
      • Non-bacterial thrombotic endocarditis
      • Libman-Sacks endocarditis
   c. Calcific aortic stenosis
   d. Myxomatous mitral valves
   e. Carcinoid heart disease
   f. Prosthetic cardiac valves
   g. Congenital
      • Bicuspid valve
      • Unicuspid valve
      • Quadricuspid valve
   h. Others
      • Metabolic (Fabry's disease)
      • Systemic lupus erythematosus
      • Ochronosis with alkaptonuria
      • Homozygous hyperlipidaemia

CALCIFIC AORTIC STENOSIS

As aging process, the cardiac valves undergo degenerative changes due to mechanical stress. Calcific aortic stenosis is the most common degenerative valve disease. It can occur in normal valves or congenital bicuspid valves.

Following are the features of aortic cusps in calcific aortic stenosis:

1. The cusps are unequal.
2. The larger cusp has raphe.
3. Calcification usually involves the valve annulus.
4. Asymptomatic until encroaches on conducting system.

Morphology

1. Heaped calcified masses on the outflow side of the cusps, these protrude into sinuses of Valsalva and impede in valve opening.
2. No commissural fusion.
3. Cusps may fibrosed or thickened.
4. Because of outflow obstruction, there is left ventricular concentric hypertrophy.

Clinical Features

1. Patient can have angina due to left ventricular hypertrophy.
2. Syncope occurs because of hypoperfusion to brain.
3. Systolic and diastolic dysfunction causes eventually cardiac decompensation.

MYXOMATOUS MITRAL VALVE

This degeneration leads to floppy or prolapse of valves during systole. This is common in females than males. Mitral valve prolapse (MVP) is the common form in myxomatous degeneration.

Morphology

1. Affected leaflets are enlarged, redundant, thick and rubbery.
2. Chordae tendineae also elongated, thinned or ruptured.

3. Along mitral valve prolapse, tricuspid valve involvement is common.

MVP is due to abnormalities of structural proteins with disease like:

a. Marfan syndrome
b. Ehlers-Danlos disease
c. Osteogenesis imperfecta
d. Pseudomyxoma elasticum

Leaflets have spongy texture and hooding during systole, producing mid-systolic click. These patients are prone for infective endocarditis and sudden death by cardiac arrhythmias.

Clinical Features

Patients with MVP are asymptomatic and incidentally detected on examination. Minority may have palpitation, dyspnoea and chest pain and on auscultation have mid-systolic click.

PROSTHETIC CARDIAC VALVES

Two types are currently used:
1. Mechanical valve
2. Bioprosthetic valve

Mechanical heart valve substitutes are durable but the patients have to be on anticoagulant therapy. These patients are prone for hazards of thromboembolism and bleeding. Mechanical heart valves induce red cell haemolysis.

Bioprosthetic valves are relatively non-thrombotic but susceptible to structural deterioration and also vary with function of valve and patient characteristics like age at implant, pressure effects and calcium levels.

Bioprosthetic valves are glutaraldehyde fixed, prepared from porcine or bovine tissue or from homograft (allograft) from cadaveric sources.

Prosthetic valves are subject to infection. Infective endocarditis involves perivascular tissue and may cause detachment as it involves suture line and perivalvular tissue. The valve and surrounding tissue may become infected. All patients with prosthetic valve with procedures including dental procedures should receive antibiotic prophylaxis.

INFECTIVE ENDOCARDITIS

Infective endocarditis (IE) is a serious infection characterised by colonisation or invasion of the heart valves or the mural endocardium by microbes often with destruction of underlying cardiac tissues. There is formation of bulky, friable vegetations composed of necrotic debris, thrombus and organisms.

Causes

- **Bacterial infections (bacterial endocarditis):** Alpha haemolytic streptococci (*Strptococcus viridans*) is the causative organism—affects 50–60% of the cases usually in damaged or abnormal valves.
  Staphylococcus aureus: 10–20% in normal or deformed valves, common in IV drug abusers.
  Coagulase-negative staphylococci (*S. epidermidis*)
- **Other microorganisms:**
  - Enterococci
  - Fungi
  - Rickettsiae
  - Chlamydiae

IE has been classified on clinical grounds into:
- Acute, and
- Subacute forms.

Acute infective endocarditis is typically caused by infection of a previously normal heart valve by a highly virulent organism (e.g. *Staphylococcus aureus*) that produces necrotizing, ulcerative and destructive lesions. These infections are difficult to cure with antibiotics and usually require surgery. Death occurs within days to weeks in many patients with acute IE, despite of treatment.

Subacute IE, the organisms are of lower virulence (e.g. *Streptococcus viridans*). These organisms cause insidious infection of deformed valves that are less destructive. In such cases, the disease may pursue a protracted course of weeks to months, and cure is expected with antibiotics.

Etiopathogenesis

Prior to endocarditis, the organisms proliferate. The entry of organisms into the bloodstream may be infection elsewhere like:
- Dental or surgical procedure which can cause transient bacteraemia.
- Injection of contaminated material by IV drug abusers.
- Occult source of infection from GIT—oral cavity/intestine, or
- Trivial injuries.

IE is common in:
- Rheumatic heart disease
- Others:
  - Mitral valve prolapse
  - Degenerative calcific valvular stenosis
  - Bicuspid aortic valve (whether calcified or not)
  - Artificial (prosthetic) valves, and
  - Unrepaired and repaired congenital defects.

Clinical Features (Fig. 26.5)

1. **Fever, chills and weakness:** Fever is the most common presentation; however, in subacute cases, fever may be absent and may have only non-specific features like fatigue, loss of weight and flu-like symptoms. Splenomegaly is common in subacute IE. Acute IE can have rapidly developing features like fever, chills, weakness and lassitude.
2. Murmers are present in 90% of the patients with left-sided lesions.
3. Petechiae, subungual haemorrhage and conjunctival haemorrhage.
4. Janeway lesions on palms and soles, these are often hemorrhagic and non-tender.
5. Osler's nodes are red purple, raised tender lesions found on fingers and toes.
6. Roth's spots in eye are white-centred retinal haemorrhages.

These hemorrhagic lesions (petechiae, subungual lesions, Janeway lesions, Osler's nodes, Roth's spots) are possibly due to immune complex mediated vasculitis or due to septic emboli.

Diagnosis is made on:

- Positive blood cultures
- ECG findings
- Clinical history
- Laboratory findings

Diagnostic Criteria for Infective Endocarditis

Pathologic Criteria

- Microorganisms demonstrated by culture or on histologic examination in a vegetation, embolus from a vegetation or intracardiac abscess.

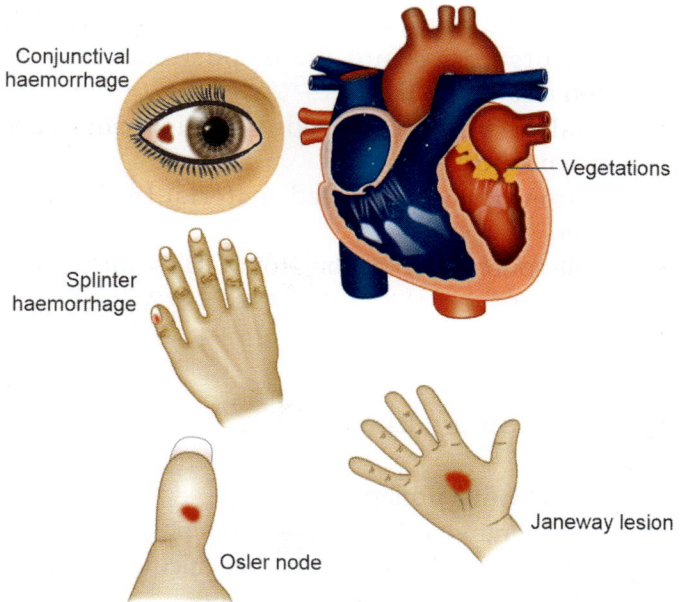

Fig. 26.5: Lesions in bacterial endocarditis (schematic)

- Histologic confirmation of active endocarditis in vegetation or intracardiac abscess.

Clinical Criteria

Major

1. Blood culture(s) positive for a characteristic organism or persistently positive for an unusual organism.
2. Echocardiographic identification of a valve-related or implant-related mass or abscess, or partial separation of artificial valve.
3. New valvular regurgitation.

Minor

1. Predisposing heart lesion or intravenous drug use
2. Fever
3. Vascular lesions including arterial petechiae, subungual/splinter haemorrhages, emboli, septic infarcts, mycotic aneurysm, intracranial haemorrhage, Janeway lesions.
4. Immunological phenomena, including glomerulonephritis, Osler nodes, Roth spots, rheumatoid factor.
5. Microbiologic evidence including a single culture positive for an unusual organism.
6. Echocardiographic findings consistent with but not diagnostic of endocarditis, including worsening or changing of a pre-existent murmur.

Gross (Fig. 26.5)

The hallmark of IE is the presence of:

- Friable, bulky, potentially destructive vegetations containing fibrin, inflammatory cells, and bacteria or other organisms.
- The vegetations may be single or multiple and may involve more than one valve.
- The aortic and mitral valves are the most common sites of infection, although the valves of the right heart may also be involved, particularly in intravenous drug abusers.
- Vegetations sometimes erode into the underlying myocardium and produce an abscess (ring abscess).
- Emboli may be shed from the vegetations at any time; because the embolic fragments may contain large numbers of virulent organisms, abscesses often develop at the sites where the emboli lodge, leading to sequelae such as septic infarcts or mycotic aneurysms.
- The vegetations of subacute endocarditis are associated with less valvular destruction than those of acute endocarditis.

Microscopy (Fig. 26.6)

- The vegetation has platelets, fibrin, and organisms.
- The underlying valve is inflamed, vascularised and shows plenty of polymorphs along with macrophages, giant cells and areas of necrosis.
- The vegetations of typical subacute IE often have granulation tissue indicative of healing at their base. With time, fibrosis, calcification, and a chronic inflammatory infiltrate can develop.

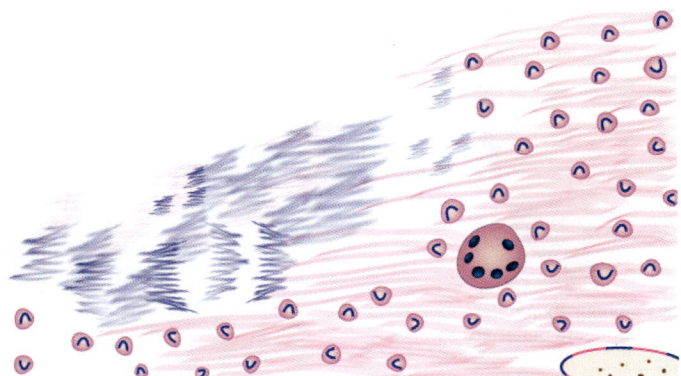

Fig. 26.6: Microscopy of vegetation in bacterial endocarditis (schematic)

Complications

1. **Cardiac complications:**
   - Valvular insufficiency/stenosis/cardia failure
   - Myocardial ring abscess
   - Perforation of aorta, interventricular septum, etc.
   - Suppurative pericarditis
   - Myocardial infarction
2. **Embolic complications**
   - *Left-sided lesions:* Brain abscess, meningitis, spleen and kindey—abscess, cerebral infarcts.
   - *Right-sided lesions:* Lung abscess, pneumonia.
3. **Renal complications:**
   - Embolic infarct
   - Focal/glomerulonephritis
   - Diffuse or multiple abscesses
4. Osteomyelitis
5. Mycotic aneurysms

RHEUMATIC FEVER AND RHEUMATIC HEART DISEASE

Rheumatic fever (RF) is an acute, immunologically mediated, multisystem inflammatory disease that occurs a few weeks after an episode of group A streptococcal pharyngitis. Acute rheumatic carditis is a frequent manifestation during the active phase of RF.

Epidemiology

This is a disease of poverty. Crowded housing, unhygienic conditions result in spread of streptococcal infection. The disease is less common in industrialized countries. Improved living condition and better hygiene and antibiotics have reduced the incidence of rheumatic heart disease (RHD) in developed and developing nations.

Incidence

Children between age 5 and 15 years are commonly affected. Recurrent episodes of acute RF are known in adolescents and adults.

Pathogenesis

- Acute rheumatic fever results from immune responses to group A streptococci, which happen to cross-react with host tissues.
- Antibodies directed against the M proteins of streptococci have been shown to cross-react with self-antigens in the heart.
- Antibodies and CD4+ T cells specific for streptococcal peptides react with self-proteins in the heart. The antibodies can activate complement and Fc receptor bearing cells and CD4 T cells produce cytokines that activate macrophages (such as those found in Aschoff bodies).
- Damage to heart tissue may thus be caused by a combination of antibody- and T cell-mediated reactions.
- Genetic susceptibility.

Evidence for preceeding group A streptococci:

1. The serological evidence with raised or rising anti-streptolysin O (ASLO) titres, hyaluronidase or anti-DNase titres
2. Positive throat swab
3. Rapid antigen test for Group A Streptococcus
4. Recent scarlet fever

Pathology of Heart in RHD (Figs 26.7 to 26.9)

The connective tissue or collagen tissue of heart is primarily affected. The heart changes can be divided into:

- **Acute rheumatic heart disease:**
  - Early exudative phase
  - Proliferative phase or granulomatous phase
  - Late phase
- **Chronic rheumatic heart disease**

In Acute Rheumatic Heart Disease

Early acute/exudative phase: This phase persists up to 4 weeks.

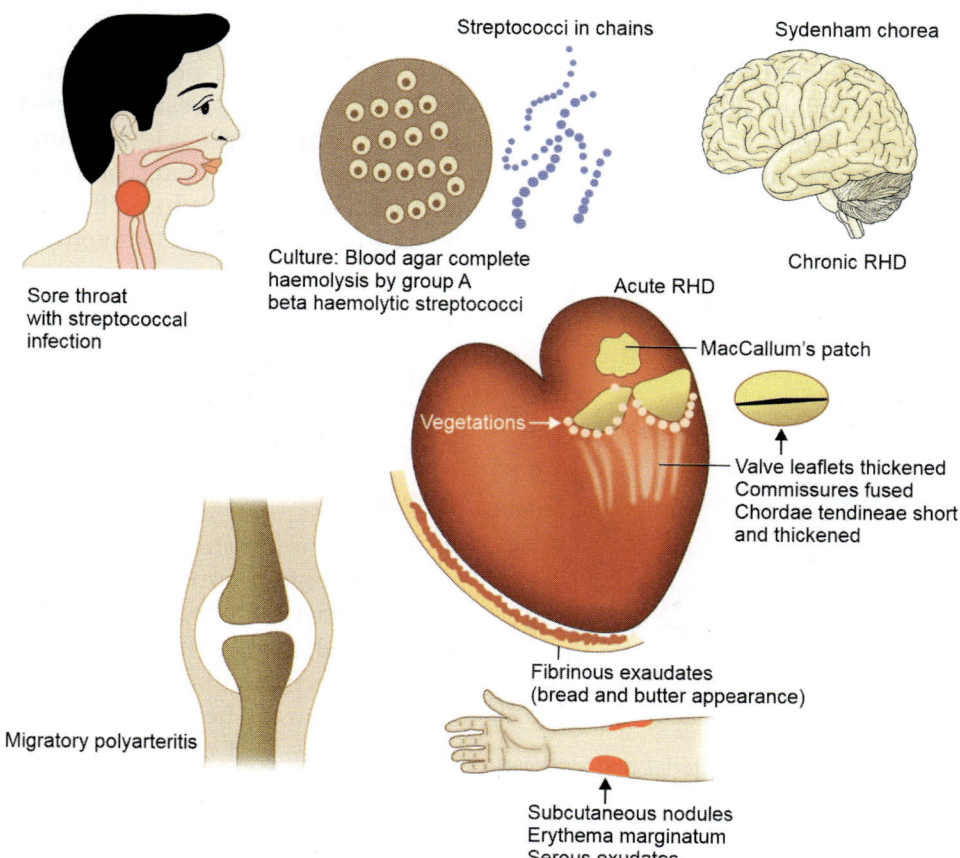

Fig. 26.7: Pathology in rheumatic heart disease (schematic)

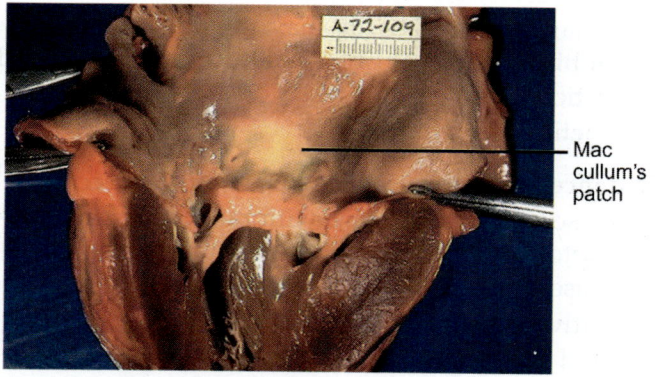

Fig. 26.8: RHD, note MacCallum's patch, thickened mitral valve, chordae tendineae and hypertrophied left ventricular wall (Gross picture) (*From* Public Heart Image Library (PHIL) ID 847)

Early exudative lesion has following features:
- Oedema
- ↑ mucopolysaccharides
- Ground substance and collagen
  - Altered
- Fibrinoid necrosis

Proliferative phase: In acute RF, the pathognomonic lesions are Aschoff bodies (Ascoff nodules). The intial lesions show perivascular focus of fibrinoid degeneration of collagen surrounded by lymphocytes, plasma cells and macrophages.

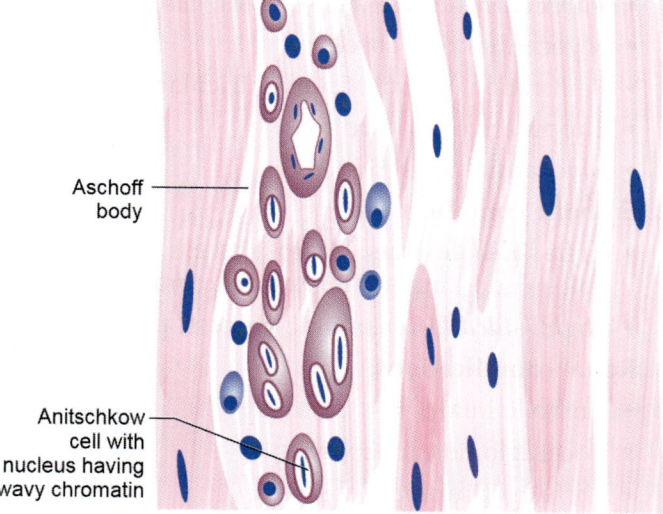

Fig. 26.9: Microscopy in RHD (schematic)

With time, the classical granulomatous lesion, the Ascoff bodies or Ascoff nodules develop. **Ascoff bodies have central area of fibrinoid necrosis, surrounded by T lymphocytes, macrophages, occasional plasma cells, plump histiocytes, i.e. Anitschkow cells.** Some altered histiocytes are multinucleated are present and these are called **Aschoff giant cells.** These **Anitschkow cells** have amphophilic cytoplasm, round to oval nuclei, chromatin is disposed in a central slender wavy ribbon giving the appearance of caterpillar. On cross-section, this appears as owl eye appearance.

Late phase: With time, the Aschoff bodies are replaced by scar tissue and merges with chronic phase (chronic rheumatic heart disease).

These lesions are found in perivascular location and are present in all three layers of the heart, causing pericarditis, myocarditis, or endocarditis (pancarditis). Inflammation of the endocardium and the left-sided valves typically results in fibrinoid necrosis within the cusps or along the chordrae tendineae.

The gross findings of heart in RHD are the following:

- *Acute rheumatic heart disease:*
  1. The heart shows pancarditis.
  2. Pericardium: Shows fibrinous pericarditis (bread and butter appearance)
  3. Myocardium: There is myocarditis.
  4. Endocardium: Shows verrucae and MacCallum's patch.
  - *Verrucae*: These develop on the valves. These are small (1- to 2-mm) vegetations, present on the focus of fibrinoid necrosis and are present along the line of closure.

    In RHD, the mitral valve is affected alone in 65 to 70% of cases, and along with the aortic valve in another 25% of cases.
  - *MacCallum's patch*: Subendocardial lesions, perhaps exacerbated by regurgitant jets, may induce irregular thickening called **MacCallum plaque,** usually in the left atrium.
- *Chronic rheumatic heart disease:*
  - Leaflet thickening
  - Commissural fusion
  - Shortening, thickening and fusion of chordae tendineae

- The thickening and commissural fusion of the valves gives rise to stenosis (fish mouth appearance) and incompetency (regurgitation) of the valves.

Clinical Features and Diagnosis

Guidelines for Diagnosis (Jones Criteria)

Major criteria
1. Migratory polyarthritis of the large joints
2. Pancarditis
3. Subcutaneous nodules
4. Erythema marginatum of the skin
5. Sydenham chorea

Minor criteria
1. Fever
2. Arthralgia
3. Elevated blood levels of acute phase reactants (e.g. CRP, ASLO, etc.) or elevated ESR or WBC count
4. ECG findings: Prolonged PR interval
   Note:
   1. ASLO titre: High titres are supportive but not diagnostic. Titres more than 400 Todd units in adults and more than 300 Todd units in children above 5 years of age is supportive evidence.
   2. Anti-streptozyme test: Sensitive in recent RHD.

The diagnosis is established by evidence of a preceding group A streptococcal infection, with the presence of:
a. Two of the major criteria, or
b. One major and two minor manifestations.

OTHER CAUSES OF VEGETATIONS

Vegetations are found in bacterial endocarditis and rheumatic heart disease. Apart from these, the other causes are (Fig. 26.10):

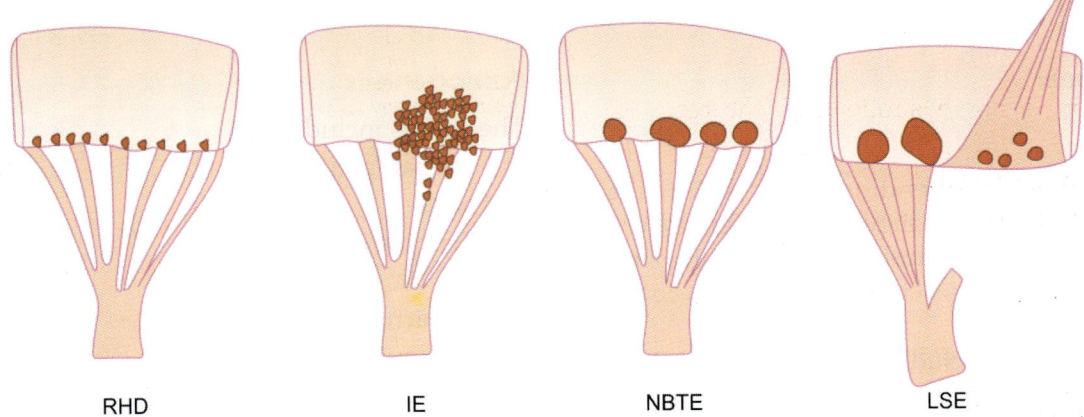

RHD   IE   NBTE   LSE

Fig. 26.10: Verrucae—differential diagnosis (RHD: Rheumatic heart disease, IE: Infective endocarditis, NBTE: Non-bacterial thrombotic endocarditis, LSE: Libman-Sacks endocarditis)

1. Non-bacterial thrombotic endocarditis (NBTE, Marantic): NBTE occurs in hypercoagulable states, like in sepsis with DIC, hyperestrogenic states, underlying malignancy; particularly mucinous carcinoma. NBTE is a part of Trousseau syndrome. Endocardial trauma due to indwelling catheter is also predisposing factor. These vegetations have following features.

1. Small, sterile masses of fibrin and other blood elements—on valve leaflets which are previously normal
2. No organisms
3. Non-destructive
4. Small (1–5 mm)
5. Single/multiple
6. No inflammation
7. Thrombus with embolisation leading to stroke
8. No valve damage
9. No new murmur

2. Libman-Sacks endocarditis: Vegetations **in Libman-Sacks endocarditis** develop on the valves in systemic lupus erythematosus. These occur presumably because of immune complex deposition and thus associated with inflammation. These vegetations have following features.

- Small (1–4 mm) and sterile
- Single/multiple
- Vegetations are on valvular endocardium including under surface and on chordae tendineae.
- There is valvulitis, fibrosis and deformity.

MYOCARDITIS

In myocarditis, there is injury to the myocardium.

Pathogenesis

The causative agents include:

- *Common:* Viral infections: Coxsackie virus A and B.

- *Less common:*
  1. CMV
  2. HIV

Many a times, the offending agent is difficult to isolate. The viruses cause direct cytolytic injury, cross-reactive antibodies or T lymphocytes. Most often injury is caused by immune reaction against virus-infected myocytes.

Non-viral myositis includes *T. cruzi* in Chagas disease. The disease occurs in endemic areas of South America.

Toxoplasma gondii also causes myocarditis especially in immunocompromised hosts.

Trichinosis is a helminthic disease associated with cardiac involvement.

Borrelia burgdorferi causes Lyme disease and myocarditis occurs in 5% of these patients.

Non-infective causes of immune origin like SLE, polymyositis and drug hypersensitivity are common causes.

Clinical Features

Clinical features may mimic MI. Arrhythmias with sudden death is known with these patients.

Fatigue, dyspnoea, palpitation, pain and fever are common clinical features.

CARDIOMYOPATHIES

Cardiomyopathies (CMPs) are cardiac diseases primarily due to intrinsic myocardial dysfunction (according to 1995 WHO/ ISFC–International Society of Federation of Cardiology). In 1980, WHO defined cardiomyopathies as diseases of unknown cause to distinguish cardiomyopathy from cardiac dysfunction due to hypertension, ischaemic heart diseases and valvular heart diseases.

American Heart Society (2006) classifies cardiomyopathies as:
1. Primary
2. Secondary

On clinical and functional basis, cardiomyopathies can be classified as:
1. Dilated cardiomyopathy
2. Hypertrophic cardiomyopathy
3. Restrictive cardiomyopathy

Among these three types, dilated cardiomyopathy is most common and restrictive is least common.

DILATED CARDIOMYOPATHY

Dilated cardiomyopathy (DCM), has progressive cardiac dilatation and contractile dysfunction.

Pathogenesis

The causes include:
1. Familial/genetic
2. Toxins
3. Thiamine deficiency
4. Viral
5. Peripartum
6. Unknown

Viruses: Coxsackie virus B and other enteroviruses are blamed for causing myocarditis and with end result of DCM.

Toxins and thiamine deficiency: Alcohol and its metabolites (especially aldehyde) have direct toxic effect on heart. Chronic alcoholism can be associated with thiamine deficiency too. Other toxins include: Chemotherapeutic agents (cobalt and adriamycin).

Familial/genetic causes: Mutation of dystrophin gene, alpha cardiac actin, desmin and nuclear lamins A and C. Mitochondrial gene deletions, and mutations in genes encoding enzymes involved in fatty acid beta-oxidation can be also responsible for causation of DCM.

Peripartum period: It occurs during late gestation or several weeks or months after delivery. Cause could be pregnancy-induced hypertension, volume overload, nutritional deficiency, metabolic derangement, etc.

Pathology

Gross: Following are the features:
1. Heart is enlarged 2 to 3 times of the normal size
2. Flabby
3. Dilatation of all the four chambers
4. Mural thrombi are common.
5. No valve pathology
6. Coronaries: No atherosclerosis

Microscopy: Following changes may be encountered:
1. Non-specific changes.
2. Myocardial fibres hypertrophied with enlarged nuclei.
3. Some myocardial fibres attenuated, stretched or irregular and may show empty spaces.
4. There is presence of focal myocyte necrosis.
5. There is variable interstitial or endocardial fibrosis, Scar formation may be present.

Clinical Features

- DCM can occur at any age. Most commonly occurs between the age of 20 and 50 years.
- It presents with slowly progressive chronic heart failure with shortness of breath, orthopnoea, dyspnoea on exertion, fatigue and dry mouth.
- There is ineffective contraction and cardiac ejection fraction is less than 25%.
- Mitral incompetence and abnormal cardiac rhythms are most common.
- Mural thrombi are frequent.
- Death is due to progressive cardiac failure or arrhythmias.
- About 50% of the patients die within 2 years and another 25% die within 5 years.

HYPERTROPHIC CARDIOMYOPATHY

Hypertrophic cardiomyopathy is also called by other synonyms like idiopathic hypertrophic subaortic stenosis.

This is characterised by myocardial hypertrophy, abnormal diastolic filling and in some cases with ventricular outflow obstruction. Heart is thick walled. It is hypercontracting and is stiff and non-compliant. Systolic function is preserved, but does not relax in diastole, thus the diastolic filling defect.

Pathogenesis

Missense point mutations of sarcomeric proteins, most commonly beta-myosin heavy chains, myocin binding protein C and troponin T are commonly affected. It has AD inheritance pattern.

There is a proposal that myocyte contraction triggers growth factor release with intense hypertrophy causing myocyte disarray and fibroblast proliferation causing interstitial fibrosis.

Pathology

Gross: Following are the features.
1. Massive myocardial hypertrophy without ventricular dilatation.
2. Disproportionate thickening of the septum relative to left ventricular free wall (asymmetrical septal hypertrophy).
3. In longitudinal section of heart, left ventricular cavity appears banana shaped.
4. There is formation of endocardial plaque in the outflow tract of left ventricle.
5. The anterior mitral leaflet is thickened.

Microscopy: Shows following features:
1. Severe myocyte hypertrophy
2. Myofibre disarray: The myocardial fibre are arranged criss-cross
3. Interstitial fibrosis

Clinical Features

- There is breathlessness on exertion, dizziness, fainting and precordial pain.
- There is massive hypertrophy of left ventricle with reduced stroke volume.
- The left ventricular chamber size is small and hence impaired diastolic filling.
- About one-fourth of the patients have outflow tract obstruction. There is systolic motion of anterior leaflet of mitral valve towards the interventricular septum. This raises the pressure in left atrium.

- In these patients, there is reduced cardiac output and increase in pulmonary venous pressure which causes exertional dyspnoea and systolic ejection murmur.
- There is frequent myocardial ischaemia, atrial fibrillation, arrhythmias, mural thrombus formation, infective endocarditis and sudden death may occur.

RESTRICTIVE CARDIOMYOPATHY

This is characterized by decrease in ventricular compliance, with impaired diastolic filling. The systolic function is normal.

Restrictive cardiomyopathy can be due to following causes:
1. Idiopathic
2. Radiation
3. Amyloidosis
4. Hemochromatosis
5. Sarcoidosis
6. In patients with inborn errors of metabolism.

Gross: The following are the features.
- The ventricles are normal in size or slightly enlarged.
- Myocardium is firm.
- Biatrial dilatation is commonly observed.

Microscopy: Shows following features.
- *Interstitial fibrosis:* Focal or diffuse, minimal or extensive.
- Endomyocardial biopsy may show amyloidosis, hemochromatosis or sarcoidosis

The important types of restrictive cardiomyopathy are:
1. *Endomyocardial fibrosis:* This is a type of restrictive cardiomyopathy occurs in children and young adults in tropical countries. There is ventricular endocardial fibrosis extending from apex to the mitral and tricuspid valves. The fibrosis restricts the volume and compliance of the affected chambers.
2. *Loeffler endomyocarditis:* This causes restrictive cardiomyopathy with endocardial fibrosis. There is associated eosinophilia, the contents of the granules, especially the major basic protein initiates endocardial damage with necrosis followed by fibrosis.

PERICARDITIS

The most common causes of pericarditis include:
1. Infections: Viral, bacterial, fungi
2. Myocardial infarction
3. Cardiac surgery
4. Irradiation to the mediastinum
5. Uremia

Less common causes include:
1. Rheumatic heart disease
2. Systemic lupus erythematosus

Pericarditis can cause:
1. Haemodymic complications
2. May resolve without leaving any sequelae
3. May progress to chronic process.

Morphological Types with Causes

1. **Fibrinous pericarditis (shaggy or bread and butter appearance):** Rheumatic heart disease, uraemia and viral infections
2. **Fibrinopurulent pericarditis:** Pyogenic bacteria
3. **Pericarditis with caseation necrosis:** Tuberculosis
4. **Fibrinous with bloody effusion:** Malignancy

With suppuration or caseation, fibrosis occurs resulting in chronic pericarditis. The fibrotic scars obliterates the pericardial sac. In severe cases, pericardial cavity may have dense fibrosis, and heart may not expand during diastole, this is termed as constrictive pericarditis.

Clinical Features

Pericarditis classically presents with chest pain, and a friction rub. When significant amount of fluid collects causes cardiac temponade.

PERICARDIAL EFFUSION

Normally about **30–50 ml** of thin clear, straw-coloured-fluid is present in the pericardial cavity.

The common causes of pericardial effusion include:
- **Serous:** CHF, hypoalbuminaemia.
- **Serosanguinous:** Blunt chest trauma, malignancy, ruptured MI, or aortic stenosis.
- **Chylous effusion:** Lymphatic obstruction.

In slowly collecting (chronic) effusions with fluid of 100 ml may remain asymptomatic.

In rapidly (acute) developing causes such as ruptured MI, ruptured aortic dissection, effusion of even 250 ml is dangerous. This can restrict diastolic filling with cardiac temponade.

SELF-ASSESSMENT EXERCISE

1. **Which of the following is an immediate consequence of myocardial infarction?**
   A. There is loss of contractibility
   B. Irreversible injury
   C. Coagulative necrosis
   D. All of the above

2. **Which of the following is the histological change seen after 24 hours?**
   A. Coagulative necrosis and neutrophilic infiltration
   B. Myofibre disintegration
   C. Deposition of collagen
   D. Granulation tissue

3. **Which of the following is the correct statement regarding bacterial endocarditis?**
   A. Commonly caused by *Staph. epidermidis* on damaged valves
   B. Commonly caused by *Staph. epidermidis* on healthy valves
   C. Commonly caused by *Staph. aureus* on damaged valves
   D. *Cryptococcus* affects damaged valves

4. **Which of the following is the correct statement?**
   A. Serous pericarditis is a consequence of uraemia
   B. Constrictive pericarditis rarely complicates suppurative pericarditis
   C. Haemorrhagic pericarditis is due to *Klebsiella* organisms
   D. Fibrinous pericarditis is due to anaemia

5. **Which of the following statements regarding myocardial infarction is wrong?**
   A. ATP depletion begins immediately
   B. Irreversible injury occurs after 20 minutes
   C. Loss of contractility occurs in less than 2 minutes
   D. Neutrophils appear after 48 hours

6. **Which of the following is not a feature of Fallot's tetralogy?**
   A. ASD
   B. VSD
   C. Overriding of VSD
   D. Subpulmonary stenosis

7. **Following lead to left ventricular hypertrophy** *except*:
   A. AS   B. MS
   C. Coarctation of aorta   D. HT

8. **Right ventricular failure causes following** *except*:
   A. Splenomegaly   B. Ankle oedema
   C. CVC liver   D. Pulmonary oedema

9. **Cor pulmonale can be caused by all the following** *except*:
   A. Interstitial lung disease
   B. Pulmonary emboli
   C. Emphysema
   D. AS

10. **Findings of left-sided failure are all** *except*:
    A. Dyspnoea   B. Orthopnoea
    C. Ascites   D. Hepatomegaly

Answers

1. A	**2.** A	**3.** A	**4.** A	**5.** D	**6.** A	**7.** B	**8.** D
9. D	**10.** D						

Gastrointestinal Pathology: Salivary Gland Lesions

NORMAL SALIVARY GLAND

There are three pairs of major salivary glands (parotid, submandibular, and sublingual) and about 500 to 1000 lobules of minor glands dispersed in the submucosa of the oral cavity.

The normal parotid gland in adults weighs 15 to 30 g. The superficial and deep lobes are separated by the facial nerve. The submandibular and sublingual glands weigh approximately 7 to 15 g and 2 to 4 g, respectively.

The parotid gland is exclusively serous, the submandibular gland mixed seromucinous, and the sublingual gland predominantly mucous; the minor glands are seromucinous or mucous depending on location. Salivary glands are exocrine glands having acini and ducts. The acini are the secretory units. The secretion reaches the oral cavity via the conducting unit, consisting of intercalated, striated, interlobular and excretory ducts.

INFLAMMATORY LESIONS

XEROSTOMIA

Xerostomia is defined as dry mouth due to decreased production of saliva.

The causes are:
1. Major cause is autoimmune disease (Sjögren's syndrome accompanied by dry eyes).
2. Radiation therapy
3. Drugs: Anticholinergic drugs, antidepressants, antipsychotic drugs, diuretics, antihypertensives, muscle relaxants, etc.

These patients have dry mucosa, atrophy of papillae of tongue with fissuring and ulceration. Patients with Sjögren's syndrome have enlarged salivary glands.

These patients have difficulty in swallowing and speaking. They are prone for candidiasis and dental caries.

SJÖGREN SYNDROME

Sjögren's syndrome is of autoimmune origin and is associated with **xerostomia, keratoconjunctivitis sicca and sialadenitis.** There is enlargement of lacrimal and salivary glands due to inflammation. These are painless. Dryness of mouth (xerostomia), and dryness of eyes are present due to less or no secretion of saliva and tears. This is referred to as **Mikulicz syndrome.**

Pathology

Parotid gland and sometimes submandibular salivary glands are unilaterally or bilaterally affected. There is periductal inflammation, extends to acini and inflammatory cells replace them with destruction of acini and ducts. The inflammatory cells are predominantly lymphocytes, with germinal centres, immunoblasts and plasma cells.

MUCOCELE

Mucocele results from blockage or rupture of salivary gland duct with leakage of saliva into the surrounding stroma. These are commonly found in the lower lip and are mainly due to trauma. These are common in all ages.

Clinically, mucoceles have bluish hue, fluctuant swelling and microscopy shows cystic lesion, lined by inflamed granulation tissue or fibrous connective tissue. The lesions are filled with mucin material and inflammatory cells. Excision is the treatment; however incomplete excision has chances of recurrence.

Ranula is an epithelium-lined cyst when the duct of the submandibular gland is damaged or blocked. It may become large with plunging ranula.

SIALOLITHIASIS

Non-specific sialadenitis involving major salivary glands, more so submandibular salivary gland is common due to obstruction by sialolithiasis. The affending organisms are *Staphylococcus aureus* and *Streptococcus viridans*. Impacted food debris, decreased secretions and dehydration may lead to stone formation and inflammation.

SIALADENITIS

Inflammation of salivary glands may be **viral, bacterial, traumatic or autoimmune origin.**

Bacterial inflammation by *Staphylococcus aureus* and *Streptococcus viridans* causes acute sialadenitis possibly secondary to obstruction by stones (sialolithiasis) or strictures of salivary ducts. The stagnant secretions act as medium for bacterial overgrowth. It may occur due to retrograde entry of bacteria from oral cavity during severe dehydration such as postoperative state. Chronic debilitating illness, immunocompromised state or medications contributing to acute dehydration increases the risk of infection. The sialadenitis is mainly interstitial, may cause focal areas of suppurative necrosis or abscess formation.

Microscopy: In acute sialadenitis, paranchyma shows suppurative necrosis and abscess formation. There is neutrophilic infiltration in the interlobular and intralobular connective tissue (Fig. 27.1).

Chronic inflammation occurs due to reduced production of saliva with subsequent inflammation, the

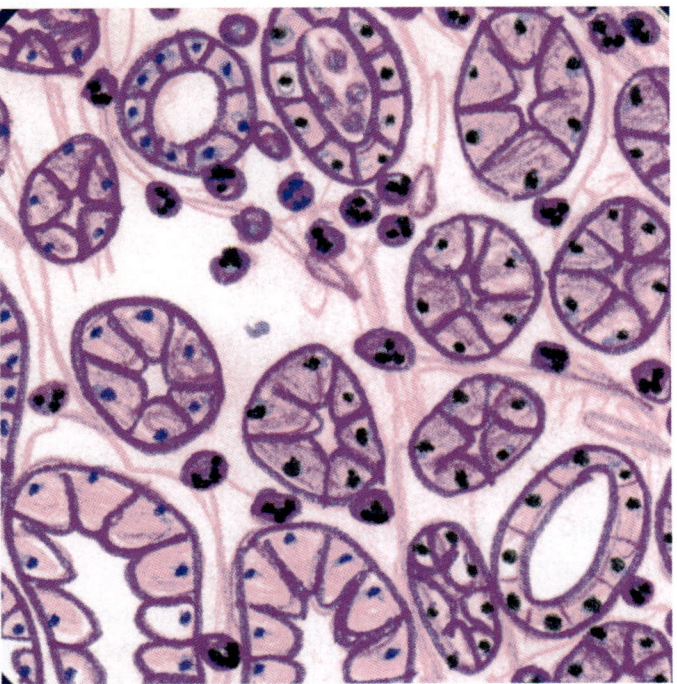

Fig. 27.1: Microscopy in acute sialadenitis (schematic)

common cause is autoimmune sialadenitis or of viral origin. This is almost always bilateral. All the major salivary glands and minor salivary glands are affected.

Mumps

This is caused by viral (paramyxovirus) infection, leads to acute enlargement of one or both salivary glands. It usually produces interstitial inflammation showing oedema and mononuclear cell infiltration, sometimes necrosis. Mumps in childhood is self-limited. In adults, it may be accompanied by pancreatitis and orchitis. The later is the cause of permanent sterility in these patients.

TUMOURS

The salivary glands give rise to a diversity of tumours. About 80% of tumours occur within the parotid gland and rest occur in other major and minor salivary glands. Males and females are affected about equally. They occur usually in the sixth or seventh decade of life. Salivary gland neoplasms are classified in Table 27.1.

PLEOMORPHIC ADENOMA (Mixed Tumour of Salivary Glands)

Because of the histologic diversity, these neoplasms have also been called *mixed tumours*. It is thought to originate from stem cells/reserve cells of ducts with epithelial or mesenchymal differentiation. There is neoplastic proliferation of glandular epithelial cells along with myoepithelial component. It accounts for 90% of the benign tumours of the salivary gland.

This tumour occurs at any age and has female predilection. The parotid gland is frequently affected. The other major and minor salivary glands also can be affected. It is slow growing, painless swelling at the angle of the jaw and readily palpable as discrete mass. Facial nerve needs to be taken care off while resecting the tumour. Recurrence is known and 2% of these tumours may undergo malignancy. A carcinoma arising in a pleomorphic adenoma is referred to as carcinoma **ex pleomorphic adenoma** or as **malignant mixed tumour.**

Gross: The tumour is capsulated, lobulated and usually measures about 5 to 6 cm in diameter. Cut section is grey white with variegated areas (Figs 27.2A and B).

Microscopy: The epithelial cells will be in the form of ducts and irregular tubules or acini. Some of these cells show squamous metaplasia. The myoepithelial cells would be arranged in sheets and show myxoid and chondroid areas. Rarely bone formation may be present (Fig. 27.3).

Table 27.1	Classification of salivary gland neoplasms[22]	
Benign epithelial tumours	**Malignant epithelial tumours**	**Soft tissue tumours**
Pleomorphic adenoma	Acinic cell carcinoma	Haemangioma
Myoepithelioma	Mucoepidermoid carcinoma	Haematolymphoid tumours
Basal cell adenoma	Adenoid cystic carcinoma	Extranodal marginal zone B cell lymphoma
Warthin tumour	Polymorphous adenocarcinoma	
Oncocytoma	Epithelial-myoepithelial carcinoma	
Canalicular adenoma	Clear cell carcinoma	
Sebaceous adenoma	Hyalinising clear cell carcinoma	
Lymphadenoma	Basal cell adenocarcinoma	
Ductal papillomas	Sebaceous carcinoma	
Sialadenoma papilliferum	Cribriform carcinoma	
Cystadenoma	Intraductal carcinoma	
Sclerosing polycystic adenosis	Cystadenocarcinoma	
Intercalated duct hyperplasia	Mucinous adenocarcinoma	
Lymphoepithelial lesion	Oncocytic carcinoma	
Nodular oncocytic hyperplasia	Salivary duct carcinoma	
	Adenocarcinoma, not otherwise specified	
	Myoepithelial carcinoma	
	Carcinoma ex pleomorphic adenoma	
	Carcinosarcoma	
	Squamous cell carcinoma	
	Small cell carcinoma	
	Large cell carcinoma	
	Lymphoepithelial carcinoma	
	Borderline tumour	
	Sialoblastoma	

Note: Simplified WHO 2017 classification of salivary gland tumours

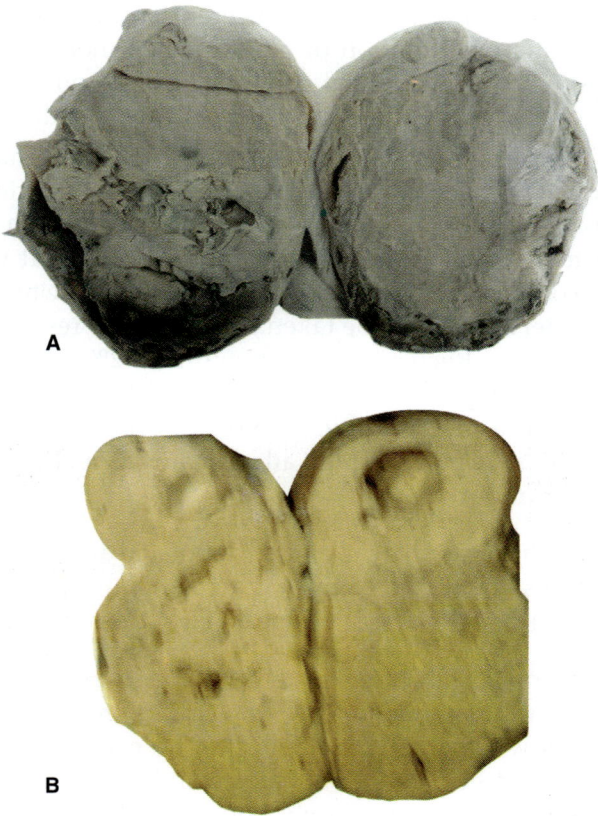

Figs 27.2A and B: Pleomorphic adenoma (gross pictures)

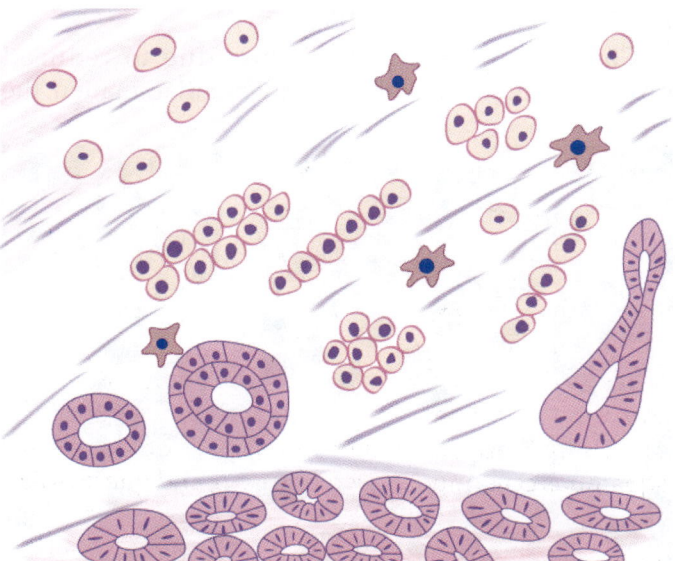

Fig. 27.3: Microscopy of pleomorphic adenoma (schematic)

WARTHIN TUMOUR (Papillary Cystadenoma Lymphomatosum/Adenolymphoma)

This is a benign neoplasm and second most common salivary gland neoplasm. It arises almost exclusively in the parotid gland (the only tumour virtually restricted to the parotid) and occurs more commonly

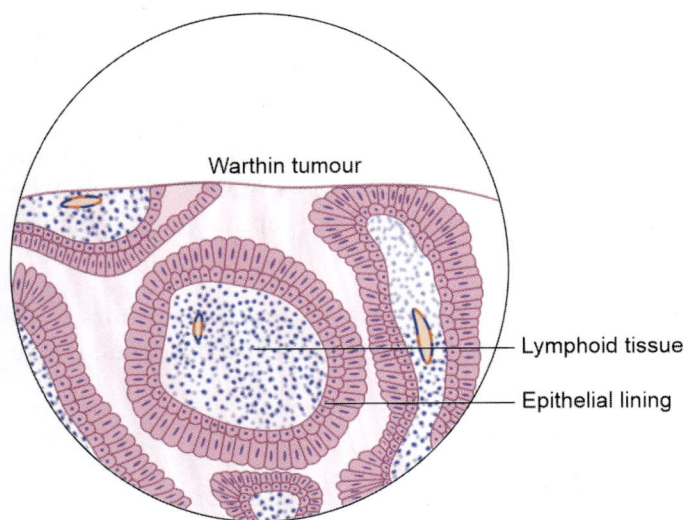

Fig. 27.4: Microscopy of Warthin tumour (schematic)

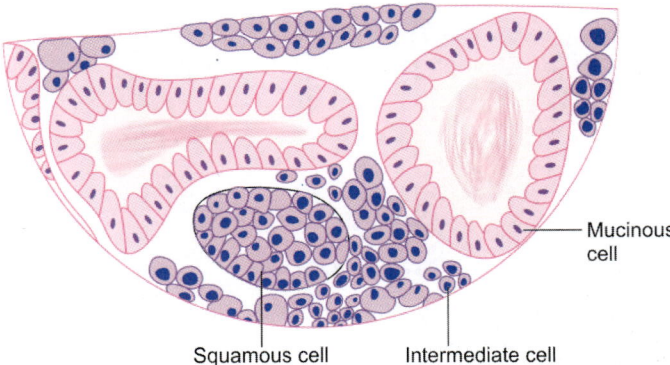

Fig. 27.5: Microscopy of mucoepidermoid carcinoma (schematic)

in males than in females, usually in the fifth to seventh decades of life. It is more common in smokers and is bilateral.

Gross: Warthin tumours are round to oval, encapsulated masses, 2 to 5 cm in diameter, usually arising in the superficial parotid gland, where they are readily palpable. Cut section reveals a pale grey surface punctuated by narrow cystic or cleft-like spaces filled with a mucinous or serous secretion.

Microscopy: There are papillary structures lined by a double layer of epithelial cells resting on a dense lymphoid stroma sometimes having germinal centres. The double layer of lining cells is distinctive; it consists of columnar cells having an abundant, finely granular, eosinophilic cytoplasm, that imparts an oncocytic appearance, which rests on a layer of cuboidal to polygonal cells. These cells form papillary structures projecting into cystic lumina (Fig. 27.4).

MUCOEPIDERMOID CARCINOMA

Mucoepidermoid carcinoma is common salivary gland tumour with potential for aggressive behaviour. These are composed of variable mixtures of neoplastic squamous cells, mucus-secreting cells, and intermediate cells. They represent about 15% of all salivary gland tumours, and they occur mainly (60 to 70%) in the parotid gland.

Gross: Mucoepidermoid carcinomas can grow as large as 8 cm in diameter and although they are apparently circumscribed or sometimes have infiltrative margins. Pale and grey-white on cut section, they frequently contain small, mucin-containing cysts.

Microscopy (Fig. 27.5): The basic histologic pattern is that of cords, sheets, or cystic configurations of squa-

mous, mucous, or intermediate cells. Mucoepidermoid carcinomas are subclassified into low, intermediate, or high grade. The low grade tumours are usually well circumscribed. The mucinous cells predominate and these cells are arranged in glandular pattern. The cells have clear cytoplasm. These are admixed with epidermoid cells which are squamous-like but lack keratinisation and intercellular bridges. The third types of cells seen are intermediate cells which are smaller than epidermoid cells.

High grade tumours are solid and have infiltrative nature. Marked atypia and frequent mitoses are not the features and when such features are present poorly differentiated adenocarcinoma or adenosquamous carcinoma is to be considered.

Prognosis: Histological grade and tumour stage affect prognosis. Higher the histological grade and stage of the tumour, perineural invasion and invasion of surgical margins have worse prognosis.

ADENOID CYSTIC CARCINOMA

These are common in minor salivary glands and are known for recurrence. Grossly, these are solid with infiltrative margins. Microscopy has typical cribriform (sieve-like) or honeycomb pattern. The nests and columns of neoplastic cells are arranged around a space (pseudocyst) and true glands which are filled with PAS positive material. Perineural spread is characteristic (Fig. 27.6).

Prognosis: This tumour has indolent growth, with recurrence and may have delayed metastasis to lungs, liver and bone.

ACINIC CELL CARCINOMA

These are relatively uncommon, representing only 2 to 3% of salivary gland tumours. Most of these tumours arise in the parotid gland; these have male preponderance and peak in 3rd decade of life.

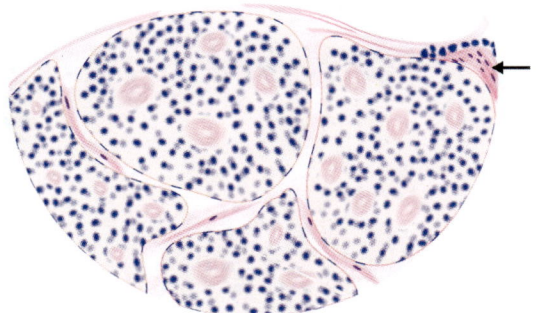

Fig. 27.6: Microscopy of adenoid cystic carcinoma. Note perineural invasion (arrow) (schematic)

Gross: Encapsulated, solid, friable, grey-white and usually are less than 3 cm. Occasionally, they present with marked cystic degeneration.

Microscopy: Shows cells with abundant cytoplasm filled with basophilic zymogen granules. They may be arranged in solid, microcystic, papillary and follicular patterns.

Prognosis: These are less aggressive tumours with good prognosis. Recurrences and metastasis are known.

SELF-ASSESSMENT EXERCISE

1. **Salivary gland stones are more common in:**
   A. Submandibular salivary gland
   B. Parotid gland
   C. Sublingual
   D. Minor salivary glands

2. **In parotid mass excision, important care has to be taken is:**
   A. Facial nerve
   B. Evaluation of lymph nodes
   C. None
   D. Both

3. **Warthin tumour is also called:**
   A. Adenolymphoma   B. Pleomorphic adenoma
   C. Carcinoma   D. All of the above

4. **Mikulicz disease is:**
   A. Inflammatory condition
   B. Autoimmune disease
   C. Viral origin
   D. Neoplastic condition

5. **Perineural spread is seen in which of the following?**
   A. Adenoid cystic carcinoma
   B. Prostatic carcinoma
   C. Both of the above
   D. None of the above

6. **A cystic lesion below the tongue, due to obstruction of salivary gland duct is:**
   A. Dermoid cyst   B. Sebaceous cyst
   C. Ranula   D. Dentigerous cyst

7. **The complication of mumps is:**
   A. Hepatitis
   B. Orchitis
   C. Myocarditis
   D. Conjunctivitis

8. **Salivary gland tumour which exclusively occurs in parotid gland is:**
   A. Mucoepidermoid carcinoma
   B. Acinic cell tumour
   C. Adenoid cystic carcinoma
   D. Warthin's tumour

9. **Cribriform or honeycomb pattern is seen in:**
   A. Mucoepidermoid carcinoma
   B. Acinic cell tumour
   C. Adenoid cystic carcinoma
   D. Warthin's tumour

10. **Pleomorphic adenoma is:**
    A. Myoepithelial or ductal reserve cell origin
    B. Teratoma
    C. Hamartoma
    D. Neuroendocrine tumour

Answers

1. A   2. A   3. A   4. B   5. C   6. C   7. B   8. D
9. C   10. A

Gastrointestinal Pathology: Oral Cavity and Esophagus

PREMALIGNANT/PRECANCEROUS CONDITIONS OF ORAL CAVITY

A **premalignant/precancerous condition** is "a generalized state associated with significantly increased risk of cancer". The term precancerous condition was coined in 1875 by Romanian physician Victor Babes.

Premalignant conditions include:
1. Oral submucous fibrosis
2. Oral lichen planus
3. Plummer-Vinson syndrome
4. Epidermolysis bullosa
5. Xeroderma pigmentosum
6. Discoid lupus erythematosus

ORAL SUBMUCOUS FIBROSIS (OSMF)

It was first described by Sushruta in 600 BC and he named it as Vidari (Sanskrit = to destroy). Joshi in 1953 gave the term oral submucous fibrosis (OSMF).

Oral submucous fibrosis is a chronic debilitating disease of the oral cavity characterised by inflammation and progressive fibrosis of the submucosal tissues (lamina propria and deeper connective tissues) usually involving oral mucosa, the oropharynx, and rarely the larynx.

The incidence of malignant change to squamous cell carcinoma in patients with OSMF ranges from 2 to 8%.

Diagnosis is made by history and clinical examination. The following features are common in OSMF:
- Trismus
- Stiff and small tongue
- Blanched and leathery floor of the mouth
- Fibrotic and depigmented gingiva
- Rubbery soft palate with reduced mobility
- Blanched and atrophic tonsils
- Shrunken uvula
- Sinking of the cheek

XERODERMA PIGMENTOSUM

Xeroderma pigmentosum (XP) is an autosomal recessive disorder, with defect in DNA repair to the DNA damage caused by UV rays of sunlight. It is characterised by:
- Hypersensitivity to UV rays
- Freckles
- Cutaneous pigmentation
- Solar keratosis
- Photophobia
- Xerosis
- Neurodegeneration

XP patients are severe predisposition to skin cancers of various types, mainly squamous cell carcinoma and basal cell carcinoma at an early age.

PREMALIGNANT/PRECANCEROUS LESIONS OF ORAL CAVITY

A **premalignant/precancerous lesion is** "a morphologically altered tissue in which oral cancer is more likely to occur than its apparently normal counterpart".

These lesions are histological continuum between normal mucosa at one end and high grade dysplasia/carcinoma *in situ*, at the other end; establishing a model of neoplastic progression.

They include:
- Leukoplakia
- Erythroplakia
- Carcinoma *in situ*
- Nicotinic stomatitis

LEUKOPLAKIA

It is a predominantly white lesion of oral mucosa that cannot be characterised as any other definable lesion; some leukoplakia will transform into cancer. This definition has no histological connotation and is used strictly as a clinical description. It is a disease of exclusion.

The total lifetime risk of malignant transformation is estimated to 4–6%.

Etiology

- Tobacco is often related with leukoplakia. Both smoking and smokeless type of tobacco are associated with leukoplakia.
- Alcohol exhibits a strong synergistic effect with tobacco.
- Sunlight (UV radiation) is well known etiologic agent for leukoplakia at vermilion border of lip.
- *Candida albicans* is often associated with nodular leukoplakia.

Clinical Features

Age: The peak incidence age is 50 years.

Gender: Strong male dominance in different parts of India.

Site: About 70% of leukoplakia lesions are found on buccal musoca, vermilion border of lower lip and gingiva. Less common sites are palate, maxillary mucosa, retromolar area, floor of mouth and tongue.

Morphology

- Presence of parakeratosis or orthokeratosis.
- May have dysplasia.
- An inflammatory reaction of lymphocytes is often present in the underlying connective tissue.
- Histopathological study of leukoplakia allows:
  - To exclude any other definable lesions
  - To establish the degree of epithelial dysplasia, if present.

Prognosis

Leukoplakia has an unpredictable tendency to undergo malignant transformation. It ranges from 0.3 to 18% over prolonged periods. This may be due to many factors like, differences in diagnostic criteria and etiological factors, such as smoking, other habits, and nutritional status, geographical areas and cultural practices.

ERYTHROPLAKIA

Erythroplakia is a clinical term that refers to a bright-red, velvety lesion on oral mucous membrane.

The prevalence is less than leukoplakia because of under reporting (less than 0.1%).

Age: 50–70 yrs.

Gender: Male predominance.

Site: Found usually in the floor of mouth or retromolar area in adults.

Etiology

Tobacco and alcohol are the etiologic factors.

Prognosis

The probability of malignant transformation is 17 times greater than that of leukoplakias. Most (90%) have *in situ* or invasive carcinoma.

Morphology

- The epithelium shows a lack of keratin, it is often atrophic.
- Connective tissue demonstrates chronic inflammation
- Dysplasia, carcinoma *in situ* or even invasive carcinoma may be present.

CARCINOMA *IN SITU*

Oral carcinoma *in situ* usually presents clinically as leukoplakia or erythroplakia. The malignant transformation has occurred in the epithelium.

There is severe epithelial dysplasia in which the whole or almost the whole thickness of the epithelium is involved. The basement membrane is intact and there is no invasion of the lamina propria.

NICOTINE STOMATITIS

In 'nicotinic stomatitis', alterations of the mucosa of the palate, secondary to the chronic exposure of the smokers to tobacco and heat are seen. The palate becomes whitish, wrinkled, and can present with fissures. Small erythematous, nodular areas can be observed, which represent inflamed minor salivary glandular ducts. Malignant transformation is relatively rare.

Morphology

The white areas show hyperorthokeratosis and acanthosis with a variable mild to moderate chronic inflammatory cell infiltrate in subepithelial area. The diagnostic feature is the swollen, inflamed duct openings of minor salivary glands with hyperkeratosis extending up to the duct orifice. The ducts may show squamous metaplasia.

CARCINOMA OF ORAL CAVITY

Squamous cell carcinoma is the commonest malignant tumour of the oral cavity.

Etiology

1. Tobacco consumption (smoking, pipe smoking, chewing pan and tobacco, betel quid consumption)
2. HPV infection
3. Genetic predisposition
4. Chronic irritation (ill-fitting dentures, jagged teeth, etc.)
5. Actinic radiation
6. Premalignant conditions: Leukoplakia, erythroplakia

Squamous cell carcinoma can arise anywhere in oral cavity but most commonly involved sites are:
- Ventral surface of tongue
- Floor of mouth
- Lower lip
- Soft palate
- Gingiva

Grossly, they may present as verrucous plaques, ulcers, **protruding masses** with irregular and indurated borders (Fig. 28.1).

Microscopically, they are similar to squamous cell carcinoma occurring elsewhere. However, the degree of differentiation does not correlate with behaviour.

Common sites of metastasis include cervical lymph nodes, mediastinal lymph nodes, lungs, liver and bones.

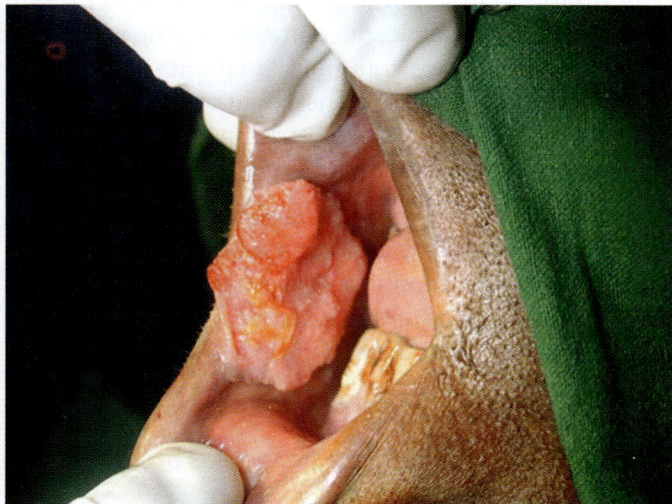

Fig. 28.1: Squamous cell carcinoma of oral cavity. Note the protruding growth in the inner aspect of cheek (*Courtesy:* Dr Basavaraj R Patil, Oncosurgeon, RB Patil Hospital, Hubli, Karnataka State, India)

ACHALASIA CARDIA

Failure to relax or incomplete relaxation of the lower esophageal sphincter is termed as achalasia cardia.

This produces a functional obstruction of the esophagus with dilatation of the proximal portion. **Failure to relax or incomplete relaxation is because of the following:**
- Aperistalsis
- Partial/incomplete relaxation of lower esophageal sphincter with swallowing.
- Increased resting tone of the lower esophageal sphincter.

Causes for Achalasia

1. **Primary causes:** The cause of primary achalasia is most often idiopathic. It may be due to loss of inhibitory innervations of the lower esophageal sphincter and smooth muscle.
2. **Secondary causes** include:
   - *Trypanosoma cruzi* (Chagas disease) destroys the myenteric plexus of the esophagus, duodenum, colon and ureter.
   - Disorders of dorsal motor neuron as in polio or autonomic neuropathy as in diabetes mellitus.

MALLORY-WEISS SYNDROME

Longitudinal tear at the esophageal-gastric junction is called Mallory-Weiss syndrome.

It occurs in:
- Chronic alcoholics
- Severe vomiting
- Hyperemesis gravidarum

Cause: This is due to inadequate relaxation of the sphincter.

Features:
- There is bleeding from the laceration.
- Tear occurs in mucosa and submucosa. The bleeding stops after 24–48 hours.

Treatment: Cauterization or epinephrin can also stop the bleeding.

BARRETT ESOPHAGUS/ESOPHAGITIS (BE)

Barrett esophagus refers to replacement of normal distal stratified squamous epithelium of esophagus by metaplastic columnar epithelium with goblet cells.

British Society of Gastroenterology defines BE as columnar epithelium lined esophagus on histology (either gastric or intestinal or both). According to 2008 updated American Gastroenterology guidelines, endoscopically and histological criteria to be met for diagnosis of BE. Endoscopically salmon pink-coloured mucosa extends proximally from gastroesophageal junction into esophagus.[24, 25]

It is a complication of gastroesophageal (GE) reflux/ gastroesophageal reflux disease (GERD). This presents with heart burn, regurgitation and dysphagia. It is a precursor lesion for *in situ* changes and adeno-carcinoma.

Risk Factors

- M:F ratio 4:1
- White and Caucasian race
- Advanced age
- Obesity
- Hiatal hernia
- Smoking

Barrett esophagus is reported in 15% of patients of gastroesophageal reflux who undergo biopsy. Prolonged and recurrent GE reflux produces inflammation and ulceration. Healing occurs by progenitor cells transforming into metaplastic columnar cells. It is believed that columnar epithelium is more resistant to damaging effects of the gastric contents (acid, pepsin and bile) than stratified squamous epithelium.

Complications

- Stricture
- Risk of dysplasia followed by development of adeno-carcinoma (30–100 times greater risk)

Barrett esophagus can be of:

1. Ultrashort segment (less than 1 cm),
2. Short segment (1 to 3 cm),
3. Long segment (4 to 10 cm), or
4. Very long segment (more than 10 cm)

Any of the above can have risk of malignancy. However, long segment Barrett's esophagus has more chances of malignancy than the short segment one.

Morphology: Grossly, metaplastic columnar epithelium looks salmon pink and velvety between the smooth pale pink stratified squamous epithelial mucosa.

Microscopy: There is columnar epithelial metaplasia with goblet cells. It is focal and variable and requires repeated endoscopic biopsy from different areas to recognize dysplastic changes.

ESOPHAGEAL TUMOURS

Most common neoplasms of esophadus are squamous cell papilloma and carcinoma.

Esophageal carcinoma can be of two types:
1. Squamous cell carcinoma
2. Adenocarcinoma

SQUAMOUS CELL CARCINOMA OF ESOPHAGUS

It is the most common carcinoma occurring in males.

Age: Peak 50–60 years of age.

It is most prevalent in African American males.

It occurs among low socioeconomic status people.

Etiology

The most common etiologies include the following:
1. Chronic irritation
2. Inflammation
3. Alcohol
4. Smoking
5. Achalasia
6. Esophageal diverticula
7. Plummer-Vinson syndrome
8. Non-epidermolytic palmoplantar keratoderma (predisposes to esophageal cancer)

Site of occurrence: The neoplasm more frequently occurs in middle third or proximal one-third portion of the esophagus.

Morphology

Gross findings: The neoplasm is grey-white fungating, ulcerating, infiltrating or stenotic mass. Tumour size may vary up to 10 cm in length. Fungating masses present as large intraluminal ulcerated masses having raised and everted margins. Less commonly may present as bulky irregular polypoid masses. The extent of infiltration does not reflect the size of the protruding mass. The eso-phageal wall is thickened with infiltration into the wall.

Microscopy: Resembles squamous cell carcinoma occurring elsewhere. Carcinoma *in situ* and high grade dysplasia are commonly observed at the periphery of the lesion. Variants of squamous cell carcinoma may be encountered including spindle cell variant.

ADENOCARCINOMA OF ESOPHAGUS

About 90% of the the adenocarcinomas occur in a pre-existing Barrett esophagus.

Clinical Features

Patients present with dysphagia, odynophagia and weight loss.

Adenocarcinoma is common in the distal one-third of esophagus as against most squamous cell carcinomas are found in middle or proximal parts of esophagus. These are detected in advanced stages.

Morphology

Gross: Adenocarcinoma presents as a flat, ulcerated, polypoid, fungating or diffusely infiltrative mass in the distal third of esophagus. The residual Barrett's mucosa is visible as velvety red lesion. The lesion may extend into the gastric cardia and in such occasions, it becomes difficult to know the primary site of origin as esophagus or cardia portion of stomach.

Microscopy: Malignant cells with glandular differentiation and mucin production are the features.

Various subtypes include:
1. Tubular
2. Papillary
3. Signet ring type
4. Adenosquamous type
5. Adenoid cystic carcinoma
6. Mucoepidermoid carcinoma.

Poorly differentiated tumours behave aggressive course than the well-differentiated ones. Hence, proper staging is necessary to assess the prognosis.

MALIGNANT MELANOMA OF ESOPHAGUS

This can occur as a primary tumour and similar to malignant melanoma occurring elsewhere.

SELF-ASSESSMENT EXERCISE

1. **Barrett's esophagus is:**
   A. Squamous metaplasia
   B. Intestinal metaplasia
   C. Intestinal dysplasia
   D. Gastric dysplasia

2. **Oral cancer is due to:**
   A. Tobacco chewing
   B. Ill-fitting dentures
   C. Sharp teeth
   D. All of the above

3. **A young male with complaints dysphagia to solid or liquid food is:**
   A. Achalasia cardia
   B. GERD

   C. Paraesophageal hernia
   D. All

4. **A young male with heart burn, regurgitation and dysphagia:**
   A. GERD
   B. Hiatus hernia
   C. Mallory-Weiss syndrome
   D. All

5. **Barrett's esophagus is premalignant lesion and produces:**
   A. Squamous cell carcinoma
   B. Adenocarcinoma
   C. Papilloma
   D. All of the above

Answers

1. B   2. D   3. A   4. A   5. B

Gastrointestinal Pathology: Stomach and Intestinal Lesions

GASTRITIS

Gastritis is defined as inflammation of the gastric mucosa. It can be acute or chronic.

Acute Gastritis

This is an acute inflammatory process which is of transient nature.

Causes

- NSAIDs
- Alcohol
- Heavy smoking
- Treatment with chemotherapeutic drugs
- Stress
- Ischaemia
- Mechanical trauma
- Reflux of bile

It can be localized or diffuse. Superficial involvement presents as acute erosive gastritis. Haemorrhage is present. Complete resolution occurs after causative agent is removed.

Chronic Gastritis

In chronic gastritis, there is presence of inflammatory changes in the mucosa leading to mucosal atrophy and intestinal metaplasia. *H. pylori* is the most important causative agent.

Morphology: There is inflammation by plasma cells and lymphocytes. Occasionally, neutrophils are present. Glandular tissue is markedly reduced and there is presence of mucosal atrophy. Lymphoid aggregates are present. There may be presence of intestinal metaplasia and dysplasia.

PEPTIC ULCER (Gastric Ulcer/Duodenal Ulcer)

Peptic ulcers are ulcers defined histologically by breach in the mucosa that extends through the muscularis mucosa into the submucosa or deeper due to the action of acid peptic juices. Often solitary and can occur in any portion of gastrointestinal tract which is exposed to action of acid/peptic juices.

Epidemiology

Amongst peptic ulcers, gastric ulcer most commonly occurs in middle aged and elderly and duodenal ulcer from 30–60 years of age. These appear with or without precipitating causes and heal after a period of weeks to months.

Common locations in order of frequency are:
- First part of duodenum
- Lesser curvature and antrum of stomach
- Gastroesophageal junction
- Margins of gastrojejunostomy (stomal ulcer)
- Stomach and/or jejunum of patients with Zollinger–Ellison syndrome
- Meckel's diverticulum containing ectopic gastric mucosa

Etiology

Following are the possible causes for peptic ulcer:
- *H. pylori*
- Chronic use of NSAIDs
- Cigarette smoking
- Alcohol
- Corticosteroid use
- Personality and psychological stress
- Heredity

- Associated diseases: Alcoholic cirrhosis, chronic obstructive pulmonary disease (COPD), chronic renal failure, hyperparathyroidism especially in duodenal ulcer.

***H. pylori* is a major factor in pathogenesis of peptic ulcers. The reason for this may be:**

1. It induces an intense inflammatory and immune response. There is production of proinflammatory cytokines such as interleukins (IL-1, IL-6, IL-8) and tumour necrosis factor (TNF). These recruit and activate neutrophils.
2. It secretes urease, phospholipase and protease enzymes. Urease breaks down urea to form toxic compounds such as ammonium chloride and monochloramine. The phospholipases and proteases damage surface epithelial cells. Thus, *H. pylori* induces defective mucosal barrier.
3. *H. pylori* enhances gastric acid secretion and impairs duodenal bicarbonate production. Thus, luminal pH is reduced which is responsible for metaplasia.
4. Evokes immunogenic response by activation of B and T lymphocytes.
5. The bacterial platelet-activating factor promotes thrombotic occlusion of surface capillaries.

H. pylori infection is found in 70–90% of the duodenal ulcers and about 70% of the gastric ulcers.

Severity of *H. pylori* depends upon cytotoxity of the organisms, Cag A genes, and presence of urease enzyme which splits urea into ammonia and carbon dioxide and produce ammonium chloride and monochloramine. Strains producing CagA and VacA produce intense inflammation, severe epithelial damage and higher cytokine production.

NSAIDs: NSAIDs are the major cause of peptic ulcer in persons who do not have *H. pylori*.

They suppress the mucosal prostaglandin synthesis and cause direct irritation, cause increased synthesis of hydrochloric acid (HCl) and reduce mucin and bicarbonate production. Loss of mucin degrades the mucosal barrier that normally prevents acid from reaching the epithelium. Synthesis of glutathione, a free radical scavenger, is also reduced.

Cigarette smoking: Impairs mucosal blood flow and healing.

Alcohol: No direct relation but alcoholic cirrhosis is associated with an increased incidence (tenfold increase).

Corticosteroid use: Causes gastritis and worsens peptic ulcer.

Personality and psychological stress: Type A personality and psychological stess are associated with peptic ulcer.

Heredity: Blood group "O" individuals and non-secretors have 2.5-fold increase in duodenal ulcer. Gastric ulcer is common in blood group "A" individuals.

Associated Diseases

Following diseases are more common in duodenal ulcers:

1. **Hyperparathyroidism:** Associated hypercalcaemia stimulates gastrin production especially in duodenal ulcer.
2. **Chronic renal failure:** Patients of chronic renal failure have ten times higher incidence of peptic ulcer.
3. **Chronic obstructive pulmonary disease (COPD):** COPD individuals have higher incidence of bleeding in peptic ulcer patients.

Pathogenesis

Imbalance between gastroduodenal mucosal defense mechanisms (Table 29.1 and Fig. 29.1) and the damaging forces particularly gastric acid and pepsin combined with environmental and other agents damage the mucosa with ulceration. The ulcers develop adjacent to epithelium containing parietal/oxyntic cells. There is close association between ulcer site and severity of gastritis. Table 29.1 shows the protective and damaging forces.

Table 29.1	Protective and damaging forces
Protective forces	**Damaging forces**
1. Stomach and duodenal epithelium secrete mucus which forms a thin layer on the epithelium	1. Gastric acidity: H ions from parietal cells
2. Bicarbonate ion secretion by the gastric/duodenal epithelium into mucosa, neutralizes the pH	2. Peptic enzymes: Produced by chief cells
3. The epithelium acts as a barrier for back diffusion of acid and leakage of other contents including pepsin	3. Ischaemia
4. The rich mucosal blood supply provides oxygen and nutrients and washes away acid which is back diffused into the lamina propria	4. *H. pylori*
5. Epithelial cells have regeneratory capacity (labile cells)	5. NSAIDs
6. Epithelial cells produce prostaglandins	6. Duodenal gastric reflux
	7. Alcohol
	8. Tobacco

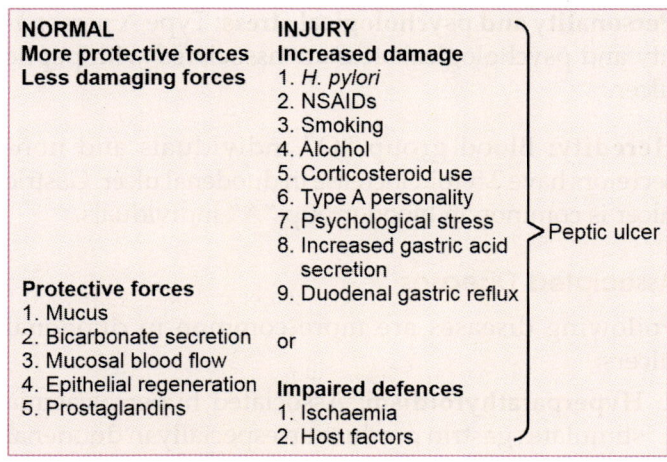

NORMAL	INJURY	
More protective forces	Increased damage	
Less damaging forces	1. *H. pylori*	
	2. NSAIDs	
	3. Smoking	
	4. Alcohol	
	5. Corticosteroid use	
	6. Type A personality	Peptic ulcer
	7. Psychological stress	
	8. Increased gastric acid secretion	
Protective forces	9. Duodenal gastric reflux	
1. Mucus		
2. Bicarbonate secretion	or	
3. Mucosal blood flow		
4. Epithelial regeneration	Impaired defences	
5. Prostaglandins	1. Ischaemia	
	2. Host factors	

Fig. 29.1: Defence mechanisms of peptic ulcer

GASTRIC ULCER

Gastric ulcers (GU) primarily result from altered/defective mucosal defenses. Most patients of gastric ulcer secrete less acid than duodenal ulcer and even sometimes lesser than normal individuals.

Factors implicated include (Fig. 29.2):

- *Back diffusion of H ions into mucosa:* The damaging factors, especially *H. pylori* and NSAIDs, weaken of intercellular junctions, and cause foveolar damage which allows H ions and pepsin to diffuse into lamina propria. The other damaging factors include alcohol and spicy food.
- *Role of NSAIDs:* Prostaglandins which play a major role in maintaining mucosal integrity are inhibited by the NSAIDs and further predispose to mucosal damage. NSAIDs also reduce mucin and bicarbonate production. The antral ulcers usually develop along lesser curvature.
- *H. pylori infection:* Causes defective mucosal barrier and intestinal metaplasia. Organisms are concentrated within the superficial mucus, luminal surface of foveolar and mucus neck cells or even may extend into gastric pits. They are most often localized to

antrum, less common in acid producing regions (fundus and body) and metaplastic epithelium.

- *Decreased number and abnormalities of parietal cells:* This suggests that hypersecretion of acid is not the cause of GU.

Sites of gastric ulcer: Lesser curvature and antrum (common), anterior and posterior wall and greater curvature (less common).

DUODENAL ULCER

Duodenal ulcers (DU) are due to increased acid production or due to the effect of acid as evidenced by the following (Fig. 29.3):

1. The gastric acid secreted depends upon the parietal cell mass. Patients of duodenal ulcer may have double of parietal cell mass and maximum acid secretion compared to controls.
2. Gastric acid secretion stimulated by food is increased in magnitude and duration in patients with duodenal ulcer.
3. Some patients of duodenal ulcer can have increased G cell response to meals and can have increased number of antral G cells.
4. Acid secretion in people with duodenal ulcer may be more sensitive to secretogogues like gastrin than the normal individuals. This is possibly due to increased vagal tone or increased affinity of parietal cells to gastrin.
5. Accelerated or rapid gastric emptying is noted in patients with duodenal ulcers. Thus acidic food enters duodenum.
6. There is hyperacidification of duodenal bulb.
7. There is decreased bicarbonate secretion.
8. Decreased retrograde motility impairs neutralization by pancreatic alkaline secretions.

Differences between gastric ulcer and duodenal ulcer are described in Table 29.2.

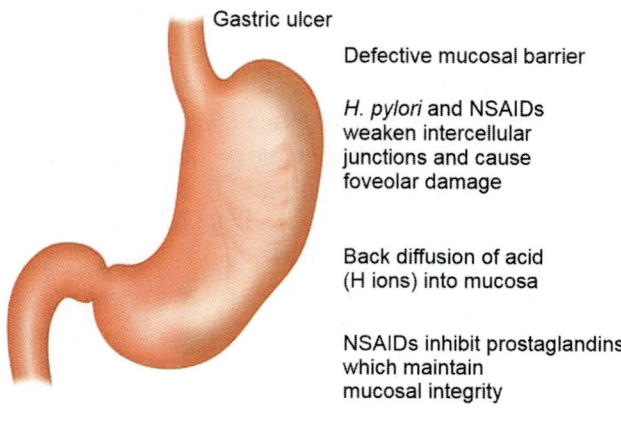

Gastric ulcer

Defective mucosal barrier

H. pylori and NSAIDs weaken intercellular junctions and cause foveolar damage

Back diffusion of acid (H ions) into mucosa

NSAIDs inhibit prostaglandins which maintain mucosal integrity

Fig. 29.2: Pathogenesis of gastric ulcer

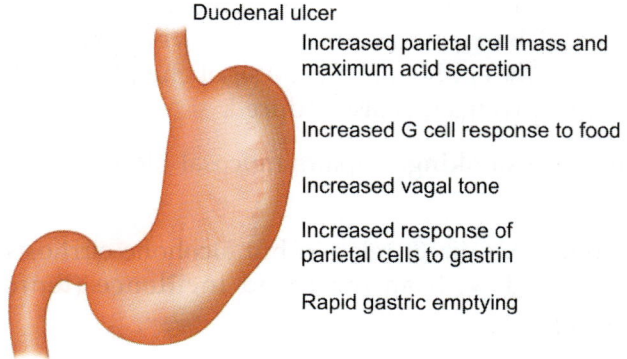

Duodenal ulcer

Increased parietal cell mass and maximum acid secretion

Increased G cell response to food

Increased vagal tone

Increased response of parietal cells to gastrin

Rapid gastric emptying

Fig. 29.3: Pathogenesis of duodenal ulcer

Table 29.2	Differences between GU and DU	
	Gastric ulcer	**Duodenal ulcer**
Incidence	Less often (25%)	More often (75%)
Association with blood group	Blood group A	Blood group O
Basal and maximum acid outputs	Normal or low	High
Etiology	Defective mucous barrier	Increased acid
Complications	Bleeding from left gastric artery, perforation, hour glass deformity	Bleeding from gastroduodenal artery, perforation, gastric outlet obstruction and pancreatitis
Malignant transformation	Common	Less common
Epigastric pain	Pain after eating	Usually 3 hours after eating

Morphology (Fig. 29.4)

1. Most commonly located in first part of duodenum (anterior wall more often affected) and stomach (more commonly on lesser curvature) usually at antral and corpus junction.
2. Majority are solitary.
3. These are usually less than 2 cm. They may penetrate the muscle tissue.
4. Round to oval, sharply punched out, with straight walls, margins are usually levelled or slightly elevated.
5. Base is smooth and clean.
6. Converging mucosal folds.
7. The blood vessels at the margins may be thrombosed.

Histology (Fig. 29.5)

In active ulcers, shows four different zones **(Askanazy zones)** from lumen outwards. They are:

1. **Zone of necrotic debris:** Superficial zone has debris.
2. **Zone of inflammation:** This zone shows dead cells and acute inflammatory cells.
3. **Zone of granulation tissue:** Composed of capillaries, fibroblasts, macrophages, lymphocytes and plasma cells.

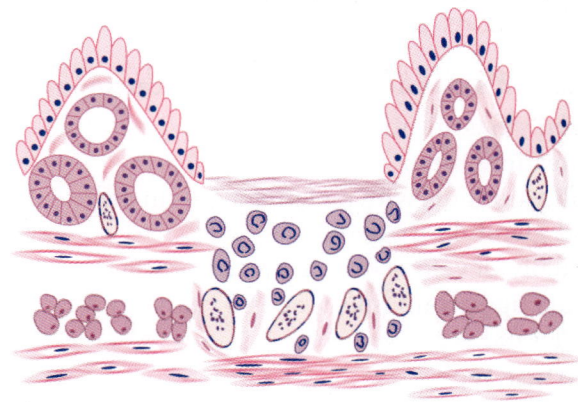

Fig. 29.5: Microscopy of peptic ulcer (schematic)

4. **Zone of fibrosis or collagenous scar:** Beneath granulation tissue, collagenous tissue is present. The ulcer may erode muscle and othe layers, causing perforation and if blood vessels are eroded, bleeding and haemorrhage.

Complications

1. Bleeding/haemorrhage
2. Perforation
3. Obstruction from oedema
4. Scarring: Can produce pyloric stenosis (duodenal ulcers) and hourglass deformity (gastric ulcers)
5. Pancreatitis
6. Rarely malignant transformation

Clinical Features

Epigastric burning or pain is a common feature. A few may have iron deficiency anaemia, haematemesis and perforation. With gastric ulcer, pain worsens after eating as gastric acid production is increased as food enters stomach, whereas in duodenal ulcer, pain is relieved by meal and manifests 2–3 hours after meal when stomach releases digested food along with acid into duodenum. Nausea, vomiting, bloating, abdominal fullness, water brush, belching, weight loss, loss of appetite, melena may be other clinical manifestations.

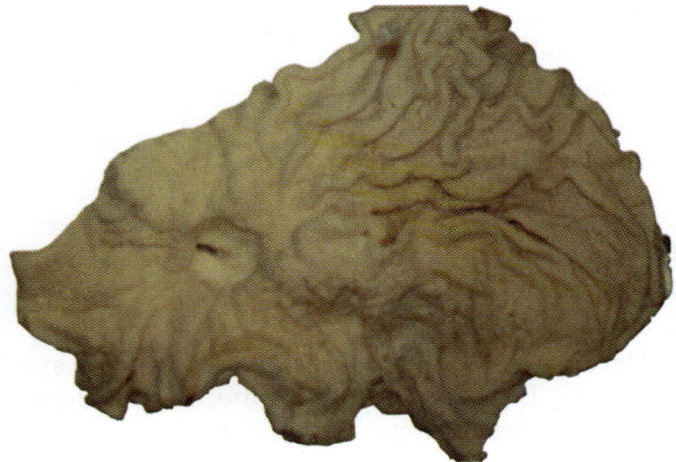

Fig. 29.4: Peptic ulcer (gross picture)

GASTRIC CARCINOMA

It is the most common malignant tumours of the stomach.

Epidemiology

Higher incidence is seen in Japan, China, Chile, Korea, Columbia, Costa Rica, Portugal, Russia and Bulgaria. Incidence is lesser in United States, United Kingdom, Canada, Australia, New Zealand, France and Sweden. It is more common in lower socioeconomic groups. It is a disease of elderly individuals and rare under the age of 30 years. Male to female ratio is 2:1.

Classifications of Gastric Carcinoma

Lauren's classification of gastric carcinoma[27]

Lauren's classification has two subtypes:

1. Intestinal type:
- Bulky tumours with malignant cells in diffuse sheets and glandular pattern
- Usually develops from a precursor lesion
- Older age group (mean age 55 years)
- M: F ratio is 2:1.

2. Diffuse type:
- Malignant cells are in diffuse sheets
- No identifiable precursor lesions present
- Affects slightly younger (mean age 48 years)
- M:F ratio is 1:1

Depending upon depth of invasion, it can be classified as:

Early gastric carcinomas: Confined to mucosa and submucosa regardless of involvement of perigastric lymph nodes (not same as carcinoma *in situ* where it is confined to the surface epithelial layer).

Advanced gastric carcinomas: Extending below the submucosa, and may infiltrate muscular wall.

WHO Classification of Gastric Tumours[28]

Epithelial tumours
1. Intraepithelial neoplasia in adenoma
2. Adenocarcinoma:
   - Papillary adenocarcinoma
   - Tubular adenocarcinoma
   - Mucinous adenocarcinoma
   - Signet ring carcinoma
   - Undifferentiated carcinoma
   - Adenosquamous carcinoma
   - Small cell carcinoma
   - Hepatoid adenocarcinoma
   - Carcinoma with lymphoid stroma (medullary carcinoma)

3. Neuroendocrine tumour/carcinoid tumour

Non-epithelial tumours
1. Leiomyoma
2. Schwannoma
3. Granular cell tumour
4. Leiomyosarcoma
5. Inflammatory myofibroblastic tumour
6. Gastrointestinal stromal tumour
7. Kaposi's sarcoma
8. Others
   Malignant lymphoma

Secondaries

Note: Simplified classification of gastric tumours from Classification of Tumours of the Digestive System, 4th Ed., 2010.

Etiology of Gastric Carcinoma

I. **Environmental factors**
   a. *Infection by H. pylori*
   b. *Diet:*
   - Nitrites and nitrates in food
   - Salt intake (dried and salted fish intake in Japan)
   - Smoked foods, pickled food, chillies and pepper
   - Lack of fresh fruit and vegetables (lack of anti-oxidants)
   c. *Low socioeconomic status*
   d. *Cigarette smoking:* This has 1.5- to 2.5-fold increases risk of stomach cancer.

II. **Predisposing gastric esophageal lesions:** Reflux of bile and pancreatic juices are implicated in causation of cancer.

Following are the conditions associated with cancer stomach:
1. Chronic gastritis
2. Atropic gastritis
3. Intestinal metaplasia
4. Autoimmune gastritis
5. Partial gastrectomy
6. Gastric adenomas
7. Barrett's esophagus

Genetic factors:
1. Blood group 'A' individuals
2. Family history
3. Hereditary: Non-polyposis colon carcinoma syndrome, Li-Fraumeni syndrome, PJ syndrome, familial adenomatous polyposis, etc.
4. Familial gastric carcinoma syndrome (E-cadherin mutation).

Pathogenesis

The following mechanisms play role:

1. Nitrates and nitrites in preserved food, smoking and salting, reduced intake of fresh vegetables and fruits (antioxidants reduce nitrosation and nitrosamides) are implicated in causation of stomach cancer. Refrigeration has reduced use of these chemicals.
2. Genetic mechanisms: Loss of alleles in various chromosomal loci, microsatellite instability of several genes.
3. Amplification of HER2/neu and increased expression of beta catenin.
4. Mutations of E-cadherin, mutations of fibroblast growth receptor family (FGFR2) and overexpression of metalloproteinases play role in causation of the disease (especially diffuse adenocarcinoma).
5. Chronic gastritis with *H. pylori* can lead to severe gastric atrophy, intestinal metaplasia followed by dysplasia and carcinoma. The Cag A strains have increased inflammatory response and risk of stomach cancer (both intestinal and diffuse types). The possible mechanism for carcinoma in *H. pylori* is:
   i. Indirect effects through inflammatory process: *H. pylori* releases ROS, can cause damage to DNA and cancer development.
   ii. Direct effects: These are caused by toxic action of virulence factors, mutation of cell cycle regulating genes and defects in DNA repair mechanisms.

Morphology

Location: Pylorus and antrum (60–65%), cardia (25–30%), and remainder in fundus and body.

Lesser curvature (40%) more involved than greater curvature (15%).

Most common on the lesser curvature of antropyloric region.

Macroscopic growth patterns:

- Exophytic
- Flat or depressed
- Excavated
- Linitis plastica (leather bottle appearance)

Histological subtypes: Intestinal and diffuse types (*refer* to Lauren's classification).

Gross: Gastric carcinoma can be early gastric cancer or advanced gastric cancer. In early gastrtic cancer, the neoplasm is limited to the mucosa and submucosa. Grossly, early gastric carcinoma can be of (a) exophytic, (b) flat or depressed, and (c) excavated types. Advanced gastric carcinoma can be of (a) exophytic (polypoid/fungating), (b) linitis plastica, and (c) excavated types.

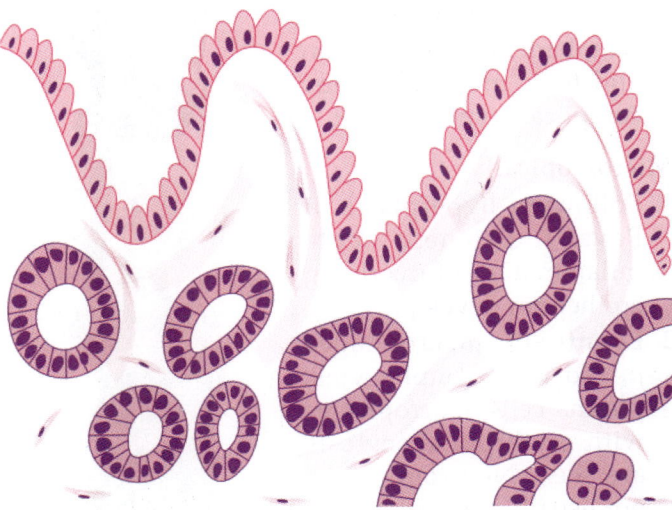

Fig. 29.6: Microscopy of adenocarcinoma stomach (schematic)

Microscopy (Fig. 29.6): In any of these types, the microscopy shows adenocarcinoma with varying degrees of differentiation. They can be of different subtypes such as papillary, tubular, mucinous, signet ring cell and undifferentiated adenocarcinoma (WHO classification). In diffusely infiltrative pattern, the neoplasm may be associated with desmoplasia.

Spread

- *Left supraclavicular lymph node* (Virchow's node, sentinel node) may be seen in even occult malignancy.
- *Sister Mary Joseph nodule:* Periumbilical metastatic nodule.
- *Local invasion:* Duodenum, pancreas, retropritoneum.
- *Metastasis to ovaries:* Kruckenberg tumour.

Clinical Features

Carcinoma stomach has insidious onset, generally asymptomatic until late in the course.

Weight loss, anorexia, abdominal pain, vomiting, altered bowel habits and anaemia are the common symptoms in gastric carcinoma. There can be clinical features of gastric outlet obstruction. Bleeding is uncommon.

INFLAMMATORY LESIONS OF INTESTINE

TYPHOID ULCER[29, 30]

Grossly (Fig. 29.7):

1. Characteristic pathology is noticed in ileum.
2. The intestine shows raised nodules representing hyperplastic Payer's patches.
3. Ulceration, linear ulcers, full thickness ulceration of surface epithelium overlying Payer's patches ensues as the disease progresses.

4. Suppurative mesenteric lymphadenitis, perforation and toxic megacolon may complicate typhoid fever.

Microscopically:

1. Following hyperplasia of Payer's patches, acute inflammation of overlying epithelium develops.
2. Eventually macrophages mixed with lymphocytes, plasma cells, macrophages with erythrophagocytosis are seen. Neutrophils are not usually present.
3. Necrosis of overlying epithelium spreads to neighbouring mucosa.
4. The ulcers are deep, with base at the level of muscularis propria.

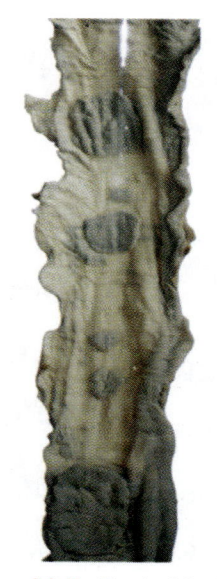

Fig. 29.7: Typhoid ulcer (gross picture)

TUBERCULOUS ULCER[29, 30]

It may primary or secondary tuberculosis. Primary is common with *M. tuberculosis, M. bovis* organisms, but the incidence has reduced with pasturisation of milk.

Grossly (Fig. 29.8):

1. Ileocaecal and jejunoileal areas are the most commonly involved areas followed by appendix and ascending colon.
2. Strictures and ulcers are the most common findings along with thickened mucosal folds.
3. Ulcerative, hypertrophic, and ulcerohypertrophic are the three morphological types.
   The ulcerative type commonly affects the ileum and jejunum. The hypertrophic and ulcerohypertrophic types commonly affect the ileocaecal region and cause obstruction or present as a mass.
4. The ulcers are often circumferential and transverse. Multiple and segmental lesions with skip areas are common.

5. Healing of ulcers leads to stricture formation, and may perforate, bleed, or form fistulas.
   Obstruction, perforation and haemorrhage are common complications.
6. Regional lymph nodes also affected.

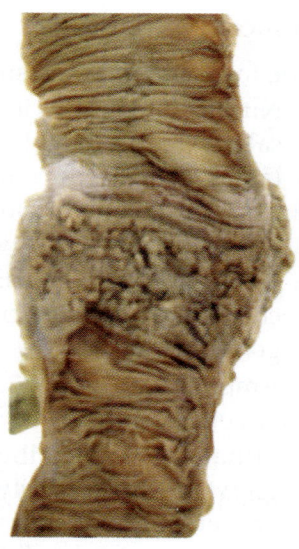

Fig. 29.8: Tuberculous ulcer intestine (gross picture)

Microscopically, shows classical granulomas with caseation necrosis surrounded by epithelioid cells, Langhan's type of giant cells and mantle of lymphocytes with surrounding fibrosis suggestive of tuberculosis are seen. These granulomas are seen mainly in the submucosal and serosal layers.

Differences between typhoid ulcer and tuberculous ulcer intestine are given in Table 29.3.

Differential diagnosis for tuberculosis:

1. Yersiniosis: Granulomas are non-caseating.
2. Crohn's: Difficult to differentiate from tuberculosis, grossly linear ulcers are present rather than circumferential ulcers; cobble stoning is typical which is not a feature in tuberculosis.
3. Fungal diseases

INFLAMMATORY BOWEL DISEASES

The inflammatory bowel diseases are group of chronic gastrointestinal tract diseases that are relapsing and remitting and involve:

1. Genetic susceptibility
2. Failure of immunological regulation
3. Triggering of microbial flora.

The different types of colitis include:

1. Ulcerative colitis
2. Crohn's disease

Table 29.3	Differences between typhoid ulcer and tuberculous ulcer intestine	
	Tuberculous ulcer intestine	**Typhoid ulcer**
Site	Anywhere in the intestine, commomly ileocaecal junction	Ileum
Ulcers	Circumferentially placed	Longitudinally placed along the Payer's patches
Gross features	Transverse and circumferential ulcers	Vertical ulcers along the Payer's patches
Microscopy	Granulomas	Erythrophagocytosis
Complications	Stricture, obstruction, adhesions	Perforation, peritonitis
Blood changes	Lymphocytosis, ESR increased	Neutropenia, widal positive

3. Collagenous colitis
4. Lymphocytic colitis
5. Ischaemic colitis
6. Radiation colitis
7. Diverticular disease associated colitis
8. Allergic proctocolitis

Ulcerative Colitis

It is a chronic idiopathic inflammatory bowel disease with episodes of bloody diarrhoea and histologically has crypt destruction, colitis with continuous involvement from rectum extending proximally.

Incidence: Uncommon, 4–20/1,00,000 population are affected.

Epidemiology

- M:F—equal
- Whites have higher incidence than other ethnic group.
- Jews have higher incidence than other religious group.
- Rare in 1st decade.
- Peak: 15–25 years of age major peak.
- 60–70 years of age minor peak.
- 25% have family history.
- These patients are associated with HLA-B27 and HLA-DRB1.
- Patients of ulcerative colitis can have ankylosing spondylitis.

Pathogenesis

- The exact cause of ulcerative colitis is not known. Viruses, bacteria, immunological disorders and environmental factors are implicated in causation of the disease.
- Though monozygotic twins have higher incidence, no distinct mode of genetic transmission is still understood.
- In these patients, there is abnormal immune response. There are increased circulating antibodies against antigens of columnar epithelial cells and cross-reacting antibodies of enterobacteria. Anti-neutrophil antibodies are found in 80% of the cases; however, it is not unique to ulcerative colitis.
- Psychological factors particularly psychological stress is associated with ulcerative colitis.

Clinical Features

Patients present with recurrent episodes of bloody diarrhoea, crampy abdominal pain, fever, tachycardia, weight loss and symptoms related to hypoalbuminaemia. They can have extraintestinal manifestations like:

1. Arthritis
2. Erythema nodosum
3. Pyoderma gangrenosum
4. Sclerosing cholangitis
5. Cholangiocarcioma
6. Uveitis
7. Ankylosing spondylitis

Gross and Endoscopic Findings

- Unremarkable serosa
- Bowel wall thickness normal
- Continuous involvement from rectum proximally
- May involve entire colon and ileum
- **Active phase:** Mucosa erythematous, bloody, friable, granular with polyps
  Toxic megacolon is a serious complication of active phase with pancolitis, characterised by segmental colonic dilatation, loss of contractile ability and rapid clinical deterioration
- **Quiescent phase:** Mucosa granular with punctate erythema with polyps
- In both phases, normal submucosal vascular network is lost.

Microscopy (Fig. 29.9)

- Crypt architecture distortion
- Active phase: Cryptitis, crypt abscesses and ulcers
- Inflammation is superficial: Mucosal and submucosal chronic inflammation, submucosa—oedema and congestion, lacks fibrosis, eosinophils may predominate.
- Lymphoid aggregate: Less common
- Regenerating epithelium (pseudopolyps) is common.
- Mucin is depleted.
- Transmural inflammation is not present unless it is deep-seated ulceration.

Prognosis: Has risk of dysplasia and adenocarcinoma.

Crohn's Disease (Regional Enteritis, Granulomatous Enterocolitis and Terminal Ileitis)

It is a chronic multifocal, relapsing and remitting progressive inflammatory disease of unknown cause that can affect any portion of GIT. It is characterised by foci of glandular destruction, aphthous (mucosal) ulcerations, serpiginous ulcers, transmural inflammation, fibrosis and granulomas in the small and large intestines.

Incidence: 2–20/1,00,000 population.

Epidemiology

- M:F—equal
- Whites have higher incidence than other ethnic group.

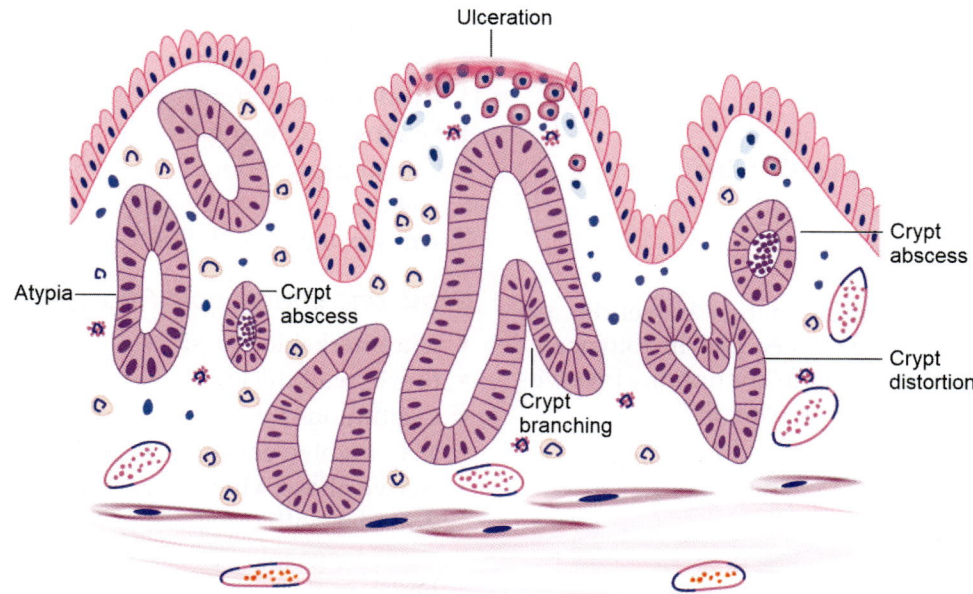

Fig. 29.9: Ulcerative colitis (schematic)

- Ashkenazi Jews have higher incidence than other religious group.
- Peak: 20–30 years of age major peak
- 60–70 years of age minor peak
- 10% have family history.

Pathogenesis

- The exact pathogenesis is not known. Infectious agents, susceptibility genes, immunological response, food allergens, environmental factors and auto-antibodies play role in causation of the disease.
- Crohn's disease patients are associated with HLA-DR4/DR7 and DQ4.
- A gene NOD2 on chromosome 16 is mutated in 25% of the cases.
- Response to bacteria with inflammation is maximum in these patients.
- One of the environmental triggers is psychological factor particularly psychological stress.

Clinical Features

- Cramping pain, non-bloody diarrhoea, fever, malaise and anorexia.
- Haemorrhage and bleeding uncommon.
- Upper intestinal involvement: Dyspepsia, weight loss, hypoalbuminaemia and iron deficiency anaemia.
- Clinical features related to fistula and stenosis of intestinal loops.
- Clinical features related to anal and perianal fistulas and fissures.
- Inflammatory changes can occur in joints, eyes, liver and skin.

Gross and Endoscopy Findings

- Aphthous ulceration
- Longitudinal ulcers (train tract and rake ulcers) and adjacent normal mucosa
- Cobble stone appearance
- Strictures
- Fissures and fistulas
- Involvement of terminal ileum
- Loss of submucosal vascular network
- Often rectal sparing
- Creeping fat—subserosal fat covers and contracted over involved area
- Firm, thick, pipe-like bowel (hosepipe-like), wall thickened
- Interloop adhesions
- Inflammatory polyps
- Multifocal
- Occasional confluent involvement

Microscopic Findings (Fig. 29.10)

- Ulcers separated by normal mucosa, transmural inflammation, variable inflammation in single biopsy, mucosal erosions with underlying lymphoid aggregate, epithelioid granuloma and submucosal fibrosis
- Duplication of muscularis mucosae
- Hyperplasia of nerve bundle
- Ulceration, fissures and fistulas

Prognosis: Has risk of malignancy.

Differences between Crohn's disease and ulcerative colitis are given in Table 29.4.

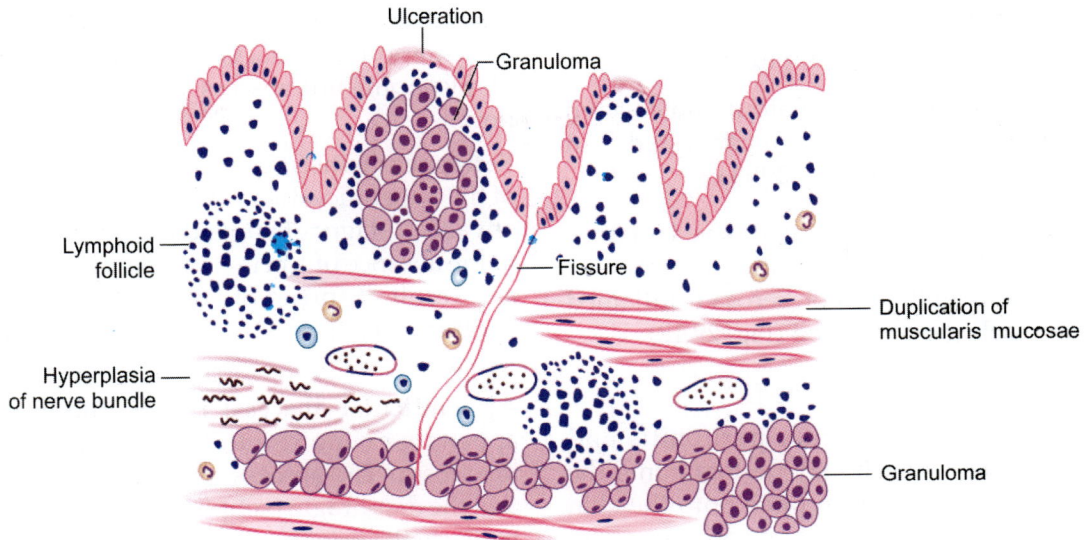

Fig. 29.10: Crohn's disease (schematic)

Table 29.4	Differences between Crohn's disease and ulcerative colitis		
		Crohn's disease	Ulcerative colitis
Macroscopy	Bowel region	Colon, ileum	Colon
	Distribution	Skip lesions	Diffuse
		Segmental involvement	
		Terminal ileum and ascending colon commonly affected	Rectum and sigmoid colon commonly affected
	Pseudopolyps	–	Common
	Strictures/fibrosis	+	Late/rare
	Wall	Thickened	Normal
	Dilatation	+	+
Microscopy	Inflammation	Transmural	Mucosal and submucosal
	Ulcers	Deep/linear	Superficial
	Submucosa	Normal/inflamed	Normal
	Cryptitis	Uncommon	Common
	Crypt abscesses	Uncommon/few	Common
	Oedema	Marked	Minimum
	Hyperaemia	Seldom prominent	Prominent
	Lymphoid reaction	Marked	Mild
	Lymphoid aggregate	+	–
	Serositis	Marked/variable	Absent/mild
	Mucin producing cells	Slightly reduced	Depleted
	Granuloma	Common (50%)	No
	Fistulas and sinuses	+	–
	Neurotic hyperplasia	Common	–
	Lymph node	Granuloma+	–
	Inflammatory pseudopolyps	Less common	Common

ACUTE AND CHRONIC APPENDICITIS

Appendiceal inflammation is associated with obstruction, usually by fecolith and less commonly by a gallstone or ball of *E. vermicularis* worms. Continued secretion of mucinous material in the obstructed appendix presumably leads to increased intraluminal pressure and ischaemia which favours bacterial growth and inflammation.

Acute Appendicitis

In early acute appendicitis, wall is oedematous; serosa shows fibrinopurulent exudate with congested vessels.

In acute suppurative appendicitis, mucosa is ulcerated. The wall is oedematous. It is infiltrated by acute inflammatory cells and foci of necrosis are present. Serosa is covered with purulent exudate.

Further vascular compromise leads to gangrenous changes creating acute gangrenous appendicitis.

Gross: Appendix is swollen, oedematous and covered with exudate, the serosal vessels are congested. Cut section, lumen shows exudate (Fig. 29.11).

Microscopy: Mucosa is ulcerated, wall is oedematous and lymphoid follicles are hyperplastic. Neutrophilic infiltrate is present in all the layers. Serosa is inflamed and the blood vessels are congested (Fig. 29.12).

Complications of Acute Appendicitis

Perforation: It can lead to diffuse peritonitis and periappendiceal abscess which may perforate into the caecum, ileum or rectum or even open onto the skin surface. Appendicitis with perforation can also result in infertility in women because of obstruction of fallopian tubes.

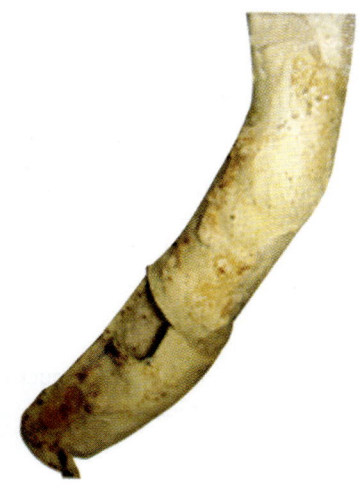

Fig. 29.11: Acute appendicitis, note oedema and exudate (gross picture)

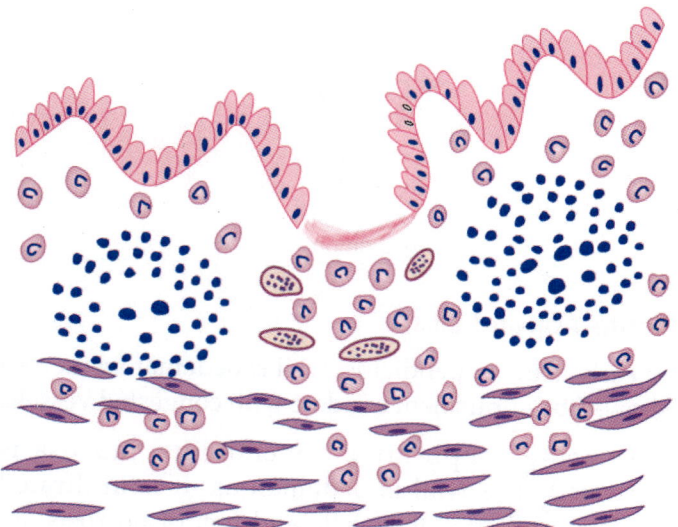

Fig. 29.12: Microscopy in acute appendicitis (schematic)

Spread of inflammation: This is via the ileocolic, upper mesenteric and portal veins to the liver with formation of 'pyelophlebitic abscess' and it is a serious complication.

Periappendicitis: It is the acute or chronic inflammation of the appendiceal serosa. It is invariably present in the advanced stages of appendicitis, but it can also be seen in the absence of a primary inflammation of this organ, as a result of spread of an inflammatory process from another site, such as infection from pelvic organs in females.

Appendicular abscess: This is due to rupture of an appendix giving rise to localised abscess in the right iliac fossa. The abscess may spread between the liver and the diaphragm (subphrenic abscess), into the pelvis between the urinary bladder and rectum and in females may involve the uterus and fallopian tubes.

Adhesions: Late complications of acute appendicitis are fibrous adhesions to the greater omentum, small intestine and other abdominal structures.

Mucocele: Distension of distal appendix by mucus following recovery from an attack of acute appendicitis is referred to as mucocele. It occurs generally due to proximal obstruction but sometimes may be due to a benign or malignant neoplasm in the appendix. Rupture of mucocele can give rise to "**pseudomyxoma peritonei**". An infected mucocele may result in formation of empyema of the appendix.

Chronic Appendicitis

The symptoms and signs of chronic appendicitis are vague. There may be collection of lymphocytes in the muscular wall of the appendix. Plasma cells or eosinophils may be admixed.

Residual changes of acute appendicitis that subsided in the past may be seen.
- If gangrene has occurred, only a stump of the appendix may remain.
- When inflammatory process has destroyed the muscle, fibrosis is present.
- If the original process was superficial and confined to the mucosa and submucosa, no residual changes may be found.
- Many cases diagnosed as chronic appendicitis represent recurrent acute appendicitis.

Gross: Appendix is shrunken in size, it is thin and cord-like.

Microscopy: The mucosa may be ulcerated or shows regenerative changes. It may sometimes show obliteration of lumen with fibrosis. There is submucosal and subserosal fibrosis. The wall shows chronic inflammatory cell infiltration.

TUMOURS OF INTESTINE

INTESTINAL POLYPS

The term polyp of the intestine refers to a protruding epithelial lesion into the lumen, from the intestinal mucosa. Polyps are usually asymptomatic but may ulcerate and bleed, cause tenesmus, if in the rectum and when very large, produce intestinal obstruction.

Polyps can be:
- Neoplastic
- Hamartomatous (Juvenile polyps, Peutz-Jeghers polyps)
- Non-neoplastic

Adenomas (adenomatous polyps): About two-thirds of all colonic polyps are adenomas. These adenomas have dysplastic foci and thus have malignant potential (Figs 29.13 and 29.14).
- *Tubular adenomas:* Tubular adenomas account for more than 80% of the colonic adenomas. They are characterised by a network of branching adenomatous epithelium. To be classified as tubular, the adenoma should have a tubular component of at least 75%.
- *Villous adenomas:* Villous adenomas account for 5 to 15% of adenomas. They are characterised by glands that are long and extend straight down from the surface to the centre of the polyp. To be classified as villous, the adenoma should have a villous component of at least 75%.
- *Tubulovillous adenomas:* These have 26 to 75% villous component. **Polyp base is** sessile–base is attached to the wall of the colon, **pedunculated** if a mucosal stalk is interposed between the polyp and the wall.

Risk factors for malignant potential of adenomatous polyps:
- Adenomatous polyps >1 cm in diameter
- Adenomatous polyps with high-grade dysplasia
- Adenomatous polyps with >25% villous histology
- Adenomatous polyps with invasive cancer

Inflammatory pseudopolyps: Inflammatory pseudopolyps are irregularly shaped islands of residual intact colonic mucosa that are the result of the mucosal ulceration and regeneration that occurs in inflammatory bowel disease.

Juvenile polyps: Juvenile polyps are hamartomatous lesions that consist of a lamina propria and dilated cystic glands rather than increased number of epithelial cells (Fig. 29.15).

Gastrointestinal Polyposis Syndromes

1. **Familial juvenile polyposis (FJP):** Mean age of occurrence <15 years and associated with APC gene mutation. FJP is associated with an increased risk for the development of colorectal cancer, and in some families, gastric cancer, especially where there are both upper and lower gastrointestinal polyps.

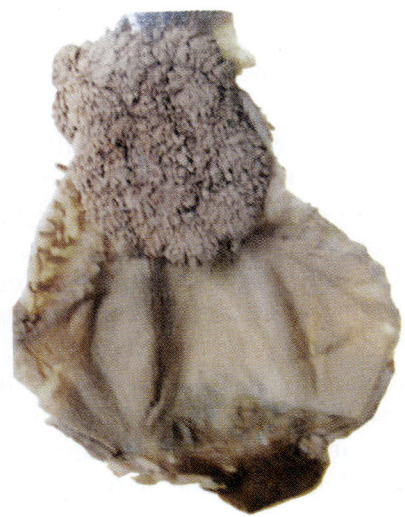

Fig. 29.13: Adenoma (gross picture)

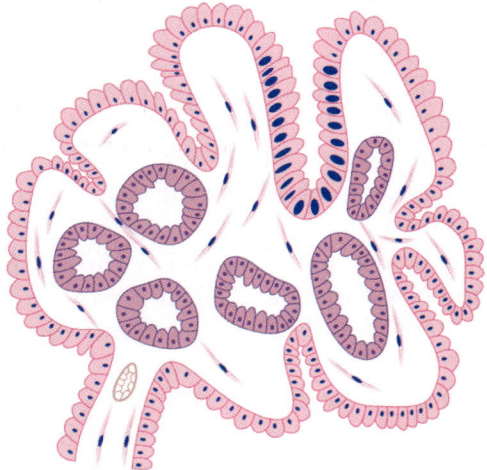

Fig. 29.14: Microscopy of adenoma (schematic)

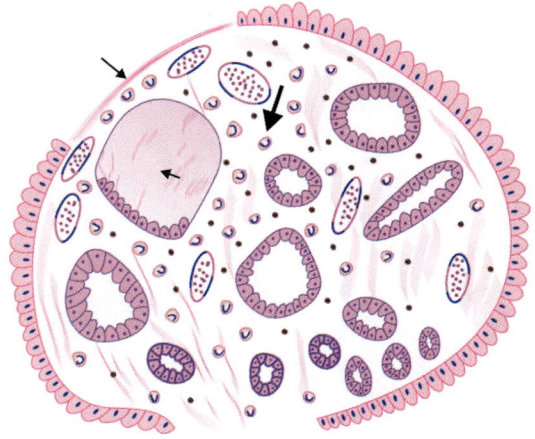

Fig. 29.15: Juvenile polyp. Thin arrow—ulceration, thick arrow—oedema and inflammation, short arrow—mucin in the glands

2. **Gardner syndrome:** It is an AD disorder, mean age of occurrence <15 years and associated with APC gene mutation. **Gardner syndrome** presents with multiple intestinal adenomas, osteomas, skin cysts (epidermoid), thyroid tumours and desmoid tumour.

3. **MYH associated polyposis (MAP):** It is an AR disorder; polyps are less than 100 in number. These have increased risk for colorectal carcinoma. When APC mutations are not present, this can be possible.

4. **Turcot's syndrome:** It is an AD disorder; the syndrome has colonic polyps with brain tumour or medulloblastoma.

5. **Peutz-Jeghers polyps** (Fig. 29.16): The Peutz-Jeghers polyp is a hamartomatous lesion of glandular epithelium supported by smooth muscle cells that is contiguous with the muscularis mucosa. Patients with Peutz-Jeghers syndrome are at increased risk of both gastrointestinal (gastric, small bowel, colon, pancreas) and non-gastrointestinal cancers with a cumulative cancer risk of about 50% by age of 60 years.

6. **Cowden syndrome:** This syndrome has hamartomatous or inflammatory intestinal polyps, lipomas, and ganglioneuromas, mean age of presentation is less than 15 years. The syndrome is associated with PTEN mutations.

7. **Cronkhite-Canada syndrome:** Mean age of occurrence >50 years, presents with hamartomatous polyps of stomach, small intestine, colon, nail atrophy, hair loss, skin pigmentation and anaemia.

8. **Muir-Torre syndrome:** It is a rare autosomal dominant cancer syndrome and subtype of HNPCC. Visceral malignancies (colonic cancer, endometrial cancer, etc.) may be associated with sebaceous adenoma, sebaceous carcinoma, keratoacanthoma. These occur at younger age. The syndrome has mutations of MLH1, MLH2, and MLH6 genes. These help in repair of damaged DNA.

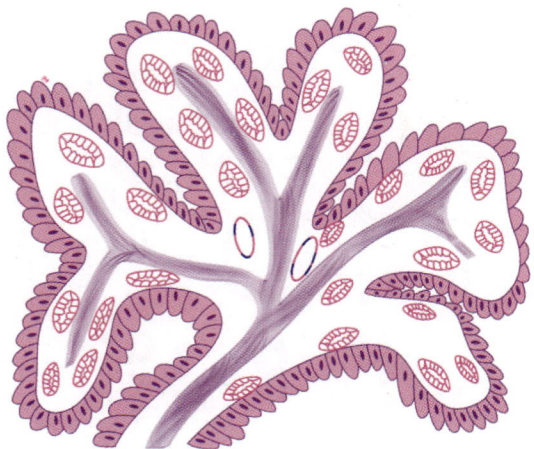

Fig. 29.16: Peutz-Jeghers polyp microscopy (schematic)

9. **Hereditary non-polyposis colorectal cancer (HNPCC)/Lynch syndrome:** This is occasionally associated with polyps, has mutation of DNA mismatch repair genes, autosomal dominant disorder and three family members are affected, one of which is first degree relative of other two or affects two successive generations. HNPCC has high risk for colonic cancer, endometrial, ovary, stomach, small intestine, renal pelvis, ureter and other organ cancers. These patients carry cancer risk around 80% and age of presentation is before 50 years.

CARCINOMA COLON

Carcinoma (adenocarcinoma) of colon is the most common cancer of gastrointestinal tract and is a major cause of morbidity and mortality worldwide.

Epidemiology

Colon cancer is highest in North America, Australia and New Zealand. Colonic carcinomain, 90% of the cases, generally affects patients >50 years of age.

Etiology

Many factors are implicated in causation of cancer. They are listed below.

1. It is associated with many hereditary conditions, syndromes or can occur sporadically.

   i. **Hereditary and familial:** Family history, younger age of onset, specific gene defects, e.g. familial adenomatous polyposis (FAP), Peutz-Jeghers syndrome, hereditary non-polyposis colorectal cancer or Muir-Torre syndrome.

   Patients having relatives with identified genetic predisposition (e.g. FAP, HNPCC) have risk, colon cancer occurs in <50 years of age and runs in families.

   • *Familial adenomatous polyposis:*
     – FAP accounts for <1% of all colorectal cancers
     – Due to mutation of the adenomatosis polyposis coli (APC) gene
     – Numerous adenomas appear as early as childhood and virtually 100% have colorectal cancer by age of 50, if untreated.

   • *Peutz-Jeghers syndrome:* Patients are at increased risk of developing GI and extra-gastrointestinal malignancies.

   • *Hereditary non-polyposis colorectal cancer/ Lynch syndrome:* Colonic cancer is more common than FAP and accounts for ~1–5% of all colonic adenocarcinomas.

   • *Muir-Torre syndrome:* 50% of these cases have colorectal cancer and 15% of the female patients have carcinoma endometrium. The median age of cancer is 50 years.

ii. **Sporadic:** In sporadic cases, there is absence of family history, affects older population and is an isolated lesion.

2. **Risk factors:** Past history of colorectal cancer, pre-existing adenoma, ulcerative colitis, radiation, etc.

3. **Diet:** Diet has special implication in causation of colonic cancer.

   i. Carcinogenic foods, diet with lack of fibre, fresh fruits and vegetables.

   ii. Fat and animal protein: Associated with obesity and increased risk for colonic cancer.

   iii. Lack of micronutrients: Associated with increased risk for colonic cancer.

4. Reduced physical activity, sedentary lifestyle, obesity: Increased risk

5. Alcohol intake: Increased risk

6. Smoking: Increased risk

7. Occupation: People working with wood, metal dust, plastics, fumes of organic solvents have increased risk.

8. Urbanisation: Increased risk

9. Radiation: Increased risk

Pathogenesis

The genetic pathways for colonic carcinoma are:

1. **APC/beta-catenin pathway:** Mutations of adenomatosis polyposis coli (APC) gene and beta catenine regulatory domain initiate majority of colorectal carcinomas. The APC gene is located on 5q21. With mutation of APC, beta catenin is available to bind to transcription factors and activation of proliferative genes takes place. Colonic carcinoma occurs in these individuals before the age of 40 years including teenage (refer to topic on neoplasia).

2. Patients with HNPCC have **mutation of DNA mismatch repair genes.**

3. Muir-Torre syndrome has **mutations of MLH1, MLH2, and MLH6 genes.** These help in repair of damaged DNA.

4. **Microsatellite instability pathway:** The individuals with mutated DNA mismatch repair (MMR) gene are known for instability during replication causing

Table 29.5	Differences between right-sided and left-sided cancer colon (Fig. 29.17)
Colorectal carcinomas begin as in situ lesions, they evolve into different morphologic patterns	
Carcinoma of proximal colon (right-sided cancer colon)	
1. Tend to grow as bulky, exophytic, polypoid masses that extend along one wall	
2. Occur typically in caecum and ascending colon	
3. Rarely result in obstruction	
4. Become quite large before clinical presentation	
Carcinoma of distal colon (left-sided cancer colon)	
1. Tend to be **annular,** encircling lesions that produce so-called **napkin-ring constriction** with narrowing of the lumen	
2. The margins are heaped up	
3. Produce ulcero-nodular lesions with invasion of the wall and desmoplastic stroma	
4. Associated with obstruction and proximal dilatation of colon with attenuation and flattening of mucosal folds. Both forms of neoplasms directly penetrate the bowel wall	

deletions and insertions. In normal health, MMR gene corrects these abnormalities. This is detected in about 15% of colorectal cancers; 3% are associated with Lynch syndrome and 12% in sporadic cases.[31]

5. KRAS, BRAF and P53 mutations may be present.

Morphology

Grossly, bulky exophytic polypoid mass or annular napkin ring like constriction with narrowing and sometimes having ulcero-nodular appearance and desmoplasia (Fig. 29.18A and B).

Most of the colorectal carcinomas occur in caecum or ascending colon, rectum and distal sigmoid, descending colon and proximal sigmoid; the remainder are scattered elsewhere. Most often carcinomas occur singly.

Microscopically, colorectal cancers are **adeno-carcinomas** which may be well-differentiated to undifferentiated and anaplastic. Many produce mucin and these secretions spread through the gut wall and facilitate cancer extension and worsen the prognosis. Cancers of the anal canal and anorectal junction can be adenosquamous or squamous cell carcinomas (Table 29.6).

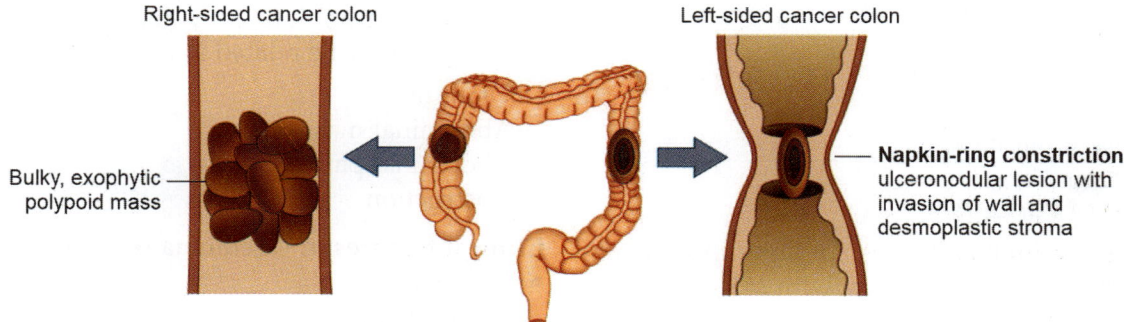

Right-sided cancer colon

Left-sided cancer colon

Bulky, exophytic polypoid mass

Napkin-ring constriction ulceronodular lesion with invasion of wall and desmoplastic stroma

Fig. 29.17: Right-sided and left-sided cancer colon (schematic)

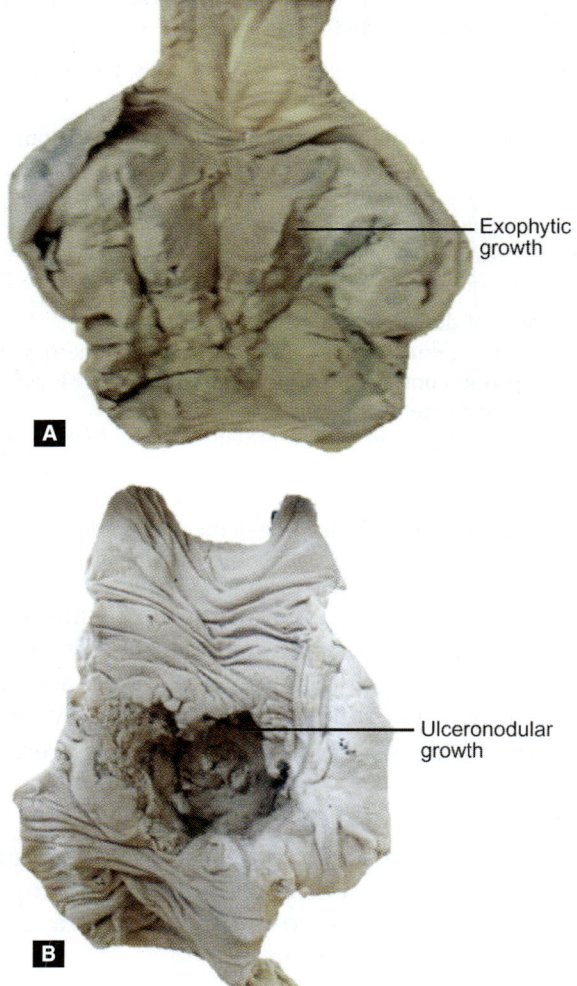

Figs 29.18A and B: Carcinoma colon (gross pictures)

Table 29.6	Histological types of colorectal carcinomas (WHO 2010 with slight modification)

- Adenocarcinoma–NOS
- Mucinous adenocarcinoma
- Signet ring cell carcinoma
- Small cell carcinoma
- Micropapillary carcinoma
- Serrated adenocarcinoma
- Cribriform comado type adenocarcinoma
- Adenosquamous carcinoma
- Squamous cell carcinoma
- Medullary carcinoma
- Undifferentiated carcinoma

Importance of Variants

1. **Mucinous carcinoma:** This is common in patients with HNPCC. Adenocarcinoma with at least 50% of the tumour component is mucinous and should be termed as mucinous adenocarcinoma.

Mucinous carcinomas are more aggressive than the non-mucinous counterparts as they show extensive involvement.

2. **Signet ring cell carcinoma:** When more than 50% of the cells are signet ring cells. These have aggressive behaviour.

Histologically, adenocarcinoma is graded as:
- **Grade I (well differentiate):** Orderly well formed glands, mainly tubular glands, no stratification, nuclei uniform and basal, no loss of polarity.
- **Grade II (moderately differentiated):** Tubules simple or complex, irregular, loss of polarity, nuclei highly pleomorphic, stratification present.
- **Grade III (poorly differentiated):** No glands, nuclei highly atypical, stratification present.

They can also graded as low and high grades:
- *Low grade:* Includes grade I and II.
- *High grade:* Includes grade III.

Clinical Features

The symptoms are related to gastrointestinal tract or constitutional in nature. Weight loss, and malaise are commonly encountered. The initial symptoms are vague and non-specific. Late symptoms produce definitive diagnosis. These symptoms depend upon the location of tumour. They may produce perforation and peritonitis due to invasion. There may be hepatomegaly due to metastasis.

Clinical features in left-sided colonic carcinoma (descending colon):
- *Early features:*
  1. Change in bowel habits
  2. Sensation of incomplete emptying
  3. Bleeding
- *Late features:*
  1. Obstruction
  2. Abdominal pain
  3. Incontinence

Clinical features in right-sided colonic cancer: These may be clinically silent and fail to produce any symptoms. Weakness, fatigue and weight loss may occur due to iron deficiency anaemia, cardiac failure and angina may be related to anaemia.

Late features
1. Abdominal mass
2. Abdominal pain
3. Obstruction

Clinical features of carcinoma rectum:
- *Early features:*
  1. Bleeding
  2. Change in stool caliber

3. Tenesmus
4. Rectal mass
- *Late features*
  1. Pain
  2. Obstruction (rare)

Diagnosis

1. Faecal occult blood
2. Colonoscopy
3. Anorectal ultrasound
4. CT and MRI—staging prior to treatment
5. Blood tests:
   - To establish type of anaemia
   - Tumour marker CEA: Useful for monitoring progress but not specific for diagnosis

CARCINOID TUMOURS

These arise from neuroendocrine cells which are present in GI tract and many other organs which synthesize and secrete variety of bioactive products and hormones. The carcinoid syndrome occurs in 1% of the tumours due to elaboration of 5-hydroxytryptamine (5-HT) and its metabolites—histamine, serotonine, bradykinin and prostaglandins. 5-hydroxyindoleacetic acid (5-HIAA) is elevated in blood and urine. In liver, 5-HIAA is converted into inactive substance. With liver metastasis, 5-HIAA cannot be inactivated and the classical syndrome occurs. The features of carcinoid syndrome are:
1. Cutaneous flushing
2. Diarrhoea
3. Abdominal cramps
4. Dyspnoea
5. Bronchospasm
6. Dementia
7. Dermatitis
8. Cardiac involvement: Increasaed heart rate, murmurs

Sites: Appendix, small intestine (ileum), rectum and colon, as paraneoplastic syndrome in lung tumours.

Gross: Intramural or submucosal polypoid lesions, rarely more than 3 cm. They are solid, yellow tan-coloured and firm because of fibrosis. In appendix occurs at the tip.

Microscopy: The cells have pink granular cytoplasm and round to oval stippled nuclei (salt-and-pepper nuclei) with minimal variation. Mitoses are infrequent or absent. The cells are arranged in trabacular, acinar, insular or solid patterns. The cells are positive for chromogranin, synaptophysin and neuron specific enolase. Larger size, recurrence and microscopy with atypia, mitoses, angiolymphatic invasion and necrosis favour malignant behaviour.

GASTROINTESTINAL STROMAL TUMOUR (GIST)

GIST arises from interstitial cells of Cajal which are present around mysenteric plexus. These are CD117 positive. C-Kit mutations are present in 85% of the GISTs. These are symptomatic or asymptomatic.

Symptoms: Dysphagia, abdominal pain, GI bleeding with anaemia and sometimes massive haemorrhage.

Sites of occurrence:
- Stomach 20–30%
- Colon 5%
- Esophagus <5%

Gross: The mass is of small-to-large size, can be exophytic or endophytic, grey white, solid with cystic degeneration, haemorrhage and necrosis may be present.

Microscopy: There are spindle to epithelioid cells with scattered T cells. These tumours can have benign-to-malignant features. Rhabdoid features may be present. In benign GIST, cells show nuclei with blunt ends or may be pointed. Mitoses are <5/50 HPF. In malignant GIST, cells have high N:C ratio. Nuclei vary in size. Necrosis is common. Mitosis are >10/50 HPF.

NICE TO KNOW

TNM classification of colon

Stage 0:	Tis N0M0
Stage I:	T1 N0M0/Dukes stage A
	T2 N0M0/Duke stage B1
Stage II:	T3N0M0/Dukes stage B2
Stage III:	T1,T, N1 or N2, M0/Dukes stage C1
	T3, T4 N1 or N2 M1/Dukes stage C2
Stage IV:	Any T, N1 or N2/ M1/Dukes stage D

Key for TNM staging

Primary tumour (T)

TX—primary tumour cannot be assessed
T0—no evidence of primary tumour

Tis—carcinoma *in situ*: Intraepithelial or invasion of lamina propria
T1—tumour invades submucosa
T2—tumour invades muscularis propria
T3—tumour invades through muscularis propria into subserosa or into nonperitonealized pericolic or perirectal tissues
T4a—tumour penetrates to the surface of the visceral peritoneum
T4b—tumour directly invades or is adherent to the organ or structure

Regional lymph nodes (N)

NX—regional lymph nodes cannot be assessed
N0—no regional lymph node metastasis

N1—metastasis in one to three regional lymph nodes
N1a—metastasis in one regional lymph node
N1b—metastasis in two to three regional lymph nodes
N1c—tumour tissue subserosa, mesentery, or non-peritonealised pericolic or perirectal tissue without lymph nodes
N2—metastasis in four or more regional lymph nodes
N2a— metastasis in four to six regional lymph nodes
N2b—metastasis in seven or more regional lymph nodes

Distant metastases (M)
MX—distant metastasis cannot be assessed
M0—no distant metastasis
M1—distant metastasis

M1a—distant metastasis to one organ
M1b—distant metastasis to more than one organ

Dukes' staging (Astler Coller modification)

Carcinoma *in situ*
Stage A: Tumour invades through muscularis mucosae into submucosa, does not reach muscularis propria
Stage B1: Tumour invades muscularis propria
Stage B2: Tumour invades serosa
Stage C: Lymph node metastasis (C1: Less than four lymph nodes; C2: More than four lymph nodes)
Stage D: Distant metastasis

SELF-ASSESSMENT EXERCISE

1. **APC gene is on:**
   A. Chromosome 17
   B. Chromosome 5
   C. Chromosome 11
   D. Chromosome 6

2. **Hirschsprung disease diagnosed by:**
   A. Rectal biopsy
   B. X-ray
   C. MRI
   D. Contrast enema

3. **In HNPCC, all are present *except*:**
   A. Extraintestinal manifestations
   B. APC gene mutations
   C. Few or no adenomas
   D. Defective DNA repair

4. **GI endoscopy in an elderly lady with heart burn is likely to be:**
   A. Hyperplasia
   B. Metaplasia
   C. Atrophy
   D. Hypertrophy

5. **Commonest gastric polyp is:**
   A. Hyperplastic polyp
   B. Inflammatory polyp
   C. Adenomatous polyp
   D. FPC

6. **Which of the following is not a premalignant lesion?**
   A. Adenomatous polyp
   B. FPC
   C. Villous adenoma
   D. Hamartomatous polyp

7. **Crypt distortion, crypt abscess with chronic diarrhea is a feature of:**
   A. Crohns
   B. UC
   C. Collagenous colitis
   D. Pseudomembranous colitis

8. **Most common site of GIT leiomyoma is:**
   A. Rectum
   B. Colon
   C. Ileum
   D. Stomach

9. **Most common site of regional ileitis is:**
   A. Distal ileum and proximal colon
   B. Transverse colon
   C. Descending colon
   D. Rectum

10. **Blood levels of CEA is increased in all *except*:**
    A. Colon cancer
    B. Breast
    C. Liver
    D. Skin cancer

11. **Following is the significant risk factor for carcinoma stomach:**
    A. Paneth cell metaplasia
    B. Intestinal metaplasia
    C. Goblet cell metaplasia
    D. Pyloric metaplasia

12. ***H. pylori* is not associated with:**
    A. Gastric symptoms
    B. Stomach cancer
    C. Peptic ulcer
    D. Gastric leiomyoma

13. **Cushing's ulcers are seen in:**
    A. Cushing's disease
    B. Stress ulcers with acute erosive gastritis seen in burns
    C. Due to aspirin
    D. All of the above

14. **Vitamin B_{12} is absorbed from:**
    A. Distal ileum
    B. Mid intestine
    C. Proximal intestine
    D. All of the above

Answers

1. B	2. A	3. B	4. B	5. A	6. D	7. B	8. D
9. A	10. D	11. B	12. D	13. B	14. A		

Liver and Hepatobiliary System

JAUNDICE

Jaundice is the yellowish discolouration of the skin and sclera resulting due to increased serum bilirubin, a common manifestation of liver disorders causing bile retention. Normal serum bilirubin range is 0.1 to 1.2 mg/dl. Bilirubin levels more than 1.2 mg/dl or for classic definition, bilirubin more than 2.5 mg/dl along with yellowish discolouration of the skin and sclera defines jaundice.

There are varied causes of jaundice depending on its pathophysiology. Hence, it is necessary to understand the normal bilirubin metabolism before considering the pathophysiology of jaundice.

Normal Bilirubin Metabolism

A large percentage of bilirubin is derived as the end product of senescent RBCs, mainly in the retico-endothelial organs like spleen and bone marrow. The rest of the bilirubin is derived from the turnover of hepatic haemproteins. Haem which is derived from senescent RBCs is oxidized to biliveridin by haem oxygenase and then reduced to bilirubin by biliverdin reductase.

Bilirubin is then released as unconjugated, water insoluble form and it then binds to serum albumin and is carried in the circulation. In this bound form, it reaches the sinusoidal plasma membrane of the hepatocytes in the liver.

The bilirubin–albumin complex now dissociates and bilirubin is transported across the plasma membrane by recognition of bilirubin by specific receptors on the plasma membrane. Once within the hepatocyte, the bilirubin binds to glutathione-S-transferases.

The conversion of water insoluble unconjugated bilirubin to water-soluble conjugated bilirubin takes place in the endoplasmic reticulum. Unconjugated bilirubin combines with glucoronic acid in the presence of uridine diphosphate glucuronyltransferase (UGT) to bilirubin diglucuronide (90%) and bilirubin mono-glucuronide.

This is the conjugated bilirubin which then diffuses through the cytosol cell membrane into the bile-canaliculi as bile by an energy-dependant process. Bile is then excreted into the small intestine. When it reaches the distal part of the small intestine and the colon, it is hydrolyzed by bacteria to form free bilirubin. A large part of this is excreted in the faeces as urobilinogen. A small part of it enters the circulation and is excreted in the urine. Another small fraction of the conjugated bilirubin is reabsorbed in the ileum and colon and is transported back in the liver and re-excreted as bile. This is called the enterohepatic circulation.

Pathophysiology of Jaundice

Jaundice occurs whenever there is an imbalance between the bilirubin production and its metabolism and clearance. There are four major mechanisms by which jaundice can occur:

1. Increased production of bilirubin (prehepatic)
2. Decreased hepatic uptake of bilirubin (prehepatic)
3. Impaired conjugation of unconjugated bilirubin (hepatic)
4. Decreased hepatocellular excretion (hepatic)
5. Impaired bile flow—intra-/extrahepatic (posthepatic)

Increased production of bilirubin: This can occur due to excessive red cell destruction which could be intra- or extravascular or due to ineffective erythropoiesis. The liver is unable to conjugate the large amount of bilirubin formed, hence leading to **unconjugated hyperbilirubinaemia.**

Causes

 i. Haemolytic anaemias: Thalassaemias, sickle cell anaemia, neonatal jaundice, etc.
 ii. Excessive internal haemorrhages: Alimentary tract or large haematomas
 iii. Ineffective haemopoiesis

This is a predominantly unconjugated hyperbilirubinaemia but when associated with parechymal liver disorders, may involve both unconjugated and conjugated bilirubin.

Decreased hepatic uptake: Any defect in the binding of bilirubin with albumin, its transportation to the liver and its binding with the receptor and cytoplasmic protein can cause jaundice which is again **predominantly unconjugated**. Causes include:

 i. Drugs: Rifampicin, probenicid
 ii. Hepatitis: Viral, alcoholic
 iii. Sepsis

Impaired conjugation: The underlying cause can be hereditary like Gilbert's syndrome and Crigler-Najjar syndrome or it could be acquired as in drugs, cirrhosis or hepatitis. Impaired conjugation is also seen in neonatal jaundice. This occurs due to deficiency or defect of the enzyme glucuronosyltransferase enzyme.

Decreased hepatocellular excretion of bilirubin: This is also called intrahepatic cholestasis and results in predominantly conjugated hyperbilirubinaemia due to regurgitation of bilirubin in the blood. The underlying pathology may be due to damage to the canalicular plasma membrane, alterations in the contractile properties of the canaliculus or alterations in the permeability of the canalicular membrane. Causes could be hereditary such as Dubin-Johnson syndrome and Rotor syndrome, drugs like oral contraceptives and cyclosporine and diffuse hepatocellular damage due to viral etiology, drug-induced or alcoholic hepatitis or cirrhosis.

Impaired bile flow—intrahepatic/extrahepatic: Intrahepatic obstruction to bile could be due to inflammatory damage to intrahepatic bile ducts as seen in primary biliary cirrhosis, graft-versus-host disease and liver transplantation.

Extrahepatic cholestasis which results in obstruction to the larger bile ducts could be due to gallstones, primary sclerosing cholangitis, tumours—both benign and malignant of the bile duct, head of pancreas and sometimes the duodenum.

NEONATAL JAUNDICE

Hyperbilirubinaemia without specific disorders in neonates results in physiological jaundice. The liver in a newborn does not have the capacity to conjugate and clear the bilirubin which is formed at a rapid rate due to increased destruction of circulating RBCs, resulting in hyperbilirubinaemia. It is more common in premature infants due to markedly reduced hepatic glucuronyltransferase enzyme activity and ligandin levels. When bilirubin levels go above 18 mg/dl, it can cross the blood–brain barrier causing kernicterus leading to brain damage. It takes 2 weeks for the bilirubin levels to reach normal adult levels. This jaundice responds well to phototherapy as the unconjugated bilirubin absorbs light and breaks down into water-soluble isomers.

OTHER RARE CAUSES OF JAUNDICE

Gilbert Syndrome

This is a genetic heterogenous inherited condition in which there is a deficiency of glucuronyltransferase enzyme. It results in mild, asymptomatic unconjugated hyperbilirubinaemia with no associated morbidity and may even go undetected for years.

Dubin–Johnson Syndrome

This is an autosomal recessive condition in which conjugated bilirubinaemia is seen. There is a defect in the transport protein responsible for excretion of conjugated bilirubin across the canalicular membrane. These patients have mild hepatomegaly along with darkly pigmented liver because of deposition of melanin-like substance. No morbidity is seen.

Crigler–Najjar Syndrome

Crigler-Najjar syndrome type I is a rare autosomal recessively inherited disorder due to complete absence of hepatic UGT activity leading to marked unconjugated hyprerbilirubinaemia. These patients have neurological problems due to brain damage by bilirubin. When there is partial decrease in UGT activity, it is known as Crigler-Najjar syndrome type II, which is a milder form of the disease.

LABORATORY WORK-UP TO DIFFERENTIATE BETWEEN VARIOUS TYPES OF JAUNDICE

There are various tests to assess the liver function in jaundice which also help us to detect whether the underlying cause of jaundice is prehepatic, hepatic or posthepatic.

Urine bile salts and pigments: These are usually not seen in the urine in prehepatic/haemolytic and some forms of congenital causes of jaundice. In case of hepatic and posthepatic causes, they are strongly present in the urine.

Serum bilirubin: According to van den Bergh/diazo reaction, bilirubin can be indirect (i.e. unconjugated), direct (i.e. conjugated) and total. Total bilirubin is increased in all types of jaundice to varying degrees depending on the severity of the underlying cause. The type of bilirubin seen in prehepatic jaundice is predominantly indirect whereas it is direct in hepatic and posthepatic/obstructive jaundice.

Liver enzymes: There are four major enzymes involved in the metabolism of liver which can be raised in varying degrees in different types of jaundice.

1. Serum glutamate pyruvate transaminase (SGPT/ALT)
2. Serum glutamate oxaloacetate transaminase (SGOT/AST)
3. Alkaline phosphatase (ALP)
4. Serum gamma-glutamyl transferase (GGT/SGGT)

SGPT and SGOT are increased in jaundice due to hepatic injury—especially viral hepatitis. SGPT levels when more than ten times the normal level indicate acute hepatocellular injury. The levels of these enzymes are not very high in intrahepatic cholestasis or post-hepatic biliary obstruction. SGOT might also be increased in myocardial infarction and muscle injury, therefore, SGPT is more specific for liver injury.

Alkaline phosphatase is normal in uncomplicated haemolytic jaundice, moderately increased in hepatic jaundice and markedly increased in posthepatic/obstructive jaundice. This is because, ALP is excreted through the biliary system in the same manner as bilirubin.

GGT/SGGT levels are raised in all forms of hepatobiliary disease and especially in intrahepatic obstructive disorders.

Some other relevant liver function tests include **serum total proteins, albumin, globulin, A/G ratio and prothrombin time.**

It is necessary to differentiate intrahepatic cholestasis from extrahepatic cholestasis. Other than radiological scans, we can differentiate between the two by doing a prothrombin time which is prolonged in extrahepatic obstructive jaundice due to malabsorption of vitamin A, D, E and K and also prolonged in intrahepatic obstructive jaundice due to hepatocellular disease. Administration of vitamin K improves the prothrombin time in obstructive extrahepatic jaundice but not in diffuse hepatocellular disease.

VIRAL HEPATITIS

Viral hepatitis is caused by hepatotrophic viruses. These are the following:

1. Hepatitis A virus (HAV), Hepatitis B virus (HBV), Hepatitis C virus (HCV), Hepatitis D virus (HDV) and Hepatitis E virus (HEV).

2. There can be other viruses causing hepatitis, e.g. virus causing yellow fever, cytomegalovirus and Epstein-Barr virus.

Yellow fever is endemic in tropical areas of Africa, Central and South America.

HEPATITIS A VIRUS

Hepatitis A virus (HAV) infection runs a self-limited course. It has an incubation period of 15 to 50 days (average 28 days). HAV does not cause chronic hepatitis, no carrier state and rarely causes fulminant hepatitis. Fatality is less common (0.1%).

Epidemiology

HAV occurs all over the world, endemic in countries with poor hygiene and sanitation. The disease tends to be mild or asymptomatic especially in children. In adults has higher morbidity.

Mode of Spread

Following are important findings as regards to how HAV spreads.

1. HAV spreads through faeco-oral route, directly from person-to-person or ingestion of contaminated water and foods.
2. Virions are shed in the stool 2 to 3 weeks before and 1 week after the onset of jaundice.
3. HAV is not shed in the body fluids like saliva, urine and semen.
4. Close contact with infected person during the period of shedding, ingestion of raw vegetables and faeco-oral contamination accounts to most of the cases and common with children in schools, play homes and nursery.
5. Viremia is transient, blood-borne infection occurs rarely. Hence, HAV is not a screening test for donated blood for blood transfusion.

HAV virion description (Fig. 30.1)**:** It is small, non-enveloped, single-stranded RNA, 27 nm in diameter,

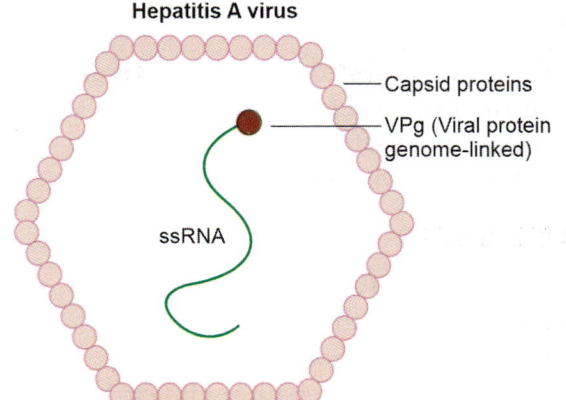

Hepatitis A virus

Capsid proteins

VPg (Viral protein genome-linked)

ssRNA

Fig. 30.1: Structure of HAV (schematic)

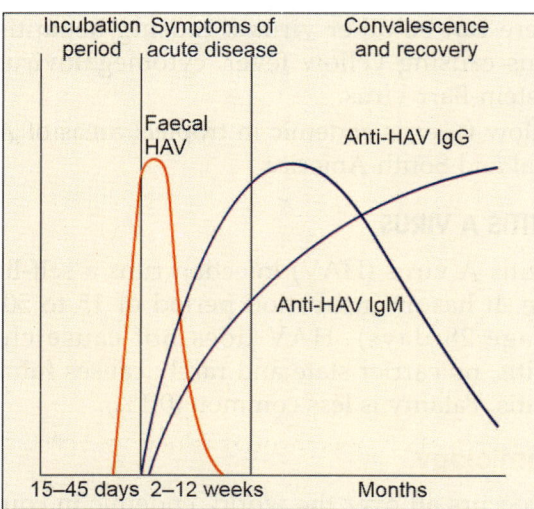

Fig. 30.2: Diagnostic markers in HAV

belongs to picornavirus group. The virions, through gut, reach hepatocytes, multiply and are shed in bile and faeces. There is damage to hepatocytes by T cells.

Diagnosis (Fig. 30.2)

1. HAV shed in stool and bile.
2. IgM antibodies against HAV (anti-HAV IgM) appear at onset of symptoms and persist for several months. This is diagnostic of current infection with HAV.
3. Anti-HAV IgG denotes past infection, persists during convalescence period and beyond and protects against re-infection.

Histopathology

HAV produces acute hepatitis, periportal inflammation and necrosis are common. Plasma cells are prominent. Perivenular cholestasis is seen. There can be fulminant hepatitis with panlobular necrosis with fatty change of surviving cells.

Clinical Course

Clinical course is characteristically mild in young individuals.

Management

1. Hygiene should be focused on disposal of human waste and personal hygiene.
2. Passive immunisation.
3. Prophylaxis with inactivated virus.

HEPATITIS B VIRUS

Hepatitis B virus (HBV) can produce:
1. Acute hepatitis with recovery
2. Non-progressive chronic hepatitis
3. Progressive chronic hepatitis with cirrhosis
4. Fulminant hepatitis

HBV Structure (Fig. 30.3)

HBV belongs to Hepadnaviridae group and is a double-stranded DNA virus. The virus also called Dane particle. It is 42 nm consists of core containing DNA and a DNA polymerase enzyme. The core is surrounded by double-shelled layers.

1. Inner nucleocapsid layer having HBcAgs.
2. Outer surface lipid envelope proteins composed of HBsAg.

The HBV has following features:
1. Core protein HBcAg retained in hepatocytes, HBeAg secreted into blood.
2. Envelope glycoprotein hepatitis B surface antigen (HBsAg) secreted in blood.
3. A DNA polymerase with reverse transcriptase activity is present inside the core.
4. HBV X, a transcriptional transactivator plays a role in hepatocellular carcinoma.

Transmission

HBV is a blood-borne disease can spread by:
1. Parenteral route: Particularly through blood and blood products, dialysis, and IV drug users.
2. It can spread through needle pricks and health care workers are at risk of infection.
3. Contact with semen, saliva, sweat, tears, breast milk, and sexual transmission can also spread the disease.

Incubation Period

45–180 days (6 weeks to 6 months). It is present in all body fluids except stool. It can withstand extremes of temperature and humidity.

Acute Phase

Follows incubation period, lasts for weeks to months.

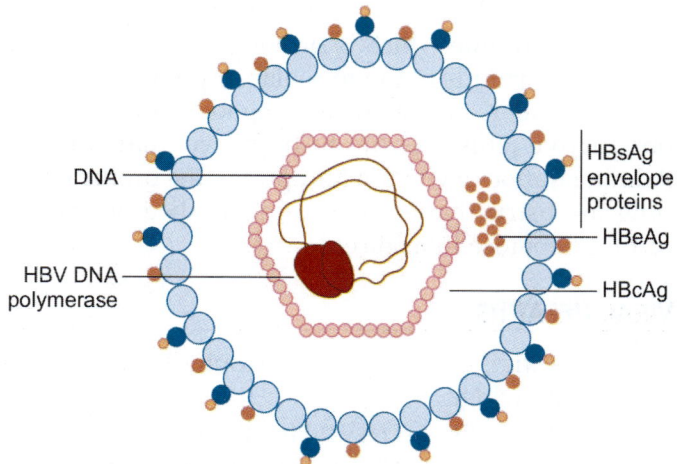

Fig. 30.3: Structure of HBV

Serum Markers in Acute Phase (Fig. 30.4)

1. HBsAg: Appears before the onset of symptoms, peaks during active phase, declines to undetectable levels in 3–6 months.
2. Anti-HBsAb: Does not appear until acute phase is over. Does not appear sometimes several months after disappearance of HBsAg. Anti-HBsAb persists for life.
3. HBeAg, HBV DNA and DNA polymerase appear in serum soon after HBsAg, these represents active viral replication. It is an indicator of viral replication, infectivity and probable progression to chronic hepatitis.
4. Anti-HBeAb: Appears when acute phase is in peak shortly after clearance of HBeAg.
5. IgM anti-C appears shortly after onset of symptoms correlate with elevated serum aminotransferase which is indicative of cell destruction.
6. With decline of IgM anti-HBc, IgM anti-HBcAb is replaced by IgG anti-HBcAb.

HBV infection can be prevented by vaccination and screening of donors of blood, organs, and tissues.

Histopathology

Histologically, the most distinctive feature of HBV infection is ground glass hepatocytes. The cytoplasm of these cells has finely granular inclusions consisting of proliferated endoplasmic reticulum containing HBsAg. These push the nucleus aside and also create halo separating the nucleus from the cell membrane.

Clinical Features

About 65% of the people are asymptomatic. Remaining may have flue-like symptoms, nausea, vomiting and jaundice. About 5% of the affected people get chronic hepatitis.

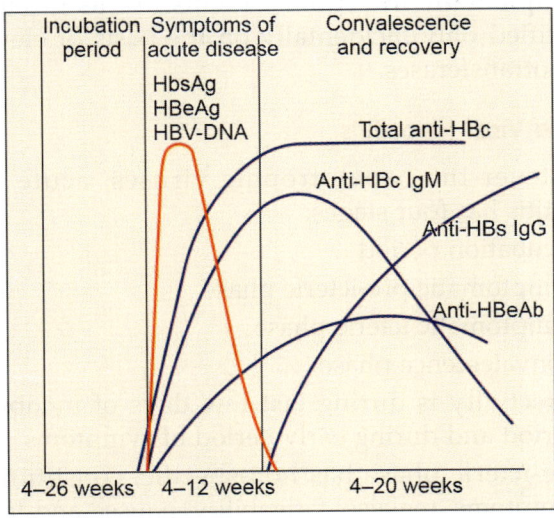

Fig. 30.4: Diagnostic markers in HBV

HEPATITIS C VIRUS

Hepatitis C virus (HCV) is a major cause of liver disease. It produces acute hepatitis, chronic hepatitis, fulminant hepatitis, cirrhosis and hepatocellular carcinoma.

HCV Structure

It is a single-stranded RNA virus and belongs to Flaviviridae group. The ssRNA is surrounded by an icosahedral protective shell, the inner glycoprotein layer and outer lipid layer (Fig. 30.5).

Transmission

Transmission of HCV is through blood and blood products. Drug abusers, health care workers, recipients of blood and blood products are at risk of the HCV. Drug abusers are the most common to get the HCV because of use of unsterilized needles. Sexual transmission and vertical transmission are rare.

Incubation period: 2–26 weeks (mean 6 to 12 weeks).

Acute Phase

The disease is asymptomatic in 75% of the cases. Following are the findings:

1. HCV RNA is detectable in blood in 1 to 3 weeks.
2. Anti-HCV antibodies develop in a few weeks to months.
   These do not confer effective immunity for infection of the disease.
3. In HCV infection, aminotransferases are elevated and represent hepatocyte injury and necrosis.
4. Persistent infection is common with subclinical infection or acute infection.
5. Cirrhosis develops in 20% of HCV cases.
6. Patients can have chronic persistent infection for years with or without progressing to cirrhosis.
7. Fulminant hepatitis is rare.

HEPATITIS D VIRUS

Hepatitis D virus (HDV) is also called hepatitis delta virus. It is replication defective and causes infection

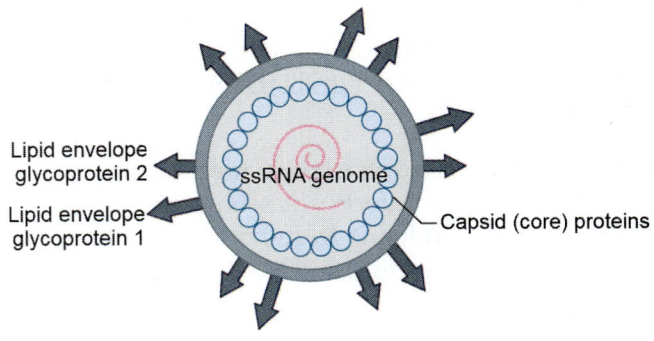

Fig. 30.5: Structure of HCV (schematic)

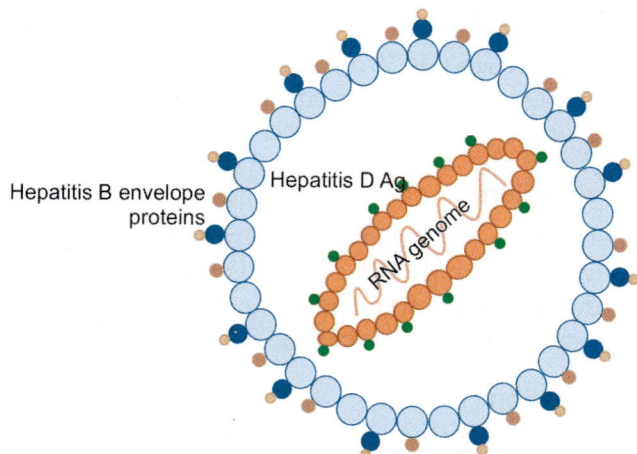

Fig. 30.6: Structure of HDV (schematic)

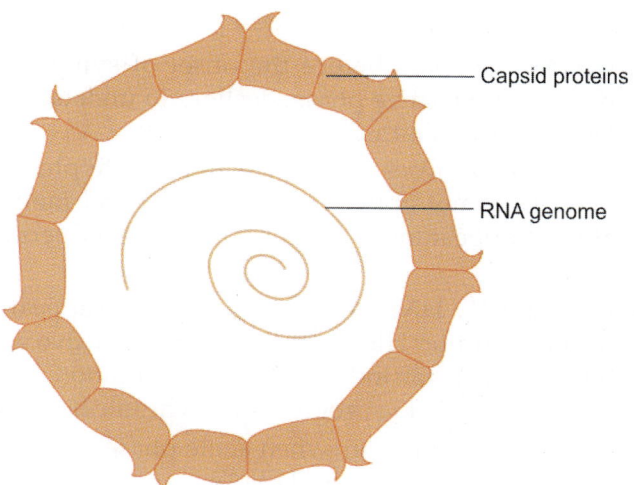

Fig. 30.7: Structure of HEV (schematic)

when encapsulated by HBsAg. Thus, the infection is dependent on coinfection.

Infection can occur when:

1. Exposure to serum infected with HDV and HBV.
2. Superinfection of chronic carrier of HBV with HDV.

HDV Structure

It is a small spherical virion, 30–40 nm in diameter, the ssRNA genome is surrounded by delta antigens and outer envelope protein layer has three HBV antigens—large, medium and small ones (Fig. 30.6).

Following are the findings:

1. In acute symptomatic disease state, HDV RNA and HDV Ag are present in the blood and serum.
2. IgM anti-HDV antibody is a reliable marker of recent infection.
3. IgG anti-HDV antibodies suggest chronicity.

HEPATITIS E VIRUS

Hepatitis E virus (HEV) is a self-limited disease associated with endemic and epidemic acute viral hepatitis in developing countries and does have chronic liver disease or persistence disease.

Structure: HEV is non-enveloped, icosahedral capsid with single-stranded RNA virus and reverse transcriptase of Hepeviridae family. Diameter of the virion is 34 nm (Fig. 30.7).

Transmission: It is a water-borne infection due to faeco-oral contamination. Infection is seen in travellers more frequently. It is endemic in India and epidemics are reported from Asia, Africa and Maxico. It is more severe in pregnant women.

Incubation period: 6 weeks (2–8 weeks).

Disease phase: Infection produces high mortality, especially in pregnant females. HEV antigen is present in hepatocytes during active infection. Virus is detected in stool. Anti-HEV IgM and IgG antibodies are detectable in infected patients.

CLINICAL FEATURES AND OUTCOMES IN VIRAL HEPATITIS

The hepatotrophic viruses produce following clinical syndromes:

1. *Asymptomatic acute infection:* During this period, only serological evidence can support the diagnosis.
2. *Acute hepatitis:* Icteric/anicteric.
3. *Chronic hepatitis* with or without progression to cirrhosis.
4. *Chronic carrier state:* This is asymptomatic without apparent disease.
5. *Fulminant hepatitis* leading to massive or submassive necrosis.

Asymptomatic infection: Patients in this group are identified only incidentally on the basis of elevated aminotransferases.

Acute Viral Hepatitis

Whatever the hepatotrophic viruses, acute viral hepatitis has four stages:

1. Incubation period
2. Symptomatic pre-icteric phase
3. Symptomatic icteric phase
4. Convalescence phase

- Infectivity is during last few days of incubation period and during early period of symptoms.
- Pre-icteric phase has non-specific, constitutional symptoms, malaise, fatigability, nausea and loss of appetite.

- Patients may have low grade fever, headache, muscle and joint aches, vomiting and diarrhoea. These symptoms subside with icteric phase. Symptoms disappear as convalescent stage begins. About 10% of the acute hepatitis B patients develop serum sickness-like syndrome with fever, rash and arthralgia due to circulating immune complexes.

Morphological Features in Acute Hepatitis

In acute hepatitis, microscopy shows:
- Diffuse ballooning degeneration of the cells. The cytoplasm looks empty. With HBV infection, the hepatocytes have ground glass appearance. (Cytoplasm is eosinophilic and finely granular. Hepatocyte cytoplasm is filled with HBsAg.)
- Hepatocytes may have sanded nuclei because of abundant intranuclear HBcAg.
- There may be cholestasis with bile plugs in the canalicul.
- There may be bile duct proliferation.
- There may be apoptotic hepatocytes. In severe cases, there is confluent necrosis with bridging necrosis connecting portal-to-portal, central-to-central and central-to-portal regions of adjacent lobules.
- There is lobular disarray with hepatocytes ballooning degeneration, necrosis and regeneration producing compression of adjacent sinusoids and loss of normal architecture.
- Kupffer cells show hyperplasia and hypertrophy, and contain lipofuscin pigment.
- Portal triads are infiltrated by mixed inflammatory cells with spillage into parenchyma to cause necrosis of periportal hepatocytes.

Following are the findings:
1. Hyperbilirubinaemia (conjugated), with liver damage unconjugated bilirubinaemia.
2. High-coloured urine with bile salts and pigments.
3. Serum aminotransferases are elevated.
4. Stools become light coloured.
5. Due to retention of bile salts, pruritus occurs.
6. On examination, liver is enlarged and tender.

Fulminant hepatitis: A small proportion of patients with hepatitis A, B, and E develop massive hepatic necrosis or submassive hepatic necrosis.

Chronic Hepatitis

In this phase, there is inflammation and necrosis.
Following are the features:
1. Patients are symptomatic, there is biochemical and serological evidence of hepatic disease. Patients can have variable symptoms, common being fatigue, malaise, loss of appetite, and mild jaundice.

2. On examination, spider angiomas, palmar erythema, mild hepatomegaly and tender liver are common features.
3. Laboratory findings reveal prolonged PT, hyper-gammaglobulinaemia, increased serum bilirubin and alkaline phosphatase levels.
4. Occasionally, in patients with HBV and HCV infections, circulating antigen–antibody complexes may produce vasculitis and glomerulonephritis.
5. Cryoglobulinaemia is found in 50% of the HCV cases.

Morphological Features in Chronic Hepatitis

In chronic hepatitis, microscopy reveals:
- Portal tract shows expansion with inflammation and formation of lymphoid follicles. The inflammatory cells in portal tract are mainly lymphocytes, macro-phages, occasional plasma cells and rare neutrophils.
- There is interphase hepatitis with spillover of inflammatory cells into parenchyma.
- Liver architecture is usually preserved.
- Periportal necrosis and bridging necrosis suggest progressive liver damage.
- Portal tract with fibrosis, periportal fibrosis, bridging fibrosis is marker of severe liver damage.
- With continued loss of hepatocytes, formation of regeneratory nodules with fibrosis results in cirrhosis.

Carrier state: A carrier is an individual who harbors the organisms and transmits to others. Carrier may not have symptoms, may have little symptoms and free from progressive liver damage. HBV and HCV have carrier state. HAV and HEV do not progress to chronic hepatitis. HAV and HEV have no carrier state.

Risk of liver cancer: HBV has risk of hepatocellular carcinoma.

ALCOHOLIC LIVER DISEASES

Alcoholic liver disease is related to alcohol consumption. Alcohol has many adverse effects. Risk of hepatic injury correlates with quantity of daily intake of alcohol and duration (at least 80 g of alcohol daily). In western countries, alcohol is the commonest cause for chronic liver disease (around 60%). About 20 to 30% of the hospitalized patients are due to alcohol abuse. WHO global status (2014) reports on alcohol consumption and health. 38.3% of the world's population consumes alcohol regularly. 30% of the Indian population consumes alcohol regularly, about 11% are moderately heavy drinkers and rural Indians consume more alcohol.

Alcoholism is one of the leading causes of liver cirrhosis and liver failure. Chronic alcoholism is the leading cause of poverty in the country. About 3.3 million deaths in India are attributed to alcohol.

Alcoholic liver diseases include:

1. Alcoholic steatosis
2. Alcoholic hepatitis
3. Alcoholic cirrhosis

Alcoholic-steatosis is the initial stage which progresses to alcoholic hepatitis followed by alcoholic cirrhosis.

Pathogenesis

Alcohol-induced liver damage is a multifactorial process. Primary mechanism is oxidative stress.

1. Alcohol is metabolized to acetate by two enzymes. Alcohol dehydrogenase and aldehyde dehydrogenase produce acetate and result in steatosis.
2. Microsomal ethanol oxidizing system: Hepatocellular damage is due to:
   a. The direct toxic effect of acetaldehyde.
   b. Oxidative stress and free radical injury: Results in mitochondrial damage.
   c. Direct effect on microtubule organization: Causing Mallory hyaline/Mallory dense bodies.
   d. Depletion of reduced glutathione (antioxidant) leading to toxicity of free radicals.
   e. Lipid peroxidation.
   f. Activation of cytochrome P450 leads to transformation of some drugs to toxic metabolites.
   g. Steatosis develops due to reduced catabolism, increased lipid biosynthesis, impaired secretion of lipoproteins and increased peripheral mobilization of fat.
   h. Abnormal cytokine regulation: Reactive oxygen species and endotoxins, derived from gut bacteria, release: TNF, IL-6, IL-8 and IL-18.

ALCOHOLIC STEATOSIS

This is the mildest form of alcoholic liver disease. Excessive drinking for 15–20 years produces alcoholic steatosis followed by alcoholic hepatitis.

Hepatic steatosis gives rise to hepatomegaly with mild increase of serum bilirubin and alkaline phosphatase. Complete resolution is possible with cessation of alcohol.

Clinical features of alcoholic hepatitis develop acutely with a bout of heavy drinking. Malaise, anorexia, weight loss, upper abdominal discomfort, tender hepatomegaly and fever are the usual symptoms.

Gross findings: Liver is enlarged, yellow, soft and greasy.

Microscopic findings: Hepatocytes contain fat vacuoles. The accumulation is more in zone 3 area, however, it may be panlobular. No inflammation of fibrosis is present.

Note: Refer to topic on fatty liver.

ALCOHOLIC HEPATITIS

Alcoholic hepatitis is the beginning stage of cirrhosis. Alcoholic hepatitis has four characteristic features:

1. **Hepatocyte swelling and necrosis:** Hepatocytes undergo ballooning degeneration and necrosis. There is fat and water accumulation in the cells.
2. **Mallory hyaline/bodies:** Tangled intermediate filaments accumulate along with other proteins visible as eosinophilic inclusion in the cytoplasm, perinuclear location in hepatocytes undergoing ballooning degeneration (Fig. 30.8). These are present in:
   • Alcoholic liver diseases
   • Biliary cirrhosis
   • Wilson's disease
   • Cholestatic syndromes
   • Hepatocellular tumours
3. **Neutrophil infiltration:** Neutrophils accumulate around degenerating hepatocytes particularly those containing Mallory bodies. Lymphocytes and macrophages also enter into the portal tract and spill into the parenchyma.
4. **Fibrosis:** There is sinusoidal and pericellular fibrosis which surrounds centrilobular hepatocytes. This is referred to as "chicken wire fibrosis". Periportal fibrosis may predominate with heavy alcohol intake.

There may be cholestasis and deposition of hemosiderin in hepatocytes and Kupffer cells.

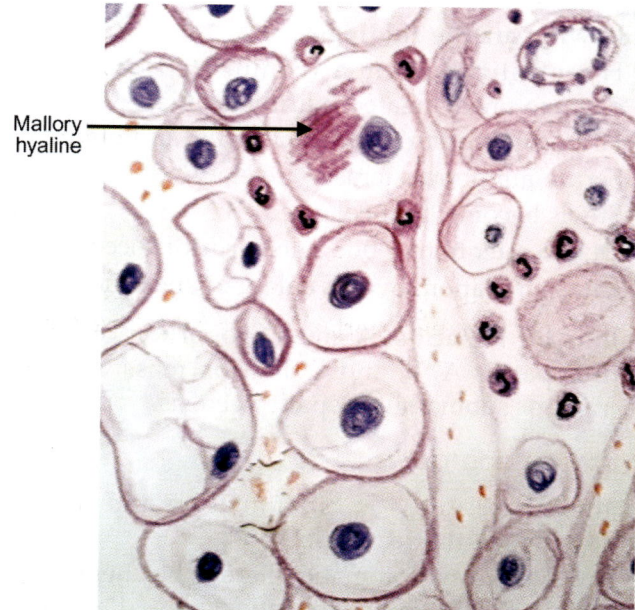

Mallory hyaline

Fig. 30.8: Microscopy in alcoholic hepatitis, note Mallory hyaline and neutrophilic infiltration around degenerating hepatocyte

Grossly, liver has bile-stained areas. Liver is either normal in size or enlarged. It may contain visible nodules.

ALCOHOLIC CIRRHOSIS

This is an irreversible stage. The disease evolves slowly and insidiously. It has following features:

1. Cirrhotic liver is tan yellow, fatty, enlarged and weighs over 2 kg. Over the years, it becomes brown, shrunken, non-fatty and may weigh less than 1 kg.
2. Initially, the fibrous septa are delicate and extend through sinusoids from central vein to portal tract and from portal tract to portal tract.
3. Regenerative activity traps parenchymal hepatocytes with uniform sized nodules. These are less than 0.3 cm in diameter. This is termed as micronodular cirrhosis.
4. The nodules become more prominent and eventually become macronodules. Thus, in a later stage, a mixed nodular pattern develops.
5. Bile stasis develops.
6. Microscopic features of cirrhosis are present. Fatty change and Mallory bodies are present.
7. Mallory bodies and fat diminish in late stages and the size shrinks progressively.

Laboratory findings:
- Bilirubin increased
- Alkaline phosphatase increased
- Neutrophilic leukocytosis
- Alanine aminotransferase elevated
- Aspartate aminotranferase elevated

CIRRHOSIS

The word cirrhosis is derived from Greek word **Kirrhos meaning tawny or yellowish**. It is chronic progressive disease.

Definition

Cirrhosis is characterised by the following.

1. It is diffuse and irreversible.
2. There is loss of normal lobular architecture.
3. There is damage to the hepatocytes with replacement of liver tissue by fibrosis (scar tissue). The fibrous scars may connect portal tract to portal tract, portal tract to central vein or central vein to central vein.
4. The viable hepatocytes divide and form regenerative nodules.
5. There is re-organisation of the vascular channels.
6. These changes lead to loss of liver function.

Tables 30.1 and 30.2 show morphological and etiological classifications of cirrhosis.

Gross findings: Cirrhotic liver is diffusely nodular, firm and variable in size, may be normal/enlarged/shrunken. Capsular surface is nodular. Cirrhosis is

Table 30.1	Etiological classification of cirrhosis	
Alcoholic liver disease		**Metabolic diseases**
Chronic hepatitis		Wilson's disease
B and C viruses		α1 antitrypsin deficiency
Autoimmune hepatitis		Tyrosinaemia
Drugs		Glycogen storage disease
Non-alcoholic fatty liver disease (NASH)		Hereditary fructose intolerance
Biliary diseases		**Indian childhood cirrhosis**
Primary biliary cirrhosis		**Cryptogenic cirrhosis**
Extrahepatic biliary obstruction		
Sclerosing cholangitis		
Haemochromatosis		
Autoimmune hepatitis		
Cystic fibrosis		
Hepatic venous outflow obstruction		

Table 30.2	Morphological classification of cirrhosis

Micronodular cirrhosis: Uniform, small nodules up to 3 mm in diameter, thin fibrous septa. Previously this was known as **Laennec's cirrhosis.**

Often caused by alcohol damage, haemochromatosis, Wilson's disease, primary biliary disease, Indian childhood disease, hepatic venous outflow obstruction.

Macronodular cirrhosis: Large irregular nodules, coarse and thick bands of connective tissue, nodules >3 mm.

Often seen following hepatitis B infection, toxins and poisoning.

Mixed micro- and macronodular cirrhosis: The causes of micronodular cirrhosis can progress to this morphological type.

firmer than normal because of fibrosis and diffuse nodularity (Fig. 30.9).

Laennec's cirrhosis may be yellowish in colour.

Depending upon the etiology, the nodules may be micro- or macronodules or mixed.

Microscopy: Shows the following features (Figs 30.10A and B):

1. Fibrosis surrounds the regenerating nodules.
2. Fibrous septa bridge PT to PT or to CV.

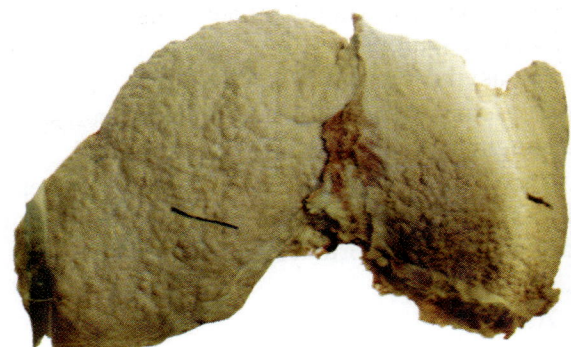

Fig. 30.9: Cirrhosis (gross picture)

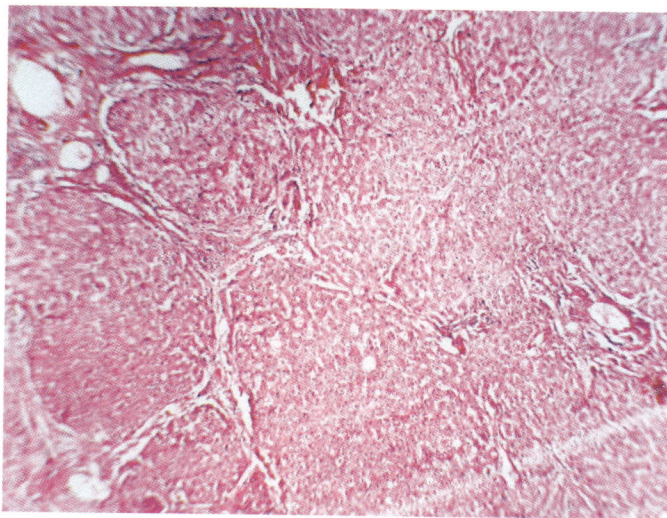

Fig. 30.10A: Microphotograph of cirrhosis

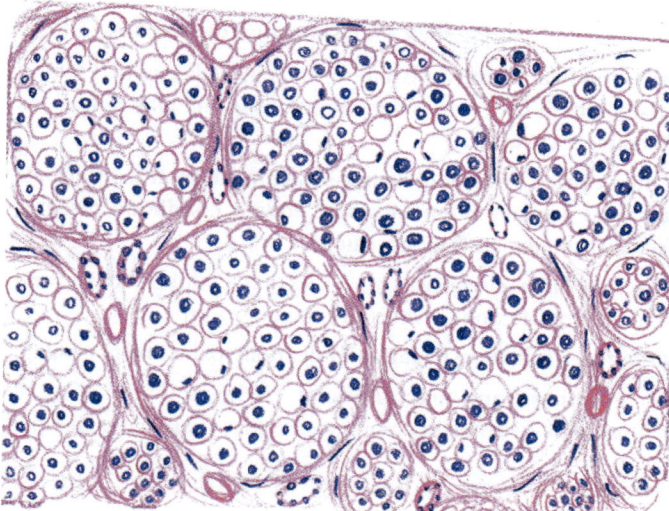

Fig. 30.10B: Microscopy of cirrhosis (schematic)

3. Variable inflammatory cells, predominantly lymphocytes, are present.
4. Bile ductular reaction in fibrous septa.

Clinical Features

The clinical manifestations are similar in all types of cirrhosis irrespective of any cause. Following are the clinical manifestations.

1. May be asymptomatic
2. May present with non-specific clinical manifestations like anaemia, weight loss and weakness.
3. Advanced cases may present with signs of hepatic cell loss with hepatic failure associated with portal hypertension and portosystemic shunts like:
   a. GI bleeding
   b. Ascites
   c. Jaundice
   d. Itching/pruritus
   e. Spider naevi/spider angioma
   f. Palmar erythema
   g. Gallstones
   h. Varices: Esophageal, haemorrhoids, leg veins
   i. Caput medusae
   j. Gynaecomastia (males)
   k. Testicular atrophy
   l. Splenomegaly
   m. Hepatic encephalopathy: Flapping tremors, confusion, delirium, stupor and coma
   n. Hepatorenal syndrome.
   o. Death in these patients is due to liver failure, complications related to portal hypertension, and development of hepatocellular carcinoma.

Pathogenesis

1. **Hepatic cell loss:** Can lead to jaundice, clotting factors disorders, deficiency of vitamine K, metabolic and hormonal disturbances.

   Impaired estrogen metabolism in males can lead to gynaecomastia and hypogonadism. Palmar erythema and spider naevi are also due to hyperestrogenic state in these patients.

2. **Effects of cirrhosis due to fibrosis and re-organisation of vasculature** (Fig. 30.11)
   - Portal hypertension is the manifestation with gastroesophageal varices, caput medusae, splenomegaly.
   - Anaemia, leukopenia and thrombocytopenia are due to hypersplenism.
   - Variceal bleeding leads to haematemesis and melena and also can be another etiological factor for causation of anaemia (iron deficiency anaemia).
   - Fetor hepaticus indicates portosystemic shunting of methyl mercaptans.

3. **Hepatocellular damage and due to portal hypertension:**
   - Ascites
   - Jaundice
   - Bleeding varices (esophageal varices and haemorrhoids)
   - Coagulation factor deficiencies

Features of hepatic encephalopathy: Gut-derived neurotoxins, specifically ammonia, are removed in liver, hence the neurological symptoms, and flapping tremors of hepatic encephalopathy.

Investigations

1. **Liver tests:** Usually elevation of serum aminotransferases, alkaline phosphatase and gammaglutamyl transpeptidase, increase in bilirubin levels, viral markers
2. Ascitic fluid examination
3. Haematological: Anaemia, leukopenia, thrombocytopenia, PT increased

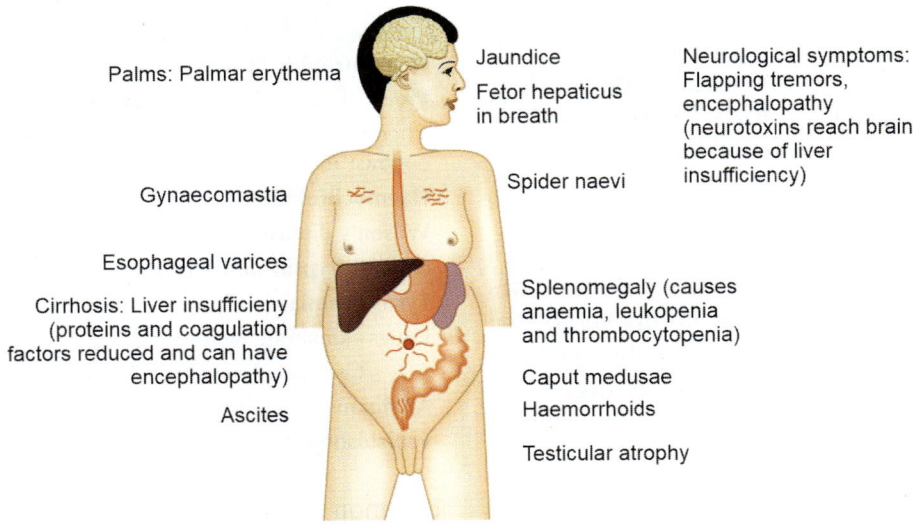

Palms: Palmar erythema

Gynaecomastia

Esophageal varices

Cirrhosis: Liver insufficieny
(proteins and coagulation
factors reduced and can have
encephalopathy)

Ascites

Jaundice
Fetor hepaticus
in breath

Spider naevi

Neurological symptoms:
Flapping tremors,
encephalopathy
(neurotoxins reach brain
because of liver
insufficiency)

Splenomegaly (causes
anaemia, leukopenia
and thrombocytopenia)

Caput medusae
Haemorrhoids

Testicular atrophy

Fig. 30.11: Effects (complications) in cirrhosis

4. **Tests for synthetic function**—serum albumin and prothrombin (reduced)
5. Endoscopy, ultrasound, CT
6. Liver biopsy

Complications

1. Portal hypertension
2. Hepatic encephalopathy
3. Hepatorenal and hepatopulmonary syndromes
4. Increased risk of HCC
5. Bleeding
6. Hypersplenism

PORTAL HYPERTENSION

Portal hypertension is defined as elevated portal venous pressure (PVP) above the normal levels. Normal PVP is 5–10 mm Hg. In PHT, pressure rises more than 10 mm Hg.

Etiopathogenesis

Portal vein is formed from the union of superior mesenteric and splenic veins. As there are no valves, raised portal pressure/vascular resistance is transmitted retrogradely to mesenteric and splenic veins resulting in congestion of spleen (splenomegaly), stomach (gastropathy) and intestine (enteropathy).

Classification of Portal HT

Classification of portal hypertension is given in Table 30.3.

Pathophysiology

As portal venous pressure is increased, there is dilatation of portal venous system resulting in congestion of spleen, congestion of GI tract, formation of collaterals between portal and systemic venous systems. The main

Table 30.3	Classification of portal hypertension according to causes
Type	**Cause**
Prehepatic (presinusoidal)	Obstruction to portal vein before entry into liver, e.g. portal vein thrombosis
Intrahepatic (presinusoidal, sinusoidal or postsinusoidal)	Cirrhosis, schistosomiasis, idiopathic, MPD/LPD, congenital, drugs (vinyl chloride), hepatic fibrosis, sarcoidosis
Posthepatic (postsinusoidal)	Blockage outside the liver— VODs, Budd-Chiari, constrictive pericarditis

collaterals are gastroesophageal junction (esophageal varices), anorectal junction (haemorrhoids), and anterior abdominal wall including around umbilicus (caput medusae). In cirrhosis, there is release of vasodilator substances which leads to peripheral and splanchnic vasodilatation.

In PHT, following are the findings:
1. Blood urea is increased.
2. Pancytopenia is due to hypersplenism.
3. Ascites due to reduced oncotic pressure because of reduced protein synthesis.

Chronic Hepatic Encephalopathy

With liver failure in chronic hepatic encephalopathy, following are encountered:
1. Fetor hepaticus develops due to accumulation of methyl mercaptans.
2. Flapping tremors with stretched hand and extended wrist.
3. Signs of cirrhosis.
4. Neurological changes.

The effects are due to neurotoxins mainly ammonia generated by enteric flora. The other neurochemicals generated by intestinal flora are: Mercaptans, oxindole, phenols, and short chain fatty acids. These accentuate the effects of ammonia such as irritability, convulsions, sedation, muscle weakness, etc.

Hepatorenal Syndrome

This is a reversible and functional renal failure occurs in patients with acute or chronic liver failure and portal hypertension and following changes are observed.

1. Liver failure also can lead to renal changes like glomerulosclerosis, interstiatial fibrosis, and tubular atrophy.
2. There is splanchnic vasodilatation with reduction in effective arterial pressure.
3. Renal vasoconstriction: Can cause acute tubular necrosis.
4. Raised serum creatinine >1.5 mg%.

NEOPLASMS OF LIVER

The neoplasms of liver can be benign or malignant. The malignant one can be primary or metastatic. Most primary tumours of the liver arise in hepatocytes and less commonly they can arise from bile duct epithelium. Table 30.4 shows WHO classification of tumours of the liver and intrahepatic bile ducts.

HEPATOCELLULAR CARCINOMA (HCC)

HCC represents 90% of the primary tumours of liver. This accounts for 5% of all the tumours, and third most

Table 30.4	Histological classification of tumours of the liver and intrahepatic bile ducts (WHO classification with modification)[32]

Epithelial tumours
Benign
- Hepatocellular adenoma (liver cell adenoma)
- Focal nodular hyperplasia
- Intrahepatic bile duct adenoma
- Intrahepatic bile duct cystadenoma
- Biliary papillomatosis

Malignant
- Hepatocellular carcinoma (liver cell carcinoma)
- Intrahepatic cholangiocarcinoma (peripheral bile duct carcinoma)
- Bile duct cystadenocarcinoma
- Combined hepatocellular and cholangiocarcinoma
- Hepatoblastoma
- Undifferentiated carcinoma

Non-epithelial tumours
Haemopoietic and lymphoid tumours
Secondary tumours

Table 30.5	Etiology of hepatocellular carcinoma

Hepatotrophic viruses—HBV, HCV
Pre-existing **cirrhosis alcohol**
Chemical carcinogens—exposure **to thorostat** as radiological contrast medium
Haemochromatosis
Wilson's disease
α-1-antitrypsin deficiency
Tyrosinaemia
Drugs—anabolic steroids
          Contraceptive pills
Aflatoxins—metabolic product of *Aspergillus flavus*
Schistosomiasis

common cause of death globally. Highest incidence is seen in geographical areas with higher incidence of Hepatitis B (most infected are Africa, Asia and pacific islands) and C virus (most infected are Mediterranean and European regions) infections. Males are at higher risk than females. Table 30.5 shows etiology of HCC.

Signs and Symptoms

- Non-specific symptoms
- Abdominal pain, fullness or with mass
- Fever with chills
- Anorexia and weight loss
- Jaundice
- Cachexia
- GI or esophageal variceal bleeding
- Liver failure and hepatic coma
- Invasion of hepatic vein and spread to inferior vena cava: Presents with right heart failure

On examination:
- Liver is enlarged
- Splenomegaly
- Ascites

Macroscopy: Three types:
1. **Unifocal:** Single large mass.
2. **Multifocal:** Many nodules of varying sizes (Fig. 30.12).
3. **Diffusely infiltrating/ spreading type:** Involves entire liver blending with underlying cirrhosis (Fig. 30.13).
   The tumour tissue is paler than normal surrounding tissue. The tumour tissue sometimes has greenish hue. Tumour emboli in portal vein is a common finding.

Microscopy (Fig. 30.14): There are four architectural and cytological types (patterns) of hepatocellular carcinoma:
1. Pseudoglandular (adenoid)
2. Pleomorphic (giant cell)
3. Clear cell
4. Fibrolamellar variant

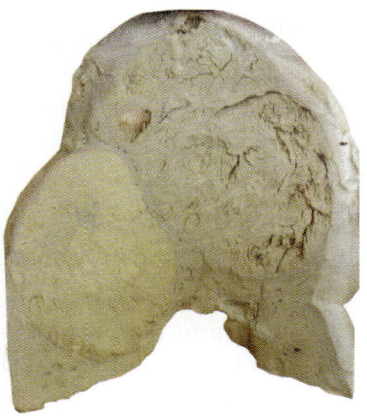

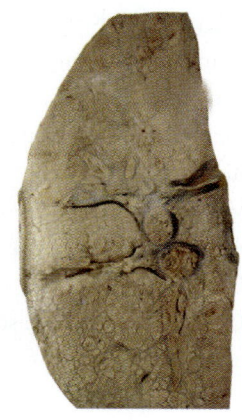

Fig. 30.12: HCC, multifocal

Fig. 30.13: Diffusely infiltrative HCC

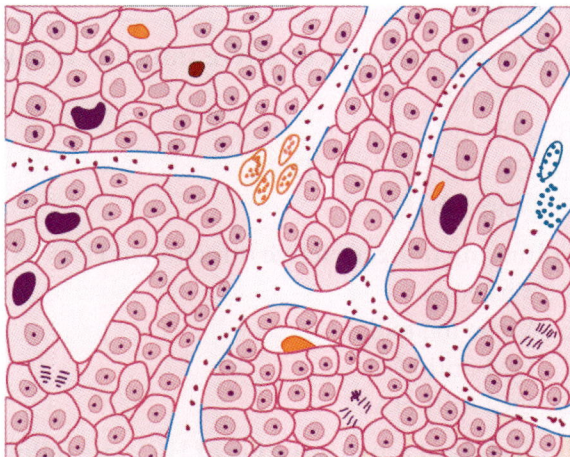

Fig. 30.14: Microscopy of HCC (schematic)

In well-differentiated forms, tumour cells resemble hepatocytes, form trabeculae, cords and nests, and may contain bile in cytoplasm.

In poorly differentiated forms, malignant epithelial cells show varying degree of differentiation. The tumour cells are discohesive, pleomorphic and anaplastic with tumour giant cells. Abnormal mitoses are frequent. Nucleoli are prominent. Cytoplasm is scanty and basophilic. The tumour cells may exhibit intranuclear pseudo-inclusions. The tumour has a scant stroma and central necrosis because of the poor vascularization.

The tumour cells have tendency to invade along the hepatic vein.

Important features that guide treatment include:
1. Size
2. Spread
3. Involvement of liver vessels
4. Presence of a tumour capsule
5. Presence of extrahepatic metastases
6. Presence of daughter nodules
7. Vascularity of the tumour

Investigations

1. Increased levels of bilirubin
2. AFP produced by 70% of HCC and it is >400 ng/ml
3. CT and MRI—localizes the mass
4. Biopsy to confirm the diagnosis
5. These patients may have hyperglycaemia, hypercalcaemia, polycythaemia, hypercholesterolaemia.

FIBROLAMELLAR VARIANT OF HCC

This distinctive variant of hepatocellular carcinoma, clinically and pathologically, occurs in young individuals between the age groups of 20 and 40 years. This has following features:

1. This has no risk factors.
2. Not associated with chronic hepatitis or cirrhosis.
3. The tumour is well circumscribed with central scar, microscopy has laminated fibrous layers with tumour cells scattered in between. The tumour cells have low nuclear cytoplasmic ratio with abundant granular eosinophilic (oncocytic) cytoplasm.
4. AFP levels normal or modestly elevated.

Prognosis: Has indolent course and 60% are surgically resectable.

HEPATOBLASTOMA

Hepatoblastoma is a common primary liver cancer in children below the age of 3 years. It mimics foetal and embryonal liver and often contains heterologous cell types. Most are sporadic but some are associated with genetic abnormalities and malformations.

Risk Factors

Beckwith–Wiedmann syndrome, Wilson's disease, porphyria cutanea tarda, familial polyposis, inborn errors of metabolism and congenital anomalies.

Clinical Features

Abdominal mass, abdominal pain, weight loss, reduced appetite, nausea and vomiting, anorexia, jaundice, fever, icterus and may present with precocious puberty.

Diagnosis

AFP—increased, CT and MRI, abdominal USG.

Gross: Solitary mass often occurs in right lobe. May become large measuring up to 20 cm. Pure epithelial hepatoblastomas are soft fleshy tan white but with predominant mesenchymal tissue it becomes firm and may be calcified. Cystic degeneration, necrosis and haemorrhage may be present.

Microscopy: The tumour cells are well-differentiated to less differentiated. Cells are with high N:C ratio. Tumour cells form cord of 2–3 cells thick and are separated by sinusoids. May present with different patterns like fetal, embryonal, trabecular, small cell and teratoid patterns (can have skeletal muscle, bone, etc.)

CHOLANGIOCARCINOMA

Cholangiocarcinoma is a relatively rare primary neoplasm of liver arising from the bile ducts classified under adenocarcinoma. Risk factors for cholangio-carcinoma are shown in Table 30.6.

Table 30.6 Risk factors for cholangiocarcinoma	
Primary sclerosing cholangitis	Smoking
Ulcerative colitis	Pancreatitis (inflammation of
Parasitic liver diseases (liver fluke)	the pancreas)
	Infection with HIV
Viral hepatitis	Exposure to asbestos
Alcoholic liver disease	Exposure to radon or other
Cirrhosis	radioactive chemicals
Congenital liver diseases	Exposure to dioxin, nitros-amines, or polychlorinated biphenyls (PCBs)

SELF-ASSESSMENT EXERCISE

1. **All are true about HBV** *except*:
   A. HBsAg is positive throughout and later period
   B. Anti-Hbs appears after disappearance of HBsAg
   C. Serum transaminases appear before HBsAg
   D. HBsAg marks the appearance of symptoms

2. **In chronic hepatitis:**
   A. Grading refers to extent of necrosis and inflammtion
   B. CAH and CPH needs be classified
   C. Fatty change is associated
   D. Common cause is HAV

3. **Non-cirrhotic portal fibrosis, following are seen** *except*:
   A. Perivenular fibrosis with PHT
   B. Inflammation of PT
   C. Splenomegaly
   D. Bridging fibrosis

4. **Fatty change is seen in:**
   A. Wilson's disease
   B. Chronic alcoholism
   C. HBV infection
   D. HCV infection

5. **Very high levels of transaminases are seen the following** *except*:
   A. Viral hepatitis
   B. Toxins
   C. Ischaemic necrosis
   D. Fatty change

6. **Risk factors for cholangiocarcinoma are all** *except*:
   A. Choledochal cyst
   B. Working with rubber industry
   C. HBV infection
   D. Liver fluke infestation

7. **Following indicates of active infection of HBV:**
   A. HBsAg
   B. HBcAg
   C. HBeAg and HBV DNA
   D. Anti-HbsAb

8. **Following indicate active infection of HAV** *except*:
   A. Viraemia
   B. Virus in stool
   C. IgM anti-HAV
   D. IgG Anti-HAV

9. **Indicators of active infection of HCV are following** *except*:
   A. HCV RNA   B. HCV antibody
   C. Elevated ALT   D. HCV DNA

10. **True about acute HCV:**
    A. Positive for HCV RNA
    B. Positive NAT HCV test
    C. Absence of HCV antibody in prior 6 months
    D. All of the above

11. **Nutmeg liver is seen in:**
    A. Biliary cirrhosis
    B. Haemochromatosis
    C. Chronic venous congestion
    D. Veno-occlusive diseases

12. **Serum amylase is increased in:**
    A. Chronic pancreatitis
    B. Fatty liver
    C. Perforation of gastric ulcer
    D. Acute appendicitis

13. **HDV cannot replicate without:**
    A. HBV   B. HAV
    C. HCV   D. All of the above

14. **Mallory hyaline (Mallory-Denk bodies) are seen in:**
    A. Alcoholic liver disease
    B. Wilson's disease
    C. Primary biliary cirrhosis
    D. All of the above

15. **Strong predictor of HBV to progress to HCC:**
    A. HBV DNA
    B. Hbs antibody
    C. HBe antibody
    D. All of the above

16. **Cirrhosis is:**
    A. Irreversible with fibrosis
    B. Irreversible with fatty change
    C. Irreversible condition with regeneratory nodules and fibrosis
    D. None of the above

17. **Which enzyme is specific for biliary tree?**
    A. ALT
    B. AST
    C. GGT
    D. Alkaline phosphatase

18. **Elevated alkaline phosphatase denotes:**
    A. Biliary tract obstruction
    B. Bone disease
    C. Placental disease
    D. All of the above

Answers

1. C	2. A	3. D	4. B	5. D	6. B	7. C	8. D
9. B	10. D	11. C	12. A	13. A	14. D	15. A	16. C
17. C	18. D						

Gallbladder

CHOLECYSTITIS

Inflammation of gallbladder is called cholecystitis. It can be classified as below:
1. **Acute:** Calculous, acalculous and emphysematous.
2. **Chronic:** Calculous, acalculous and xanthogranulomatous.

ACUTE CALCULOUS CHOLECYSTITIS

The precipitating cause for acute calculous cholecystitis is obstruction of neck of gallbladder or a cystic duct by gallstone.

There is increase in intraluminal pressure and oedema of the wall of gallbladder.

The main causes for cholecystitis include:
- **Mucosal ischaemia** resulting from dilatation of gallbladder.
- **External compression** of cystic artery by an impacted stone.
- **The phospholipases** released by the injured cells convert lecithin into lysolecithin which is toxic to the mucosa.

Morphology

Grossly and microscopically gallbladder has following features.

Gross
- Gallbladder enlarged
- Tense, oedematous and hyperaemic
- Bright red or green black discolouration
- Serosal layer has exudate in severe cases
- Bile is cloudy or turbid.
- When gallbladder contains pus, it is referred to as empyema of gallbladder.
- When colour of gallbladder is green black and necrotic it is called gangrenous cholecystitis.

Microscopy
- Mucosa may be necrosed.
- Wall is oedematous.
- Neutrophilic leucocyte infiltration in the wall.
- Vascular congestion and haemorrhage are seen.
- Abscess and gangrenous necrosis may be seen.

Clinical Features
- Female
- 40–70 years
- Right upper quadrant pain
- Abdominal rigidity
- Local tenderness

These symptoms may be absent, mild or severe. When patient inhales deeply, right upper quadrant pain is felt (Murphy's sign). Some may be febrile, jaundiced and show leukocytosis.

Complications
- Empyema
- Gangrene
- Perforation
- Pericholecystic adhesions
- Abscess formation
- Bacteraemia and sepsis

ACUTE ACALCULOUS CHOLECYSTITIS

The gallbladder here does not have stones. These individuals have other associated conditions:
- History of trauma
- Incomplete emptying of gallbladder
- Non-biliary surgical procedure
- Sepsis
- Burns
- Dehydration

- Vascular compromise and bacterial contamination
- Ventilation-dependent patients

Morphology

Gross: Has similar features as that of calculus chole-cystitis, but does not show gallstones.

Microscopy: Shows following features:
1. Bile infiltration is deeper into the wall.
2. Neutrophilic leucocyte infiltration in the wall.
3. Mucosal ischaemic changes are frequent.

ACUTE EMPHYSEMATOUS CHOLECYSTITIS

This is an uncommon type of acute cholecystitis caused by bacterial infection with gas producing organisms.

Blood cultures are positive for clostridial organisms and in a few cases *E. coli* or *Bacteroids fragilis* infection.

CHRONIC CALCULOUS CHOLECYSTITIS

Gallstones are present. This type has recurrent attacks of epigastric and right upper quadrant pain. Nausea, vomiting and intolerance to fatty food are frequent complaints.

Morphology

Following gross and microscopic features may be observed.

Gross
1. Gallbladder is shrunken with inflammation and fibrosis.
2. Serosal adhesions may be present.
3. Wall is thickened/thinned.
4. Mucosal ulcers with impacted stones may be present.

Microscopy
- Mononuclear inflammatory call infiltration in lamina propria. When neutrophils are present, it suggests activity.
- Fibrosis
- Metaplastic changes
- Occasionally lymphoid follicles are present. When lymphoid follicles are diffuse it is termed as follicular cholecystitis.

CHRONIC ACALCULOUS CHOLECYSTITIS

These patients do not have gallstones. The possible cause for cholecystitis is gallbladder has incomplete emptying or other associated conditions already mentioned in acute acalculous cholecystitis.

Grossly, gallbladder is shrunken in size, mucosa is opaque and microscopy has following features.
1. Muscularis propria is thickened and shows abundant Rokitansky-Aschoff sinuses.
2. Eosinophils and lymphocytes are the inflammatory cells.

XANTHOGRANULOMATOUS CHOLECYSTITIS

This is a type of chronic cholecystitis with gallstones. Grossly, gallbladder wall appears yellowish. Microscopy shows lipid-laden macrophages, plasma cells and fibrosis. Cholesterol clefts, foreign body giant cells and Touton type of giant cells are also seen.

GALLSTONES (Cholelithiasis)

Gallstones or cholelithiasis accounts for more than 95% of the gallbladder diseases. About 10–20% of the adult population is affected by the gallstones. Gallstones are collections of cholesterol, bile pigment or a combination of the two, which can form in the gallbladder or within the bile ducts. In the West, cholesterol stones are more common.

Cholesterol stones form due to an imbalance in the production of cholesterol or the secretion of bile. Pigmented stones are primarily composed of bilirubin, which is produced as a result of normal breakdown of red blood cells. Bilirubin gallstones are more common in Asia and Africa but are seen in diseases that damage red blood cells such a sickle cell anaemia.

Gallstones, as they are formed in the gallbladder, they can cause blockage of the bile ducts, which normally drain bile from the gallbladder and liver. Blockage of the bile ducts may cause symptoms such as abdominal pain, nausea and vomiting. If the bile duct remains blocked, bile is unable to drain properly, jaundice and infection of gallbladder may also develop.

Occasionally, the gallstones can also block the flow of digestive enzymes from the pancreas since both the bile ducts and pancreas ducts drain through the same small opening (called the ampulla of Vater) which is held tight by a small circular muscle called the sphincter of Oddi. This results in inflammation of the pancreas. This is known as gallstone pancreatitis.

Pathogenesis and Risk Factors for Gallstones

Pathogenesis of Cholesterol Stone Formation

Bile contains cholesterol, lecithin and bile salts. Cholesterol is water insoluble and rendered water soluble in combination with lecithins and bile salts secreted in the bile. There is formation of mixed micelles which are aggregation of cholesterol, bile salts and lecithins.

When bile contains excess cholesterol and when cholesterol concentrations exceed the solubilising capacity of bile (supersaturation), cholesterol can nucleate into solid cholesterol monohydrate crystals.

The excess cholesterol is carried as vesicles. These are unstable and fuse as multilamellar vesicles. The bile with excess cholesterol is called lithogenic bile. When cholesterol to lecithin ratio is more than 1, cholesterol crystallizes at the surface and later into stone formation. Thus, the steps of gallstone formation are (Fig. 31.1):

1. Excess cholesterol as compared to lecithins and bile salts.
2. Establishment of nucleation site by microprecipitation of calcium salts.
3. Crystal formation.
4. Stone formation.

The stone formation requires time and also simultaneously occurs in other conditions. The other factors which influence stone formation are:

- **Hypomotility** of gallbladder which causes stasis of lithogenic bile and promotes nucleation.
- **Mucus hypersecretion** can trap the crystals and can enhance formation of stone.
- **Females with increased level of hormones** in pregnancy, those who are on oral contraceptive pills and estrogen therapy are prone for stone formation.

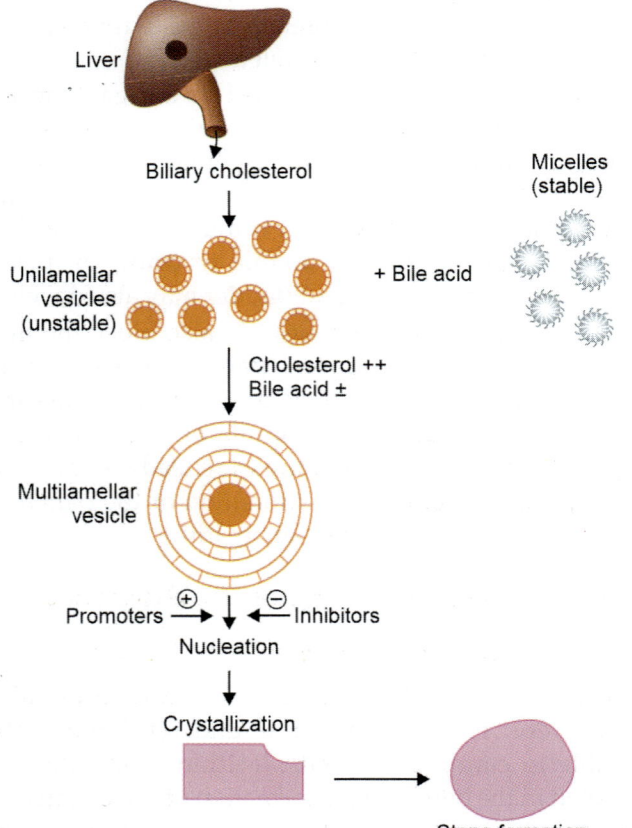

Fig. 31.1: Mechanism of gallstone formation

Pathogenesis of Pigment Stone (Calcium Bilirubinate) and Calcium Carbonate Stone Formation

The process of pigment stone is complex. There is an increased amount of unconjugated bilirubin in the biliary tree. Unconjugated bilirubin is solubilised by bile salts into mixed micelles and later combines with calcium to form calcium bilirubinate. Thus, the conditions with elevated levels of unconjugated bilirubin predispose to pigment stone formation, e.g. haemolytic anaemia. Biliary infection causes bile stasis and predisposed to pigment stone formation. Mucosal infection interferes with acidification of bile resulting in increased biliary pH and subsequent calcium carbonate precipitation.

The major risk factors are the following:

1. **Age and gender:** People over the age of 40 are more likely to develop gallstones than younger people. Women are more likely to develop gallstones than men.
2. **Ethnic and geographical region:** American natives have increased risk of developing cholesterol stones and the prevalence is related to cholesterol hypersecretion in bile.
3. **Heredity:** People with a family history of gallstones have a higher risk. These individuals may have mutation in human cholesterol 7-alpha hydroxylase (CYP7A1) gene and deficiency of this enzyme leading to hypercholesterolaemia and cholesterol gallstones.
4. **Estrogen excess:** Estrogenic influences including oral contraceptives and pregnancy have increased risk.
5. **Obesity:** People who are obese, especially women, have increased risk of developing gallstones. Obesity increases the amount of cholesterol in bile, which can cause stone formation.
6. **Rapid weight loss:** As the body breaks down fat during prolonged fasting and rapid weight loss, the liver secretes extra cholesterol into bile. Rapid weight loss can also prevent the gallbladder from emptying properly.
7. **Diet:** Diets which are high in calories, refined carbohydrates and low in fibre increase the risk of gallstones.
8. **Intestinal diseases:** Diseases that affect normal absorption of nutrients, such as Crohn's disease, are associated with gallstones.
9. **Metabolic syndrome, diabetes mellitus with insulin resistance:** These conditions increase the risk of gallstones. Metabolic syndrome also increases the risk of gallstone complications. Metabolic syndrome is a group of traits and medical conditions linked to being overweight or obese that puts people at risk for heart diseases and type 2 diabetes mellitus.
10. **Liver diseases:** Cirrhosis and infection of bile duct are associated with increased risk.

11. **Patients of haemolytic anaemia:** The red blood cells are broken down with release of bilirubin and these patients are at risk of gallstones usually the pigmented ones.

12. **Pneumonic for gallstones:** 5Fs. These are female, family history, forty, fat (obese) and fertile.

Morphology of Gallstones

Pure cholesterol stones are pale yellow, several and faceted (result from opposition to each other) (Fig. 31.2).

These are radiolucent; around 20% may contain calcium to make them radio-opaque.

Pigment gallstones are black- or brown-coloured; the stones contain calcium salts of unconjugated bilirubin, lesser amounts of other calcium salts, mucin glyco-proteins and cholesterol. Black-coloured pigment stones are usually small, in large numbers and break easily. These are radio-opaque due to calcium carbo-nates and phosphates. Brown-coloured pigment stones are a few in number, soft, greasy due to fatty acid salts (calcium soaps) and these are radiolucent (Fig. 31.3).

Clinical Features

About 70 to 80% of the people with gallstones are asymptomatic or they remain silent, gallstones. Silent gallstones do not interfere with the function of the gallbladder, liver, or pancreas.

If gallstones block the bile ducts, pressure increases in the gallbladder, causing a gallbladder inflammation. The pain is excruciating and constant or colicky. Inflammation of gallbladder along with stones also causes pain.

A gallstone in the common bile duct is called choledocholithiasis and may cause intermittent or constant discomfort. The pain of choledocholithiasis is

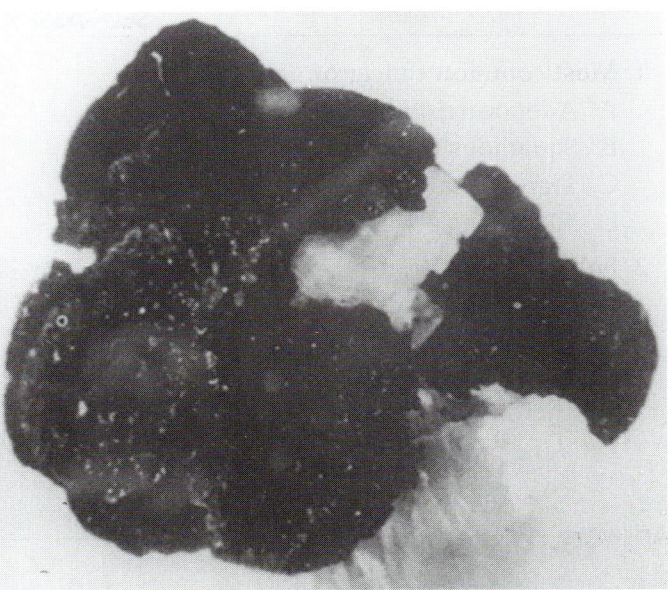

Fig. 31.3: Pigment gallstones

usually localized in the upper abdomen, and can radiate (be felt in another location) in the right shoulder, may last many minutes to hours, and be associated with sweating, nausea and vomiting.

Complications

These include empyema, perforation, fistulae, inflamma-tion of the biliary tree, obstructive cholestasis and pancreatitis. The larger stones are safer than the small ones including gruvel which commonly block the bile duct.

GALLBLADDER NEOPLASMS

These can be benign or malignant. The benign ones are adenomas. Adenomas have to be carefully looked for *in situ* changes. Carcinoma of the gallbladder is the most common malignancy occurring in gallbladder.

The disease is common in USA, Chile and India. It is more common in females than males. The important risk factor for gallbladder carcinoma is gallbladder stones apart from gender and ethnicity. The patients are diagnosed in advance stages and in surgically unresectable stages.

Grossly, two patterns are well recognized:
1. Infiltrative growth pattern
2. Exophytic growth pattern

The infiltrative pattern is common and infiltrates the wall with diffuse mural thickening. It may ulcerate and penetrate into liver and there can be fistula formation. The masses are hard or schirrhous in nature.

Microscopically, 95% are adenocarcinomas and 5% can be squamous cell carcinoma or adenosquamous carci-noma. Minority can be carcinoids or carcinosarcomas.

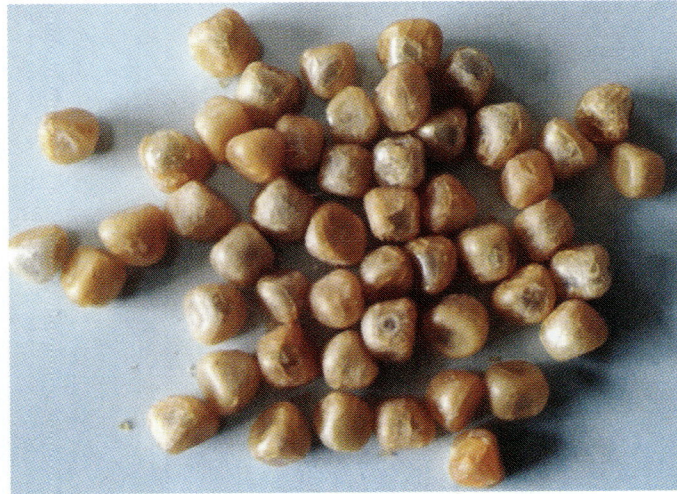

Fig. 31.2: Cholesterol gallstones (yellow-white, faceted and uniform size)

SELF-ASSESSMENT EXERCISE

1. **Most common cancer of gallbladder is:**
   A. Adenocarcinoma
   B. Squamous cell carcinoma
   C. Transitional cell carcinoma
   D. All of the above

2. **Following pattern of carcinoma gallbladder is more common:**
   A. Infiltrative pattern
   B. Exophytic pattern
   C. Microinvasive pattern
   D. None of the above

3. **For gallstone formation, all are true *except*:**
   A. Females   B. Obesity
   C. Estrogen excess   D. High fibre diet

4. **Rokitansky-Aschoff sinuses are present in:**
   A. Gallbladder   B. Urinary bladder
   C. Pelvis of kidney   D. None of the above

5. **Following are causes for lithogenic bile *except*:**
   A. Hypomotility of gallbladder
   B. Mucus hypersecretion
   C. OC pills
   D. High fibre diet

Answers

1. A   2. A   3. D   4. A   5. D

Pancreas

PANCREATITIS

Pancreatitis is defined as inflammation of the exocrine pancreas. Acute pancreatitis can be a reversible condition, if the underlying cause of the pancreatitis is removed; however, chronic pancreatitis is an irreversible loss of exocrine pancreatic parenchyma. The clinical manifestations range in severity from a mild, self-limited disease to a life-threatening acute inflammatory process. The duration of the disease can range from a transient attack to a permanent loss of function.

ACUTE PANCREATITIS

Acute pancreatitis is defined as a reversible inflammation of exocrine pancreatic parenchyma.

Etiology

Alcoholism and biliary tract disease together comprises about 80% cause of acute pancreatitis. Alcoholism is the major cause in male (M:F::6:1) while biliary tract diseases in female (M:F::1:3). Gallstones are present in 35 to 60% of cases of acute pancreatitis. The various causes are listed in Table 32.1.

Hereditary pancreatitis: Hereditary pancreatitis is characterised by repeated attacks of severe pancreatitis usually beginning in childhood (Table 32.2).

Pathogenesis (Fig. 32.1)

The three main mechanisms of acute pancreatitis are:
1. Primary acinar cell injury

Table 32.1	Etiologic factors in acute pancreatitis			
Metabolic	**Genetic**	**Mechanical**	**Vascular**	**Infectious**
Alcoholism Hyperlipoproteinaemia Hypercalcaemia drugs, e.g. diuretics, azathioprine	Genetic mutations in the cationic trypsinogen (PRSS1) and trypsin inhibitor (SPINK1) genes	Gallstones, blunt abdominal trauma, iatrogenic injury, operative injury during ERCP (endoscopic retrograde cholangiopancreaticography) procedures with dye injection	Shock thrombosis, atheroembolism, vasculitis such as polyarteritis nodosa	Mumps, coxsackie-virus, cytomegalo-virus

Table 32.2	Information of mutations in cationic trypsinogen gene and serine protease inhibitor Kazal type 1 gene
Mutations in cationic trypsinogen gene	**Mutations in serine protease inhibitor Kazal type 1 gene**
• Also known as PRSS1 • Germline (inherited) mutations • Autosomal dominant • These mutations alter a site on the cationic trypsinogen molecule that is essential for the inactivation of trypsin by trypsin itself • When this site is mutated, trypsin becomes resistant to inactivation by another trypsin molecule • Thus, if a small amount of this trypsin is inappropriately activated in the pancreas, it can activate other digestive proenzymes, resulting in the development of pancreatitis • Only one mutated allele is required for disease presentation	• Also known as SPINK1 • Autosomal recessive • The gene codes for a pancreatic trypsin inhibitor that inhibits trypsin activity • Pancreatic trypsin inhibitor helps to prevent the autodigestion of the pancreas by activated trypsin • Both the alleles must be inactivated for disease presentation

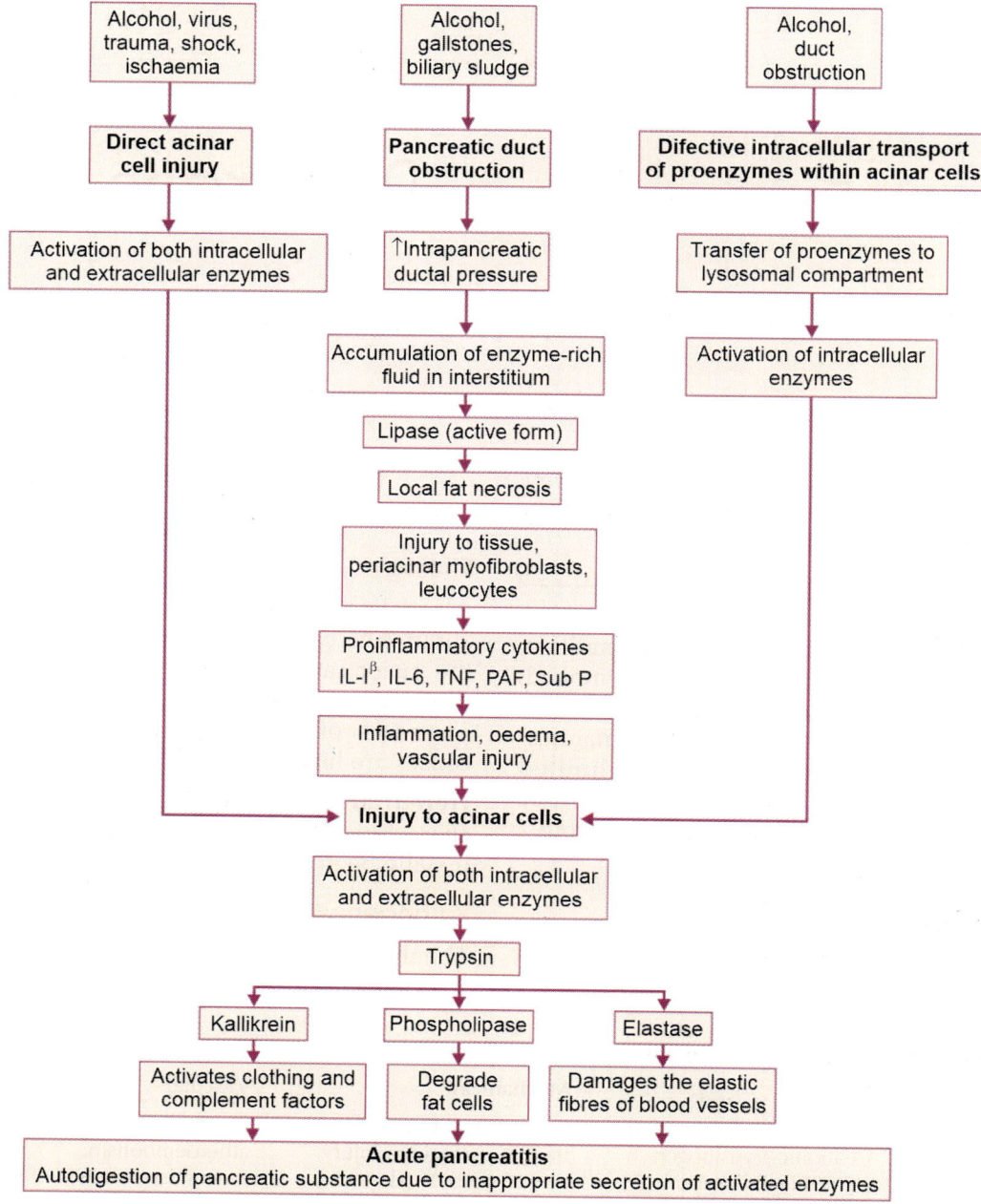

Fig. 32.1: Pathogenesis of acute pancreatitis

2. Pancreatic duct obstruction
3. Defective intracellular transport of proenzymes within acinar cells

These will eventually lead to acinar cell injury causing the activation of pancreatic enzymes. The pancreatic enzymes, including trypsin, are synthesised in an inactive proenzyme form. Once trypisin is activated, it can in turn activate other proenzymes such as proelastase and prophospholipase. Elastase enzymes mainly degrade the elastic fibres of blood vessels and causes haemorrhage; while the phospholipase degrades fat cells and causes fat necrosis. Trypsin also converts prekallikrein to its activated form, thus activating the kinin system, the clotting and complement systems. Thus, the inappropriate activation of trypsinogen is an important triggering event in acute pancreatitis.

Morphology

The morphological features of acute pancreatitis range from trivial interstitial inflammation to severe extensive hemorrhagic necrosis of the pancreas.

The morphological features are:
1. Microvascular leakage
2. Fat necrosis
3. Acute inflammation

4. Proteolytic destruction of pancreatic parenchyma
5. Destruction of blood vessels leading to interstitial haemorrhage

Acute interstitial pancreatitis: This is a mild form of the disease. The pancreas shows minimal inflammation, mild interstitial oedema and focal areas of fat necrosis. Fat necrosis results from enzymatic activity of lipase. The released fatty acids combine with calcium to form insoluble salts that impart a granular blue microscopic appearance to the fat cells.

Acute necrotizing pancreatitis: This is a more severe form of the disease. The entire pancreas including the islets of Langerhans shows haemorrhagic necrosis. Grossly, the pancreas shows areas of red-black haemorrhage interspersed with foci of yellow-white, chalky fat necrosis. Fat necrosis may be seen in omentum and the mesentery of the bowel, and even outside the abdominal cavity, such as in the subcutaneous fat.

Clinical Features

- Acute abdominal pain is the chief presentation of acute pancreatitis. The pain is constant, severe intense and is often referred to the upper back and left shoulder. The severity increases from mild to severe and incapacitating.
- It is associated with nausea and vomiting.
- Acute pancreatitis is a medical emergency. It leads to systemic inflammatory response syndrome (SIRS) causing haemolysis, disseminated intravascular coagulation (DIC), acute respiratory distress syndrome (ARDS), shock with acute renal tubular necrosis and death.

Laboratory Diagnosis

Marked elevation of serum amylase levels during the first 24 hours and levels return to normal within 3 to 5 days unless extensive, there is an extensive necrosis. Serum lipase levels also rise within 72 to 96 hours. Glycosuria occurs in a few patients. Ultrasound shows an enlarged inflamed pancreas. Leucocytosis is also seen. Hypocalcaemia may occur due to precipitation of calcium at sites of fat necrosis.

Complications

Most of the patients recover from acute pancreatitis; only 5% develop shock and die due to complications such as ARDS, DIC or acute tubular injury. A few develop sterile pancreatic abscess or a pancreatic pseudocyst. Recurrent attacks can lead to chronic pancreatitis.

Management

The main principle in the management of acute pancreatitis is "resting" the pancreas. The patients are kept nil per oral with total parenteral nutrition, analgesic, fluids and supportive therapy.

CHRONIC PANCREATITIS

Chronic pancreatitis is defined as inflammation of the pancreas with irreversible destruction of exocrine parenchyma, fibrosis, and, in the late stages, the destruction of endocrine parenchyma.

Etiology

- The most common cause of chronic pancreatitis is long-term alcohol abuse.
- Chronic obstruction of the pancreatic duct by pseudocysts, calculi, trauma, neoplasms, or pancreas divisum.
- Hereditary pancreatitis, caused by mutations in PRSS1 (cationic trypsinogen gene) or SPINK1 (serine protease inhibitor Kazal type 1 gene).
- Cystic fibrosis is caused by mutations in the cystic fibrosis transmembrane conductance regulator (CFTR) gene.
- Idiopathic.

Pathogenesis (Fig. 32.2)

- Repeated episodes of acute pancreatitis.
- Ductal obstruction: Agents such as alcohol is known to increase the protein concentrations in the pancreatic juice. These proteins form ductal plugs which may later calcify.
- Toxin: Alcohol and its metabolites exert a direct toxic effect on acinar cells.
- Oxidative stress: Alcohol-induced oxidative stress may generate free radicals in acinar cells, leading to membrane lipid oxidation and the activation of transcription factors, which induce the expression of chemokines that attract mononuclear cells.

Morphology

Grossly, the pancreatic gland may be hard, shrunken in size and fibrosed with areas of calcification.

Microscopically, chronic pancreatitis is characterised by:
- Chronic inflammatory infiltrate around the pancreatic lobules and ducts
- Pancreatic parenchymal fibrosis
- Reduced number and size of acini
- The epithelial lining of the ducts can be atrophied or hyperplastic or show squamous metaplasia.

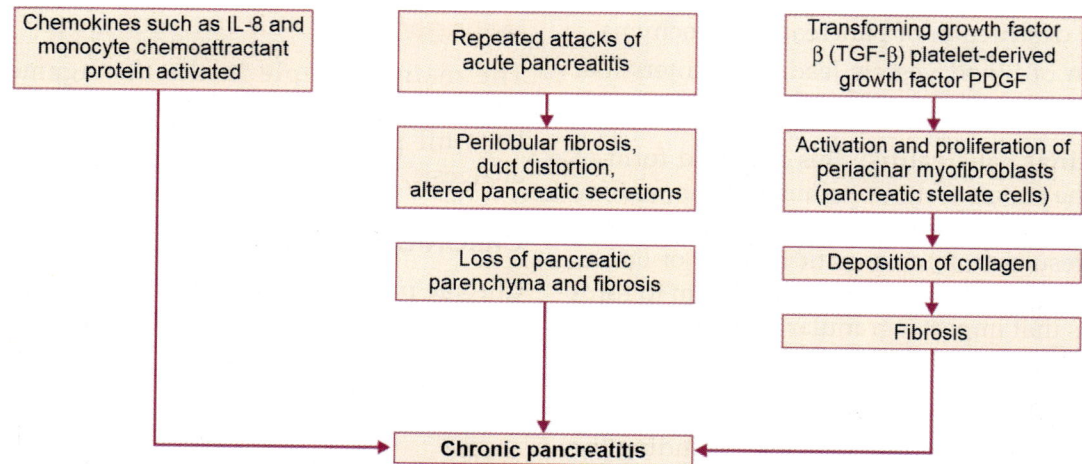

Fig. 32.2: Pathogenesis of chronic pancreatitis

- The interlobular and intralobular ducts are dilated and contain protein plugs in the lumen.
- Relative sparing of the islets of Langerhans initially. In late stages, there is fibrosis of the islet cells leading to diabetes mellitus.

Clinical Features

- Repeated attacks of acute pancreatitis consisting of abdominal pain which can be mild to moderately severe pain, or continuous abdominal and back pain.
- It can be silent until late stages of pancreatic insufficiency and until diabetes mellitus develops.
- Recurrent attacks of jaundice.
- Attacks are triggered by alcohol abuse, overeating or the use of opiates and other drugs that increase the tone of the sphincter of Oddi.

Laboratory Diagnosis

- Diagnosis requires a high degree of suspicion.
- Mild-to-moderate elevations of serum amylase
- Mild hyperbilirubinaemia
- Elevated serum levels of alkaline phosphatase
- Computed tomography and ultrasonography may show calcifications within the pancreas.
- Diabetes mellitus can develop due to destruction of islets cells.
- Severe pancreatic exocrine insufficiency can lead to indigestion and chronic malabsorption

The 20- to 25-year mortality rate for chronic pancreatitis is 50%.

PANCREATIC CARCINOMA

Pancreatic cancer is the fourth leading cause of cancer deaths, preceded only by lung, colon and breast cancers. Pancreatic cancer has one of the highest mortality rates amongst all cancers.

The precursor lesions of pancreatic adenocarcinomas are called "pancreatic intraepithelial neoplasias" (PanINs). Multiple genes are altered in pancreatic cancer. The important molecular alterations in pancreatic carcinogenesis are KRAS, p16/CDKN2A, TP53 and SMAD4.

Risk Factors

- Seen in elderly in the 6th to 8th decade
- Cigarette smoking
- Consumption of a diet rich in fats
- Chronic pancreatitis and diabetes mellitus
- Genetic mutations such as BRCA2 mutations and mutations in CDKN2A (p16)
- Strong family history (3 or more relatives) of pancreatic cancer
- Hereditary pancreatitis and Peutz-Jeghers syndrome are also associated with pancreatic carcinoma.

Morphology

Site: Head (60%), body (15%), tail (5%) and diffuse involvement of entire pancreas (20%).

Grossly, the tumour is hard, stellate, gray-white, poorly defined masses.

Majority of pancreatic carcinomas are ductal adenocarcinomas. Pancreatic malignancies are highly aggressive and invasive in early stages and they produce a desmoplastic response to tumour. Desmoplastic reaction is an intense non-neoplastic host reaction composed of fibroblasts, lymphocytes and extracellular matrix.

Microscopically, the tumour is moderately to poorly differentiated adenocarcinoma, composed of tumour cells arranged in cell clusters, abortive tubular structures or deeply infiltrative growth pattern. The tumour elicits a dense desmoplastic response. Perineural invasion is an important finding in these tumours.

Lymphatic and large vessel invasions are commonly seen. The malignant glands are poorly formed and are usually lined by pleomorphic cuboidal-to-columnar epithelial cells.

Pancreatic cancers can invade into the adjacent organs and retroperitoneum. Peripancreatic, gastric, mesenteric, omental and portahepatic lymph nodes are frequently involved. Distant metastases occur, mainly to the liver, lungs, and bones.

Clinical Features

Carcinomas involving the head of pancreas will obstruct the distal common bile duct resulting in obstructive jaundice. Hence, they are diagnosed at an early stage, whereas, carcinomas of the body and tail do not impinge on the bile duct and usually grow to large size with distant metastasis before they are discovered.

- Obstructive jaundice is usually associated with carcinoma head of pancreas.

- Pain is usually the first symptom.
- Weight loss, anorexia, generalized malaise and weakness tend to be signs of advanced disease.
- Migratory thrombophlebitis, known as the Trousseau sign, is seen in patients with pancreatic carcinoma.

Laboratory Diagnosis

- Tumour markers such as carcinoembryonic antigen and CA19–9 antigen are often elevated, while they are used mainly to analyse the patient's response to treatment.
- Imaging techniques, such as endoscopic ultrasonography and computed tomography, have proved of great value in establishing the diagnosis.

The course of pancreatic carcinoma is progressive and highly aggressive. Fewer than 20% of pancreatic cancers overall are resectable at the time of diagnosis. The 5-year survival rate is dismal, less than 5%.

SELF-ASSESSMENT EXERCISE

1. Malabsorption of fat manifests only when:
   A. With 25% destruction of pancreas
   B. With 50% destruction of pancreas
   C. With 10% destruction of pancreas
   D. With 90% destruction of pancreas

2. Serum amylase rise by:
   A. 24 hours
   B. 6 hours
   C. 72 hours
   D. 3 to 5 days

3. How long serum amylase remains elevated in acute pancreatitis?
   A. Up to 24 hours
   B. Up to 5 days
   C. Up to 10 days
   D. Up to 4 weeks

4. Amylase is found in:
   A. Salivary gland
   B. Small intestine
   C. Pancreas
   D. All of the above

5. In acute pancreatitis, all are true except:
   A. Injury to pancreatic acini
   B. Activation of trypsin
   C. Coagulative necrosis
   D. Acute abdomen

Answers

1. D   2. A   3. B   4. D   5. C

Systemic Pathology II

Lesions of Breast

NORMAL ANATOMY AND HISTOLOGY OF BREAST

The female mammary gland (breast) is covered by skin, subcutaneous fat and lies on pectoralis muscle from which it is separated by a fascia. The glandular unit of breast is made up of terminal duct lobular unit (TDLU) and large duct system (Fig. 33.1).

The TDLU has lobule and terminal ductule, together also called acinus and this is a secretory portion.

The large duct system has subsegmental duct, segmental duct and collecting duct (lactiferous duct) which empties into nipple. The fusiform portion between the segmental duct and collecting duct is lactiferous sinus.

The lobular and duct system has two layers of cells, inner being cuboidal or columnar and outer cells are myoepithelial cells. This is surrounded by a specialized hormonally responsive loose and moderately cellular connective tissue. The interlobular stroma is dense.

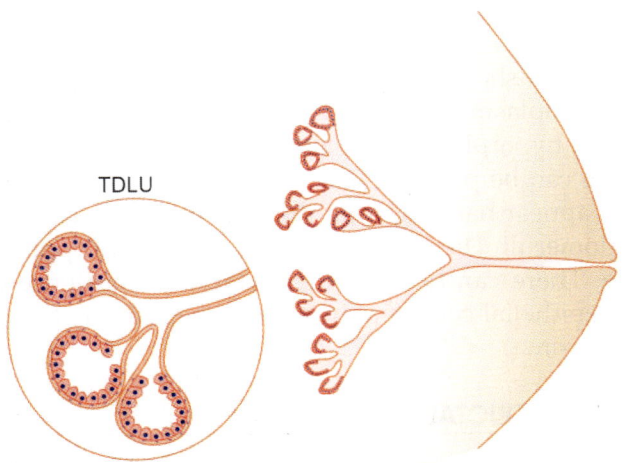

Fig. 33.1: Terminal duct lobular unit and large duct system (schematic)

CONGENITAL ANOMALIES

Supernumerary/accessory nipples or breasts: These can be found along the milk line, anywhere from axilla to inguinal region and subject to changes similar to normal breast tissue including risk of cancer.

Ectopic breast tissue: This can be found in other locations like face, foot, lumbar region, etc. apart from milk line.

INFLAMMATORY AND RELATED CONDITIONS

Galactocele

This is a cystic dilatation of an obstructed duct which usually occurs during lactation. This is painful, may rupture and invite local inflammatory reaction and induration and this is a differential diagnosis for malignancy.

Mammary Duct Ectasia

This is referred to as granulomatous mastitis, periductal mastitis and in the past as plasma cell mastitis.

Other Inflammatory Conditions

Breast abscesses, lymphocytic mastitis, tuberculosis, actinomycosis, sarcoidosis, foreign body reactions, breast infarct and thrombophlebitis (Mondor's disease, involving breast and thoracoabdominal wall) are known.

MALE BREAST AND GYNAECOMASTIA

Male Breast

This is composed mainly of ducts and connective tissue stroma. Gynaecomastia and carcinoma breast can occur in male breast.

Gynaecomastia

Gynaecomastia is the enlargement of male breast resulting from hypertrophy and hyperplasia of both glandular and stromal components.

Causes

- Increased estrogen activity—exogenous or endogenous
- Decreased androgen activity: Before the age of 25 years, it is usually related to hormonal pubertal changes. Later ages, it may be because of following causes:
  1. Hormonally active tumours: Leydig cell tumours of testis, HCG secreting germ cell tumours, carcinoma lung or others
  2. Cirrhosis
  3. Medication: Digitalis, phenytoin

Clinical Features

The mass lies below the nipple. It may be unilateral or bilateral.

Pathology

Gross: It is an oval mass and has elastic consistency with well circumscribed borders.

Microscopy: There is ductal and stromal hyperplasia surrounded by myxoid stroma with halo effect containing large amounts of mucopolysaccharides (hyaluronic acid).

FIBROCYSTIC DISEASE

Fibrocystic disease (FCD) is an important lesion as it may simulate the clinical, radiographical, and gross appearance of carcinoma and also its possible association with carcinoma. Alternative terms like fibrocystic change, mammary dysplasia, etc. have been used. FCD usually has the following morphological changes:

a. Epithelial hyperplasia with or without atypia
b. Apocrine change
c. Cyst formation
d. Chronic inflammation
e. Fibrosis
f. Fibroadenomatoid change
g. Calcification

Epithelial hyperplasia with or without atypia: The lobules, ducts and ductules may be filled with proliferated cuboidal epithelium. Sometimes papillary excrescences project into the lumen which is termed as ductal papillomatosis. Epithelial hyperplasia can be with or without atypia. The degree of hyperplasia can be mild, moderate or severe. The epithelium may show atypical changes in the lobular or ductular hyperplasia, the recognition of which is very important. These are associated with fivefold increase in risk of developing carcinoma. When associated with family history, the risk increases by 10-fold.

Apocrine change: This is very common change and is observed in dilated and cystic structures.

Cyst formation: These can be microscopic or grossly visible cysts. They usually contain cloudy yellow or clear fluid. The cysts may rupture and elicit an inflammatory response in the stroma with abundant foamy macrophages and cholesterol clefts. The cysts may have flattened epithelium or may only have a fibrous wall with or without the epithelium.

Chronic inflammation: This is common but secondary feature in FCD. This is related to rupture of the cysts and release of secretions in the stroma. Lymphocytes, plasma cells and foamy histiocytes are the predominant cells.

Fibrosis: This change is often present, but varies in degree. This is probably due to secondary reaction to rupture of the cysts.

Fibroadenomatoid change: This has microscopic picture reminiscent of fibroadenoma, but lacking the sharp circumscription and is less common change in FCD.

Calcification: This is less common.

DUCTAL HYPERPLASIA/USUAL DUCTAL HYPERPLASIA

Epithelial hyperplasia is also referred to as epitheliosis. This is of ductal or lobular origin. In **ductal hyperplasia** also referred as **usual ductal hyperplasia,** the degree of hyperplasia can be mild, moderate and florid and may be having atypical features.

The nuclei are oval in shape and appear normal. The nuclei may show streaming effect (parallel arrangement). The cytoplasm is acidophilic and finely granular. The tufts of hyperplastic epithelium projects into the lumen. There can be presence elongated clefts and epithelial cells appear hanging from the wall like vascular tufts of glomeruli. There can be bridges connecting opposite side. There can be apocrine metaplasia, presence of myoepithelial cells, foamy macrophages in the lumen and stroma.

ATYPICAL DUCTAL HYPERPLASIA

Atypical ductal hyperplasia should be used for the cells having atypical features, but short to label as duct carcinoma *in situ* (DCIS).

ATYPICAL LOBULAR HYPERPLASIA

Atypical lobular hyperplasia is the term used to describe hyperplasia that is cytologically similar to lobular carcinoma *in situ*, but fall short of features.

For details of DCIS and LCIS, please refer to non-invasive breast carcinomas.

INTRADUCTAL PAPILLOMA

This is a neoplastic papillary growth within a duct. It presents with mass which may be:

1. Solitary/central papilloma
2. Peripheral/multicentric papilloma, or
3. Sclerotic papilloma

These occur in all age groups. Central papillomas are subareolar in location, few cm in size and present with bloody discharge. These usually remain benign. The peripheral or multiple papillomas sometimes become malignant and papillary carcinomas must be excluded. The myoepithelial component is lacking in these lesions.

FIBROADENOMA

This benign tumour is common in reproductive age. It is common between 20 and 35 years of age.

Etiology: It increases in size during puberty and pregnancy and regresses as the age of patient advances. This shows the hormonal influence especially of estrogen.

Gross: These are sharply circumscribed, freely mobile masses and usually measure about 1 to 2 cm or even larger in diameter. The borders of the mass slip under the palpating fingers and hence called "mouse in the breast" (Fig. 33.2).

Microscopy (Figs 33.3 and 33.4): There is proliferation of glandular and stromal tissue. The ducts are round

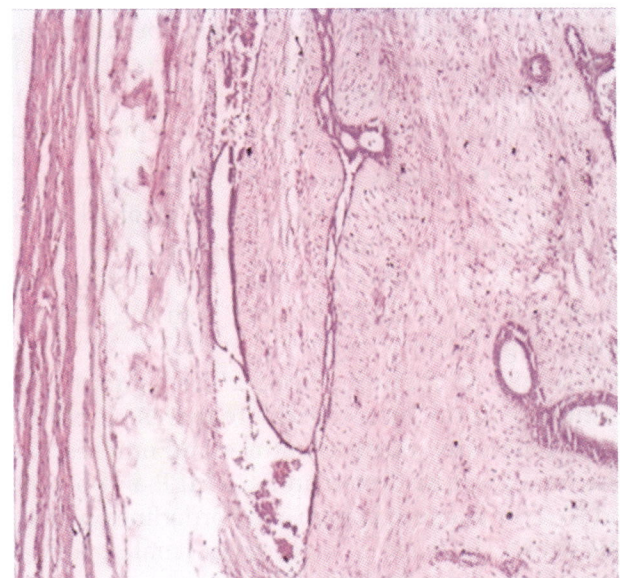

Fig. 33.3: Microphotograph of fibroadenoma, note stromal and glandular proliferation

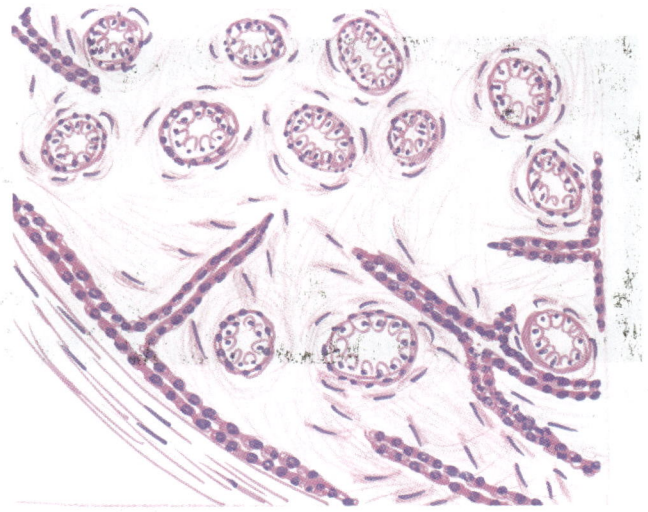

Fig. 33.4: Microscopy of fibroadenoma (schematic)

to tubular, lined by single or multilayered epithelium (pericanalicular pattern) or compressed into slit-like spaces having active proliferation of stroma (intra-canalicular pattern).

Fibroadenoma may show hyalinisation, calcification, ossification, myxoid change, apocrine metaplsia, lactational changes and hyperplasia as in juvenile fibroadenoma. Malignant transformation is rare and seen in 0.1% of the cases.

PHYLLODES TUMOUR

The term **phyllodes tumour** was previously called cystosarcoma phyllodes. Phyllodes tumour generally occurs in older age groups than fibroadenoma.

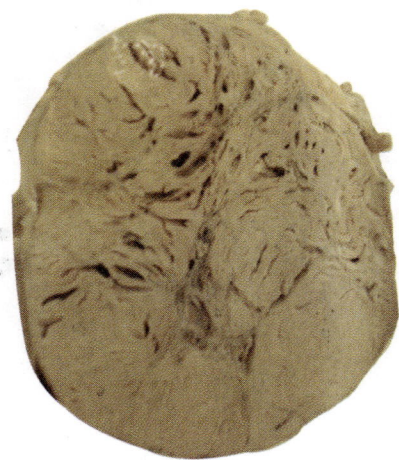

Fig. 33.2: Fibroadenoma (gross picture)

Gross: These attain large sizes than fibroadenomas. These are fast growing tumours. Cut section, the glands exhibit leaf-like clefts and slits (Fig. 33.5A), hence the name phyllodes (in Greek—*phyllodes* means leaf-like).

Microscopy: Phyllodes tumour has features similar to fibroadenoma, but has predominant stromal hyper-cellularity. Thus, the tissue is composed of epithelial and stromal components. There is predominant proliferation of periductal stroma than the glandular element (Fig. 33.5B).

These can be benign, borderline or malignant depending upon histological features, including stromal cellularity, nuclear features and mitoses. Most of the times, mitosis less than 5/10 HPF and between 5 and 10/HPF suggests benign and borderline phyllodes, respectively. The features suggestive of malignancy are:
1. Mitotic activity >10/10HPF
2. Atypia of stroma
3. Stromal overgrowth
4. Infiltrating margins
5. Haemorrhage and necrosis

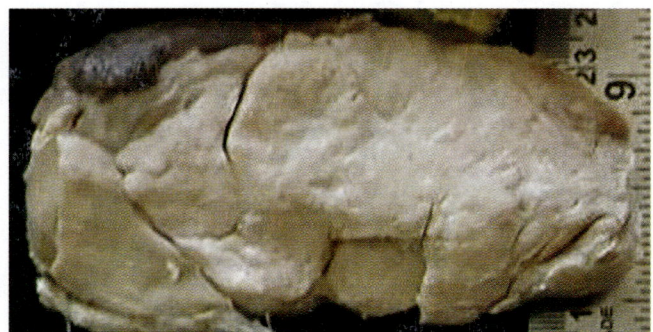

Fig. 33.5A: Phyllodes tumour (A), note extensive stromal proliferation with slits or leaf-like clefts (gross picture) (*Courtesy:* HOD and staff of Pathology, SDM College, Dharwad)

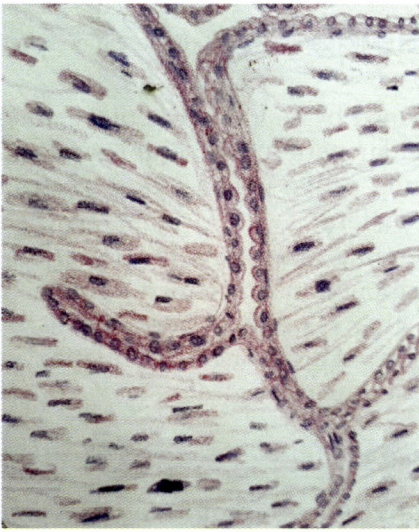

Fig. 33.5B: Microscopy of phyllodes tumour with predominant stromal proliferation

Metaplasia in stroma is more frequent than fibro-adenomas. Stromal metaplasia to fatty tissue, bone, cartilage and skeletal muscle are known. Epithelium can show hyperplasia and squamous metaplasia. Apocrine metaplasia is less frequent than fibroadenoma.

Most of the benign phyllodes tumours remain localized and can be cured by wide excision. About 15% of the malignant tumours may metastasize to distant sites.

PAGET'S DISEASE OF NIPPLE

Paget's disease is a crusted lesion of nipple and was described by Sir James Paget in the year 1874.

This is caused by extension of underlying duct carcinoma *in situ* (DCIS) up to the lactiferous ducts or into the contiguous skin. In 50% of these cases, invasive carcinoma will also exist underneath this lesion. Clinically, Paget's disease presents as eczema-like lesion.

Microscopically, the tumour cells disrupt the normal epidermal barrier and are seen in the epithelium. These cells are large, cytoplasm is clear with atypical nuclei. They are concentrated along the basal layer. They are seen singly, in clusters or small glandular structures (Fig. 33.6). Occasionally, the cytoplasm of these cells may have melanin granules.

The prognosis depends upon the underlying lesion whether DCIS or invasive malignant tumour.

NON-INVASIVE BREAST CARCINOMAS

These are non-invasive malignant tumours involving ducts and lobules. There is no breach of the basement membrane.

Duct carcinoma *in situ* (DCIS): This has different achitectural patterns like solid, comedo, cribriform, papillary, micropapillary and clinging types. Necrosis may be present (Fig. 33.7). The nuclear features may be of low grade to high grade.

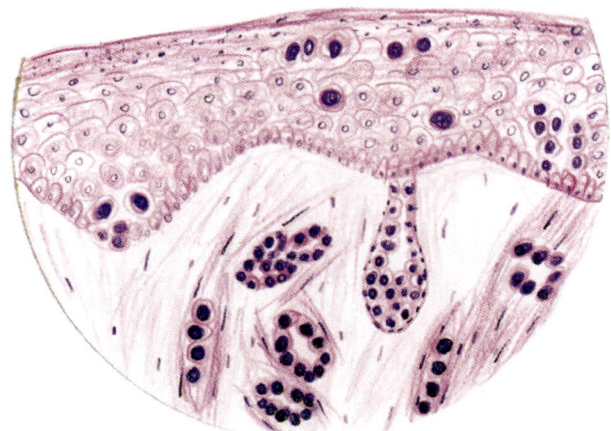

Fig. 33.6: Paget's disease of nipple with underlying duct carcinoma (schematic)

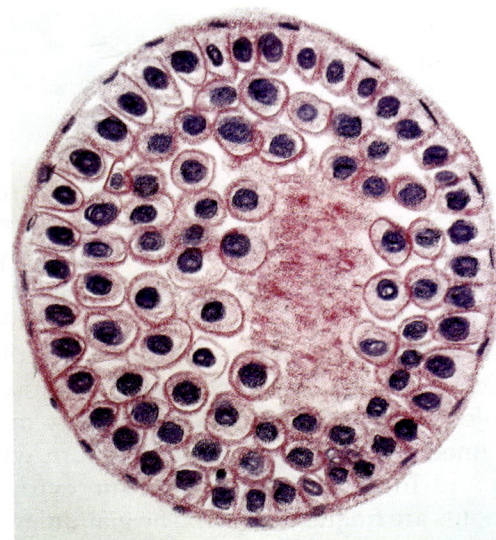

Fig. 33.7: Microscopy in duct carcinoma *in situ* (DCIS), note intact basement membrane and necrosis

Comedo type of DCIS: This has high grade nuclear features with central extensive necrosis. The resected tissue sample when pressed, the necrotic material protrudes like toothpaste or worm. Calcification is frequently seen. The progrosis of DCIS is excellent after simple mastectomy.

Lobular carcinoma *in situ* (LCIS): This has uniform monomorphic cells with bland, round nuclei and occur in loosely cohesive clusters inside the lobules. Signet ring cells are common. No calcificatios is present. LCIS will eventually develop into lobular carcinoma.

BREAST CARCINOMA

It is familial and has about 1.5 to 2 times higher risk in women who are having first degree relatives with breast carcinoma. Mutations of p53 gene are present. Estrogen is known to play a role. Women who are on oral contraceptives, those with increased length of reproductive life and also nulliparous women have increased risk of breast carcinoma. BRCA1 and 2 have increased risk of breast cancer. 17q21 (BRCA1) and 13q12–13 (BRCA2) are the breast carcinoma susceptibility genes and there is amplification of erbB/neu gene in these patients.

WHO classification of tumours of breast is given in Table 33.1.

INFILTRATING (INVASIVE) CARCINOMA

The most common histological type of invasive breast carcinoma is invasive ductal carcinoma. The salient features of these are described below.

Infiltrating Duct Carcinoma—Not Otherwise Specified EB (IDS-NOS)/No Special Type (IDS-NST)

Majority of invasive duct carcinomas fall into this type. This is also called **scirrhous carcinoma.**

Table 33.1	**Histological typing of tumours of the breast**[33]

Benign epithelial tumours: Sclerosing adenosis, apocrine adenosis, adenomas
- Intraductal proliferation: Ductal hyperplasia, atypical ductal hyperplasia
- Precursor lesions: Duct carcinoma *in situ*, lobular carcinoma *in situ*, atypical lobular hyperplasia
- Papillary lesions: Intraductal papilloma, intraductal papillary carcinoma, solid papillary carcinoma
- Epithelial myoepithelial: Pleomorphic adenoma, adenoid cystic carcinoma

Malignant epithelial tumours
- Invasive carcinoma: No special type/not otherwise specified
- Invasive lobular carcinoma: Classic, solid, alveolar, pleomorphic
- Tubular carcinoma
- Mucinous carcinoma
- Cribriform carcinoma
- Medullary pattern: Medullary carcinoma, atypical medullary carcinoma, invasive carcinoma no special type with medullary feat
- Carcinoma with apocrine differentiation
- Carcinoma with signet ring differentiation:
- Secretory carcinoma
- Invasive papillary carcinoma
- Salivary gland tumours

Neuroendocrine tumours
Metaplastic carcinoma with mesenchymal differentiation
- Adenosarcoma
- Squamous cell carcinoma
- Spindle cell carcinoma with mesenchymal differentiation

Mesenchymal tumours
Fibroepithelial tumours
Malignant lymphomas
Metastatic tumours

Note: Modified WHO (2012) classification of tumours of the breast

Gross: The gross appearance of this is typical with irregular and stellate outline. They are delimited, firm or hard, about 1 to 2 cm masses and they infiltrate into the surrounding tissue with fixation to the chest wall. Cut section of the tumour is retracted below the cut surface and it is gritty to cut (Figs 33.8A and B).

Microscopy: The malignant cells are in cords, solid cell nests, tubules and glandular pattern. Depending upon the nuclear atypia, tubule formation and mitosis, they are categorized into well, moderately or poorly differentiated varieties (Fig. 33.9).

Some of the Invasive Breast Carcinomas with Favourable Prognosis

1. Tubular carcinoma
2. Mucinous carcinoma
3. Cribriform carcinoma
4. Medullary carcinoma
5. Secretory carcinoma

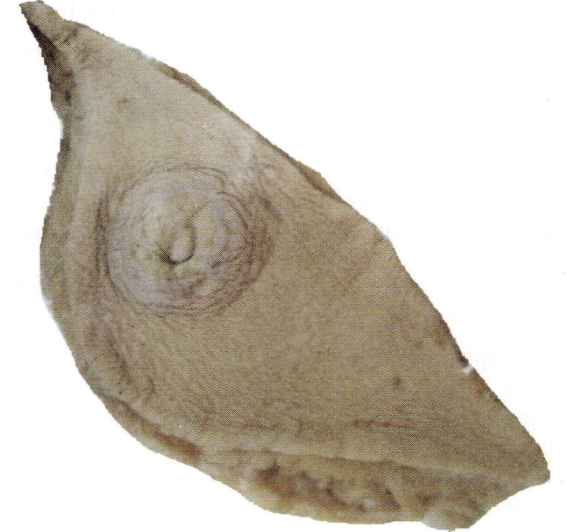

Fig. 33.8A: Infiltrating duct carcinoma breast, note retracted nipple (gross picture)

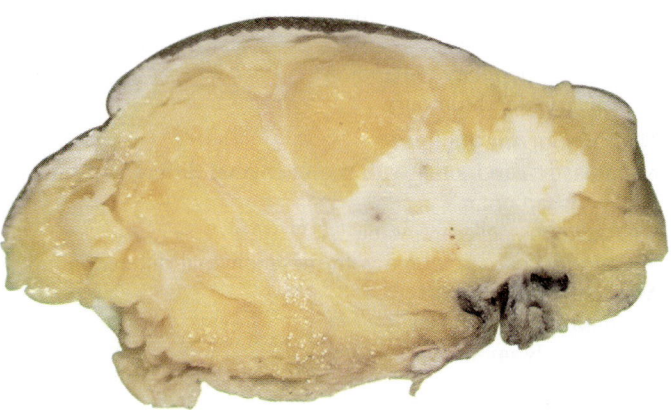

Fig. 33.8B: Infiltrating duct carcinoma breast (gross picture—C/S)

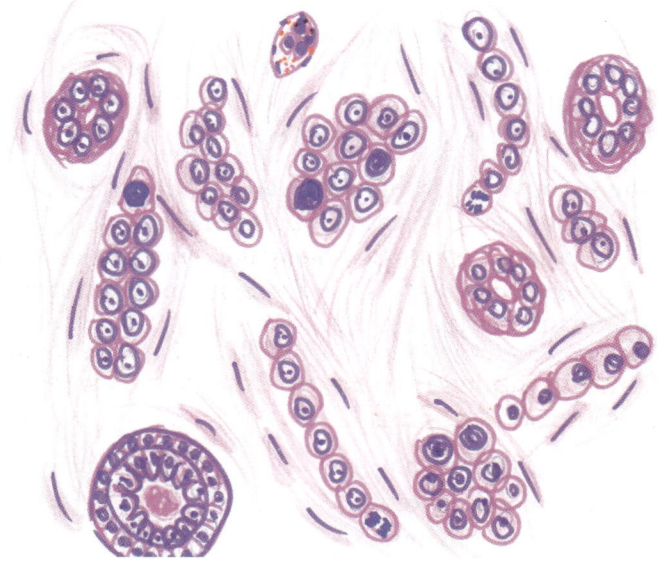

Fig. 33.9: Microscopy of infiltrating duct carcinoma breast (schematic)

Other breast carcinomas:
1. Metaplastic carcinoma
2. Inflammatory carcinoma

Tubular Carcinoma

The average age of the patients for tubular carcinoma is around 50 years. These are well-differentiated tumours and have favourable prognosis. Grossly, these do not differ much from IDC-NOS. They are less than 2 cm, hard in consistency and poorly circumscribed margins. Microscopically, the glands are well differentiated, there is absence of necrosis, no mitoses, and scanty pleomorphism. There are irregularly arranged tubules lined by single layer of epithelium with low mitoses and little pleomorphism. The cytoplasmic apical snouts are frequently seen. The glandular lumina is open and have angulated outlines. The intervening stroma is fibroblastic. The tubular carcinoma should be called only when tubular component is more than 90%.

Mucinous Carcinoma

This is also called mucoid, colloid and gelatinous carcinoma. This usually occurs in postmenopausal women. Grossly, well circumscribed, crepitant on palpation, and contains jelly-like material. Foci of haemorrhage are frequent. This variant has favourable prognosis.

Microscopically, it has small cluster of malignant tumour cells showing little pleomorphism and low mitoses; and these cells are floating in a sea or pool of mucin which is surrounded by bands of fibrous connective tissue. Intracellular mucin may be seen.

Medullary Carcinoma

This occurs usually in patients of less than 50 years of age. It is well circumscribed, soft in consistency and often large. Cut section is solid, homogenous, and gray with small foci of necrosis. These have favourable prognosis. Microscopy has following features:
1. Syncytial growth pattern, with cells in sheets.
2. The malignant cells are large with marked nuclear pleomorphism, prominent nucleoli and frequent mitoses. Tumour giant cells may be present. Stroma is sparse.
3. There is lymphocytic and plasma cell infiltration in the stroma and necrosis is frequent.
4. The neoplasm has pushing margins.
5. The plasma–lymphocytic infiltrate and syncytial growth pattern of cells are important to designate the tumour as medullary carcinoma. This pattern should be more than 75% of the tumour to call as medullary carcinoma.

Prognostic Factors

1. Age of the patient: Age of the patient lesser than 50 years has better prognosis.

2. Histologic types: Special types of invasive carcinomas (tubular, mucinous, papillary and secretory) have long survival.
3. Tumour grade: With Bloom-Richardson grading, well-differentiated grade 1 tumours have long survival (Table 33.2).
4. Estrogen and progesterone receptors: Tumour cells with positive hormone receptors have better prognosis. 80% tumours with estrogen and progesterone receptors respond to hormone manipulation. Tumours with estrogen/progesterone receptors negativity are less likely respond to hormone manipulation.
5. During pregnancy and lactation: Aggressive behaviour.
6. HER 2/neu over expression is associated with poor prognosis.
7. Lymphovascular invasion: Poor prognosis.
8. Tumours with high proliferation rate (S phase fraction, Ki 67): Worse prognosis.
9. DNA content: Aneuploid tumours, abnormal DNA indices have a slightly worse prognosis.
10. BRCA 1 and 2 mutations are associated with worse overall survival.
11. Early diagnosis with small tumours and devoid of lymph node metastasis have lesser stage and favourable survival.
12. Size of breast carcinoma less than 1 cm and associated with negative lymph nodes have better prognosis.

Table 33.2   Modified Bloom-Richardson grading

Tubule formation, nuclear features and mitosis	Score
Tubule formation	
More than 75%	1
10–75%	2
Less than 10%	3
Nuclear pleomorphism	
Small, regular, uniform	1
Moderately increased, variable size	2
Marked variation	3
Mitotic count	
0–9	
10–19	
More than 20	
Leitz or ortholux 25x objective or field diameter of 0.59 mm	
Grade	
3–5 points Grade I Well differentiated	
6–7 points Grade II Moderately differentiated	
8–9 points Grade III Poorly differentiated	

13. Tumours with pushing margins have better prognosis.
14. Tumour necrosis, increased lymph node metastasis and high grade tumours have decreased survival.
15. Increased microvessel density around the tumour has aggressive course.

NICE TO KNOW

Molecular Classification

Major histological subtypes:

Luminal A: The breast carcinoma of luminal A type is ER/PR positive, luminal CK positive, HER2 negative (50%), respond to hormone therapy and response to chemotherapy variable. This includes tubular, cribriform, low grade infiltrating duct carcinoma—NOS and classic lobular carcinoma. This type of breast carcinoma has good prognosis.

Luminal B: Luminal B type of breast carcinoma is ER/PR variable, luminal CK positive and HER2 variable. This type has higher proliferative activity than luminal A, of higher histological grade, includes high grade infiltrating duct carcinoma—NOS and micropapillary carcinoma, response to hormone therapy is not as good as luminal A, response to chemotherapy is variable and prognosis is not good when compared to luminal A type of breast carcinoma.

HER2 positive: HER2 postive breast carcinomas are P53 positive, high grade and respond to herceptin and anthracyclin based chemotherapy. This includes high grade infiltrating duct carcinoma—NOS.

Basal like: This type of carcinoma is positive for basal epithelial genes (cytokeratin 5/6 and others, EGFR), ER/PR negative, HER2 negative, P53 positive, BRCA1 mutations positive. Most are triple negative. This includes high grade infiltrating duct carcinoma—NOS, Metaplastic carcinoma and medullary carcinoma. This type of tumour does not respond to herceptin (transtuzumab). This occurs in young women. It is sensitive to platinum-based chemotherapy, relapse is rapid and has poor prognosis.

Note: Even though medullary carcinoma is included in this type, it may have better prognosis.

Following is the ER/PR and HER2 status with relation to age of occurrence, survival, recurrence, etc.
1. **ER positive, HER2 negative:** These have low proliferation rate, occur in older females, detected by mammography, bone metastasis is 70%, viscera 25% and brain less than 10%, associated with long survival and relapse is later than 10 years.
2. **ER positive/negative and HER2 positive:** Occurs in young females, associated with P53 mutations, relapse is short and has survival less than 10 years.
3. **Triple negative (ER negative, PR negative, HER2 negative):** These occur in younger females, associated with BRCA1 mutations and have short survival.

SELF-ASSESSMENT EXERCISE

1. **Following breast carcinomas have good prognosis** *except*:
   A. Scirrhous carcinoma   B. Mucinous carcinoma
   C. Papillary carcinoma   D. Tubular carcinoma

2. **Old lady, small breast lump, mammogram calcifications +, biopsy on pressing paste like material comes. The possibility is:**
   A. Comedo carcinoma
   B. Medullary carcinoma
   C. Paget's disease
   D. Infiltrating lobular carcinoma

3. **Young female with breast carcinoma and family history of ovarian carcinoma, possible gene mutation is:**
   A. P53   B. Her2/neu
   C. BRCA2   D. Cmyc

4. **Fibroadenoma, the etiology is:**
   A. Increased estrogen
   B. Increased progesterone
   C. Increased testosterone
   D. All

5. **22 years lady, nipple discharge, subareolar mass, possibility is:**
   A. Intraductal papilloma B. Papillary carcinoma
   C. Secretory carcinoma   D. Apocrine carcinoma

6. **Breast mass, syncytial cells in sheets and periphery of the mass has lymphoid cells. The possibility is:**
   A. Medullary carcinoma   B. Paget's disease
   C. Lobular carcinoma   D. Apocrine carcinoma

7. **Bulls eye pattern of tumour cells around normal acini and ducts:**
   A. Lobular carcinoma *in situ*
   B. Duct carcinoma *in situ* (DCIS)
   C. Phyllodes
   D. Paget's disease

8. **Clefts and slits are typically in:**
   A. Phyllodes   B. Fibroadenoma
   C. Both of the above   D. None of the above

9. **Breast enlargement in pregnancy and lactation is mainly due to:**
   A. Hyperplasia of glandular tissue
   B. Proliferation of stroma tissue
   C. Due to edema
   D. Fibrosis

10. **Painless lump breast can be all** *except*:
    A. Fibroadenoma   B. Fibrocystic disease
    C. Papilloma   D. Mastitis

11. **Fat necrosis breast is characterised by all** *except*:
    A. Mimics malignancy
    B. Frequent in obese females
    C. Related to trauma
    D. Has risk of malignancy

12. **Most common breast lesion in females is:**
    A. FA   B. Carcinoma
    C. Papilloma   D. Fat necrosis

13. **Freely mobile benign breast lesion is:**
    A. FA
    B. Phyllodes
    C. Fibroadenomatous lesion
    D. Adenoma

14. **Breast carcinoma with dense collagenous tissue and clumps of malignant cells is:**
    A. Infiltrating duct carcinoma—NOS
    B. Medullary
    C. Secretory
    D. Papillary

15. **Paget's disease of breast has:**
    A. Only eczema of skin
    B. Underlying breast cancer
    C. Sclerosing adenosis
    D. Estrogen stimulation

16. **Early diagnosis of breast carcinoma includes all** *except*:
    A. Ultrasonography
    B. Self palpation
    C. FNA
    D. CT and MRI

17. **Nipple papilloma, common clinical presentation is:**
    A. Bloody nipple discharge
    B. Painless lump
    C. Painful lump
    D. All

18. **Mammogram with foci of calcification is:**
    A. Comedo carcinoma or IDC
    B. Fibroadenoma
    C. Fibrocystic disease
    D. Phyllodes

Answers

1. A	2. A	3. C	4. A	5. A	6. A	7. A	8. C
9. A	10. D	11. D	12. A	13. A	14. A	15. B	16. D
17. A	18. A						

Female Genital System: Cervix

GROSS ANATOMY

The uterus is divided into the corpus, isthmus, and cervix. The cervix (term taken from the Latin, meaning neck) is the most inferior portion of the uterus, protruding into the upper vagina. The transition between the endocervix and the lower portion of the uterine corpus is termed the isthmus or lower uterine segment. The vagina is fused circumferentially and obliquely to the distal part of the cervix. The cervix measures 2.5–3 cm in length in the adult nulligravida, and when normally positioned, is angled slightly downward and backward. The vaginal portion (portio vaginalis) of the cervix, also referred as the exocervix or ectocervix. The portion may be divided into anterior and posterior lips. In the center of the exocervix is the external os. The external os is circular in the nulligravida and slit-like in the parous woman. The external os is connected to the isthmus of the cervical canal (endocervix). The canal is an elliptical cavity, measuring 8 mm in its greatest diameter.

NON-NEOPLASTIC LESIONS

Metaplasia

Squamous and other metaplasia (like tubal, intestinal, transitional, goblet cell, etc.) of mucous secreting glandular epithelium is known. Squamous metaplasia is common. It can be focal or extensive metaplasia.

Nabothian cysts develop due to blockage of the endocervical glands with secondary changes associated with inflammation.

Microglandular hyperplasia of endocervical glands is common with oral contraceptive users and less frequently during pregnancy.

Arias-Stella reaction as seen in endometrial glands during pregnancy and can also be observed in endocervical glands.

Mesonephric duct rests can undergo cystic dilation with hyperplastic and atypical changes.

Decidual change of stromal cells can be seen as a response to hormones.

Endometriosis of cervix presents with blue or reddish nodules and may result in abnormal vaginal bleeding.

INFLAMMATIONS

CERVICITIS: ACUTE AND CHRONIC

Inflammation of the cervix is common and is related to constant exposure to bacterial flora in the vagina. Acute and chronic cervicitis results from infection with many micro-organisms, particularly endogenous vaginal aerobes and anaerobes, *Streptococcus*, *Staphylococcus*, and enterococcus. Other specific organisms include *Chlamydia trachomatis*, *Neisseria gonorrhoeae*, and occasionally by herpes simplex virus.

Pathology

In acute cervicitis, the cervix is grossly red, swollen and oedematous, with copious pus from the external os.

Microscopically, the tissues exhibit an extensive infiltrate of polymorphonuclear leucocytes and stromal oedema.

In chronic cervicitis, which is more common, the cervical mucosa is hyperaemic and there may be true epithelial erosions.

Microscopically, the stroma is infiltrated by mononuclear cells, principally lymphocytes and plasma cells.

Metaplastic squamous epithelium of the transformation zone may extend into endocervical glands, forming clusters of squamous epithelium with slightly enlarged nuclei.

ENDOCERVICAL POLYP

Endocervical polyps are the most common benign exophytic growths within the endocervical canal and the mass vary from being sessile to polypoidal, less than 3 cm in the greatest dimension. The polyps typically manifest as vaginal bleeding or discharge. The lining epithelium is mucous-secreting tall columnar-epithelium with varying degrees of squamous metaplasia and underlying fibromyxomatous stroma. Simple excision or curettage is curative. Cancer rarely arises in an endocervical polyp.

PREMALIGNANT AND MALIGNANT LESIONS OF CERVIX

CERVICAL INTRAEPITHELIAL NEOPLASIA

Cervical intraepithelial neoplasia (CIN) is the precursor of invasive cancer. CIN is defined as a spectrum of intraepithelial changes that begins with minimal atypia and progresses through stages of more marked intraepithelial abnormalities to invasive squamous cell carcinoma.

CIN, dysplasia, carcinoma *in situ* (CIS), and squamous intraepithelial lesion (SIL) are commonly used interchangeably. Dysplasia in the cervical epithelium carries a risk for malignant transformation.

Sequence of Histologic Changes from CIN 1 to CIN 3

CIN 1 (Mild Dysplasia)

- Indistinguishable from condyloma.
- Dysplastic changes are seen in the basal third of the epithelium.
- Cytoplasmic differentiation is present in the upper two-thirds of the epithelium.
- Koilocytotic changes which are seen as perinuclear halos in suprabasilar cells may be seen.
- Cells display mild dysplasia. There is mild to moderate variation in nuclear size, slight irregularities in nuclear shape and contour and hyperchromasia is present with nuclei having coarse chromatin.
- The exfoliated cells are detected as abnormal in Pap smears.

CIN 2 (Moderate Dysplasia)

- Abnormal cells are present in the lower two-thirds of the epithelium.
- Highly associated with HPV types 16 and 18 and other types.

- Koilocytotic changes may be seen.
- Cytodifferentiation occurs in cells in the upper third.
- Cells display moderate dysplasia.
- The exfoliated cells are detected as abnormal in Pap smears.

CIN 3 and CIS (Severe Dysplasia and Carcinoma *in situ*)

- The cells in the superficial (upper) epithelium disclose some, albeit minimal, differentiation.
- Highly associated with HPV types 16 and 18 and other types.
- Koilocytotic changes may be seen.
- Cells display severe dysplasia. There are marked variation in nuclear size with increased N: C ratio, marked irregularities in nuclear shape and contour and markedly increased hyperchromasia having irregular coarse chromatin.
- The exfoliated cells are detected as abnormal in Pap smears.

The Bethesda System for Reporting Cervical/ Vaginal Cytology

The Bethesda system of reporting uses terms like low-grade squamous intraepithelial lesion (LSIL) and high-grade squamous intraepithelial lesion (HSIL) (Table 34.1).

LSIL reflects conditions that rarely progress in severity and commonly disappear (CIN 1, mild dysplasia). This regresses spontaneously, occasionally may progress to HSIL.

HSIL corresponds to more severe histologic lesions (CIN 2 and CIN 3). HSIL may progress to invasive squamous cell carcinoma.

Pathogenesis

Role of human papillomavirus (HPV) in the pathogenesis of cervical neoplasia: The critical factor is HPV infection, which correlates with multiple sexual

Table 34.1	Grading of cervical intraepithelial neoplasia (CIN) or squamous intraepithelial lesion (SIL)—low and high grade
CIN 1, low grade SIL	Dysplastic cells in lower one-third of the epithelium
CIN 2, high grade SIL	Dysplastic cells in lower two-thirds of the epithelium
CIN 3, high grade SIL	Dysplastic cells extending beyond the lower two-thirds of the epithelium
CIS/CIN	Dysplastic cells full thickness of the epithelium

partners and early age at first coitus. Thus, CIN is essentially a sexually transmitted disease. Infection with species high-risk types of HPV plays a critical role in the development of high grade CIN (HSIL) and cervical cancer.

The normal process by which cervical squamous epithelium matures is disturbed in CIN, as evidenced morphologically by changes in cellularity, differentiation, polarity, nuclear features and mitotic activity.

Clinical Features

- SIL is seen at any age following the onset of sexual activity.
- HPV infection is ubiquitous in young, sexually active women.
- Other risk factors: Age, defects in immunity (HIV), tobacco use.

GLANDULAR INTRAEPITHELIAL NEOPLASIA

Glandular intraepithelial neoplasia is the precursor to most invasive cervical adenocarcinomas. This is based upon:

1. The association with high-risk HPV types (16 and 18)
2. Mean age at diagnosis for glandular intraepithelial neoplasia predates that for invasive adeno-carcinoma.

Pathological Features

- Glandular intraepithelial neoplasia almost always arises at the squamocolumnar junction (transformation zone).
- Extent of lesion may vary from focal to diffuse circumferential cervical involvement.
- In 30–50% of cases, associated with squamous intraepithelial lesions.

Microscopy

Normal cervical glandular architecture is preserved with glands being lined by crowded cells with enlarged, hyperchromatic, stratified or pseudostratified nuclei. An abrupt transition from normal to neoplastic change within gland is characteristic. Nucleoli are usually small and inconspicuous, occasionally may be prominent. Mitotic figures present, typically on luminal side.

Histologic Subtypes

- Endocervical
- Intestinal
- Stratified
- Ciliated

CARCINOMA OF CERVIX

The carcinoma cervix has relatively long natural history. Premalignant lesions occur before Frank cancer develops (Figs 34.1 and 34.2). The intervention and treatment in premalignant stage is highly effective. As cervix can be easily approachable organ and availability of simple tests for detecting cancer have made it for mass screening programmes and cure rate can be 100%, if treated in premalignant stage. The premalignant lesions are mentioned above.

Epidemiology

Cervical cancer remains the fourth most common cancer amongst all malignancies in women (WHO, 2012). Estimated new cases of carcinoma cervix worldwide by 2018 are **500000**. Higher incidences of carcinoma

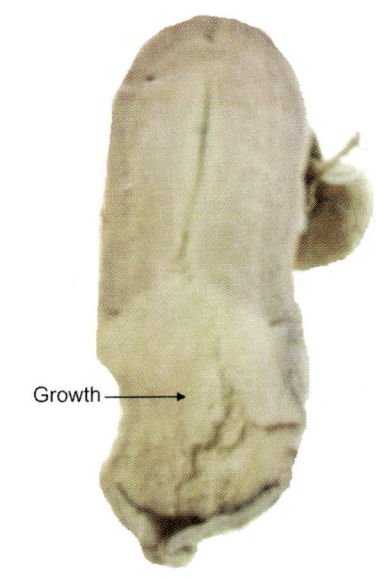

Growth

Fig. 34.1: Squamous cell carcinoma cervix (gross picture)

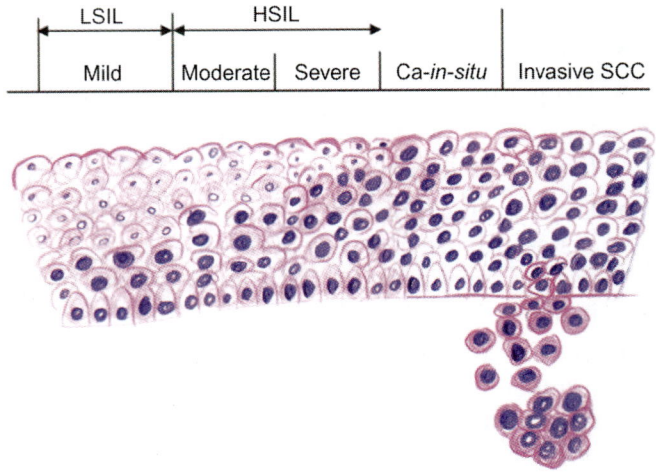

LSIL	HSIL			
Mild	Moderate	Severe	Ca-*in-situ*	Invasive SCC

Fig. 34.2: Carcinoma *in situ* and malignant transformation (schematic)

cervix are found in developing countries and in India it ranks second most frequent cancer in women (IOC/IARC information on HPV and Cancer, 2017). In developing countries, as cytologic screening is not regularly practiced, squamous cell carcinoma of cervix is still a major cause of cancer death.

Etiology and Pathogenesis

1. About 99.7% of the cancers and pre-malignant lesions are associated with oncogenic HPV subtypes. More than 90% of cervical carcinoma contains DNA sequences of specific HPV types, especially HPV 16 and HPV 18. The distribution of HPV types in invasive cervical cancers shows only minor geographic variations. Globally, HPV 16 is most frequently detected in invasive cervical cancer, followed by HPV 18. HPV types 31, 33, 35, 45, 52, and 58 are the next most common types found incervical cancers.

   A cervical cancer vaccine has recently been approved and recommended for females between the ages of 9 and 26, which in clinical trials has decreased the risk of cervical cancer. Vaccinated women developed neither HPV-associated precancer nor invasive cervical cancer.[34]

2. The other sexually transmitted diseases like herpes simplex virus may play concurrent role.

3. **Other risk factors:**

   - Lower education attainment, older age, obesity, smoking, poverty (socio-economical status), parity, use of oral contraceptives, sexual activity and lowered immunity (immunosuppression) are independently related to high rates of cancer.

   - **Cigarette smoking:** Both passive and active have higher risk. HPV infection along with smoking has two- to threefold increased risk.

   - **Alcohol**

   - **Drug abuse**

   - **Parity:** Increased parity has more risk. Nulliparous females have reduced risk.

   - **Oral contraceptives (OC) and progesterone use:** Long-term use of combination OC or progesterone use has increased risk. HPV with OC association increases risk fourfold.

   - **Sexual activity:** HPV infection is related to number of sexual partners. Early age of first intercourse (at the age of 20–21 years) increases the risk of HPV infection and carcinoma cervix.

   - **Immunity:** Immunocompromised women have more risk of cervical cancer.

Mechanism of Cancer Development

The molecular mechanisms involved in carcinogenesis are complex and not fully understood. Increasing evidence suggests that HPV oncoproteins are the critical components of cancer cell proliferation. The high-risk HPV oncoproteins gets integrated into the host DNA. The early viral replication proteins E1 and E2 makes the virus to replicate within the cervical cells. The E6 oncoprotein degrades the P53 gene and inhibits apoptosis, while E7 oncoprotein binds to RB gene and degrades it. Thus, both of these are involved in proliferation and survival of the transformed cells. Markers of actively of dividing cells like Ki-67, P-16, a cyclin dependent kinase inhibitor are over expressed in upper layers of the epithelium. Ki-67 and P-16 staining is highly correlated with high grade HPV infection. In addition, E6 upregulates the expression of telomerase, which leads to immortalization of the cells.

Pathology

Squamous cell carcinoma is the most common histologic subtype accounting for 70–80% of invasive carcinomas. **Adenocarcinoma and adenosquamous carcinoma** comprise 10–15% of all cases.

INVASIVE SQUAMOUS CELL CARCINOMA

- Often seen in younger women, with peak incidence around 45 years of age.
  Around 10 to 15 years after detection of the precancerous lesion; this needs regular follow-up with biopsies.
- Related to HPV infection
- Patients most commonly presents with abnormal vaginal bleeding
- Bleeding following intercourse
- Serosanguinous discharge
- Weakness/pallor/weight loss
- More advanced tumours may be polypoid, fungating or ulcerative.

Gross

- Early lesions may be focally indurated, ulcerated, or present as a slightly elevated, granular area that bleeds readily.
- Approximately 98% of early carcinomas are localized within the transformation zone.
- Most advanced tumours are endophytic or exophytic. Endophytic carcinomas are ulcerated or nodular; they tend to develop within the endocervical canal and invade deeply into the cervical stroma to produce an enlarged, hard, barrel-shaped cervix.
- The exophytic varieties of cervical carcinoma have a polypoid or papillary appearance.

Microscopy

- Keratinizing squamous cell carcinoma is the common histological type encountered.
- This type shows conspicuous evidence of keratinization in the form of keratin pearls.
- Cytoplasm shows keratohyaline granules.
- Individual keratinized cells are commonly seen.
- Nests of well-differentiated squamous cells with keratinization are common features.
- The cells display atypia, increased and abnormal mitoses.

Microscopic Grading

The tumour cells with keratinization, formation of squamous pearls, nuclear atypia and a number of mitoses are taken into account. There are different grading systems. The one which is commonly used is given below.

The histologic grading divides keratised squamous cell carcinomas into three groups:
1. Well differentiated (grade 1),
2. Moderately differentiated (grade 2), and
3. Poorly differentiated (grade 3).

Most are moderately differentiated (grade 2), followed by poorly differentiated (grade 3) and well differentiated (grade 1).

Other Histological Types of Squamous Cell Carcinoma

Large Cell Non-Keratinizing

- Composed of histologically recognizable squamous cells, which are large and polygonal with eosinophilic cytoplasm and indistinct cell borders.
- Lack keratin pearl formation or nests of squamous cells with keratinization.
- Greater degree of nuclear pleomorphism.
- Infiltrative border with associated inflammation is often seen.

Small Cell Non-Keratinizing

- Composed of tumour cells with high N:C ratio.
- Minimal evidence of histologically recognizable squamous differentiation.
- Generally classified as poorly differentiated.

ADENOCARCINOMA CERVIX

Prevalence

- Increasing among the younger women
- Particularly among the age group 40 years

Etiology

- HPV and oral contraceptives

- Other risk factors mentioned for squamous cell carcinoma

Pathology

Gross: Mostly papillary/polypoid, some are nodular and may ulcerate the cervix. Some are high in the endocervical canal and so difficult to visualize on clinical examination. Diffusely infiltrate and enlarge the cervix resulting in "barrel cervix".

Microscopy: The glands exhibit different histological types, the most common are of endocervical and endometrioid differentiation. The cells are columnar with elongated, hyperchromatic nuclei that may show marked atypia with nuclear pleomorphism and coarse chromatin. The cells are often stratified and contain amphophilic or eosinophilic apical cytoplasm. The glands may be widely spaced or densely arranged in a complex racemose pattern. A cribriform pattern is very common and papillae commonly project into gland lumens.

Microscopic grading:
- Well-differentiated tumours are defined as those in which <10% of the tumour volume is composed of solid sheets of cells, the remainder of the tumour being glandular.
- A moderately differentiated tumour, 11–50% of the tumour is composed of solid sheets of cells.
- Poorly differentiated tumours, >50% of the tumour cells are in solid sheets.
- Measurement of the depth of invasion is more difficult than for squamous cell carcinomas because of the difficulty in determining the point of origin.

Clinical Features

- May be asymptomatic
- Symptomatic:
  - Early stage: Watery blood-tinged vaginal discharge, or
  - Intermittent vaginal bleeding with coitus or vaginal douching, or
  - Rarely uncontrolled bleeding from tumour can occur.

Examination Findings

- Exophytic or endophytic growth
- Bleeds on touch
- Watery/bloody/purulent discharge may be seen.
- Uterus may be enlarged because of invasion and growth.
- Hematometra or pyometra with obstruction to the cervical canal and distension of the cavity above the obstruction level.

- Disease may spread to vagina and posteriorly to rectovaginal septum which is thick, hard and irregular.
- With advanced disease: Inguinal, supraclavicular LNs enlarged, lower leg oedema, low back pain radiating to posterior part of leg suggests compression of sciatic nerve root, lymphatics, veins or ureter by expanding tumour.
  Obstruction of ureter leads to hydronephrosis, uraemia and renal failure.

Prognosis

The prognosis of squamous cell carcinoma is related to following parameters.

1. Clinical stage: The most important prognostic predictor
2. Nodal status
3. Size of primary tumour
4. Depth of invasion
5. Size of largest lymph node
6. Endometrial extension
7. Parametrial extension
8. Microscopic grade
9. Microscopic type
10. Cell proliferative index
11. HPV serotypes

Spread and Metastases

Carcinoma of the cervix spreads principally by direct local invasion to adjacent tissues and through lymphatics and less commonly through blood vessels.

Spread

1. Local extension into surrounding tissues (parametrium) results in ureteral compression and ultimately renal failure which is the most common cause of death (50% of patients). Bladder and rectal involvement may lead to fistula formation.

2. Metastases to regional lymph nodes involve para-cervical, hypogastric, and external iliac nodes.
   The Pap smear remains the most reliable screening test for detecting cervical cancer. In the earliest stages of cervical cancer, patients complain most often of vaginal bleeding after intercourse or douching.

The clinical stage of cervical cancer is the best prognostic index of survival. The overall 5-year survival rate is 60% and decreases to 10% in widely disseminated disease.

Radical hysterectomy is favoured for localized tumour, especially in younger women; radiation therapy or combinations of the two are used for more advanced tumours.

Investigations

Laboratory Investigations

1. Haemogram
2. CBC: To identify type and severity of anaemia
3. Urine analysis: To look for haematuria
4. Biochemistry profile: Electrolyte abnormality
5. Liver function tests: Liver metastasis
6. Creatinine and urea: To assess renal impairment

Radiological Investigations

1. Chest X-ray: Lung metastasis
2. Intravenous pyelogram: Hydronephrosis
3. CT scan abdominal: Nodal or distant organ metastasis
4. MRI: Parametrial involvement

Procedural Investigations

1. Cystoscopy: To know bladder involvement
2. Proctoscopy: To know rectal involvement
3. Examination under anaesthesia: To know tumour spread for staging
4. Pap smears: To detect malignant cells
5. Biopsy: To confirm malignancy
6. Demonstration of HPV-DNA (by hybrid capture technique and PCR).

NICE TO KNOW

Other Histological Types of Squamous Cell Carcinoma

Basaloid squamous cell carcinoma: Basaloid appearance with nests of tumour cells having peripheral palisading of nuclei with variable amounts of squamous differentiation.

Verrucous squamous cell carcinoma:
- This is extremely rare subtype, clinically, verrucous carcinoma appears as a large, sessile tumour that grossly resembles a condyloma.

- It is composed of broad-based papillae lined by squamous epithelium with little to no cytologic atypia.
- Tumour shows pushing margins of uniform epithelial stromal interface. No stromal invasion is seen.

Warty/condylomatous squamous cell carcinoma:
- Refers to exophytic squamous cell carcinomas that have koilocytotic surface epithelial changes characteristic of HPV infection.

(contd.)

- Unlike verrucous carcinoma, warty carcinomas demonstrate features of a typical squamous cell carcinoma at the deep margin. In addition, many of the malignant cells have cytoplasmic vacuolization and nuclear changes closely resembling koilocytotic atypia.

Papillary squamous cell carcinoma: Characterised by papillary growth pattern.

Lymphoepithelioma-like squamous cell carcinoma:
- The Epstein-Barr virus (EBV) has been suggested as a potential causative agent and has been detected in 75% of cervical lymphoepithelioma-like carcinoma.
- Consists of poorly defined aggregates of non-keratinizing tumour cells with large vesicular nuclei, prominent nucleoli, moderate amount of eosinophilic cytoplasm with indistinct cytoplasmic border.
- The nests of undifferentiated cells are surrounded by a marked chronic inflammatory infiltrate composed of lymphocytes, plasma cells and eosinophils.

Histological classification of invasive carcinomas of the uterine cervix[35]

Squamous cell carcinoma

Microinvasive (early invasive) squamous cell carcinoma

Invasive squamous cell carcinoma
- Keratinizing
- Non-keratinizing
- Basaloid
- Verrucous
- Warty
- Papillary
- Squamotransitional
- Lymphoepithelioma-like carcinoma

Adenocarcinoma
- Usual type adenocarcinoma
- Mucinous adenocarcinoma
- Endocervical type
- Intestinal type
- Signet-ring type
- Minimal deviation
- Villoglandular
- Endometrioid adenocarcinoma
- Clear cell adenocarcinoma
- Serous adenocarcinoma
- Mesonephric adenocarcinoma

Other epithelial tumours
- Adenosquamous carcinoma
  - Glassy cell variant
  - Clear cell variant
- Adenoid cystic carcinoma
- Adenoid basal carcinoma

Neuroendocrine tumours
- Carcinoid
- Atypical carcinoid
- Small cell carcinoma
- Large cell neuroendocrine carcinoma

Undifferentiated carcinoma

(WHO classification with modification)

Carcinoma of the cervix: FIGO Staging (FIGO, revised 2009)[36]

IA1 Confined to the cervix, diagnosed only by microscopy with invasion of <3 mm in depth and lateral spread <7 mm

IA2 Confined to the cervix, diagnosed with microscopy with invasion of >3 mm and <5 mm with lateral spread <7 mm

IB1 Clinically visible lesion or greater than A2, <4 cm in the greatest dimension

IB2 Clinically visible lesion, >4 cm in the greatest dimension

IIA1 Involvement of the upper two-thirds of the vagina, without parametrial invasion, <4 cm in the greatest dimension

IIA2 >4 cm in the greatest dimension

IIB With parametrial involvement

IIIA Not extended to pelvic wall, lower third vagina involved

IIIB Extended to pelvic wall or hydronephrosis, or non-functioning kidney

IVA Spread of growth to adjacent pelvic organs

IVB Spread to distant organs

SELF-ASSESSMENT EXERCISE

1. **In case of frank invasive carcinoma on gross appearance, following is suggested:**
   A. Cone biopsy
   B. Colposcopy directed biopsy
   C. Pap smear sufficient for diagnosis
   D. Wedge biopsy

2. **Young female with high grade CIN, HSIL or carcinoma *in situ* requires, who wants to preserve fertility:**
   A. LEEP, i.e. loop electrosurgical excision procedure
   B. Hysterectomy with node dissection
   C. Wethiem's hysterectomy
   D. Follow-up for carcinoma

3. **Bleeding per vagina and postcoital bleeding can be present in:**
   A. Endometrial carcinoma
   B. Cervical carcinoma
   C. Carcinoma *in situ*
   D. Endometrial hyperplasia

4. **Ca cervix is caused by:**
   A. HPV 16, 18, 33
   B. HPV 16, 18, 21
   C. HPV 18, 21, 33
   D. HPV 6, 11, 16

5. **ASC-US, all are true *except*:**
   A. Repeat smears after 4–6 months
   B. HPV DNA testing
   C. Loop electrosurgical excision procedure (LEEP)
   D. Colposcopy

6. **Screening programme with Pap smears for cancer cervix should be done for:**
   A. Women younger than 30 years
   B. Women older than 30 years
   C. All patients
   D. Only elderly patients more than 60 years

7. **In which part of cervix, commonly carcinoma starts?**
   A. Ectocervix   B. Endocervix
   C. T zone   D. All of the above

8. **Estimated new cases of carcinoma cervix world wide by 2018 is:**
   A. 36000   B. 500000
   C. 1 million   D. 50000

9. **How can a woman reduce chances of carcinoma cervix?**
   A. Delay of sexual activity
   B. Practice of safe sex
   C. Multiple partners
   D. A and B

Answers

1. B	2. A	3. B	4. A	5. C	6. B	7. C	8. B
9. D							

Female Genital System: Uterus and Gestational Trophoblastic Diseases

UTERUS

Myometrium (muscular wall of uterus) and endometrium (mucosal lining) of uterine cavity are the two components of uterus.

ENDOMETRIAL CHANGES DURING MENSTRUAL CYCLE

Endometrium undergoes cyclical changes during menstrual cycle, in response to steroidal sex hormones produced from the ovary. Endometrium of the body and fundus of the uterus are usually uniform and merge with epithelium of fallopian tube at its upper extremity and with endocervical epithelium at its lower end. Endometrium has two different zones—stratum basalis (basal layer, lower one-third) and stratum functionalis (functional zone, upper two-thirds). Basal layer is adjacent to myometrium and does not show changes during menstrual cycle. It is not responsive to hormones.

Cyclical change of the endometrium is due to rise and fall in the levels of estrogen and progesterone, under the influence of FSH and LH secreted by the pituitary. The ovum develops in the follicles and enlarging ovarian follicle produces estrogen. The action of estrogen lasts for two weeks with a peak just before ovulation. After ovulation, the ruptured follicle is converted into corpus luteum which secretes progesterone which acts on the endometrium during second half of the cycle just before menstruation, there is a fall in the levels of both hormones.

Normal endometrial cycle has 28 days and is customarily divided into:
1. Menstrual phase
2. Proliferative phase
3. Secretory phase.

Proliferative Phase

Synonyms: Estrogenic phase, follicular phase and pre-ovulatory phase.

This phase lasts for two weeks or 14 days in a 28-day cycle. It is under the control of estrogen, secreted from follicular cells of ovary. Proliferative phase is further divided into early, mid and late proliferative phase. During this phase, endometrial glands are straight and tubular, lined by tall columnar epithelium having oval dense nucleus. The lining becomes pseudo-stratified in late proliferative phase. Endometrial stroma is composed of spindle cells with scanty cytoplasm. Numerous mitoses are seen in stroma and lining cells.

Secretory Phase

Synonyms: Post-ovulatory phase, progesterone or luteal phase.

This phase is mediated by progesterone and lasts for 14 days following ovulation. Histological features are appearance of subnuclear vacuoles in the early phase. Cells lining the endometrial glands show presence of clear vacuoles because of glycogen which indicates secretory activity. Secretory changes become more prominent in the late stages; basal vacuoles progressively move towards the surface of the cell. Glands are dilated, tortuous and show a serrated margin, resembling sawtooth appearance. Stromal changes are more prominent than glandular changes. Stroma shows oedema and spiral arterioles by 21st to 22nd day of the cycle. Stromal cells show hypertrophy and acquire more eosinophilic cytoplasm. This is referred to as predecidual change. Stroma shows infiltration of lymphocytes and neutrophils. Dating of the endometrium (assigning the correct day after ovulation) is possible only in secretory phase as this phase is constant lasts for 14 days.

Menstrual Phase

Corpus luteum undergoes dissolution in the absence of pregnancy. There is drop in progesterone levels. Stratum functionalis degenerates. There is bleeding into the stroma and shedding marking the onset of menstrual cycle.

FUNCTIONAL ENDOMETRIAL DISORDERS

Abnormal Uterine Bleeding (AUB)/ Dysfunctional Uterine Bleeding (DUB)

AUB/DUB is a term used by gynaecologists for abnormal uterine bleeding in which no gross anatomic lesion is present to account for the bleeding.

There are various causes for abnormal uterine bleeding ranging from hormonal disturbances to organic (structural) abnormality (Table 35.1).

ANOVULATORY CYCLES

DUB due to anovulatory cycles is common at menarche (due to temporary defect in hypothalamic-pituitary-ovarian axis) and perimenopausal age. Since ovulation does not occur, corpus luteum fails to form and there is no progesterone production. So, there is no secretory activity. Endometrium proliferates. If the unruptured follicle involutes quickly, estrogen level drops rapidly and there is break through bleeding.

Anovulatory cycles also occur in association with obesity, malnutrition, thyroid disorders, pituitary tumours, adrenal diseases, polycystic ovaries, etc.

ENDOMETRITIS

Inflammation of endometrium is less common because of endocervical barrier. Acute endometritis is rare and occurs as a complication of pregnancy, and due to bacterial infection. Chronic endometritis occurs in association with pelvic inflammatory disease, intrauterine contraceptive devices, and postpartum period.

Tuberculosis of endometrium is due to systemic infection or tuberculous salpingitis and is one of the causes for infertility in developing countries.

Infiltration of plasma cells is the criteria for diagnosing chronic endometritis as they are not normally present in endometrium.

ENDOMETRIOSIS

It is characterised by endometrial glands and stroma, in a location outside the endometrium and myometrium. It occurs in as many as 10% of women in their reproductive years and in nearly half of women with infertility. It is a common cause of dysmenorrhoea and pelvic pain and may present as a pelvic mass filled with old haemorrhage (chocolate cyst).

It is frequently multifocal and may involve tissue in the pelvic organs and tissues (ovaries, pouch of Douglas, uterine ligaments, fallopian tubes and rectovaginal septum), surgical scars particularly of caesarean section, less frequently in more remote sites of the peritoneal cavity and about the umbilicus and uncommonly lymph nodes, lungs, and even heart, skeletal muscle, or bone.

Three possibilities/theories:

1. The **regurgitation theory**, proposes menstrual backflow through the fallopian tubes with subsequent implantation. Indeed, menstrual endometrium is viable and survives when injected into the anterior abdominal wall; however, this theory cannot explain lesions in the lymph nodes, skeletal muscle, or lungs.

2. The **metaplastic theory** proposes endometrial differentiation of coelomic epithelium, which is the origin of the endometrium itself. This theory, too, cannot explain endometriotic lesions in the lungs or lymph nodes.

3. The **vascular** or **lymphatic dissemination theory** can explain extrapelvic or intranodal implants.

Table 35.1	Causes of abnormal uterine bleeding
Age	**Causes**
Prepuberty	Precocious puberty (hypothalamic, pituitary or ovarian origin)
Adolescence	Coagulation disorders Anovulatory cycles
Reproductive age	Pregnancy complications (miscarriage, retained products incomplete abortions, trophoblastic diseases—hydatidiform mole, invasive mole, choriocarcinoma) Anatomic lesions—leiomyoma, adenomyosis, endometrial polyps, endometrial hyperplasia, endometrial carcinoma. Anovulatory cycles—hormonal disturbance
Perimenopausal	Endometrial hyperplasia, carcinoma, polyp, leiomyoma, hormonal disturbances
Postmenopausal	Endometrial hyperplasia, carcinoma polyp, endometritis
Other causes Iatrogenic	Exogenous administration of hormones
Dysfunction of ovaries	Polycystic ovaries, hormone producing ovarian tumours (granulosa, theca cell tumour)
Systemic causes	Blood dyscrasia with thrombocytopenia, haemophilia, von Willebrand disease, infectious diseases

Gross: Endometriosis appears as bluish cystic nodules often surrounded by fibrosis. Sometimes may appear polypoid simulating neoplastic process.

Microscopy: Endometrial glands and stroma are often embedded in the fibrous stroma. The lesion may have fresh or old haemorrhage with haemosiderin-laden macrophages.

ADENOMYOSIS

Adenomyosis refers to presence of glands and stroma deep within the myometrium, one low power field below the basalis of endometrium.

Gross: The uterus is enlarged and globular because of myometrial hypertrophy. The enlargement is asymmetrical, cut section has depressed cystic spaces embedded in bulged myometrial tissue and may contain hemorrhagic foci.

Microscopy: Glands and stroma are seen in the myometrium at a distance of at least one low power field from the endometrial and myometrial junction. The endometrial glands are in proliferative phase.

ENDOMETRIAL HYPERPLASIA

Definition

An excess of estrogen relative to progesterone, if sufficiently prolonged, will induce exaggerated endometrial proliferation/hyperplasia. There is increased proliferation of the endometrial glands relative to the stroma. This results in increased gland to stromal ratio (glands are more compared to stroma).

It is one of the important causes for abnormal uterine bleeding. It can occur at any age during reproductive period, but common age is around 4th to 5th decade, predominantly at extremes of reproductive life (peri- and post-menopausal period). Hyperestrinism with prolonged estrogenic stimulation of the endometrium results in continued proliferation and hyperplasia of the glands.

Causes for Excessive Estrogen

1. Failure of ovulation, such as seen around the menopause.
2. Obesity (peripheral conversion of androgens to estrogens).
3. Tumours of the ovary producing estrogen (viz granulosa cell tumour, thecoma).
4. Polycystic ovarian syndrome (including Stein-Leventhal syndrome), follicular cysts of ovary, ovarian cortical stromal hyperplasia.
5. Prolonged administration of estrogen (iatrogenic estrogen replacement therapy) during menopause.
6. Excessive adrenocortical function.

There are different classifications. Following is one of the recommended classifications. In this, the severity of hyperplasia is classified based on crowding and cytologic atypia of endometrial glands into:
- Simple hyperplasia
- Complex hyperplasia
- Atypical hyperplasia

The latter two can be also classified as:
- Complex hyperplasia without atypia
- Complex hyperplasia with atypia

WHO (2014)[37] classifies endometrial hyperplasia as below:
1. Hyperplasia without atypia
2. Atypical hyperplasia with atypia

Hyperplasia was thought to represent a continuum of morphological changes due to estrogen excess. The risk of developing carcinoma is dependent on the severity of the hyperplastic changes and associated cellular atypia. When atypical hyperplasia is discovered, it must be carefully evaluated for the presence of cancer and must be monitored by repeated endometrial biopsy. However, some studies suggest that:
1. Endometrial hyperplasia and neoplasia are two biologically different diseases.
2. Important feature is presence or absence of cellular atypia.

Simple hyperplasia carries a negligible risk, while a person with atypical hyperplasia with cellular atypia has a 28% risk of developing endometrial carcinoma.[38]

Simple hyperplasia is a hyperplasia with increase in endometrial bulk, it is a diffuse process involving basal and functional zones. The glands show proliferative endometrium. The glands vary in size. Some are small, some large and some are cystically dilated. The stroma is cellular; however, gland to stroma ratio is normal.

Complex hyperplasia is focal, mainly involves glandular component. The glands are variable in size, larger, more numerous, closely packed or crowded, irregular in contour with reduction in the intervening stroma. The glands show out-pouching or budding. The glandular epithelium is tall columnar or cuboidal with basal or central nuclei, multilayering is minimal, no loss of nuclear polarity, mitoses are numerous.

Atypical hyperplasia is focal and involves glandular component. The glands are closely packed or crowded with reduction in the intervening stroma. The glands show back to back arrangement and similar to complex hyperplasia are irregular in shape, show out-pouching or budding and intraluminal tufting. The glandular epithelium is tall columnar or cuboidal with basal or central nuclei, multilayering (stratification) is marked with loss of nuclear polarity, mitoses are numerous. There is nuclear atypia and N:C ratio is increased.

LEIOMYOMA

This is the most common benign tumour of the uterus. They are common in the reproductive age group. They are rare before 20 yrs of age. Overall incidence is 4 to 11%. They are known to shrink after menopause. Cell of origin is smooth muscle of uterine myometrium. Higher levels of estrogen receptors are present in the myometrium harbouring leiomyoma.

Clinical Features

These tumours may be asymptomatic or may cause abnormal uterine bleeding, pain and pressure symptoms due to compression of surrounding structures and infertility. Malignant transformation is extremely rare.

Morphology (Figs 35.1 and 35.2)

Gross: The size of the tumour varies from small nodules to massive tumours filling the entire pelvis. They may be single or multiple and sharply circumscribed but lack a true capsule. They are discrete, firm and grey white. Cut section shows a characteristic whorled appearance. Based on their location in the uterus, they are classified as:

1. Intramural—tumours present within the myo-metrium.
2. Submucosal—tumours projecting into the uterine cavity and present beneath the endometrium.
3. Subserosal—tumours present beneath the serosa and projecting outwards.

   Pedunculated—subserosal and submucosal leiomyomas may have a pedicle or stalk.

Microscopy: The tumour is composed by whirled, interlacing bundles of smooth muscle cells separated by vascularised connective tissue. The muscle cells are uniform in size and shape, have oval nucleus and long slender bipolar cytoplasmic processes. Mitoses are sparse.

The histological variants are:
1. Cellular leiomyoma
2. Atypical, bizarre, symplastic or pleomorphic leiomyoma
3. Mitotically active leiomyoma
4. Leiomyolipoma
5. Pallisaded leiomyoma

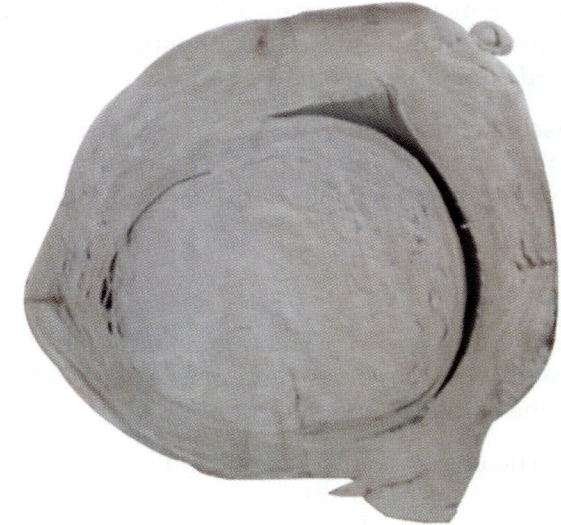

Fig. 35.1: Leiomyoma uterus (gross picture)

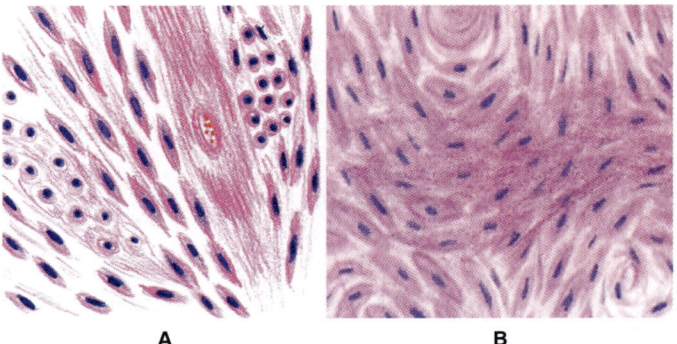

A   B

Fig. 35.2A and B: Microscopy of leiomyoma uterus (schematic)

6. Epithelioid (clear cell) leiomyoma
7. Parasitic leiomyoma
8. Angioleiomyoma

Sites of leiomyomas are:
1. Myometrium
2. Cervix
3. Broad ligament
4. Other sites:
   i. Skin (origin is arector pylorus)
   ii. Blood vessels: Angioleiomyoma.
   iii. Gastrointestinal tract.

Secondary Changes in the Leiomyomas

1. Hyaline change: Eosinophilic homogenous areas seen in between the smooth muscle cells.
2. Myxomatous areas.
3. Calcification: Bluish granular deposits, sometimes the calcification may be extensive occupying the entire tumour associated with ossification referred to as wombstone.
4. Cystic change.

5. Red degeneration seen in pregnancy and oral contraceptive usage. There is coagulative necrosis. Occurs in large tumours. Cut section is dark red.
6. Lipoleiomyoma: Contains an admixture of smooth muscle and mature adipose tissue.
7. Sarcomatous change—very rare.

ENDOMETRIAL CARCINOMA

A primary malignant epithelial tumour, usually with glandular differentiation, arising in the endometrium has the potential to invade into the myometrium and spread to distant sites.

Epidemiology and Pathogenesis

While the disease affects mainly post-menopausal women frequently between the ages of 55 and 65, approximately 20% of the cases occur in premenopausal women. It is a most common malignant tumour of female genital tract. It occurs commonly in:

- Developed countries
- Obese, diabetic, nulliparous, hypertensive females

Estrogen-dependent tumours (about 80–85%) are of low grade, well/moderately differentiated, predominantly endometrioid type and occur in premenopausal or perimenopausal women.

Non-estrogen-dependent tumours (about 10–15%) are of higher grade, serous/clear cell carcinoma and occur in older postmenopausal women.

Risk Factors for Endometrial Cancer

- Early menarche (age <12)
- Late menopause (age >52)
- Infertility or nulliparous
- Obesity, diabetes, caucasian women, diet high in animal fat
- Treatment with tamoxifen for breast cancer
- Estrogen replacement therapy (ERT) after menopause
- Age greater than 40 yrs
- Family history of endometrial cancer or hereditary non-polyposis colon cancer (HNPCC)
- Personal and family history of breast or ovarian cancer
- Prior radiation therapy for pelvic cancer

Symptoms of Endometrial Cancer

- Heavy bleeding, postmenopausal bleeding or discharge
- Dysuria
- Pain and/or mass in pelvic area
- Weight loss
- Back pain

Pathology

Endometrial cancer includes:

1. Those arising in the endometrial lining (endometrial carcinoma)—these make up about 95% of all uterine cancers.
2. Those arising in the uterine stroma or myometrial cells (uterine sarcomas).

Gross (Fig. 35.3): Endometrial cancer is seen as raised, rough, polypoid lesion which protrudes into the cavity and also infiltrates the wall. With extensive infiltration, there can be uterine enlargement. The infiltration of the tumour appears as firm grey white tissue with linear extensions from the base of the tumour. Myometrial invasion may be visible to the naked eye. The invasion of myometrial wall whether less than half or more than half has to be documented which helps in staging of the endometrial carcinoma. The size of the uterus may remain normal too. It often arises in the fundal region of the uterus. Mass may arise from body, isthmus and cornual part of uterus.

Microscopy: Endometrial carcinomas are adenocarcinomas characterised by glandular pattern resembling normal endometrial epithelium. The glandular/villoglandular structures are lined by simple to pseudostratified columnar cells with their long axis perpendicular to basement membrane with elongated nuclei polarized in the same direction. Grade of endometrioid carcinoma is based on architectural pattern, nuclear features or both.

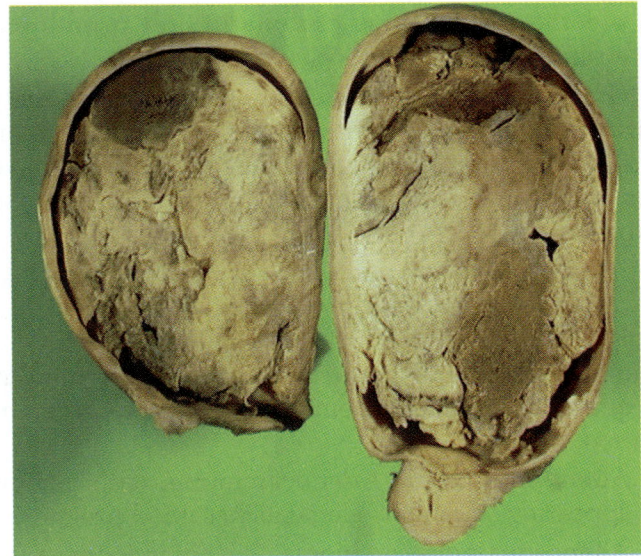

Fig. 35.3: Cut section showing endometrial carcinoma filling the endometrial cavity (gross picture)

Histological Subtypes of Endometrial Cancer

- Endometrioid adenocarcinoma
- Adenosquamous carcinoma
- Serous papillary carcinoma
- Carcinosarcomas
- Clear cell carcinoma

The other variants include:

- Adenoacanthoma
- Glassy cell carcinoma
- Secretory carcinoma
- Ciliated carcinoma
- Mucinous carcinoma
- Undifferentiated carcinoma
- Small cell (neuroendocrine) carcinoma
- Squamous cell carcinoma
- Endometrial carcinoma with trophoblastic differentiation

The most frequent histological type is endometrioid carcinoma or conventional adenocarcinoma. The histological (microscopic) grading is done based on the architectural pattern and nuclear features. The histological grading of the tumour tissue is given below.

- *Grade 1:* Tumour has 5% or less non-squamous solid growth, nuclei are oval, mildly enlarged and has evenly dispersed chromatin (well differentiated).

- *Grade 2:* Tumour tissue has 6–50% non-squamous solid growth, nuclear features are in between grade 1 and 3 (moderately differentiated).

- *Grade 3:* Tumour tissue has more than 50% non-squamous solid growth, nuclei markedly enlarged, pleomorphic, coarse chromatin and prominent eosinophilic nuclei (poorly differentiated).

Grade 1 and 2 (well differentiated and moderately differentiated) cancers have a better prognosis than Grade 3 cancers. Mitoses have less than 5/HPF have good outcome and more than 10/HPF have worse prognosis.

Endometrioid Carcinoma with Squamous Differentiation

Squamous elements should constitute 10% of a tumour to qualify an adenocarcinoma with squamous differentiation.

1. **Adenoacanthoma:** Adenocarcinoma with benign appearing squamous elements has good prognosis
2. **Adenosquamous carcinoma:** Adenocarcinoma with malignant appearing squamous epithelium has worse prognosis.

GESTATIONAL TROPHOBLASTIC DISEASES

Gestational trophoblastic disease is a spectrum of disorders with abnormal proliferation and maturation of villous or trophoblastic tissue, as well as neoplasms derived from trophoblast that originate in the placenta.

Classification

1. Hydatidiform mole
   Complete and
   Partial mole } non-invasive mole
2. Invasive hydatidiform mole
3. Placental site trophoblastic tumour
4. Choriocarcinoma

HYDATIDIFORM MOLE (Vesicular Mole)

Hydatidiform mole is a non-invasive abnormal placental neoplasm characterised by voluminous mass of swollen enlarged, oedematous and vesicular chorionic villi accompanied by variable amounts of proliferated trophoblastic epithelium. Moles are common before the age of 20 or after the age of 40 (Fig. 35.4).

The incidence is 1 to 1.5 in 2000 pregnancies. Higher incidence is seen in Asian countries.

Two categories:

- Complete hydatidiform mole
- Partial hydatidiform mole

Complete Hydatidiform Mole

1. Characterised by hydropic swelling of all the villi and a variable degree of trophoblastic proliferation.
2. Does not permit embryogenesis. Fetal tissue is not usually present.

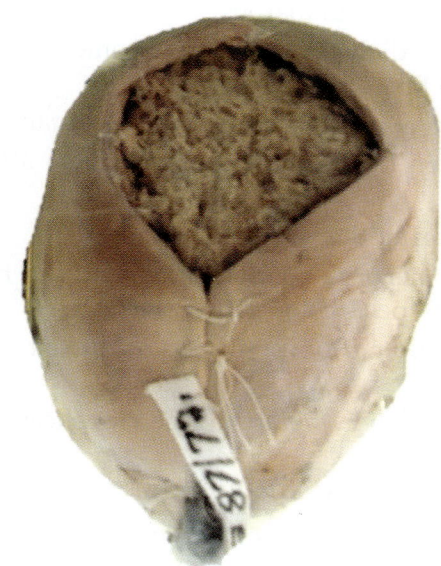

Fig. 35.4: Vesicular mole (gross picture)

Cytogenetics

Complete mole results from fertilization of an empty ovum that lacks functional maternal DNA. Most commonly, a haploid (23X) set of paternal chromosomes introduced by monospermy duplicates to 46XX, but dispermic 46XX and 46XY moles also occur. Because the embryo dies at a very early stage before placental circulation has developed, a few chorionic villi develop blood vessels and fetal parts are absent.

Clinical Features

1. Usually discovered between 12 and 14 weeks of gestational age.
2. Vaginal bleeding with passage of vesicles after a period of amenorrhoea.
3. Uterus is abnormally enlarged and soft.
4. Hyperemesis gravidarum and pregnancy-induced hypertension (PIH) may be associated.
5. USG abdomen shows "snowstorm appearance".
6. Serum β-hCG levels are elevated.

Pathological Features

Gross: Oedematous villi forming characteristic grape-like transparent vesicles (Fig. 35.4).

Lack of fetal tissue is characteristic.

Microscopy (Fig. 35.5):
1. Diffuse hydropic swelling of majority of villi with central acellular cistern formation.
2. The villi are avascular.
3. Diffuse, irregular, circumferential, exuberant, focal, or minimal proliferation of trophoblasts.
4. Trophoblast proliferation is almost always associated with cytological atypia.
5. Absent fetal parts

Diagnosis

Elevated serum β-hCG levels and absence of fetal parts or absence of fetal heart sounds are diagnostic.

Sequelae: 2–3% of these cases go for choriocarcinoma.

Partial Hydatidiform Mole

It occurs between 9 and 34 weeks of gestation. Uterine size is generally small for gestational age. Abnormal uterine bleeding is common feature. Missed or spontaneous abortion is common in cases of incomplete molar pregnancy. Serum β-hCG levels are in the normal or low range for gestational age.

Pre-eclampsia occurs in some cases.

Cytogenetics

Partial hydatidiform mole is a distinct form of mole that almost never evolves into choriocarcinoma. These moles have 69 chromosomes (triploidy), of which one haploid set is maternal and two are paternal in origin. This abnormal chromosomal complement results from fertilization of a normal ovum (23X) by two normal spermatozoa, each carrying 23 chromosomes, or a single spermatozoon that has not undergone meiotic reduction and bears 46 chromosomes. This, results from fertilization of a haploid ovum and duplication of the paternal haploid chromosomes or from dispermy (single ovum and two sperms 23X or 23Y). Thus, in partial mole, karyotype is triploid. 69XXY is most common karyotype (70–80%) followed by 69XXX (20–25%) and rarely 69XYY may also be encountered. The fetus associated with a partial mole usually dies after 10 weeks gestation, and the mole is aborted shortly thereafter. In contrast to a complete mole, fetal parts may be present.

Gross: Villi may be evident as vesicles. Fetus or fetal parts are always present.

Microscopy (Fig. 35.6):
1. Normal villi and villi with hydropic changes
2. Inconspicous/no central cistern formation
3. Trophoblastic hyperplasia is focally present but without atypia.
4. Fetal parts present

Complications

May rarely develop into choriocarcinoma.

Table 35.2 describes comparative features of complete and partial hydatidiform mole.

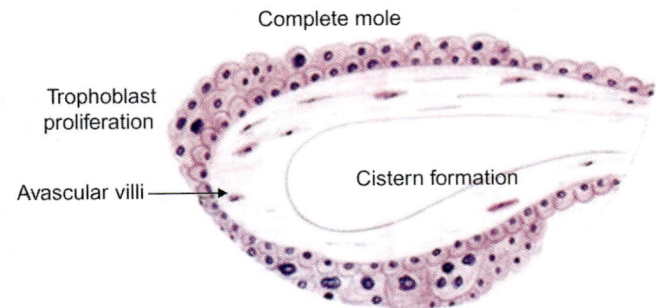

Fig. 35.5: Microscopy of vesicular mole, complete mole (schematic)

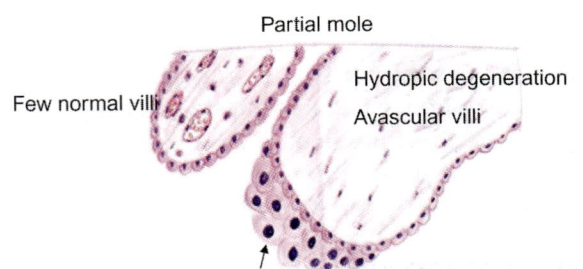

Fig. 35.6: Microscopy of vesicular mole, note changes in partial mole (schematic)

Table 35.2	Comparative features of complete and partial hydatidiform mole	
Features	**Complete mole**	**Partial mole**
Karyotype	46XX and rarely 46XY	Triploid 69XXY or 69XXX, rarely 69XYY
Parental origin of haploid genome sets	Both paternal	1 maternal, 2 paternal
Preoperative diagnosis	Mole	Missed abortion
Marked vaginal bleeding	Marked	Mild
Uterus size	Large for gestational age	Small for gestational age
Serum hCG	Markedly elevated	Less elevated than complete mole
hCG in tissue	3+	1+
Hydropic villi	All	Some
Trophoblastic proliferation	Diffuse	Focal
Atypia	Minimal	Minimal or absent
Embryo	No	Fetal parts may be present
Blood vessels	Absent	Present
Nucleated erythrocytes	No	Sometimes seen
Choriocarcinoma	2% after mole	No choriocarcinoma

INVASIVE HYDATIDIFORM MOLE

It is defined as a mole that penetrates the underlying myometrium or even perforates the uterine wall.

Pathology

There is microscopic invasion of the myometrium by hydropic chorionic villi along with proliferation of both cytotrophoblasts and syncitiotrophoblasts. Local spread is through parametrial tissues and blood vessels. Haematogenous spread is to the lungs and brain. Unlike choriocarcinoma, distant deposits of an invasive mole do not penetrate beyond the confines of the blood vessels in which they are lodged and death from such spread is unusual. The clinical distinction between invasive mole and choriocarcinoma is often difficult. Patients present with vaginal bleeding and irregular uterine enlargement.

Laboratory Finding

Diagnostic finding is persistently elevated serum hCG.

Microscopy: Invasive moles show less hydropic changes than complete moles. Trophoblastic proliferation is usually prominent. The villi are each 1 to 3 mm in diameter and appear grape-like. Individual molar villi have cavitated central cisterns and exhibit considerable trophoblastic hyperplasia and atypia. The blood vessels of the villi will either become atrophic or disappear. Uterine perforation is a major complication, but occurs in only a minority of cases.

PLACENTAL SITE TROPHOBLASTIC TUMOURS

Placental site trophoblastic tumours (PSTT) account for 3% of the gestational trophoblastic diseases.

Grossly, they can be circumscribed or poorly demarcated and project into the myometrium.

Microscopy of PSTT is composed of intermediate trophoblastic cells. Myometrium is invaded by these cells. The cells are arranged in nests or masses or singly. They are large and polygonal. There is no necrosis. Calcification is absent. Mitoses 0 to 6/HPF, chorionic villi are absent.

CHORIOCARCINOMA

Gestational choriocarcinoma is a malignant tumour derived from trophoblast.

Sites:
- Uterine
- Extrauterine

Clinical Features
- Abnormal foul-smelling uterine bleeding is the most frequent initial indication that heralds choriocarcinoma.
- Occasionally, the first sign relates to metastases to the lungs or brain.
- In some cases, it may become evident in 10 or more years after the last pregnancy.

Gross: The uterine lesions of choriocarcinoma range from microscopic foci to huge necrotic and hemorrhagic areas. Viable tumour is usually confined to the rim of the neoplasm.

Microscopy: The tumour contains population of cyto-trophoblast and syncytiotrophoblast, with varying degrees of intermediate trophoblast. By definition, tumours containing any villous structures, even if metastatic, are considered to be a hydatidiform mole and not choriocarcinoma.

Metastasis

Choriocarcinoma invades primarily through venous sinuses in the myometrium. It metastasizes widely by the haematogenous route, especially to lungs, brain, gastrointestinal tract, liver, and vagina.

With currently available chemotherapy, recognition of risk factors and early treatment, most patients are cured.

Survival rates exceed 70% for tumours that have metastasized and virtually 100% remission is expected, if a tumour is localized. Serial serum hCG levels monitor the effectiveness of treatment.

NICE TO KNOW

Clinicopathological Classification of Endometrial Carcinoma

Clinicopathological analysis classifies endometrial carcinoma into two broad categories:

• Type I: Endometrioid carcinoma
• Type II: Serous, clear cell, mixed mullerian tumour

Endometrial cancer is seen in two different clinical settings. In perimenopausal women with estrogen excess, the cancer is of endometroid type (Type I), well to moderately differentiated and early stage disease. Type I are associated with mutation of PTEN, beta catenin, K-Ras and microsatellite instability. Conversely tumours of elderly patients with endometrial atrophy are more likely to be clear cell or serous carcinomas (Type II) have more advanced disease at the time of diagnosis. P53 mutations are common with non-endometriod endometrial carcinoma.

The FIGO staging of uterine cancer was redefined in 2009, with positive cytology previously allocated to Stage III disease, now abandoned in the staging process. However, it is recommended to continue to collect peritoneal washings for cytological evaluation.

As part of staging agreed, preoperative investigations are chest X-ray and MRI/CT. Besides these investigations, cystoscopy, sigmoidoscopy and an examination under anaesthetia are all permitted under staging. Endometrial cancer can be staged both clinically and surgically with surgical staging being most commonly employed.

Distinguishing features of type I and type II endometrial cancer

Factor assessed	Type I	Type II
Age	Premenopausal age or perimenopausal	Postmenopausal age
Estrogen excess	H/o unopposed estrogen excess present	No association
Fertility	Anovulatory/subfertile	No disturbance
Obesity	Present	Absent
Diabetes mellitus	Present	Absent
Background endometrium	Endometrial hyperplasia	No changes
Histological type	Low grade; endometrioid type	High grade tumour; serous or clear cell
Tumour grade	Grade 1 or 2	Grade 3
Myometrial invasion	Superficial	Deep
Lymph node metastases risk	Low	High
Sensitivity to estrogens and progestogens	High	Low
Associated cancers	Ovary, breast, colon	None identified
Genetics	Mutation of PTEN, beta catenin, K-Ras and microsatellite instability	P53
Prognosis	Favourable	Poor

FIGO surgical staging of endometrial carcinoma[39]

Stage I: Tumour confined to the uterus
IA: No or less than half of the myometrium involved
IB: Equal or more than half of the myometrium involved

Stage II: Tumour invades cervix

Stage III: Local or regional spread
IIIA: Tumour invades serosa of uterus and /or adenexa, positive cytology
IIIB: Vaginal and parametrial involvement
IIIC1: Positive pelvic lymph nodes
IIIC2: Para-aortic with or without pelvic lymph nodes
IVA: Bladder and/or bowel mucosa
IVB: Distant metastasis

SELF-ASSESSMENT EXERCISE

1. **Swiss cheese endometrium is seen in:**
   A. Metropathia haemorrhagica
   B. Carcinoma endometrium
   C. Proliferative phase
   D. Secretory phase

2. **Risk of complex hyperplasia with atypia progressing for malignancy in an elderly lady is:**
   A. 3%   B. 8%
   C. 15%   D. 28%

3. **Percentage of CGH going for malignancy:**
   A. 0.1%   B. 2%
   C. 1%   D. 10%

4. **Endometrial hyperplasia is seen in all *except*:**
   A. HRT treatment
   B. Tamoxifen for breast carcinoma
   C. Granulosa cell tumours
   D. Brenner tumour

5. **Risk of endometrial carcinoma is the highest in:**
   A. Endometrial hyperplasia with atypia
   B. Endometrial hyperplasia without atypia
   C. Simple hyperplasia
   D. All of the above

6. **Pregnant lady, beta hCG positive, USG fetus present, uterine height not correlating with gestational age. Possibility is:**
   A. Complete mole   B. Partial mole
   C. Both of the above   D. None of the above

7. **Uterine enlargement can be because of all *except*:**
   A. Adenomyosis   B. Leiomyoma
   C. Carcinoma cervix   D. Pregnancy

8. **Fifteen-year-old girl with irregular cycles, possibility is:**
   A. Polycystic ovarian tumour (PCOS)
   B. Adenomyosis
   C. Leiomyoma
   D. Ovarian thecoma

9. **Patient of breast cancer on tamoxifen, complains of irregular cycles. Possibility are:**
   A. Endometrial hyperplasia
   B. Secretory phase
   C. Atrophic endometrium
   D. All

10. **Risk factors for endometrial hyperplasia are all *except*:**
    A. HRT   B. Nulliparity
    C. Obesity   D. Progesterone

11. **Intermediate trophoblasts invading myometrium:**
    A. Placental site trophoblastic tumour
    B. Vesicular mole
    C. Choriocarcinoma
    D. All of the above

12. **No fetal parts, hydropic villi with raised beta hCG:**
    A. Complete mole
    B. Partial mole
    C. Both of the above
    D. None of the above

13. **Infertility case, semen analysis done. Normal sperm count to be:**
    A. Minimum 15 million sperms/ml
    B. 1–4 lakh cells/cmm
    C. 3–4 million cells/cmm
    D. 10–150 million cells/ml

14. **Endometriosis can have all *except*:**
    A. Endometrial glands and stroma
    B. Haemosiderin-laden macrophages
    C. Smooth muscle tissue
    D. Haemorrhage

15. **For endometriosis, all are true *except*:**
    A. Ovary is the common site
    B. Most common presentation: Infertility, dysmenorrhoea
    C. Important investigation: USG
    D. Estimation of beta hCG

Answers

1. A	2. D	3. C	4. D	5. A	6. B	7. C	8. A
9. A	10. D	11. A	12. A	13. A	14. C	15. D	

Female Genital System: Ovarian Lesions

NORMAL OVARY

The ovaries are paired pelvic organs, lie one either side of the uterus along the posterior surface of the broad ligament, inferior to the fallopian tubes and anterior to the rectum.

The ovaries are the sites of ova production in women. They are also the main source of the hormones estrogen and progesterone in premenopausal age. There are three types of ovarian tissue that can produce cancers: Epithelial cells, which cover the ovary; stromal cells, which produce hormones; and germ cells, which form ova. Most of the ovarian cancers are of epithelial origin.

OVARIAN TUMOURS

Histogenesis

Most of the surface epithelial tumours are derived from ovarian surface epithelium.

Serous tubal intraepithelial carcinoma (STIC) is gaining importance as a precursor lesion for serous high grade tumours. Other tumours are from germ cells or sex-cord stromal origin (Table 36.1).

Etiology

Several hypotheses are proposed for development of ovarian cancer. These are the following:

1. **Incessant ovulation hypothesis:** During ovulation, the surface epithelium of the ovary is damaged with repair which increases the opportunity for developing mutations that promote carcinogenesis.
2. **Gonadotropin over stimulation hypothesis:** Over stimulation of the ovarian surface epithelial cells by gonadotropins (follicle-stimulating hormone and luteinizing hormone) increases cell division and mutations that promote carcinogenesis.
3. **Hormonal stimulation:** High concentrations of androgens promote carcinogenesis and progestins decrease the risk.

4. **Inflammatory response:** Ovulation is accompanied by release of inflammatory mediators which promote malignant transformation.
5. **Genetic and familial predisposition:** BRCA1 (located in the long arm of chromosome 13) or BRCA2 (located in the long arm of chromosome 17) mutations produce high-grade carcinomas, with a poor prognosis.

Risk Factors Associated with Ovarian Carcinoma

1. Low parity, delayed child-bearing, early age at menarche and late age at menopause are associated with increased number of ovulations.
2. Oral contraceptives, breastfeeding and multiparity are the factors with reduced ovulation and decreased risk of cancer.
3. Infertile women treated with clomiphene, age, family history and obesity have increased risk.
4. Hormone replacement therapy (HRT) and endometriosis have increased risk.
5. Smoking has increased risk of ovarian tumours.

Epidemiology

Benign tumours are common in the age range of 20–40 years and over 70% of ovarian cancer occurs after the age of 50 years. Ovarian cancer ranks third, next to breast and cervix cancers.

Clinical Features

Epithelial ovarian cancer (EOC) presents with a wide variety of non-specific symptoms. These are:

1. Abdominal pain, pelvic pain, abdominal bloating, increased abdominal size, difficulty in eating and feeling full quickly after eating.
2. Torsion or rupture of the tumour can result in acute abdominal symptoms.

Table 36.1	WHO histological classification of tumours of the ovary (WHO, 2014)[35]

Surface epithelial–stromal tumours

Serous tumours:
- Benign: Cystadenoma, adenofibroma, cystadenofibroma
- Borderline tumour: Serous borderline tumour, micropapillary variant
- Malignant: Low grade and high grade adenocarcinoma

Mucinous tumours:
- Benign: Cystadenoma, adenofibroma, cystadenofibroma
- Borderline tumour
- Malignant: Adenocarcinoma
- Mucinous cystic tumour with pseudomyxoma peritonei

Endometrioid tumours including variants with squamous differentiation

Clear cell tumours

Transitional cell tumours
- Malignant: Transitional cell carcinoma (non-Brenner type), nalignant Brenner tumour
- Borderline
- Benign: Brenner tumour

Seromucinous tumours
- Benign: Cystadenoma, adenofibroma
- Borderline: Borderline seromucinous tumour
- Malignant: Seromucinous carcinoma

Squamous cell tumours

Mixed epithelial tumours (specify components)

Undifferentiated and unclassified tumours

Germ cell tumours
1. Dysgerminoma
2. Yolk sac tumour
3. Embryonal carcinoma
4. Polyembryoma
5. Non-gestational choriocarcinoma
6. Mixed germ cell tumour (specify components)
7. Immature teratoma
8. Mature teratoma with malignant transformation—solid, cystic (dermoid cyst)
9. Monodermal teratoma and highly specialized types

Thyroid tumour group—struma ovarii, benign and malignant carcinoid group

Sex cord-stromal tumours
- Pure sex cord tumours: Granulosa cell tumour (GCT)
- Sertoli cell tumour
- Sex cord tumour with annular tubules
- Pure stromal
  - Fibroma/sarcoma
  - Thecoma
  - Sclerosing stromal tumour
  - Leydig cell tumour
  - Steroid cell tumour
- Gonadoblastoma
- Mixed germ cell-sex-cord-stromal tumour

Tumours of the rete ovarii

Miscellaneous tumours

Tumour-like conditions

Lymphoid and haematopoietic tumours

Secondary tumours

(WHO 2014 classification with slight modification)

3. Ovarian cancer is bilateral in 25% of cases.
4. Presence of ascites is mostly suggestive of carcinoma.
5. Patients with functional sex cord stromal tumours may be with features related excess estrogen or androgens.
6. Granulosa cell tumours occurring in a young girl may have precocious puberty.

Ovarian mass in a female over the age of 45 years should raise the suspicion of ovarian cancer and should be evaluated. The identification of solid or complex mass by ultrasonography is worrisome.

SEROUS CYSTADENOMA OVARY

Gross: The surface is smooth and occasionally papillary excrescences are observed over the surface. These tumours contain thin watery fluid. The inner surface of the cyst wall is smooth and may display papillary structures (Fig. 36.1).

Microscopy: This tumour shows single layer of ciliated or non-ciliated columnar epithelium lining the cyst wall and the papillae (Fig. 36.2).

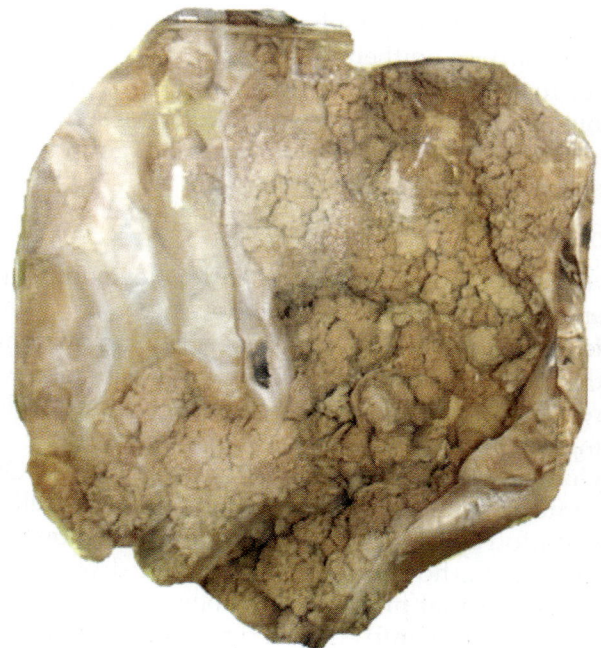

Fig. 36.1: Papillary serous cystadenoma (gross picture)

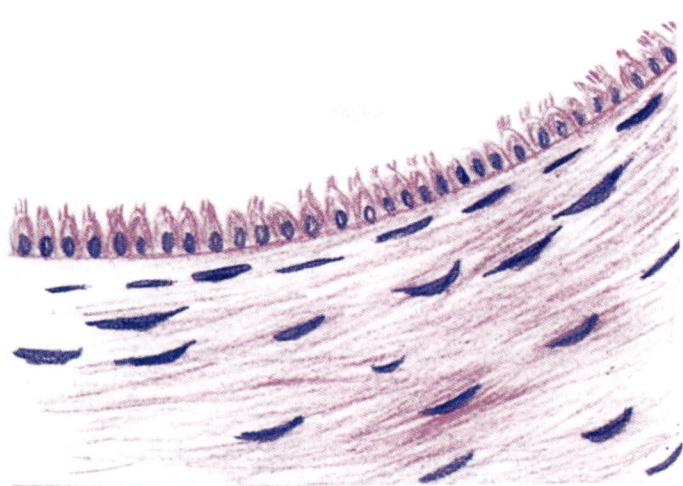

Fig. 36.2: Microphotograph of serous cystadenoma, note tall columnar ciliated epithelial cells

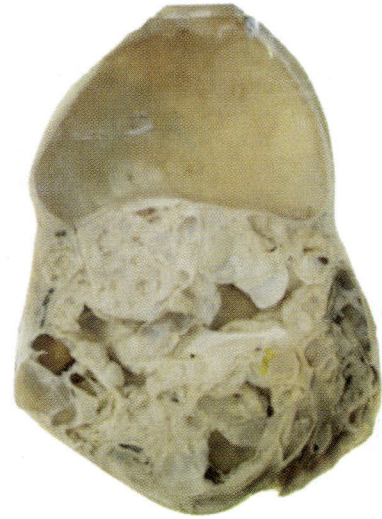

Fig. 36.3: Mucinous cystadenoma (gross picture)

Serous borderline or low malignant potential tumours represent 15% of serous tumours. It is important to separate these tumours from malignant tumours as these have better prognosis. These tumours have papillary excrescences lined by an architecturally complex epithelium.

Serous adenocarcinomas, grossly these consist of large masses of friable papillary areas, and solid areas, often with foci of haemorrhage and/or necrosis. Microscopically, serous adenocarcinomas may show destructive stromal invasion by irregularly shaped glands, or stratification of cells with an associated desmoplastic stromal response. Psammoma bodies are often present in 70% of well-differentiated tumours and these well differentiated tumours have low grade cytological features.

MUCINOUS CYSTADENOMA OVARY

Gross: These are round, ovoid or irregularly lobulated masses. They have smooth outer surface with a whitish or bluish colour. The content of the cyst is a viscid fluid, sometimes very thick or thin. These tumours are frequently multiloculated (Fig. 36.3).

Microscopy: The tumour microscopy shows single layer of non-ciliated tall columnar epithelium with pale stained cytoplasm. The nuclei are placed at the base. Paneth cells, goblet cells and endocrine cells may be noticed in these tumours (Fig. 36.4).

MUCINOUS BORDERLINE OR LOW MALIGNANT POTENTIAL TUMOURS

These present grossly as multiloculated cysts with papillary excrescences. Microscopically, most border-line tumours have stratification not more than four layers; mild to moderate nuclear atypia is present.

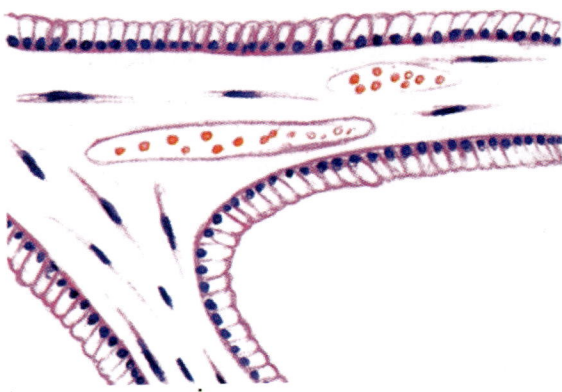

Fig. 36.4: Schematic diagram of mucinous cystadenoma, tall columnar mucin-secreting epithelium with basal nuclei

Glandular stromal invasion is uncertain, and destructive stromal invasion is not present.

MUCINOUS ADENOCARCINOMAS

These present as multiloculated cysts with cell atypia, increased layer of cells, greater complexity of glands and papillae. These tumours often show solid areas, haemorrhage, and necrosis. A diagnosis of adeno-carcinoma can be made when destructive stromal invasion is present or when complex back-to-back epithelium without intervening stroma.

ENDOMETRIOID TUMOURS OF THE OVARY

Endometrioid tumours of the ovary co-existent with endometriosis. Grossly, endometrioid adenocarcinoma may present as cystic or solid mass. These tumours usually resemble endometrial adenocarcinoma.

CLEAR CELL TUMOURS

Clear cell adenocarcinomas present as white-tan to yellow mixed solid and cystic masses, associated with haemorrhage and necrosis. Microscopically, clear cell carcinoma shows many growth patterns including solid, tubulocystic, and papillary. Cytologically, the tumour cells are large with abundant clear cytoplasm that may contain hyaline globules. These cells exhibit a high degree of nuclear atypia with hobnail nuclei.

BRENNER AND TRANSITIONAL CELL TUMOURS

These have a white to tan-yellow whorled cut surface. In benign Brenner's tumour, microscopy shows small solid to cystic nests of bland transitional epithelial cells with longitudinal nuclear grooves, surrounded by abundant fibrous stroma. Borderline or low malignant potential Brenner tumours are grossly cystic with papillary excrescences. Microscopically, the cysts and papillae are lined by stratified transitional cells resembling the cells of non-invasive papillary urothelial carcinoma.

In malignant Brenner tumours, the epithelium shows desmoplastic stromal invasion, although areas of benign or borderline Brenner tumour are still identifiable.

Transitional cell carcinomas of the ovary, microscopically, they are composed of stratified, cytologically atypical epithelium, and closely resemble transitional cell carcinoma of the bladder and no benign Brenner component is present.

CARCINOSARCOMA OVARY

This also known as malignant mixed mullerian tumour. The tumour usually occurs in postmenopausal women and has a poor prognosis, shows both malignant epithelial and malignant mesenchymal elements.

MATURE CYSTIC TERATOMA OVARY

Gross: This tumour has a thick capsule, usually unilocular and contains a pale yellow greasy material composed of frequently keratin, sebum and hair. There is often a solid portion at one pole of the cyst, which contains the bulk of the cellular elements. Teeth are found in many of the cases (Fig. 36.5).

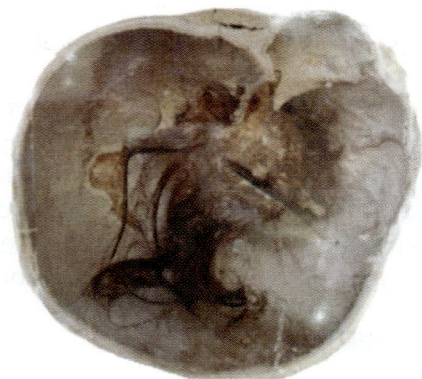

Fig. 36.5: Mature teratoma (dermoid cyst) (gross picture)

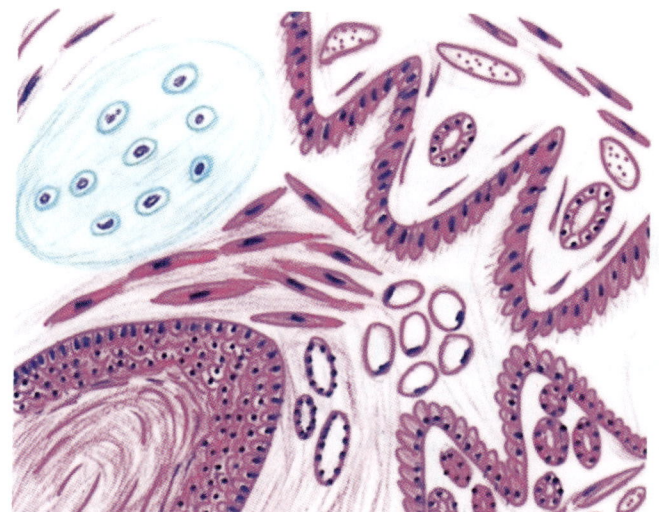

Fig. 36.6: Mature teratoma, note skin with its appendages and other mature elements (schematic)

Microscopy: The mature elements derived from mesoderm, endoderm and ectoderm are observed. Skin and its appendages are frequently present followed by neural tissue, cartilage, respiratory epithelium and gastrointestinal epithelium (Fig. 36.6).

IMMATURE TERATOMA

Immature teratoma usually presents in children and adolescents. It is composed of mixture of embryonal cells and well-developed tissues derived from all the three germ cell layers.

The main component is neuroepithelium, but mesodermal and endodermal derivatives are also present. GFAP is positive.

Grossly, immature teratoma is solid with cystic areas.

Prognosis depends upon the immature component. Depending upon the presence of primitive neuroectodermal elements and it is graded as shown below.

- *Grade I:* Abudant mature tissues with loose mesenchymal tissue, immature cartilage present.
- *Grade II:* Fewer mature tissue, rare foci of neuroectodermal elements, with mitosis, not exceeding 3 low magnification (×40) fields in any one slide.
- *Grade III:* No mature tissue, numerous neuroepithelial elements, four or more low magnification fields.

MONODERMAL (SPECIALIZED) TERATOMA

These are rare and include:
a. Struma ovarii and
b. Carcinoid tumour

Struma Ovarii

It refers to mature teratoma, which is entirely composed of visible amount of mature thyroid tissue. Rarely thyroid tissue may hyperfunction causing hyperthyroidism or can have thyroid carcinoma.

Carcinoid Tumour

It arises from the intestinal epithelium in a teratoma. This may produce 5-hydroxytryptamine (5-HT), leading to development of carcinoid syndrome.

Struma-carcinoid: It is a rare combination of struma ovarii and ovarian carcinoid.

DYSGERMINOMA

This is a most common germ cell tumour of ovary. About 80% develop in females younger than 30 years of age. Bilateral in 10% of the cases.

Pathology

Gross: They have an average diameter of 15 cm, solid lobulated, soft and fleshy, C/S cream coloured, grey-pink or tan-coloured. Cystic change, areas of haemorrhage and necrosis occasionally present. Streak ovary may be present at the periphery of the tumour.

Microscopy: Shows large, uniform rounded cells with clear (glycogen rich) cytoplasm, round nuclei with prominent nucleoli. The cells are in diffuse sheets, alveolar, insular patterns. Thin to broad septa with collagen runs in between which has lymphocytic infiltrate and 20% of the cases have sarcoid-like granulomas and 5% contain syncytiotrophoblasts. Serum β-hCG level is raised in these tumours.

YOLK SAC TUMOUR

These tumours are common below the age of 20 years. Serum alpha-fetoprotein (AFP) level is always raised. These are positive for alpha-1 antitrypsin and pankeratin.

Pathology

Gross: They are large tumours and median diameter is 15 cm. External surface is smooth and glistening. Cut section is soft, friable, yellow to grey, extensive areas of haemorrhage and necrosis present. Cystic degeneration is common.

Microscopy: The tumour cells are primitive cells arranged in reticular, solid, papillary and other patterns. There are **Schiller-Duval bodies**, wherein the cells are arranged around a vessel. Intracellular and extracellular hyaline can be present which is AFP. These hyaline globules are PAS positive and diastase resistant. Yolk sac tumour is common component with other germ cell tumours (mixed germ cell tumours).

EMBRYONAL CARCINOMA

This is a rare tumour of ovary. It accounts for 3% of germ cell tumours. These tumours occur in children and young adults. Serum hCG and alpha-fetoproteins are raised.

Pathology

Gross: The size of the tumour is around 15 cm, external surface smooth and glistening. Cut section solid and variegated with white/tan grey/yellowish-coloured areas, soft and areas of haemorrhage and necrosis present.

Microscopy: Shows cells in sheets, glands and papillae. The neoplastic cells are large primitive cells with amphophilic or vacuolated cytoplasm. Nuclei have one or more nucleoli and mitoses are numerous.

CHORIOCARCINOMA

Choriocarcinoma represents 1% germ cell tumours. They occur before puberty and are associated with other germ cell tumours. Serum β-hCG is raised in these tumours.

Pathology

Gross: Cut section of the mass is solid and friable. Areas of haemorrhage and necrosis are common.

Microscopy: Shows mixture of cytotrophoblasts, syncytiotrophoblasts and intermediate trophoblasts with haemorrhage and necrosis. The nuclei of these cells are highly pleomorphic and show increased mitosis. Choriocarcinoma can be gestational or non-gestational. Gestational has better prognosis than non-gestational ones.

Tumour markers in different germ cell tumours are given in Table 36.2.

SEX CORD STROMAL TUMOURS

These may be functional or non-functional tumours. Grnulosa cell tumour (GCT) and thecomas produce hyperestrogenic conditions like bleeding per vagina, in children precocious puberty, Sertoli-Leydig cell tumours can produce androgen and patients with this

Table 36.2	Tumour markers in germ cell tumours of ovary	
Histology	**AFP**	**hCG**
Dysgerminoma	–	±
Yolk sac tumour	+	–
Immature teratoma	±	–
Choriocarcinoma	–	+
Embryonal carcinoma	+	+
Mixed germ cell tumour	±	±
Polyembryoma	±	±

tumour can have features like hirsutism, male hairline and atrophy of breast.

GRANULOSA CELL TUMOUR

This can be produced before puberty, in child-bearing age and during menopausal age. About 3/4th of these tumours are associated with hyperestrinism. When these tumours occur in young girls they may produce precocious puberty. Metrorrhagia and menorrhagia are produced in adult females including menopausal female patients.

Pathology

Gross: These tumours are smooth, lobulated, solid grey to yellow coloured.

Microscopy: These tumours show variable histological morphology, the cells arranged in microfollicular pattern with Call-Exner bodies is the more frequent histological type. The neoplastic cells have nuclei with grooves (coffee bean nuclei). When theca cell component is also present, the tumour is called granulosa-theca cell tumour.

The other variants include macrofollicular pattern, trabacular, insular, watered silk, solid and pseudo-papillary patterns.

THECOMAS

Thecomas present usually after menopause in 65% of the cases. They are unilateral. This tumour has to be differentiated from fibroma ovary. These patients may present with symptoms of excess estrogen including postmenopausal patients.

Pathology

Gross: These tumours vary in size, capsulated and firm. Cut section of these tumours is solid and yellowish.

Microscopy: The comas have fascicles of spindle cells with centrally placed nuclei and moderate amount of cytoplasm. The intervening tissue has collagen deposition with hyaline plaque formation. With "oil red O stain", the cells show abundant intracytoplasmic neutral fat and silver stain demonstrates reticulin fibres around each cells. These features are not observed in fibromas.

FIBROMAS

Fibromas are unilateral and usually seen in after puberty. Ovarian fibroma may be associated with right-sided pleural effusion, i.e. Meig's syndrome. Ovarian fibroma with basal cell naevus is called **Gorlin syndrome**.

Pathology

Gross: They are solid, lobulated, firm, whitish coloured. They measure around 6 cm or more. Myxoid change may be seen. Sometimes cystic changes are encountered.

Microscopy: They have spindle cells arranged in storiform pattern. Hyaline deposition, oedema and hyaline globules may be seen.

SERTOLI–LEYDIG CELL TUMOUR
(Androblastoma, Arrhenoblastoma)

These consist of mixture of Sertoli cells and Leydig cells in varying proportion. They occur in young patients and rare after menopause. About 50% of these tumours are accompanied by signs of androgen excess.

Following can be androgenic effects:
1. Defaminisation: Atrophy of breast, amenorrhoea, loss of subcutaneous fat
2. Musculinisation: Clitoral hyperplasia, deepening of voice, hirsutism

Pathology

Gross: These tumours are predominantly solid with cystic areas.

Microscopy: These tumours have tubulr structures having Sertoli cells and in between the tubules Leydig cells. These tumours can be well differentiated, moderately differentiated or poorly differentiated.

The prognosis depends upon the stage of the tumour and degree of differentiation.

LEYDIG CELL TUMOURS

These tumours produce steroid hormones. They are unilateral and originate in the hilum. They are common in postmenopausal age group. They cause hirsutism/virilisation in 80% of the patients. The serum testosterone and urinary 17-ketosteroids are elevated.

Pathology

Gross: They are yellow to yellow-brown coloured and lobulated.

Microscopy: Shows polyhedral cells in sheets, cords and nests. They are uniform cells with large central nucleus with one more prominent nucleoli. Cytoplasm is vacuolated and may show crystals of Reinke.

Prognosis: The tumour has good prognosis.

GYNANDROBLASTOMA

• These are rare sex cord stromal tumours.

- There is combination of patterns of both granulosa-theca cell tumour and Sertoli-Leydig cell tumour. The term gynandroblastoma stands for combination of female (gyn) and male (andro).
- Present at mean age of 30 years with estrogenic or androgenic effects.
- They may be functional with estrogen or androgen hormones.
- These are with low malignant potential.
- Recurrences are known.

LIPID CELL TUMOURS

- These account for 5% of sex cord stromal tumours.
- These contain cells of steroid hormone secretion.
- The cells can be theca cells/Leydig cells or adrenal cortical rests of hilum.
- A few contain crystalloids of Reinke.
- These can occur at any age.
- These can be hormonally active with androgen excess/cortisol excess with Cushing syndrome.

Pathology

Gross: Uniform, yellow or yellow brown tumours, nodular separated by fibrous septa.

Microscopy: Shows rounded or large polyhedral cells with pale or vacuolated cytoplasm.

With malignancy, size increases with areas of haemorrhage and necrosis.

METASTATIC TUMOURS

Constitute 3% of ovarian tumours. Women in the age group of 30–60 years are commonly affected. Metastasis may occur by lymphatic or hematogenous route but direct extension from adjacent organs (uterus, fallopian tube and sigmoid colon) also occur. Bilaterality of the tumour is an important clue for diagnosis of metastatic tumour.

Source: Primary malignancy may be from stomach, large intestine, appendix, pancreas, biliary tract, breast and haemopoietic malignancies.

KRUKENBERG TUMOUR

It is a distinctive bilateral tumour metastatic to the ovaries by transcoelomic spread, usually secondary to gastric carcinoma. Breast carcinoma and other GI malignancies including those of biliary tract and pancreas can also produce Krukenberg tumour of ovary.

Gross: Both ovaries show large round or kidney-shaped, firm multinodular masses.

Microscopy: Characterised by mucin-filled signet ring cells which may lie singly or in clusters. Stroma also shows cellular proliferation in storiform pattern.

NICE TO KNOW

MOLECULAR CLASSIFICATION OF EPITHELIAL OVARIAN TUMOURS/CANCER (EOT/EOC)

Recent advances in pathology and genetics have shown that different histologic subtypes of EOCs have distinctive risk factors, genetic abnormalities, and oncologic pathways that determine biologic behaviour, response to chemotherapy, and prognosis. Based on histopathology, immune-histochemistry and molecular genetic analysis, at least five main types of epithelial ovarian tumours are recognized. They are:
1. High grade serous carcinoma (HGSC)
2. Endometrioid carcinoma
3. Clear cell carcinoma
4. Mucinous carcinoma
5. Low grade serous carcinoma

Most HGSCs react for p53, BRCA1, WT1, and p16. They also exhibit a high proliferation index as indicated by an increased nuclear expression of Ki-67. Estrogen receptor (ER) is expressed in approximately two-thirds of cases of HGSCs. Low grade serous carcinomas have KRAS, BRAF, ERBB2 and PTEN mutations.

Kurman and Shih have classified malignant epithelial ovarian tumours into Type 1 and Type 2 categories. Type 1 tumours are low grade indolent tumours. These lack P53 mutations, arise step-wise *de novo* from benign, borderline and later into malignant tumours. These include low grade serous carcinoma, low grade endometrioid carcinoma, mucinous carcinoma, clear cell carcinoma, and Brenner's tumour. Type 2 category tumours are more aggressive tumours, display P53 mutations and include high grade serous carcinoma, undifferentiated carcinoma and malignant mixed mullerian tumours. Transitional cell carcinoma is related to high grade serous carcinoma.

FUNCTIONAL/HORMONE-SECRETING OVARIAN TUMOURS

Sex-cord stromal tumours: Nearly 90% of hormone-producing ovarian tumours are sex-cord stromal tumours. These can be:
  I. *Pure stromal tumours:*
  - Thecoma (estrogens)
  - Leydig cell tumour (androgens)
  - Steroid cell tumours
  II. *Pure sex-cord tumours:*
  - Granulosa cell tumour (estrogens, rarely androgens)
  - Sertoli cell tumour (androgens, rarely estrogens)

III. *Mixed sex-cord stromal tumours:*
- Sertoli-Leydig cell tumours also called gynandroblastoma or arrhenoblastoma.
- Sex-cord stromal tumours (not otherwise classified).

The other hormone-secreting ovarian tumours are:
- *Carcinoid tumours of ovary:* These can be primary or metastatic (mainly from GIT). These secrete variety of neurohumoral substances including serotonin, histamine, brachykinin, bradykinin, prostaglandins, etc.
- *Struma ovarii:* Rare monodermal teratoma with predominant presence of thyroid tissue and sometimes may be functional.
- *Choriocarcinoma of ovary:* Aggressive tumour of trophoblastic cells and secrete beta-hCG.

FIGO staging of ovarian tumours[40]

Stage I: The cancer is limited to the ovaries

IA Limited to one ovary and the outer ovarian capsule is not ruptured. There is no tumour on the external surface of the ovary and there is no ascites and/or the washings are negative.

IB Cancer is present in both ovaries, but the outer capsule is intact and there is no tumour on external surface. There is no ascites and the washings are negative.

IC The cancer is either Stage IA or IB level but the capsule is ruptured or there is tumour on the ovarian surface or malignant cells are present in ascites or washings.

Stage II: Cancer involves one or both ovaries with spread to other pelvic organs or surfaces

IIA Extension or implants onto the uterus and/or fallopian tube. The washings are negative and there is no ascites.

IIB Extension or implants onto other pelvic tissues. The washings are negative and there is no ascites.

IIC Pelvic extension or implants like Stage IIA or IIB but with positive pelvic washings.

Stage III: Cancer spread outside the pelvis to the abdominal area, including metastases to liver surface

IIIA Tumour is grossly confined to the pelvis but with microscopic peritoneal metastases beyond pelvis to abdominal peritoneal surfaces or the omentum.

IIIB Same as IIIA but with macroscopic peritoneal or omental metastases beyond pelvis less than 2 cm in size.

IIIC Same as IIIA but with peritoneal or omental metastases beyond pelvis, larger than 2 cm, with or without retroperitoneal lymph node metastases.

Stage IV: Metastases or spread to the liver or outside the peritoneal cavity to areas such as the chest or brain including regional lymph nodes and lymph nodes outside of abdominal cavity.

(Simplified FIGO Ovarian Cancer Staging 2014)

SELF-ASSESSMENT EXERCISE

1. **Schiller-Duval bodies are seen in:**
   A. Embryonal carcinoma
   B. Yolk sac tumour
   C. Granulosa cell tumour
   D. Teratoma

2. **Immature neuroepithelial elements are seen in:**
   A. Teratocarcinoma   B. Struma ovarii
   C. Immature teratoma   D. Dermoid cyst

3. **CA125 is associated with:**
   A. Ca colon
   B. Serous carcinoma ovary
   C. Teratoma ovary
   D. Fibroma ovary

4. **A lady with ovarian tumour, X-ray shows radio-opaque shadow. Possible ovarian tumour is:**
   A. Serous tumours   B. Mucinous tumours
   C. Dermoid cyst   D. Granulosa cell tumour

5. **True about dysgerminoma:**
   A. Bilateral
   B. Radiosensitive
   C. Occurs in postmenopausal age
   D. Increased alpha-fetoprotein

6. **Meigs syndrome:**
   A. Aggressive in nature
   B. Associated with yolk sac tumour
   C. Ascites and pleural effusion
   D. Associated with epithelial tumour

7. **Meigs syndrome has all *except*:**
   A. Ascites and pleural effusion
   B. Solid benign tumour
   C. Excision of tumour has cure
   D. CA125 raised

8. **Pseudomyxoma peritonei is seen in:**
   A. Serous carcinoma   B. Yolk sac tumour
   C. Mucinous carcinoma D. Dermoid cyst

9. **In Krukenburg tumour, all are true *except*:**
   A. Bilateral
   B. Signet ring cells
   C. Metastasis from GI malignancy
   D. Mucinous carcinoma ovary

10. **Ovarian tumours commonly arise from:**
    A. Surface epithelium
    B. Germ cell
    C. Stromal cells
    D. Germ cells and stromal cells

11. **Most common ovarian tumour in children:**
    A. Serous tumour
    B. Granulosa cell tumour
    C. Germ cell tumour
    D. Mucinous tumour

12. **Call-Exner bodies are seen in:**
    A. Thecoma
    B. Granulosa cell tumour
    C. Dysgerminoma
    D. Fibroma

13. **Reinke crystals are found in:**
    A. Leydig cell tumour
    B. Granulosa cell tumour
    C. Thecoma
    D. Dysgerminoma

14. **Krukenburg tumour, all are true _except_:**
    A. Secondaries to ovary
    B. Primary colon
    C. Signet ring cells on microscopy
    D. Primary adenocarcinoma

15. **Struma ovarii is predominant element of:**
    A. Fibrosis
    B. Thyroid tissue
    C. Neuroendocrine cells
    D. All of the above

Answers

1. B	2. C	3. B	4. C	5. B	6. C	7. D	8. C
9. D	10. A	11. C	12. B	13. A	14. D	15. B	

Male Genital System: Scrotum, Testis, Epididymis, Penile Lesions and Prostate

SCROTUM

Skin of scrotum may be affected by many inflammatory lesions including fungal infections.

Neoplasms of scrotal sac are less common. Squamous cell carcinoma of scrotal skin, as an environmental or occupational health hazard as described by Sir Percival Pott in chimney sweepers, is reduced nowadays.

Lymphatic obstruction of scrotum and lower limbs by filariasis may cause elephantiasis.

TESTIS AND EPIDIDYMIS

CRYPTORCHIDISM

This represents testicular non-descent into the scrotum. Normally, testes develop in relation to lumbar region, they reach the iliac fossa during 3rd month and deep inguinal ring by 7th month of intrauterine life. By the end of 8th month, they reach the scrotal sac.

Cryptorchidism is present in 1% of the male population. About 10% of these are bilateral. Hormonal abnormalities, testicular abnormalities, mechanical problems like obstruction of the inguinal canal may interfere with testicular descent. It is seen with Prader-Willi syndrome.

The cause is not known in many of the cases. Unilateral or bilateral cryptorchidism causes sterility and atrophy. Unilateral cryptorchidism may be associated with atrophy of other side testis which is descended and also contributes to infertility.

Unilateral or bilateral cryptorchidism is associated with 5-fold increased risk of malignancy. Orchidopexy (placement of undescended testis into scrotum before puberty) reduces likelihood of testicular atrophy and risk of cancer.

Pathology

The affected cryptorchid testis is normal in size in early life or may be reduced at the time of puberty. There is tubular atrophy by 5–6 yrs of age and hyalinization by puberty. Following are the important features:

- Loss of tubules
- Thickened basement membrane
- Hyperplasia of Leydig cells
- Foci of intratubular germ cell neoplasia may be observed in cryptorchid testes.

Atrophic changes similar to cryptorchid testes may be seen in chronic ischaemia, trauma, radiation, chemotherapy or with increased levels of estrogen as seen in cirrhosis. This may not develop intratubular neoplasia.

INFLAMMATORY LESIONS

Infections are more common in epididymis than testis. The most common inflammatory lesions include: Tuberculosis, leprosy, sarcoidosis or Crohn's disease, malakoplakia, pyogenic epididymo orchitis, gonorrhoea, non-specific epididymo-orchitis and mumps infection.

- Testicular tuberculosis begins as an epididymitis and later involves testes.
- Gonorrhoea causes acute prostatitis, orchitis and epididymitis.
- Infarct of the testes is usually due to torsion of the spermatic cord or due to venous thrombosis secondary to pyogenic epididymo-orchitis.

TESTICULAR TUMOURS

Many types of testicular tumours originating from germ cells or sex cord stromal tumours are known.

Etiology

1. **Undescended testis (cryptorchidism):** 10% of testicular tumours are associated with cryptorchidism.
2. **Environmental factors:** Pesticides and non-steroidal estrogen (diethylstilbesterol or DES) exposure *in utero* is known with testicular dysgenesis syndromes (cryptorchidism, hypospadiasis and poor germ quality).
3. **Genetics:** Familial association is known in testicular tumours.

Pathogenesis

Most tumours arise from precursor lesion called intratubular germ cell neoplasia. The exception to this is paediatric tumours (yolk sac tumours, mature teratoma) and spermatocytic seminoma. The term carcinoma *in situ* was used earlier to this lesion.

Table 37.1 shows the classification of testicular tumours.

Table 37.1	Classification of testicular tumours[41]

Germ cell tumours derived from germ cell neoplasia *in situ*
- Non-invasive germ cell neoplasia
  - Germ cell neoplasia *in situ*
  - Specific forms of intratubular germ cell neoplasia
- Tumours of single histological type
  - Seminomatous germ cell tumours
    - Seminoma
  - Non-seminomatous germ cell tumours
    - Spermatocytic seminoma
    - Embryonal carcinoma
    - Yolk sac tumour
    - Trophoblastic tumours
      - Choriocarcinoma
      - Non-choriocarcinomatous trophoblastic tumours
      - Placental site trophoblastic tumour
      - Epithelioid trophoblastic tumour
    - Teratoma—post-pubertal type
    - Germ cell tumours of more than one histological type
    - Mixed germ cell tumours

Sex cord stromal tumours
- Pure tumours
  - Leydig cell tumours
  - Sertoli cell tumour
  - Granulosa cell tumour
  - Fibroma–thecoma
- Mixed
  - Gonadoblastoma
  - Unclassified

Miscellaneous tumours

Haematolymphoid tumours

(WHO 2016 classification with modification)

GERM CELL NEOPLASIA *IN SITU*

This was earlier termed as intratubular germ cell neoplasia or testicular intratubular germ cell neoplasia. Now has been known as germ cell neoplasia *in situ* **(GCNIS)**. Many germ cell tumours of testis arise from this precursor lesion. This can be classified as below.
1. Differentiated seminomatous GCNIS
2. Differentiated non-seminomatous GCNIS
3. Undifferentiated GCNIS

Microscopy: In seminomatous GCNIS, the affected tubules are expanded and filled with large polygonal cells with large nucleus having prominent nuclei and clear cytoplasm (seminoma-like cells). Placental alkaline phosphatase and OCT3/4 are positive. In non-seminomatous GCNIS, intratubular embryonal carcinoma, intratubular yolk sac tumour, intratubular teratoma, etc. can occur.

SEMINOMA TESTIS

This is the most common testicular tumour. Typical (classical) seminoma accounts for 85–90% of the cases and occurs in the age range of 35–45 years. It is rare in old age as well as in young age. It is associated with cryptorchidism. The testis is enlarged with or without pain. The serum levels of hCG and PLAP may be increased. About 75% of the seminomas are confined to the testis at the time of presentation in contrast to about 50–70% of the non-seminomatous germ cell tumours which can have metastasis by the time they are diagnosed.

Gross: The tumour is well demarcated, homogenous, firm, grey white and lobulated (Fig. 37.1).

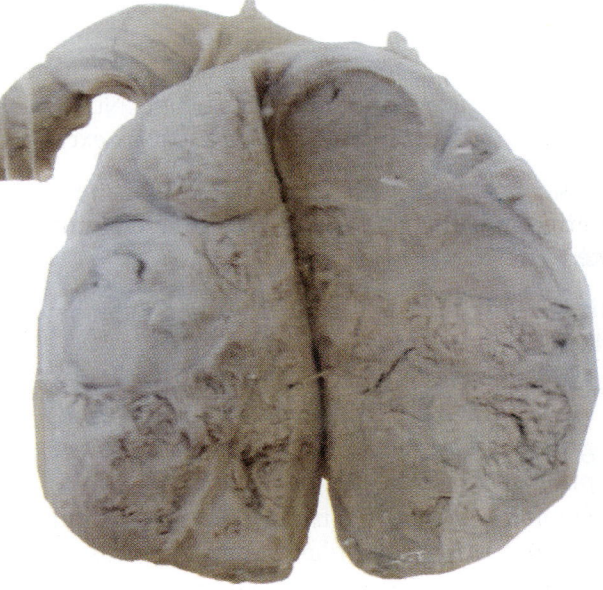

Fig. 37.1: Seminoma testis (gross picture)

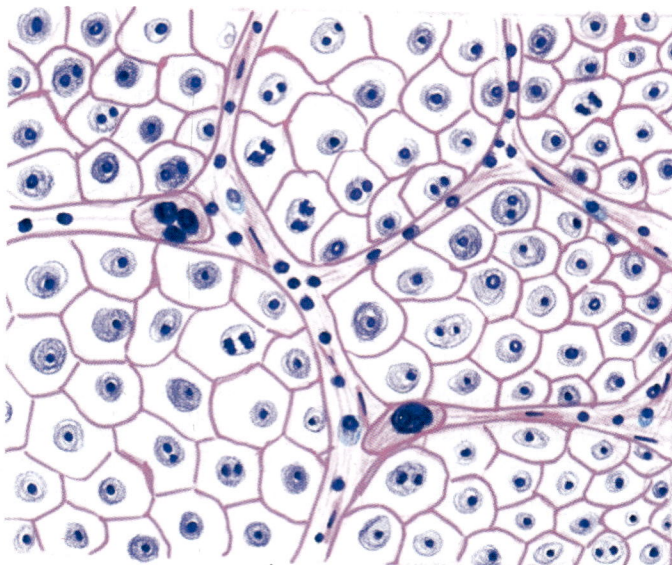

Fig. 37.2: Seminoma (schematic)

Microscopy: There is a diffuse proliferation of large uniform tumour cells which are arranged in sheets, nests, and cords. The tumour cells are separated into lobules by supporting stroma which contains variable number of lymphocytes. They have distinct cell membrane. The nuclei are centrally placed; they are large and round with sharp nuclear membrane and they have prominent nucleoli. The cytoplasm is abundant and usually clear/eosinophilic/amphophilic. Mitoses are common. The stroma may show scattered syncytiotrophoblastic giant cells. The PAS stain demonstrates glycogen in the cytoplasm of these tumour cells (Fig. 37.2).

SPERMATOCYTIC SEMINOMA

Spermatocytic seminoma is a rare slow growing germ cell tumour affecting older people. It is distinctive tumour, not related to seminoma clinically and histologically. It represents 1 to 2% of all testicular tumours. Affects around 65 years of age. No metastasis is seen in these tumours and prognosis is excellent.

Gross: Soft, pale grey, cut section is mucoid or gelatinous with cystic areas. Extension beyond testis is rare.

Microscopy: Spermatocytic seminoma contains intermixed three cell types.
1. Medium sized cells (15 to 20 μ in size) are the most numerous. These have round nucleus, finely granular chromatin and moderate amount of eosinophilic cytoplasm.
2. Smaller cells (6 to 8 μ in size), these containing scant narrow rim of cytoplasm, homogenous, pyknotic nucleus with dense chromatin, resemble secondary spermatocytes.

3. Scattered large cells (uninucleate or multinucleate giant cells) are less in number.

Medium-sized cells and large cells can have filamentous and spireme chromatin similar to spermatocytic cells seen in meiotic phase.

Spermatocytic seminoma lacks glycogen in its cytoplasm, lymphocytic infiltrate, granulomas, trophoblastic cells in the stroma, and extra-testicular origin. No admixture of other germ cell tumours.

TERATOMA TESTIS

Teratoma refers to various cellular or organoid components derived from more than one germ layer. These tumours may occur at any age from infancy to adult life, pure forms are common in infants and children and these are second in frequency to yolk sac tumours. In adults, pure forms are rare. Teratoma in combination with other germ cell tumours is common.

Gross: Teratoma testis is a large tumour measuring about 5 to 10 cm in diameter. The cut section is heterogenous with solid to cystic and cartilagenous areas. Haemorrhage and necrosis are common features (Fig. 37.3).

Microscopy: Teratomas comprise different tissues like neural tissue, muscle, islands of cartilage, squamous epithelium, thyroid tissue, respiratory epithelium, intestinal epithelium and so on. These elements may be mature or immature. Malignant transformation of any of these elements can be present. There can be combination of other germ cell tumours too (Fig. 37.4).

Tumour markers in germ cell tumours: The following markers are helpful in detection of the germ cell tumours: (i) Alpha-fetoproteins for yolk sac tumour,

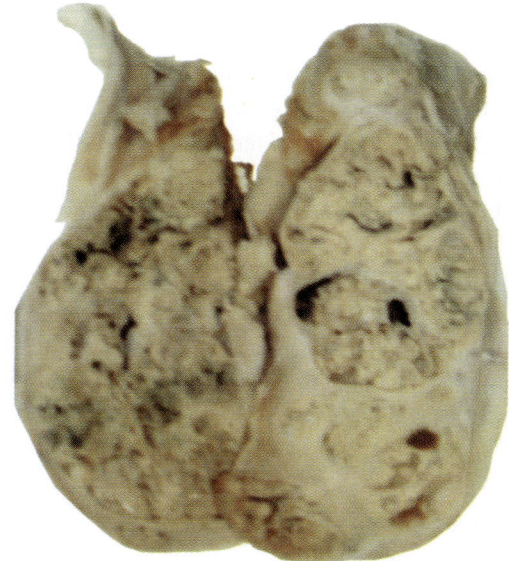

Fig. 37.3: Teratoma testis (gross picture)

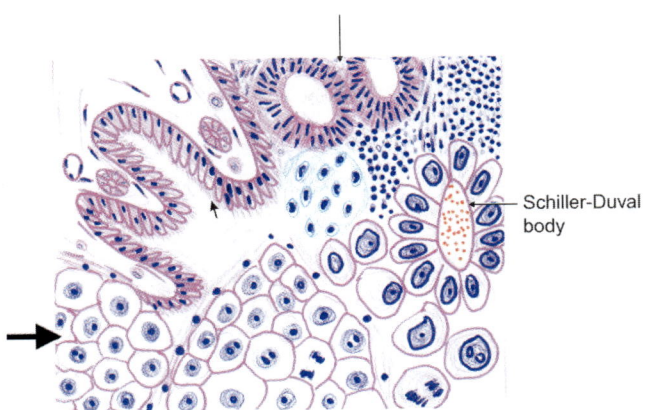

Fig. 37.4: Microscopy of teratoma testis (*Note:* Mixed germ cell tumour components—seminoma component (thick arrow), immature (thin arrow) and mature teratoma (short arrow) components and yolk sac tumour component with Schiller-Duval body (schematic)

(ii) hCG for choriocarcinoma, (iii) hCG, placental alkaline phosphatase and placental lactogen for seminoma, and (iv) lactate dehydrogenase for tumour burden.

The tumour markers are helpful in: (i) Histological typing of the tumour, (ii) for staging of the testicular germ cell tumours, (iii) assessing tumour burden, and (iv) in monitoring response to therapy.

EMBRYONAL CARCINOMA

This tumour commonly occurs in the age group of 20 to 30 years. These are aggressive tumours characterised by rapid growth. It is rare in pure form and common with mixed germ cell tumours. It shares some markers of seminoma such as PLAP.

Gross: These tumours may or may not occupy the entire testis. They are often variegated, have areas of necrosis and haemorrhage. The tumour has poorly demarcated margins. Extension of tumour through tunica albuginea into epididymis and cord are frequently seen. Lymphatic and vascular metastasis with lymph node involvement and spread to liver and lungs is common.

Microscopy: The undifferentiated cells are in sheets, alveolar, tubular, and papillary patterns. The nuclei are hyperchromatic with prominent nucleoli. The cell borders are indistinct. Mitosis and tumour giant cells are frequently seen.

YOLK SAC TUMOUR

It is a most common tumour in children below the age of 2 years. In this age, it has good prognosis. In adults, pure form is less common. Yolk sac tumours commonly occur with embryonal carcinomas. These tumours are positive for alpha-fetoproteins.

Gross: These are non-encapsulated, homogenous, yellow white and mucinous tumours.

Microscopy: Tumour tissue has medium-sized cuboidal cells or falttened cells reticular network, papillary structures and solid sheets. The cells are also seen around the vessel giving the appearance of Shiller-Duval body. Within the cytoplasm and out side the cells, eosinophilic hyaline globules are seen and these represent alpha-fetoproteins.

CHORIOCARCINOMA

It is highly malignant tumour. Pure form is rare and occurs along with mixed germ cell tumours. These secrete β-hCG. These may be small and detected as palpable nodules. These spread rapidly by haematogenous route. Lungs and liver metastasis commonly seen.

Gross: Small-sized tumours with areas of haemorrhage and necrosis.

Microscopy: Shows two types of cells cytotrophoblasts and syncytiotrophoblasts.

Cytotrophoblasts are polygonal cells with distinct borders and clear cytoplasm. These are seen in cords and sheets with single nucleus. Syncytiotrophoblasts are large multinucleated cells with abundant eosinophilic vacuolated cytoplasm.

MIXED GERM CELL TUMOURS

About 60% of the testicular tumours are having mixture of pure forms. Common combinations are: Teratoma with embryonal and yolk sac tumour, seminoma with embryonal carcinoma, and teratoma with embryonal carcinoma.

Lymphatic spread is common with spread to retroperitoneal para-aortic lymph nodes. Mediastinal and supraclavicular lymph nodes may also be involved. Lungs, liver, brain and bone may be involved by haematogenous spread.

PENILE LESIONS

Penis may be affected by malformations, infections and neoplasms. The malformations include abnormalities in the location of distal urethral orifice.

Hypospadias: This occurs in 1:250 live male births and the opening of urethra is along the ventral aspect of the penis.

Epispadias: In this, the orifice is located on the dorsum of the penis. Both these malformations predispose to lower urinary tract infections. Epispadias may be associated with bladder extrophy.

Infections: Balanitis (inflammation of the glans penis) and balanoposthitis (inflammation of glans penis and prepuce) occur due to poor local hygiene in uncirumcised penis. Smegma acts as an irritant.

Phimosis represents a condition wherein the prepuce cannot be retracted over the glans penis.

When stenotic prepuce is retracted forcibly over the glans penis, circulation to glans penis is compromised resulting in congestion, swelling, and pain of distal penis. This is called paraphimosis.

Fungi and candidiasis may affect penis. Candidiasis presents with erosive, painful, pruritic lesion involving glans penis, scrotum and adjacent areas.

NEOPLASMS OF PENIS

Squamous cell carcinoma and its precursor lesions are most important penile lesions.

Precancerous Lesions (Precursor or Intraepithelial Lesions) of Penis

Precancerous lesions of penis include the following:
1. Bowen's disease
2. Erythroplasia of Queyrat
3. Bowenoid papulosis

Risk factors: These are similar to penile carcinoma.

Bowen's Disease

This has sharply demarcated scaly erythematous plaques on skin of shaft. Epithelium shows dysplasia.

Erythroplasia of Queyrat

This presents as shiny velvety erythematous plaque on glans or prepuce. The lesions may even flat, papules or macules other than plaque lesions. These usually occur in elderly individuals. Microscopy has increased numbers of layers of epithelial cells with elongated and anastomosing rete ridges with epithelial pearl formation. Atypia is present. Parakeratosis is frequent.

Bowen's disease and erythroplasia of Queyrat harbor carcinoma *in situ* changes. These lesions may represent a well-differentiated invasive SCC, if a though search is undertaken.

Bowenoid Papulosis

This is histologically similar to Bowen's disease but occurs in young adults and has small soft multiple reddish to violaceous papules or macules on the shaft of glans or less frequently on glans sulcus or foreskin. This is HPV-related penile lesion and most often high-risk HPV 16.

Microscopy reveals squamous cell carcinoma *in situ*. There is proliferation of epithelial cells with hyperchromatic nuclei with increased N: C ratio.

PENILE CARCINOMA

Penile carcinoma affects elderly individuals. According to National Cancer Tumour Registry, penile carcinoma is the second most urological malignancy after prostatic carcinoma. High incidence is found in Latin America, Africa, and Asia. Low incidence is found in the United States of America and Europe. In India, there is variation in prevalence. The risk factors include:
1. Uncircumcised men (poor hygiene)
2. Phimosis
3. HPV infection
4. Smoking
5. Tobacco
6. Radiation/UV rays
7. Exposure to arsenic

Penile lesions can be classified according to patterns of growth, and histological features. The classification which is mainly based on histolological features is given in Table 37.2.

Depending upon the growth patterns, following can be different types:
1. Superficial spreading
2. Vertical growth pattern
3. Squamous cell carcinoma of verruciform growth pattern

Table 37.2   Classification of penile tumours[41]
Malignant epithelial tumours
• Squamous cell carcinoma
• Non-HPV-related squamous cell carcinoma
– Squamous cell carcinoma usual type
– Pseudohyperplastic carcinoma
– Pseudoglandular carcinoma
– Verrucous carcinoma
– Carcinoma cunuculatum
– Papillary squamous cell carcinoma—NOS
– Adenosquamous carcinoma
– Sarcomatoid carcinoma
– Mixed squamous cell carcinoma
• HPV-related squamous cell carcinoma
– Basaloid squamous cell carcinoma
– Papillary basaloid carcinoma
– Warty carcinoma
– Warty basaloid carcinoma
– Clear cell squamous carcinoma
– Lymphoepithelioma-like carcinoma
• Precursor lesions
– Penile intraepithelial neoplasia
– Warty/basaloid/warty-basaloid
Melanocytic tumours
Mesenchymal tumours
Malignant tumours including tumours of uncertain malignant potential
Lymphoma
Metastatic tumour

(WHO 2016 classification with slight modification)

4. Squamous cell carcinoma of multicentric growth pattern
5. Squamous cell carcinoma of mixed growth pattern

Squamous cell carcinoma occurs on the glans or shaft as an ulceronodular infiltrative lesion which grossly and histologically similar to squamous cell carcinoma occurring in other sites. They spread to inguinal lymph nodes and rarely to distant sites. The important features in different growth patterns are mentioned below.

1. The superficial spreading pattern has raised and grey white lesion. The lesion grows horizontally initially involving glans, sulcus and foreskin. This is followed by vertical growth in advanced cases.
2. The vertical growth has large, ulcerated and fungating mass, cut section is solid with invasive nodular appearance.
3. Verruciformis pattern grows slowly, has more of exophytic lesion, with well-differentiated hyperkeratotic to papillary configuration. The lesion is superficial and rarely invasive in nature.
4. In multicentric pattern, two or more independent foci separated by benign tissue are present.

LESIONS OF PROSTATE

PROSTATITIS

Prostatitis represents inflammation of prostate. It may be acute or chronic which is based upon clinical features, culture of fractionated urine samples obtained before or after prostatic massage. *E. coli* is associated with acute prostatitis. There is inflammation of urethra and bladder, as it is an ascending infection.

Chronic prostatitis follows acute prostatitis or may develop insidiously without episodes of acute infection. It can be of bacterial origin or sometimes bacteriological findings are negative (chronic abacterial prostatitis). The causes for this abacterial prostatitis include nongonococcal urethritis, *Chlamydia trachomatis* and *Ureaplasma urealyticum*.

Pathology

In acute prostatitis, there is presence of neutrophilic infiltrate congestion and oedema. Inflammatory cells are present within the glands and may destroy the glandular epithelium and extends into surrounding stroma with formation of microabscesses. There may be extensive areas of necrosis in diabetic patients.

In chronic prostatitis, there is variable infiltration of mononuclear cells, frequently accompanied by acute inflammatory cells. There is tissue destruction and areas of fibrosis.

Chronic granulomatous prostatitis is a variant of chronic prostatitis which can be encounted in tuberculosis, sarcoidosis, fungal infections and Wegener's granulomatosis. It may occur as a reaction to inspissated prostatic secretions too.

Foamy macrophages, lymphocytes and multinucleated giant cell and eosinophils are the cells which are encountered in these lesions. In tuberculosis, caseations, necrosis and epithelioid cells are evident.

Clinical Features

These patients of acute prostatitis have dysuria, urinary frequency, low back pain, and suprapubic pain. The prostate is enlarged and tender, accompanied by fever and leucocytosis.

Chronic prostatitis may be asymptomatic or silent and is a reservoir of organisms and in turn causes recurrent urinary tract infection.

NODULAR HYPERPLASIA OF PROSTATE

Usually called **benign prostatic hypertrophy (BPH)**, recently it is termed as **nodular hyperplasia of prostate (NPH)** by Moore[42] as the disease presents with nodular enlargement of the gland caused by hyperplasia of glandular and stromal components.

Pathogenesis

About 20% of men at the age of 40 years have nodular hyperplasia of prostate which increases to 70% by the age of 60 years and to 90% by the age of 70 years.

The exact cause is not understood. However, the following mechanisms are explained:

1. Androgen seems to play role. The proliferation is related to dihydrotestosterone (DHT) which is synthesized from testosterone by the action of an enzyme 5α-reductase type 2. DHT binds to nuclear androgen receptors and stimulates the growth of prostate. Both the glands and stroma proliferate.
2. Estrogens also play role. As age advances, there is increase in estrogen levels which stimulate production of DHT receptors and thus estrogens too stimulate proliferation of glands and stroma of prostate.
3. Alpha 1 adrenergic receptors are over-expressed in hyperplasia of prostate and blocking these receptors can relax the smooth muscle of prostate and reduce the obstructive symptoms.

Clinical Features

Symptoms related to lower urinary tract are more common as inner portion is more involved in proliferation than the peripheral portions. Urinary symptoms include:

1. Hesitancy—difficulty in starting the stream of urine
2. Frequency

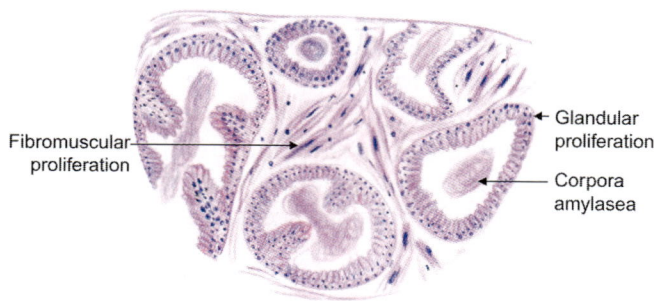

Fig. 37.5: Microphotograph of nodular hyperplasia of prostate showing proliferation of glands and stroma

3. Intermittent interruption
4. Nocturia
5. Complete blockage of urine with painful distension of bladder
6. Chronic obstruction leads to urinary tract infection (UTI)

Gross: Prostate is enlarged, weighs up to 200 g. Cut section is nodular with milky white ooze. When predominantly fibromuscular, it is firm, pale-grey and has less fluid.

Microscopy: There is glandular and fibromuscular proliferation. The glandular element shows cystically dilated glands lined by two layers—inner columnar and outer cuboidal to flattened epithelium. The epithelium is thrown into papillae. The lumen shows corpora amylacea and foci of squamous metaplasia. The stroma may show chronic inflammation, abscesses or infarction (Fig. 37.5).

PROSTATIC INTRAEPITHELIAL NEOPLASIA (PIN)

It is a **precursor lesion** of prostate cancer. It has rearrangement involving ETS genes which are also found in invasive prostate cancer. Both PIN and invasive cancer typically predominate in the **peripheral zone**. Prostates containing cancer have a higher frequency and greater extent of PIN and often seen in proximity to cancer.

Morphology

It consists of prostatic acini or ducts lined by cytologically atypical cells with enlarged nuclei, having prominent **nucleoli,** and show marked crowding. PIN glands are surrounded by a patchy layer of basal cells and an intact basement membrane.

Prostatic intraepithelial neoplasia was originally graded from 1 to 3, currently divided into two grades depending upon degree of atypia, i.e. the nuclear features regardless of architecture:
1. Low grade
2. High grade

Grade 1 is considered as low-grade PIN, whereas grades 2 and 3 are currently considered together as high-grade PIN.

Low-grade PIN has more architectural complexity than hyperplasia, occasional enlarged and hyperchromatic nuclei, rare nucleoli.

High grade of PIN is associated with cytologically atypical cells with enlarged nuclei, having prominent **nucleoli** and progressive disruption of the basal cell layer. Architecturally, four main patterns of high-grade PIN have been described; they are tufting, micropapillary, cribriform, and flat. High grade is always associated with adenocarcinoma.

PROSTATIC CARCINOMA

Carcinoma prostate is the most common malignancy in men after carcinoma lung. It occurs in old age of more than 50 years, and peaks between 65 and 75 years of age. Occult malignancy is more common in prostate.

Etiology and Pathogenesis

The risk factors can be endogenous or exogenous origin. The environmental factors are considerd as exogenous and endogenous factors include cadmium, family history, hormones, race, aging, diet, oxidative stress, smoking, agricultural fertilizers, pesticides, etc. Some of the important risk factors are discussed below.

Family history: If first degree relatives are affected, the risk increases two- to elevenfold depending upon number of first degree relatives affected.

Hormones: Androgens (testosterone and its metabolite dihydrotestosterone) for increased duration have risk of malignancy.

Diet: Fat especially polyunsaturated fats have positive corelation. Vitamin D deficiency has increased risk. Reduced levels zinc and selenium have higher incidence of prostatic cancer.

Environmental factor: Cadmium has higher risk.

Clinical Features

Prostatic carcinoma may not have specific symptoms and may remain silent. They may be incidentally detected in BPH/NPH specimens. It may cause following symptoms.
1. Urinary obstruction similar to nodular hyperplasia.
2. Prostatism (discomfort and lower urinary obstruction).
3. Bony pain is common feature because of bony metastasis (osteoblastic) more to the spines (axial skeleton).

Investigations

In men over 40, digital rectal examination may show firm, nodular prostate.

Serum prostate specific antigen (PSA) level is more than 4 ng/ml.

Pathology

In about 70% of the cases, carcinoma prostate arises in the peripheral zone of the gland, classically in a posterior location.

Gross: On cut section, the mass is gritty and firm. Milky ooze is absent or minimal.

Microscopy: Prostatic carcinoma is an adenocarcinoma with following features (Figs 37.6 and 37.7):

1. Glands lined by single layer of uniform cuboidal to columnar cells.
2. Basal layer is absent.

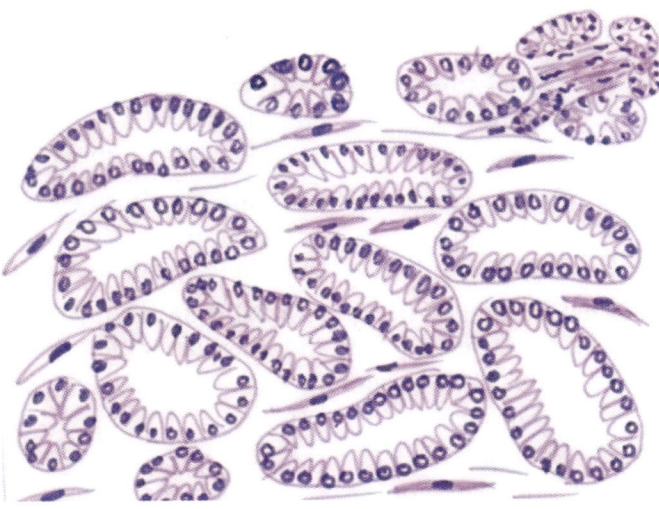

Fig. 37.6: Microphotograph of prostatic carcinoma

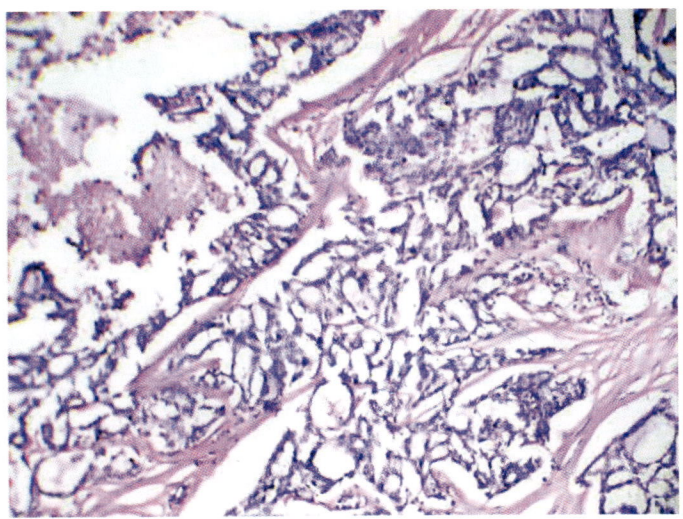

Fig. 37.7: Microscopy of prostatic carcinoma (schematic)

Table 37.3	Gleason's microscopic grading of prostatic carcinoma
Grade	**Description**
1	Single, separate, uniform glands in closely packed masses with a definite, usually rounded edge limiting the tumour
2	Single, separate, slightly less uniform glands, loosely packed with less sharp edge
3a	Single, separate, much more variable glands, may be closely packed but irregularly separated, ragged poorly defined edge
3b	Like 3a, but very small glands or tiny cell clusters
3c	Sharply or smoothly circumscribed rounded masses of papillary or cribriform tumour
4a	Raggedly outlined, raggedly infiltrating, fused glandular tumour
4b	Like 4a, with large pale cells(Hypernephroid)
5a	Sharply circumscribed, rounded masses of of almost solid cribriform tumour, with central necrosis (comedocarcinoma)
5b	Ragged masses of anaplastic carcinoma with only enough gland formation, or vacuoles to identify as adenocarcinoma

3. The glands are crowded and the cytoplasm is pale to clear or amphophilic.
4. The nuclei lining these glands are large with some variation in size and shape, having one or more nucleoli.
5. There is perineural invasion.
6. Microscopic findings can be graded according to Gleason's grading of prostatic carcinoma (Table 37.3).
7. There is increased microvessel density.
8. Vascular and lymphatic invasion correlates with higher grade and stage.

Gleason's score: This is sum of most common microscopic grades and higher score has worst grade.

2014 WHO/ISUP grading[43]

Grade group 1: Gleason's score less than 6 (well formed glands)

Grade group 2: Gleason's score 3 + 4 = 7 predominantly well formed glands with few poorly formed glands)

Grade group 3: Gleason's score 4 + 3 = 7 Poorly formed/cribriform/fused glands with lesser well-formed glands.

Grade group 4: Gleason's score 4 + 4 = 8, 3 + 5 = 8, 5 + 3 = 8 Predominantly poorly formed/cribriform/fused glands with lesser well-formed glands.

Grade group 5: Gleason's score 9 – 10 (4 + 5, 5 + 4, 5 + 5), Lack gland formation with necrosis with or without poorly formed/cribriform/fused glands.

Gleason's patterns

Gleason's pattern	Description
Gleason's pattern 3	Well-formed glands, closely packed glands, variable sized, few poorly formed glands at high magnification
Gleason's pattern 4	Cribriform glands, glomeruloid glands, presence of poorly formed glands
Gleason's pattern 5	Sheets and individual tumour cells, solid nests, comedo-necrosis

SELF-ASSESSMENT EXERCISE

1. **Which of the following does not progress to carcinoma?**
   A. Bowen's disease   B. Balanitis
   C. Leukoplakia   D. Erythroplakia

2. **Intratubular germ cell neoplasia can progress to:**
   A. Seminoma
   B. Teratoma
   C. Spermatocytic seminoma
   D. Embryonal carcinoma

3. **Testicular biopsy to be sent to histopathological examination in:**
   A. Bouin's fluid   B. Normal saline
   C. 95% alcohol   D. Methyl alcohol

4. **Testicular mass, cut section firm, and lobulated, possibility is:**
   A. Seminoma   B. Yolk sac tumor
   C. Teratoma   D. Embyronal carcinoma

5. **35 years male with left inguinal mass, left testis not in its place, right testis normal location. The possibility is:**
   A. Left inguinal mass to be removed and right testis to be biopsied
   B. Left cryptorchid testis, can be placed in its place by orchidoplexy
   C. Radiation to left inguinal mass
   D. All of the above

6. **Carcinoma prostate is more common in:**
   A. Peripheral portion
   B. Central portion
   C. Between central and periphery
   D. All of the above

7. **Possible risk factor for carcinoma penis is:**
   A. Phimosis
   B. HSV
   C. EBV infection
   D. Lichen simplex chronicus

8. **Genital warts and cancers of penis can by:**
   A. HPV   B. EBV
   C. HSV   D. Klebsiella

9. **Bag of worms feel of spermatic cord with infertility can be because of:**
   A. Spermatocoel   B. Parasitic infection
   C. Varicocoel   D. All of the above

10. **BPH most commonly involves:**
   A. Posterior lobe   B. Median
   C. Lateral lobes   D. None of the above

11. **Gonorrhoea with urethritis commonly causes:**
   A. Epididymis   B. Balanitis
   C. Orchitis   D. None of the above

12. **Testicular swelling with AFP 86 ng/ml, hCG 5 IU/l, cut section soft and haemorrhagic:**
   A. Embryonal carcinoma
   B. Seminoma
   C. Teratoma
   D. Choriocarcinoma

13. **Pelvic pain, tender prostate in a 35 years male is possibly due to:**
   A. Non-specific prostatitis
   B. *C. trachomatis* infection
   C. HIV infection
   D. None

14. **Which cells produce testosterone?**
   A. Sertoli cells   B. Sustentacular cells
   C. Leydig cells   D. All

15. **Which is not a testicular marker?**
   A. HCG   B. AFP
   C. LDH   D. CEA

Answers

1. B	2. A	3. A	4. A	5. A	6. A	7. A	8. A
9. C	10. C	11. A	12. A	13. B	14. C	15. D	

Endocrine Pathology

THYROID LESIONS

THYROID GLAND

Thyroid gland has two lateral lobes connected by the isthmus. It is located below and anterior to larynx. Weight of normal thyroid gland is 15 to 25 g. In response to thyrotropin-releasing hormone (TRH) from hypothalamus, TSH is released from the anterior pituitary and this raises the T_3 and T_4. Elevated levels of T_3 and T_4 in turn suppress TRH and TSH (Fig. 38.1).

FORMATION OF THYROID HORMONES

Thyroglobulin, secreted by the follicular cells, is rich in tyrosine. Iodinisation of tyrosine later gets converted into T_3 and T_4 and following steps are involved. Iodide circulating in blood is taken up and this is called iodine trapping. This undergoes oxidation from iodide to iodine.

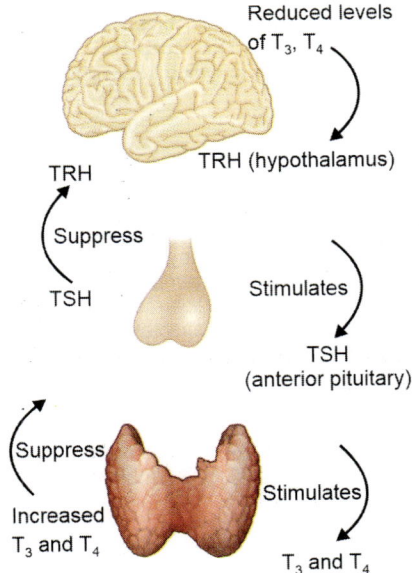

Fig. 38.1: Regulation of thyroid hormones

$$\text{Iodide} \xrightarrow[\text{Peroxidase enzyme and hydrogen peroxide}]{} \text{Iodine}$$

Iodine binds to thyroglobin $\longrightarrow$ organification/hormone formation.

Tyrosine is iodised to monoiodotyrosine and then to diiodotyrosine. Two molecules of diiodotyrosine forms T_4. One molecule of monoiodotyrosine and one molecule of diiodotyrosine forms T_3. It is T_3 that has 10 times more affinity than T_4 for thyroid hormone receptors (THR).

THYROIDITIS

Inflammation of thyroid gland is mainly due to autoimmune diseases and common amongst these are:
1. Acute thyroiditis
2. Hashimoto thyroiditis
3. Granulomatous (de Quervains) thyroiditis
4. Palpation thyroiditis
5. Subacute lymphocytic thyroiditis

Hashimoto Thyroiditis

Hashimoto thyroiditis is the most common type of thyroiditis. It is an autoimmune disease with destruction of thyroid gland having gradual and progressive failure of thyroid function. This is the commonest cause of hypothyroidism with normal iodine levels.

In the year 1912, Hashimoto described this disease in patients with goitre, showing intense lymphocytic infiltration and destruction of thyroid follicles. It is prevalent in the age group of 45 to 65 years. Women are frequently affected than men in the ratio of 10:1 or 20:1.

Etiology

Breakdown of self-tolerance to thyroid autoantigens seen in Hashimoto's thyroiditis is thought to be due to combination of genetic susceptibility and environmental factors like viral or bacterial infection.

Risk factors for Hashimoto thyroiditis include:
1. Family history
2. Smoking

Pathogenesis

In Hashimoto disease, there is breakdown in self-tolerance and following different mechanisms can cause damage to the thyroid gland (Fig. 38.2).

1. Activation of CD4 T lymphocytes which are sensitized by thyroid antigen. The activated lymphocytes secrete IF-gamma and with this there is activation of macrophages and damage to the follicles.
2. T cell-mediated cytotoxicity: The CD4 T lymphocytes in turn activate CD8 T lymphocytes which attack thyrocytes.
3. Antibody-dependent cell-mediated cytotoxicity: There can be formation of anti-thyroid antibodies by the plasma cells. These bind to the antigens on thyroglobulin (Tg) and thyroid peroxidase (TPO) and damage them.

Gross: The gland is firm, diffusely and symmetrically enlarged, weighs 25 to 250 g. The normal thyroid lobulations are accentuated by interlobular fibrosis (Fig. 38.3).

Microscopy: The thyroid follicles are small and atrophic. Colloid is scanty or absent. There is epithelial metaplasia most often to Hurthle cells. The stroma has lymphoplasmacytic infiltrate with prominent germinal centres. There is variable degree of interlobular fibrosis. The lymphocytes are T or B cell type. Foci of neoplasia either papillary carcinoma or non-Hodgkin lymphoma may be present (Fig. 38.4).

Clinical Features

The patient is a middle-aged female, has painless enlargement of thyroid gland with some degree of hypothyroidism. Symmetric and diffuse enlargement of thyroid is common feature. Any localized nodularity should raise the suspicion of neoplasia. Hypothyroidism develops gradually. Patients with Hashimoto thyroiditis are at increased risk of developing neoplasia usually papillary carcinoma and non-Hodgkin lymphomas. These patients are also at increased risk of developing other autoimmune diseases such as diabetes mellitus, SLE, myasthenia gravis and Sjögren's syndrome.

Investigations

T_3 and T_4 levels are reduced, TSH is high and serum has antibodies to thyroglobulin and peroxidase enzyme.

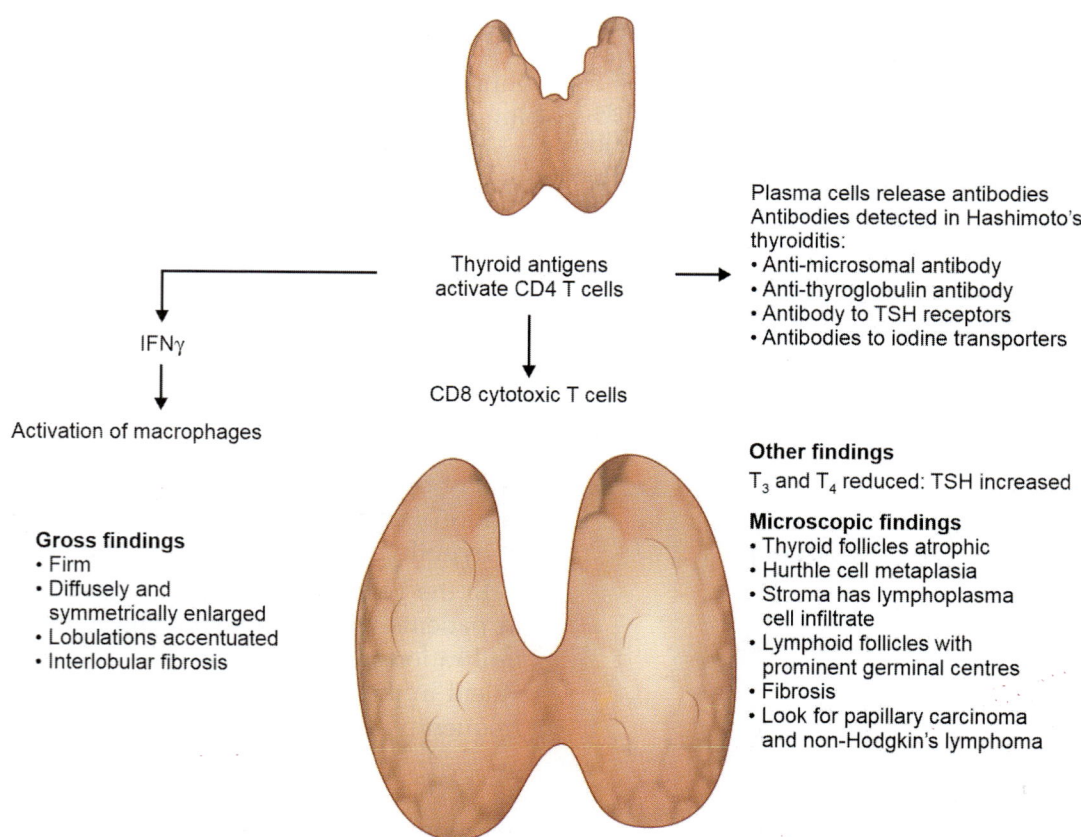

Fig. 38.2: Pathogenesis in Hashimoto disease (schematic)

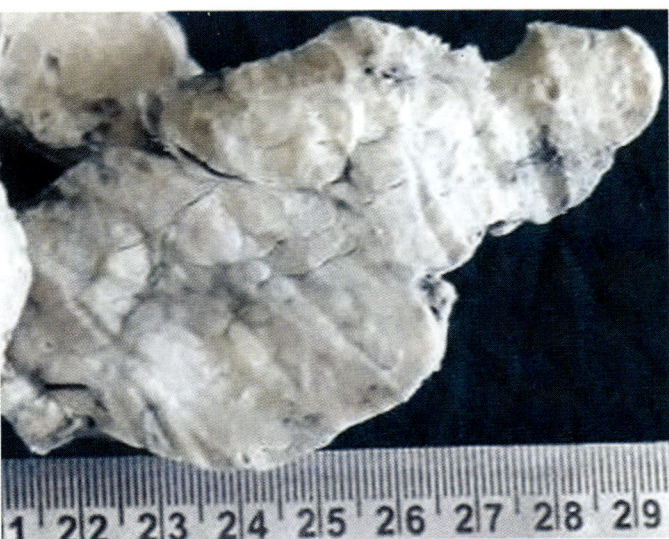

Fig. 38.3: Gross appearance in Hashimoto disease. Note the pale-grey appearance of the lobular cut surface of the thyroid (*Courtesy:* HOD and Staff, SDM Medical College, Dharwad)

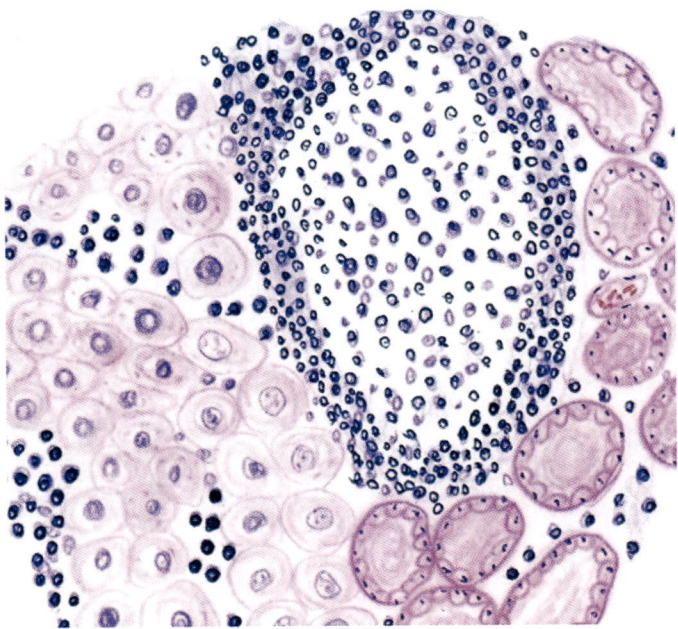

Fig. 38.4: Microscopy in Hashimoto disease, the section shows a dense infiltrate of lymphocytes with prominent germinal centre.

THYROTOXICOSIS

The causes for thyrotoxicosis with or without hyperthyroidism are the following.

Thyrotoxicosis with hyperthyroidism:
- Graves disease
- Toxic multinodular goitre
- Toxic adenoma
- Iodine-induced hyperthyroidism
- Neonatal Graves
- TSH-secreting pituitary adenoma

Thyrotoxicosis not associated with hyperthyroidism:
- Granulomatous (De Quervain's) thyroiditis
- Subacute lymphocytic thyroiditis
- Struma ovarii (ovarian teratoma with predominant thyroid tissue)
- Exogenous thyroxine intake

Graves Disease/Diffuse Toxic Goitre

Synonym: Basedow disease (Europe).

It is an autoimmune disorder. The disease has triad of clinical findings.
1. There is diffuse goitre with hyperthyroidism.
2. Infiltrative ophthalmopathy giving rise to exophthalmos.
3. Localised infiltrative dermopathy giving rise to pretibial oedema.

It is a most prevalent disease in US affecting 0.5 to 1% of the population under the age of 40 years (peak 20–40 years of age). Women are affected 10 times more than the men.

Etiology

Genetic and environmental factors are involved although no single gene responsible for the disease. Family history is the important risk factor. About 30–50% of the monozygotic twins are affected. HLA Class II molecules (HLA-DR3 and DQ genes) have susceptibility foci for Graves disease.

Pathogenesis

There is formation of IgG antibodies in the body and these bind thyroid stimulating hormone receptors on the follicular cells. Most (90%) of the antibodies are thyroid stimulating immunoglobulins rather than the blocking ones. This stimulates TSH and further T_3 and T_4 are elevated. Thus, there is thyroid hyperplasia and excessive vascularity of the tissue (Fig. 38.5).

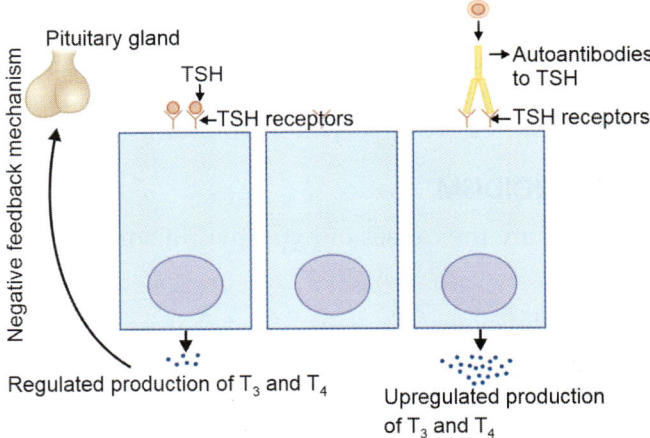

Fig. 38.5: Pathogenesis of Graves disease

Pathology

The thyroid gland is symmetrically enlarged. It weighs 35 to 100 g. It is firm, meaty and dark red in colour and highly vascular.

Microscopy: Thyroid is diffusely hyperplastic and highly vascular. The epithelial cells are tall columnar, often arranged in papillae. The papillae lack fibrovascular core. The colloid is depleted and appears scalloped. The interstitium has lymphoid infiltrate consisting of T cells along with B cells and plasma cells. Germinal centres are common.

Clinical Features

Exophthalmos seen in Graves disease is due to oedema, excessive retro-orbital connective tissue (hydrophilic glycosaminoglycans such as hyaluronic acid and chondroitin sulphate), extraocular muscles and increased adipose tissue along with lymphocytic infiltration. Sympathetic overactivity produces staring gaze and lid lag. The extraocular muscles are weak and patients may have corneal injury.

Graves' dermopathy is due to oedema and deposition of glycosaminoglycans usually pretibial and skin over the shin is warm and moist.

Patients have palpitation, tachycardia, anxiety, tremors, weakness, weight loss and are intolerant to heat. They tend to seek cooler areas and sweat profusely. The heart rate is increased. They may have hypertrophic heart with ischaemic changes. The patients may develop congestive cardiac failure. These patients are at risk of developing other autoimmune diseases.

Investigations

T_3 and T_4 levels are elevated and TSH is depressed. There is presence of autoantibodies to the TSH receptors (thyroid-stimulating immunoglobulins). Radioiodine scans show diffuse uptake of iodine.

Treatment

Beta blockers, administration of thionamides to decrease thyroid hormone synthesis, radioiodine ablation are given and thyroidectomy is done with large thyroid mass having compressive effects on surrounding structures.

HYPOTHYROIDISM

Following are the causes of hypothyroidism.

Primary:
- Iodine deficiency: Endemic/food faddism
- Congenital biosynthetic defects (dyshormonogenetic goitre)
- Postablative: Surgery, radiation therapy, external irradiation
- Autoimmune: Hashimoto thyroiditis
- Drugs: Lithium, iodides, p-aminosalicylic acid

Secondary:
- Pituitary failure
- Hypothalamic failure

Colloid Goitre and Multinodular Goitre

Enlargement of the thyroid gland is called goitre which is caused by impaired synthesis of thyroid hormones due to deficiency of iodine.

Goitre occurs as:
1. Endemic goitre
2. Sporadic goitre

Endemic Goitre

This is common in geographical areas where soil, water and food contain low content of iodine. When 10% of the population is affected, the term endemic goitre is used. Such condition is more common in mountainous areas. There is lack of iodine in water and there is decreased production of thyroid hormones and increased levels of TSH leading to hypertrophy and hyperplasia and goitrous enlargement. With dietary supplementation of iodine, the severity of goitre has been reduced in recent years.

Goitrogens also can induce a state of deficiency of iodine with interference with thyroid hormone synthesis. The vegetables belonging to Brassicaceae (Crucifereae) family which includes cabbage, cauliflower, brussels, sprouts, turnips, cassava root, etc. are goitrogenic.

Sporadic Goitre

This is less common than the endemic goitre. This is common in females, usually adolescents or young adults.

This is caused by:
1. Ingestion of substances that interfere with hormone synthesis.
2. Hereditary enzyme defects which interfere with hormone synthesis (dyshormonogenetic goitre).

The colloid goitre, also called simple goitre, has **hyperplastic phase** and **involution phase**. In hyperplastic phase, the thyroid gland is diffusely and symmetrically enlarged. The follicles vary in size; some are large and some are small. These are lined by cuboidal to columnar epithelium which piles up at places. When the dietary iodine increases or the demand for thyroid hormone decreases or the euthyroid stage is reached, the stimulated follicular epithelium involutes. In the involution phase, the follicles are large and are lined by cuboidal epithelium. The lumen contains abundant colloid.

Thus grossly, in colloid goitre, the thyroid is symmetrically enlarged, weight does not increase 100 to 150 g, the cut section shows brownish translucent material of colloid.

The episodes of hyperplasia and involution produce **multinodular goitre**. At this stage grossly, the thyroid gland is multilobulated, asymmetrical and at some instances, the nodules may be prominent (Fig. 38.6). Variable amount of colloid, areas of fibrosis, haemorrhage, calcification and cystic degeneration are present. Microscopy shows colloid-rich follicles lined by flattened epithelium and areas of follicular epithelial hyperplasia (Fig. 38.7). A prominent capsule which is present in follicular adenoma does not surround these hyperplastic nodules.

In multinodular goitre, grossly, the thyroid gland weighs around 2000 g, multinodular, brownish, translucent because of colloid and may have haemorrhage, fibrosis, calcification and cystic change.

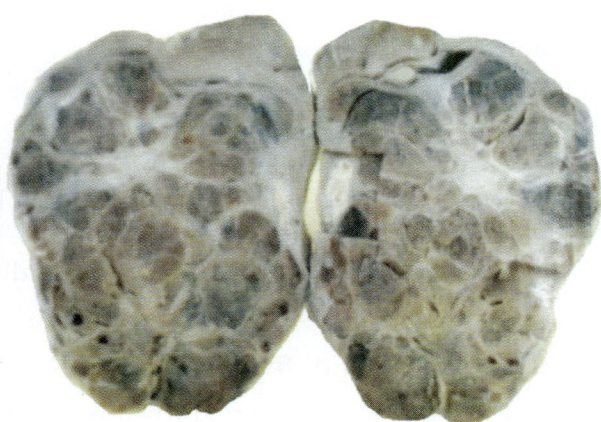

Fig. 38.6: Multinodular goitre (gross picture)

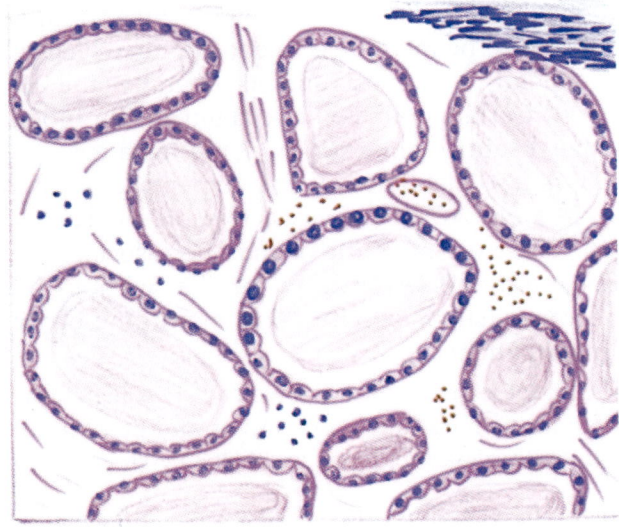

Fig. 38.7: Microscopy of multinodular goitre, note haemorrhage and calcification (schematic)

NEOPLASMS OF THYROID

These include:

Benign:
- Follicular adenoma
- Hurthle cell adenoma

Malignant:
- Papillary carcinoma
- Follicular carcinoma
- Medullary carcinoma
- Anaplastic carcinoma

Follicular Adenoma

These present as solitary nodules, rarely may synthesize excess T_3 or T_4 and appear as hot nodules on isotope scan and some times cause thyrotoxicosis.

Gross:
1. Follicular adenomas are well circumscribed masses.
2. Solid, encapsulated capsule is complete, compresses surrounding normal thyroid tissue.

Microscopy (Fig. 38.8):
1. Compact micro- or macrofollicles with little colloid
2. No capsular or vascular invasion

Papillary Carcinoma Thyroid

This is the most common primary carcinoma of thyroid. Commonly found in 20–50 years of age group.

Gross:
1. Well circumscribed, non-encapsulated, solitary or multifocal infiltrative masses
2. Occasionally capsulated
3. Firm and white due to fibrosis and calcification

Microscopy (Figs 38.9 and 38.10):
1. Branching papillae with fibrovascular core

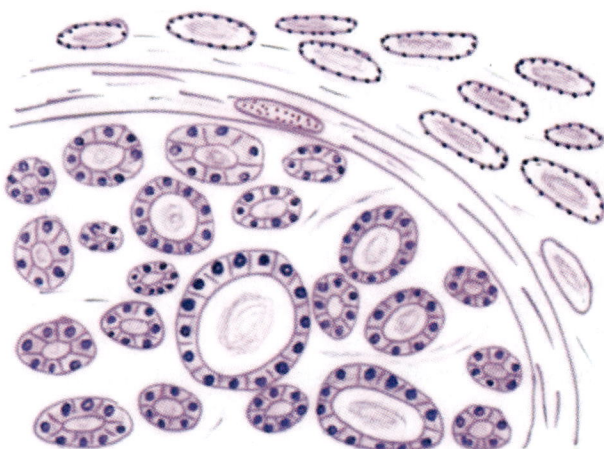

Fig. 38.8: Microscopy of follicular adenoma (schematic)

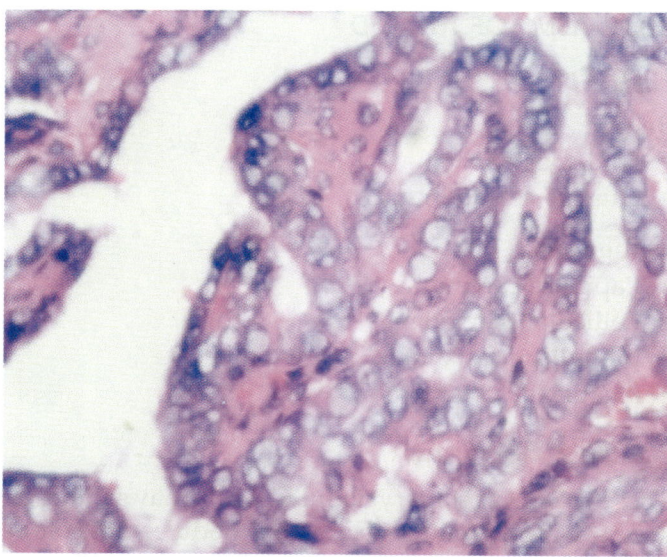

Fig. 38.9: Microscopy of papillary carcinoma thyroid

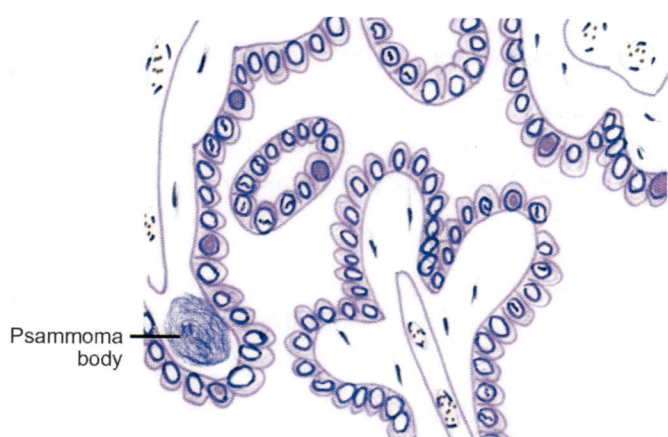

Psammoma body

Fig. 38.10: Microscopy of papillary carcinoma thyroid, note psammoma body, nuclei with peripheral clumping of chromatin, nuclear overlapping, nuclear grooves and intranuclear eosinophilic cytoplasmic inclusions (schematic)

2. Single or stratified lining of cuboidal or columnar cells

3. Nuclei large with ground glass or peripheral clumping of chromatin (**Orphan Annie eye nuclei**)

4. Eosinophilic inclusions in the nuclei (cytoplasmic invaginations)

5. Nuclear grooves and nuclear overlapping (eggs in the basket appearance)

6. Psammoma bodies in the stroma are commonly present.

These tumours metastasize via lymphatics. Variants include follicular variant, tall cell variant, diffuse sclerosing and papillary microcarcinoma (size of tumour <1 cm).

Follicular Carcinoma

This is the second most common primary thyroid cancer. These tumours account for 15–30% of the thyroid tumours. They are:

- Common above the age of 40 years.
- F : M = 3 :1.
- Common in endemic areas with iodine deficiency.
- Presents as solitary nodule.

Gross:

1. Vary in size
2. Yellow-tan coloured
3. Thick fibrous capsule with invasion
4. Haemorrhage, necrosis and cystic degeneration present.
5. These can be minimally or widely invasive, depending upon capsular invasion.

Microscopy:

1. Microfollicles and macrofollicles.
2. Haemorrhage and necrosis present.
3. Mitoses common.
4. No papillae are seen.
5. Capsular and/or vascular invasion is the sign of carcinoma and differentiates from follicular adenoma.
6. These tumours metastasize via hematogenous dissemination.

Medullary Carcinoma of Thyroid

Medullary carcinoma (MC) of thyroid, a neuroendocrine neoplasm originates from parafollicular cells or C cells of thyroid. These account for 5% of the thyroid neoplasms. About 70% of these are sporadic (old age) and 30% are familial. These are autosomal dominant nature. These neoplasms secrete calcitonin which helps in preoperative diagnosis and postoperative follow-up as well. Carcinoembryonic antigen in the blood is another useful biomarker. In some instances, these tumours also elaborate other polypeptide hormones like serotonin, ACTH and vasoactive intestinal peptides (VIP). These are sporadic or may be associated with MEN syndrome 2A or 2B or familial without MEN syndrome. The ones with MEN syndrome occur in younger patients.

RET proto-oncogene is known to play role in familial and sporadic medullary carcinomas and these occur in adults with peak incidence in 40 to 50 years of age.

Gross: The sporadic MC usually presents as solitary nodule whereas the familial ones are associated with bilaterality and are multicentric. Areas of haemorrhage and necrosis are present and tumour may extend beyond the capsule. The tumour is firm, pale-grey to tan and has infiltrative margines.

Microscopy: Medullary carcinomas are composed of polygonal to spindle-shaped cells and the cells are arranged in nests, trabaculae, and follicles. The cytoplasm is granular amphophilic/eosinophilic, nucleus has fine granular chromatin and inconspicuous nucleoli. Some anaplasia may be present in the cells. The stroma shows a cellular amyloid deposits derived from calcitonin polypeptides.

Clinical course: These patients present with mass in the neck, dysphagia and hoarseness of voice. Patients can present with diarrhoea due to VIP and Cushing syndrome due to ACTH.

Investigations: Calcitonin levels and carcinoembryonic antigen and neuroendocrine markers in the blood are useful biomarkers.

The familial syndromes with MEN2A and 2B are associated with medullary carcinoma. MEN2A is the most common type and is associated with MC, phaeochromocytoma and hyperparathyroidism. MEN2B patients develop MC at an early age with phaeochromocytoma but no hyperparathyroidism.These patients have multiple neuromas, ganglioneuromatosis of GIT and megacolon.

Anaplastic (Undifferentiated) Carcinoma

Anaplastic carcinoma, which is also called undifferentiated carcinoma, accounts for less than 5% of the cases. These are aggressive tumours and occur in older patients with mean age of 65 years. It is the most aggressive tumour with a mortality rate approaching near 100%.

Microscopy: The neoplastic cells are highly anaplastic with large pleomorphic giant cells, occasional osteoclast like multinucleate giant cells, spindle cells with sarcomatoid features. Foci of papillary carcinoma or follicular carcinoma may be present.

The neoplastic cells are negative for thyroid markers. The tumour cells express epithelial markers like cytokeratin.

PARATHYROID GLAND

There are four parathyroid glands and they are composed of chief cells and oxyphil cells. Chief cells produce parathyroid hormone (PTH) and regulate calcium homeostasis. Oxyphil cells are larger and lighter stained than the chief cells with little function. PTH is released in response to decreased serum calcium, causes efflux of calcium from bones and increased reabsorption by the kidneys and it is degraded in liver and kidney.

PTH has following effects:
1. Increases the renal tubular reabsorption of calcium.
2. Inhibits renal reabsorption of phosphates and bicarbonates.
3. Converts vitamin D to its active dihydroxy form in the kidneys.
4. Increases GI absorption of calcium.
5. PTH activates osteoclasts.

PRIMARY HYPERPARATHYROIDISM

Underlying parathyroid lesions can be adenomas (80–90%)/carcinomas (1%) or primary hyperplasia (15%). Oxyphil adenomas are the most common. Primary hyperplasia is characterised by chief cell hyperplasia with water clear cells involving all four glands.

SECONDARY HYPERPARATHYROIDISM

Chronic hypocalcaemia leads to compensatory over-activity of the parathyroid glands. Chronic renal failure is the most common cause. The parathyroid glands are hyperplastic with chief cells. The patients manifest with skeletal abnormalities like osteoporosis, osteitis fibrosa cystica (von Recklinghausen's disease of bone) and brown tumours.

In primary or secondary hyperparathyroidism, there is excess of bone resorption as a greater number of osteoclasts become active. Decrease in the bone mass makes the person more susceptible to bone deformity, fractures and joint problems.

- Primary or secondary untreated hyperparathyroidism manifests with osteoporosis or brown tumour (osteitis fibrosa cystica).
- Osteoporosis is most commonly noted in cortical bones. Medullary bones are also affected.
- Increased osteoclastic activity may dissect the trabeculae leading to dissecting osteitis. Surrounding marrow spaces are replaced by fibrovascular tissue.

  This is also called by name Brown tumour because of its brownish colour due to haemorrhage and hemosiderin. Refer to topic on "Bone Lesions" for details.
- Radiologically, the erosive lesion is first evident in phalanges. Lesion also noted in vertebrae and mandible.

TERTIARY HYPERPARATHYROIDISM

There is persistent hypersecretion after a long period of secondary hyperparathyroidism. This usually occurs in patients with chronic renal failure after renal transplant.

HYPOPARATHYROIDISM

Causes

1. Surgery induced
2. Autoimmune
3. Familial
4. Congenital absence of parathyroid gland

Clinical Manifestations

1. **Tetany:** This has neuromuscular irritability like numbness or paraesthesiae, carpopedal spasm, laryngospasm, generalized seizures. Chevstek sign elicited with tapping of facial nerve which induces contraction of eye, mouth and nose. Trousseau sign has carpal spasms.
2. **Mental instability:** There are anxiety, depression, confusion, and hallucinations.
3. **Intracranial manifestations:** Calcification of basal ganglia, Parkinson like movements disorders, and increased ICP with papilloedema.
4. **Ocular manifestations:** Calcification of lens and cataract formation.
5. **Cardiovascular manifestations:** Conduction defects with prolonged QT interval on ECG.
6. **Dental abnormalities:** Dental hypoplasia, failure of eruption, defective enamel, root formation and caries teeth.

DIABETES MELLITUS

Diabetes mellitus (DM) is a metabolic disease characterised by hyperglycaemia resulting from inherited and/or acquired deficiency in production of insulin by the pancreas, or by the ineffectiveness of the insulin produced.

Criteria for DM

WHO criteria (2014): A fasting glucose level of 126 mg/dl (7 mmol/l) or higher (fasting is no calorie for at least 8 hours) and 2 hours plasma glucose levels of 200 mg/dl (11.1 mmol/dl) or higher is DM. American diabetic association (ADA) criteria is given in Table 38.1.

Table 38.1	American Diabetic Association (ADA) criteria (2016) for diabetes mellitus
HbA1c: >6.5% (DM)	
FPG: >126 mg/dl (7.0 mmol/l) or	
2-hour plasma glucose: ≥200 mg/dl (11.1 mmol/l)	
Oral GTT: ≥200 mg/dl (11.1 mmol/l)	
Pre-diabetics	
HbA1c: 5.7 to 6.4%	
FPG: 110–125 mg/dl (5.6 to 6.9 mmol/l)	
2-hour plasma glucose: 140–199 mg/dl (7.8 to 11.0 mmol/l)	

Following are the principal forms of diabetes mellitus:
1. **Type I** diabetes mellitus
2. **Type II** diabetes mellitus
3. The rare and third form includes monogenic form of DM. This includes maturity onset diabetes of young (MODY) and DM due to insulin receptor mutations.

Type I diabetes mellitus, also called insulin-dependent diabetes mellitus (IDDM), occurs in childhood and is associated with severe deficiency or total absence of insulin production. This is an autoimmune reaction with destruction of beta cells.

Type II diabetes mellitus, also called maturity onset diabetes, is due to unresponsiveness of target cells to insulin. The unresponsiveness may be due to:
1. Inadequate secretion because of decreased number of insulin receptors, or antibodies against insulin receptors, or
2. Decreased response of peripheral tissues to insulin, especially tissues like liver cells, skeletal muscle cells and adipose cells.

Before going into DM of both types, let us briefly review glucose regulation and actions of insulin.

Glucose Regulation and Metabolic Actions of Insulin

Glucose homeostasis is regulated by three processes:
1. Glucose production by liver.
2. Glucose uptake and utilization by peripheral tissues (skeletal muscle, cardiac muscle, fat and other tissues).
3. Insulin is produced in beta cells of islets of pancreas as precursor proteins and cleaved in golgi complex to release mature hormone and C-peptide. Both insulin and C-peptide are stored in secretory granules (Fig. 38.11).

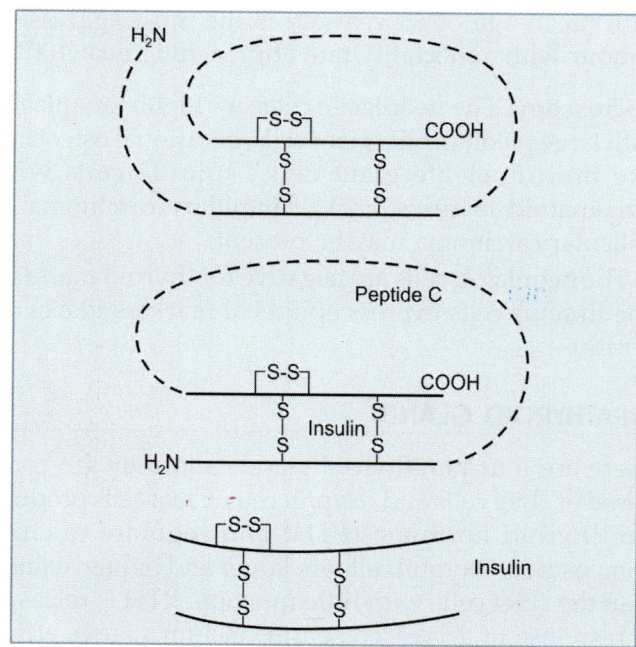

Fig. 38.11: C peptide and insulin hormone production from precursor proteins

4. Stimulus for insulin release is glucose itself. Glucose enters beta cells by GLUT 2 (insulin-dependent glucose transporter). Beta cells have ATP sensitive K channels and sulfonylurea receptors. ATP inhibits K channel, leading to membrane depolarization, influx of calcium and insulin release.

Actions (Fig. 38.12)

1. Actions of insulin and counter-regulating hormones including glucagon influence glucose uptake and catabolism.
2. Insulin helps in uptake of glucose inside the cells. Glucose is needed to generate ATP and excess glucose is stored as glycogen in muscle and as lipid in fat tissue. Insulin inhibits lipolysis in adipocytes and promotes protein synthesis and inhibits its catabolism. In liver, insulin inhibits gluconeogenesis, increases glycogen synthesis and lipogenesis.

Pathogenesis of Type I Diabetes Mellitus

In type I DM, there is autoimmune destruction of beta cells of pancreas which involves genetic and environmental factors.

Genetic susceptibility: Higher concordance rate for diabetes mellitus is seen in monozygotic twins than dizygotic twins. Over a dozen of susceptibility loci for type 1 diabetes are known. Most important is the HLA locus on chromosome 6p21.

Environmental factors: Viral infections may be involved in triggering islet cell destruction in type 1 diabetes mellitus. Epidemiological association has been seen with type 1 diabetes mellitus and infection with mumps, rubella, coxsackie B or cytomegalovirus and others.

Both genetic and environmental factors (viruses—coxsackie, mumps, rubella, etc.) are important factors.

Mechanism of destruction: In type I DM, there is failure of self-tolerance of T cells specific for islet cell antigens. It may be a result of:
1. Defective clonal deletion of self-reactive T cells in thymus
2. Defects in functions of regulatory T cells or
3. Resistance of effector T cells to the suppressive activity by regulatory T cells

The autoreactive T cells survive. Multiple T cell population have been implicated. The Th1 cells secrete cytokines like INF-γ and TNF which injure the beta cells and CD8 T cells kill beta cells directly. The islet cell antigens of immune attack are: Insulin, beta cell enzyme glutamic acid decarboxylase and islet cell autoantigen 512.

Pathogenesis of Type II Diabetes Mellitus

Type II DM involves interplay of genetic factors and environmental factors. There is no autoimmune basis.

Environamental factors such as sedentary lifestyle and dietary habits play a major role.

Genetic factors are also involved in the pathogenesis as evidenced by the disease concordance rate of 35 to 60% in monozygotic twins compared with nearly half that in dizygotic twins. Lifetime risk for type II DM in an off-spring is more than double, if both parents are affected.

Mechanism of Type II DM

The two metabolic defects that characterise type II diabetes are:
1. Insulin resistance: A decreased response of peripheral tissues to insulin.
2. Beta cell dysfunction: This is manifested as inadequate insulin secretion due to insulin resistance and hyperglycaemia.

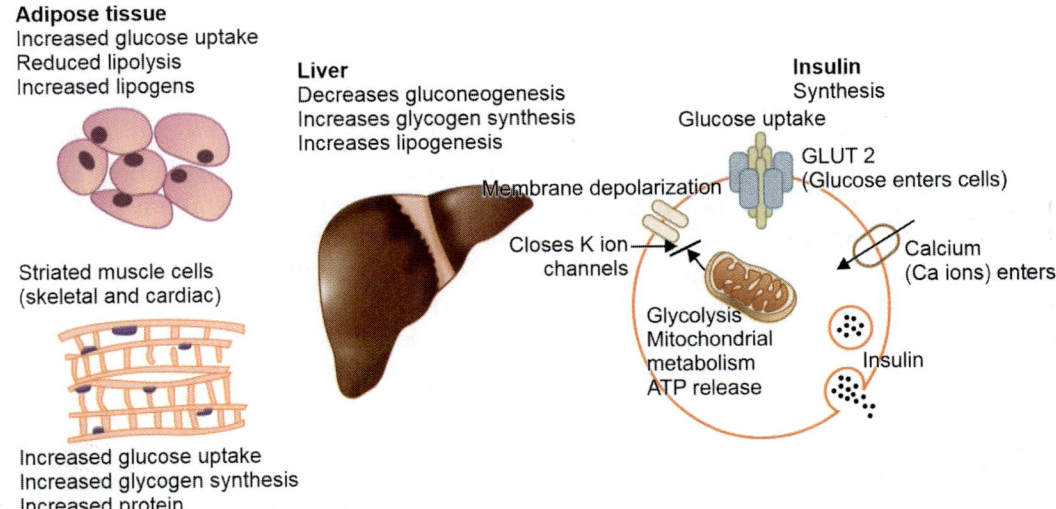

Adipose tissue
Increased glucose uptake
Reduced lipolysis
Increased lipogens

Striated muscle cells
(skeletal and cardiac)

Increased glucose uptake
Increased glycogen synthesis
Increased protein

Liver
Decreases gluconeogenesis
Increases glycogen synthesis
Increases lipogenesis

Membrane depolarization

Closes K ion channels

Glycolysis
Mitochondrial metabolism
ATP release

Insulin
Synthesis
Glucose uptake

GLUT 2
(Glucose enters cells)

Calcium
(Ca ions) enters

Insulin

Fig. 38.12 Regulation and actions of insulin (schematic)

Insulin Resistance

Insulin resistance is failure of target tissue to respond normally to insulin. Liver, skeletal muscle and adipose tissue are the important cells involved.

Insulin resistance results in:

1. Failure to inhibit hepatic gluconeogenesis
2. Decreased uptake of glucose in the skeletal muscle
3. Failure of glycogen synthesis
4. Reduced fatty acid oxidation in liver with increase in circulating free fatty acids which again exaggerates the state of insulin resistance.

Obesity and insulin resistance: Obesity is important factor which contributes to insulin resistance. Risk of DM increases as body mass index increases. Obesity has adverse role in insulin sensitivity in different ways. The adipokines, increased FFA and inflammation contribute to insulin resistance.

- As the insulin receptor signaling pathway is at fault, insulin cannot inhibit gluconeogenesis and the first responsible enzyme is phosphophenol pyruvate carboxylase enzyme.
- Excess FFA, inhibit enzymes of glycolysis, thus exaggerating the hyperglycaemia state. One of the adipokines which decreases blood glucose is reduced in obesity.
- Excess FFA and hyperglycaemia induce pro-inflammatory cytokines. IL-1 and other cytokines are released into circulation and these promote insulin resistance.

Beta Cell Dysfunction

This leads to overt DM. Initially beta cell function increases as a compensatory measure to insulin resistance and reaches euglycaemia state and later period of the disease, pancreas is not able to produce sufficient insulin and cannot adapt to the long-term demand of insulin resistance and a state of insulin deficiency arises.

Monogenic Forms of DM

Two forms of genetic defects can rarely cause DM.

1. About 1 to 2% of the DM cases harbor a genetic defect in the beta cell function, which occurs without beta cell loss. Maturity onset diabetes of young (MODY) belongs to this group. Germ line loss of function with mutations of genes of glucose metabolism, the most important amongst these mutations being mutation of glucokinase. Glucokinase is a rate limiting step in oxidative glucose metabolism.
2. Insulin receptor mutations can affect insulin binding, tyrosine kinase activity and can cause severe insulin resistance, hyperinsulinaemia and DM. These patients have acanthosis nigricans (hyperpigmentation), additionally females have polycystic ovaries and elevated androgens.

Table 38.2	Differences between type I and type II diabetes mellitus	
	Type I	**Type II**
Age of onset	Young age <20 years	Old age >50 years
Obesity	Absent	Present
Insulin	Dependent on insulin	Not dependent on insulin
Blood insulin	Reduced	Normal/increased
Autoantibodies	Present	Absent
Ketonuria	Present	Absent
HLA	Association +	Not present
β cells	Reduced	Normal/reduced
Islet cell antibodies	+	Absent

Differences between type I and type II diabetes mellitus are given in Table 38.2.

Clinical Features of DM

Type I DM was earlier thought to occur only in younger age, but now known to can occur at any age. Initially, for 1 to 2 years, the exogenous insulin requirement is minimal, but later beta cell reserve gets exhausted and insulin requirement will increase. Type II DM occurs in individuals older than 40 years of age and in obese individuals.

The triad of symptoms are: Polyphagia, polydipsia and polyuria. In DM, not only glucose metabolism is affected but also fat and protein metabolism are affected. There is unopposed action of glucagon, growth hormone and epinephrine. Glucose utilization by tissues especially skeletal muscle is greatly diminished. Glycogen storage is reduced. The hyperglycaemia induces osmotic diuresis and polyuria. The renal water loss and hyperosmolarity triggers osmoreceptors and thirst centres are stimulated. Protein and fat catabolism follow and produce negative energy balance which leads to increased appetite. There is weight loss and muscle weakness.

Pathological Changes in Different Organs

Insulin deficiency leads to catabolic state. The following are important changes taking place in patients with diabetes mellitus.

1. The levels of glucagon, growth hormone and epinephrine are increased.
2. Glucose uptake diminished.
3. Glucose reserves depleted.
4. There is hyperglycaemia leading to:
   - Osmotic diuresis giving rise to polyuria.
   - Intracellular water is depleted: Osmoreceptors are stimulated and this is the reason for intense thirst in these patients (polydipsia).

- Proteins and fat are broken down with increased appetite (polyphagia).

The various pathological changes due to complications in diabetes mellitus can be:

1. **Acute metabolic complications:** The complication in the form of diabetic ketoacidosis is due to:
   i. With insulin deficiency, there is stimulation of glucagon leading to neoglucogenesis.
   ii. Insulin deficiency stimulates lipoprotein lipase. There is increased FFA, ketone bodies are produced in excess. This leads to fatigue, nausea and vomiting, abdominal pain, fruity odour, Kussmal's breathing and coma.

2. **Late systemic complications of diabetes mellitus:** The important morphologic changes are related to late complications. The changes are seen in both type I and type II diabetes.

The chronic complications are caused mainly by lesions involving both large- and medium-sized muscular arteries (macrovascular disease) and capillary dysfunction in target organs (microvascular disease) (Fig. 38.13).

Macrovascular complications
- Accelerated atherosclerosis
- Myocardial infarction
- Gangrene of lower extremities
- Peripheral vascular disease and foot ulcer

Microvascular complications
- Diabetic retinopathy
- Diabetic nephropathy
- Diabetic neuropathy

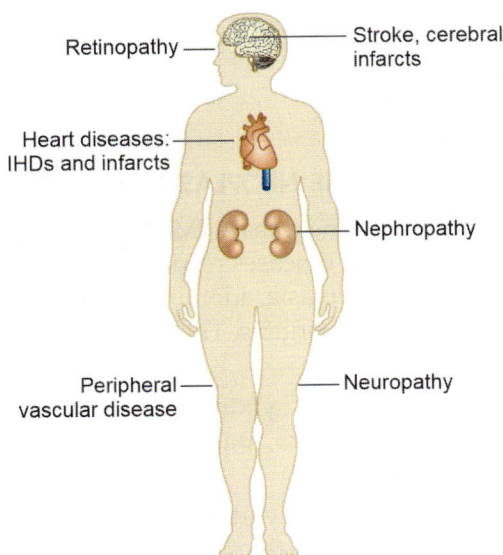

Fig. 38.13: Complications in DM

The pathogenesis of the long-term complications of diabetes mellitus is multifactorial, although persistent hyperglycaemia (glucotoxicity) seems to be a key mediator. Following are important factors for pathogenesis:

1. The assessment of long-term glycaemic control in the patients is based on the percentage of glycosylated haemoglobin, also known as HbA1c, which is formed by non-enzymatic covalent addition of glucose moieties to haemoglobin in red cells. Unlike blood glucose levels, HbA1c provides a measure of glycaemic control over the lifespan of red cells (120 days) and is little affected by day-to-day variations. Early stage stable product is called Amarodi–Lysine product which undergo further irreversible chemical reaction to advanced glycation end products (AGEs) which are formed as a result of non-enzymatic reactions between intracellular glucose derived dicarbonyl precursors (glyoxal, methylglyoxal, and 3-deoxyglucosone) with the amino groups of both intracellular and extracellular proteins including plasma proteins and collagen and with some other endogenous molecules including lipids and nucleic acids. The natural rate of AGE formation is greatly accelerated in the presence of hyperglycaemia and play an important role in the pathogenesis of diabetic complications like retinopathy, nephropathy, neuropathy along with other diseases.

2. Release of cytokines and growth factors, including transforming growth factor β (TGFβ), which leads to deposition of excess basement membrane material, and vascular endothelial growth factor (VEGF), implicated in diabetic retinopathy.

3. Generation of reactive oxygen species (ROS) in endothelial cells.

4. Increased procoagulant activity on endothelial cells and macrophages.

5. Enhanced proliferation of vascular smooth muscle cells and synthesis of extracellular matrix.

6. Hyperosmolar hyperglycaemic state.

Consider screening asymptomatic patients for diabetes type II, if:

1. BMI >25 kg/m^2
2. All patients at the age of 45 years

Investigations

1. Glycosuria: Benedict's test/reagent strip test.
2. To detect ketone bodies in urine: Rothera's test/reagent strip test.
3. Fasting blood glucose: After at least 8 hours of the last meal.
4. Random blood glucose.

5. Postprandial blood glucose levels
6. Glucose tolerance test:
   - 75 g of glucose is given to a patient with 300 ml of water after an overnight fast, after taking fasting blood sample.
   - Blood samples are drawn 1, 2 and 3 hours after taking the glucose.
   - This is more accurate test for glucose utilization, if the fasting glucose is borderline.

ADRENAL GLAND

Adrenal glands, paired organs above the kidney are endocrine glands which produce variety of hormones. The adrenal cortex has three zones, namely zona glomerulosa, zona fasciculata and zona reticularis from outside to inside (Fig. 38.14).

Hormones Produced by Adrenal Gland

Following are the hormones released from the adrenal cortex:

1. Mineralocorticoids (aldosterone) from zona glomerulosa.
2. Glucocorticoids (corticosterone and cortisol) primarily from zona fasciculata and to lesser extent from zona reticularis.
3. Dehydroepiandrosterone (DHEA) which is precursor for testosterone and estrogen from zona reticularis.

The adrenal medulla produces catecholamines (epinephrine, norepinephrine and small amounts of dopamine).

The syndromes associated with hyperfunctioning of adrenal gland are the following:
1. Hypercortisolism/Cushing syndrome
2. Hyperaldosteronism
3. Adrenogenital syndromes

Hypofunction/adrenocortical insufficiency is associated with following syndromes or conditions:
1. Waterhouse-Friderichsen syndrome
2. Addison's disease (reduced glucocorticoids and mineralocorticoids).

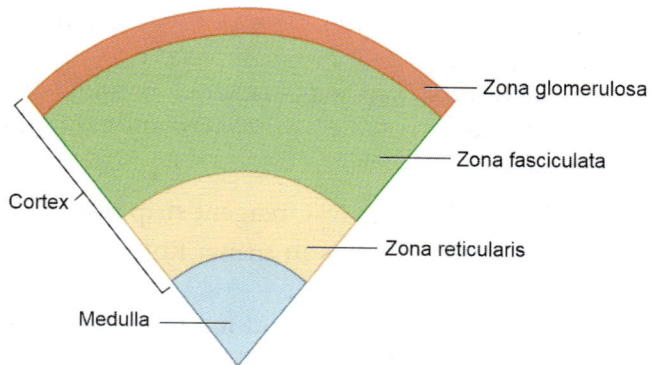

Fig. 38.14: Different parts of adrenal gland (schematic)

The most common cause for primary adrenal insufficiency in developed countries is autoimmune adrenalitis whereas in India, it is tuberculous adrenalitis.

Waterhouse-Friderichsen Syndrome (WFS)

There is adrenal gland failure due to bleeding into adrenals, commonly caused by severe bacterial infection. This can occur at any age, but most commonly in children. This syndrome has the following features:
1. There is hemorrhagic infarction, most often of both the glands. It is typically caused by *Neisseria meningitidis* organism.
2. There is profound shock with hypotension
3. DIC with skin rash and purpura
4. Hyponatraemia
5. Hypoglycaemia

Prompt recognition and treatment is required, otherwise the condition is fatal.

Addison's Disease

The adrenal gland produces less cortisol and aldosterone. There is extreme fatigue, weight loss, reduced appetite, hyperpigmentation of skin, irritability and depression.

Addisonian crisis occurs suddenly with loss of consciousness, hyponatraemia, hyperkalaemia, hypotension, vomiting and diarrhoea leading to dehydration. Hyperpigmentation of skin in Addison's disease is caused by increased precursor of ACTH proopiomelanocortin (POMC) which produces ACTH and alpha melanocyte stimulating hormone (MSH).

NEOPLASMS OF ADRENAL GLAND

Adrenal cortex:
1. Adrenocortical adenomas
2. Adrenocortical carcinomas

Adrenal medulla:
1. Pheochromocytoma

MULTIPLE ENDOCRINE NEOPLASIA SYNDROMES

Multiple endocrine neoplasia (MEN) syndromes are genetically inherited diseases resulting in proliferative lesions such as hyperplasia, adenomas, and carcinomas of multiple endocrine organs. The three main types are the following:

1. MEN type 1 (Werner syndrome) is associated with parathyroid tumours, pancreatic tumours and pituitary tumours.
2. MEN type 2a (Sipple syndrome) is associated with medullary carcinoma thyroid, pheochromocytoma and parathyroid tumours.

3. MEN type 2b is associated with medullary carcinoma thyroid, pheochromocytoma and neuromas.

MEN Type 1 (Werner Syndrome)

This is a rare inherited AD disorder with prevalence of 2/100,000 population. It involves mnemonic 3Ps: Pancreas, parathyroid and pituitary. Primary hyperparathyroidism is the most common manifestation and appears by the age of 40 to 50 years. There is hyperplasia and adenomas of parathyroid glands. Endocrine tumours of pancreas are aggressive tumours with metastasis and associated with high morbidity and mortality. Zollinger-Ellison syndrome (ZE syndrome) and insulinomas are most common. Insulinoma patients have recurrent hypoglycaemia. ZE syndrome patients have peptic ulcers and PTH-induced hypercalcaemia causing nephrolithiasis.

Mutation of MEN 1 tumour suppressor gene which encodes 610 amino acid protein called 'menin' is commonly encountered in MEN type1 disorder. With MEN1 gene mutations, the 50% of the first degree relatives of the family can be affected.

MEN Type 2a (Sipple Syndrome)

MEN type 2a has medullary carcinoma thyroid, pheochromocytoma and parathyroid tumours. Medullary carcinoma can occur in all patients MEN2a and foci of C cell hyperplasia are associated in adjacent areas. This is clinically aggressive. About 40 to 50% of the MEN 2a have pheochromocytoma which are bilateral or may arise in extra-adrenal location. These are associated with RET proto-oncogene gain of function mutations. RET gene is located on chromosome 10 (10q11.2) encodes a receptor tyrosine kinase. Those patients having RET gene abnormalities are advised prophylactic thyroidectomy.

MEN2b

This overlaps with MEN 2a and is associated with medullary carcinoma thyroid, pheochromocytoma and neuromas. Mucosal neuromas of lips and tongue, intestinal ganglioneuromas and distinctive facial features of marfanoid facies are characteristic. This is more aggressive than MEN2a and usually multifocal. This is not associated with hyperparathyroidism. MEN2b also shares similar gene mutations as that of MEN2a.

CUSHING'S SYNDROME (Hypercortisolism)

This disorder is caused by a conditions that produce elevated glucocorticoid levels.

Etiopathogenesis

The causes can be exogenous or endogenous. The vast majority are due to exogenous (iatrogenic) causes.

Exogenous Causes

Iatrogenic Cushing's syndrome due to prolonged administration of high doses of glucocorticoids or ACTH may result in Cushing's syndrome, e.g. in organ transplant recipients and in autoimmune diseases.

Endogenous Causes

1. **Pituitary Cushing's syndrome:** About 60–70% cases of Cushing's syndrome are caused by excessive secretion of ACTH due to a lesion in the pituitary gland, most commonly a corticotroph microadenomas. All cases with pituitary Cushing's sydrome are characterised by bilateral adrenal cortical hyperplasia and elevated ACTH levels. These cases show therapeutic response on administration of high doses of dexamethasone which suppresses ACTH secretion with fall in plasma cortisol level. In low doses, this cannot be suppressed.

2. **Adrenal Cushing's syndrome:** Approximately 20–25% cases of Cushing's syndrome are caused by disease in one or both adrenal glands. These include adrenal cortical adenoma, carcinoma and cortical hyperplasia. These show increased levels of cortisol with low levels of ACTH.

3. **Ectopic Cushing's syndrome:** About 10–15% cases of Cushing's syndrome have an origin in ectopic ACTH elaboration by non-endocrine tumours. Most often, the tumour is small cell carcinoma of the lung but other lung cancers, carcinoids; medullary carcinoma thyroid, malignant thymoma and pancreatic islet cell tumours have also been implicated. The plasma ACTH level is high in these cases and cortisol secretion is not suppressed by high or low levels of dexamethasone.

Pathology

The lesions are found in the **pituitary or adrenal glands**. Pituitary shows changes regardless of the cause. The most common alteration resulting from high levels of endogenous or exogenous glucocorticoids is termed as Crooke's hyaline change. The normal granular, basophilic cytoplasm of the ACTH-producing cells in the anterior pituitary becomes homogenous and paler. This alteration is the result of the accumulation of intermediate keratin filaments in the cytoplasm. Depending on the cause of the hypercortisolism, the adrenals show one of the following abnormalities:

1. Cortical atrophy
2. Diffuse hyperplasia
3. Macronodular/micronodular hyperplasia
4. Adenoma or carcinoma

Cliinical Features

Cushing's syndrome occurs more often in patient between the age of 20 and 40 years with three times higher frequency in women than in men. The classical features are as follows:

1. Central or truncal obesity contrasted with relatively thin arms and legs, buffalo hump due to prominence of fat over the shoulders, and rounded oedematous moon-face.
2. Increased protein breakdown resulting in wasting and thinning of the skeletal muscles, atrophy of skin and thinning of skeletal muscles, atrophy of the skin and subcutaneous tissue with formation of purple striae on the abdominal wall, osteoporosis and easy bruising of the thin skin from minor trauma.
3. Systemic hypertension present in 80% of the cases because of associated retention of sodium and water.
4. Impaired glucose tolerance and diabetes mellitus are found in 20% of cases.
5. Amenorrhoea, hirsutism, and infertility in many women.
6. Insomnia, depression, confusion and psychosis.

Diagnosis

The diagnostic tests which may help to pinpoint the cause are:
1. The 24-hour cortisol concentration
2. Loss of diurnal variation of cortisol secretion
3. To know the cause: Serum ACTH and urinary steroid excretion after administration of dexamethasone (dexamethasone suppression test).

Treatment

Treatment for Cushing syndrome is designed to lower the high level of cortisol levels. Treatment options include:
1. Reducing corticosteroid use
2. Surgery
3. Radiation therapy
4. Medication: Ketoconazole (Nizoral), mitotane (Lysodren) and metyrapone (Metopirone).

PHEOCHROMOCYTOMA (Chromaffin Tumour)

Pheochromocytoma is a rare tumour derived from chromaffin cells, also known as pheochromocytes, develops in adrenal medulla. About 10% tumours can be extra-adrenal. Its name is derived from its characteristic dark brown black appearance caused due to oxidation of catecholamines. The tumour releases excess of epinephrine and norepinephrine. Increased level of their metabolites like Vanillylmandelic acid (VMA) and metanephrin are present. Tumour arising from extra-adrenal chromaffin cells is called paraganglioma. About 10% of the tumours are malignant.

Clinical Course

Pheochromocytoma occurs at any age, but most patients are 20–60 years old. It has the most benign course in 90% of the cases and is slow growing. The traditional "10% rule" for pheochromocytoma is 10% malignant, 10% bilateral, 10% children, 10% extra-adrenal and 10% familial (multiple endocrine neoplasia (MEN) having association with medullary carcinoma of thyroid, hyperparathyroidism, pituitary adenoma, mucosal neuromas, and Von Recklinghausen's neurofibromatosis).

Clinical Features

Features are predominantly due to secretion of catecholamines, both epinephrine and norepinephrine. The most common feature is fluctuating hypertension (paroxysmal or episodic) and tachycardia. Patient is resistant to antihypertensive therapy.

Other clinical manifestations include—hyperglycaemia, aortic dissection, cerebral haemorrhage, pulmonary oedema, myocardial infarction, congestive heart failure, malignant hypertension (encephalopathy, papilloedema, proteinuria) and even death.

Pathology

Gross: The tumour is soft and spherical in shape. The cut-section shows grey, dusky brown colour with areas of haemorrhage, necrosis, calcification, and cystic changes. On immersion of the tumour in dichromate fixative, it turns brown-black due to oxidation of catecholamines in the tumour, hence the name chromaffin tumour.

Microscopy: Tumour cells are arranged characteristically as well-defined nests (zellballen pattern), solid columns, sheets, trabeculae or clumps, separated by abundant fibrovascular stroma. The cells are large polygonal with abundant granular cytoplasm with eccentric nuclei. The tumour cells stain positively with neuroendocrine substances such as neuron-specific enolase (NSE) and chromogranin.

Diagnosis

Urine analysis: Urinary vanillylmandelic acid (VMA), a norepinephrine metabolite, is markedly elevated in pheochromocytoma.

Gene testing: Pheochromocytoma is linked to mutation in the RET oncogene, a transmembrane receptor of the tyrosine kinase family.

Management

Minimally invasive laparoscopic adrenalectomy should be performed for most adrenal pheochromocytomas, with open resection reserved for very large or invasive pheochromocytomas. Surgical resection of the tumour is the treatment of choice for pheochromocytoma and usually results in cure of the hypertension. Careful preoperative management is required to control blood pressure, correct fluid volume, and prevent intraoperative hypertensive crises.

HYPERALDOSTERONISM

There is excess production of aldosterone resulting in reduced production of renin. Most patients have high blood pressure, poor vision and headache. It may be because of the following:

1. Primary: Hyperplasia, adrenocortical neoplasms (adenomas and rarely carcinoma), glucocorticosteroid remediable hyperaldosteronism.
2. Secondary: Decreased renal perfusion (nephrosclerosis, renal artery stenosis), hypovolaemia and oedema (CCF, cirrhosis, nephrotic syndrome), pregnancy (estrogen-induced increase in plasma renin substance).

Primary hyperaldosteronism/Conn's syndrome: Hyperaldosteronism produced due to solitary aldosterone producing adenoma or hyperplasia is called Conn's syndrome. The disease occurs in adults in middle age and most commonly females are affected than the males.

Patients have high blood pressure and low potassium levels. Adrenalectomy is the treatment of choice in these neoplasms.

PITUITARY GLAND

Hormones Producd by Pituitary Gland

The anterior pituitary gland constitutes 80% of the gland. It produces:

1. Somatotrophs: Growth hormones
2. Mammosomatotrophs: GH and prolactin
3. Corticotrophs: ACTH, POMC, MSH
4. Thyrotrophs: TSH
5. Gonadotrophs: FSH and LH

The clinical effects in pituitary diseases are related to deficiency, due to excess production of these hormones or due to mass effects.

Posterior pituitary gland produces ADH and oxytocin which are actually synthesized in the hypothalamus and stores in the axon terminals in posterior pituitary. ADH conserves water by restricting diuresis and oxytocin helps for cervical dilatation during uterine labor. The posterior pituitary syndromes are related to ADH.

Hyperpituitarism

The causes are the following:

1. Pituitary adenomas
2. Hyperplasia
3. Carcinoma
4. Hypothalamic disorders

Hypofunctioning of Pituitary Gland

Hypofunctioning of pituitary is seen in the following conditions.

1. Non-functioning adenomas replacing normal pituitary
2. Traumatic brain injury
3. Injury during surgery
4. Radiation
5. Pituitary apoplexy: Due to sudden haemorrhage
6. Ischaemic necrosis (Sheehan syndrome): Necrosis during pregnancy, DIC, SCA, increased intracranial pressure, traumatic injury and shock.
7. Hypothalamic lesions

With hypofunctioning, the following effects can be present.

1. GH deficiency: Dwarfism
2. Gonadotropin deficiency (LH and FSH):
   - Females: Amenorrhoea, infertility
   - Males: Loss of libido, impotence, loss of pubic hair and axillary hair
3. Hypothyroidism
4. Hypoadrenalism
5. Prolactin deficiency: Failure of postpartum lactation
6. Loss of melanocytes

Diabetes Insipidus

Deficiency of ADH causes diabetes insipidus. This is characterised by excessive urination as the tubules fail to reabsorb water from the filtrate. The urine is dilute, with lower specific gravity than normal. Serum sodium and osmolarity are increased with loss of excessive water in urine resulting in thrust and polydipsia.

Syndrome of Inappropriate ADH (SIADH)

ADH excess causes reabsorption of water resulting in hyponatraemia.

Following are causes for SIADH:

1. Ectopic ADH secretion by the malignat tumours, e.g. small cell tumours of lung
2. Drugs
3. CNS disorders including infections and trauma

NEOPLASMS OF PITUITARY GLAND

Pituitary adenomas are the most common tumours and carcinoma occurs only in 1% of pituitary tumours.

Pituitary Adenomas

These are found in adults. Age incidence is between 35 and 60 years. Depending on the size, they are called microadenomas (less than 1 cm) or macroadenomas (more than 1 cm). Non-functional adenomas attain larger size as they are detected late. Most of the adenomas are silent and microadenomas.

Gross: Well circumscribed, small ones are confined to sella turcica, with expansion erode sella turcica and anterior clinoid process. Superiorly compress the optic chiasma and adjacent structures like cranial nerves.

About 30% of the adenomas are not capsulated and invade the sinuses, dura, and sometimes brain. These are called invasive adenomas.

Microscopy: Adenomas are composed of uniform, polygonal cells arranged in sheets and cords. Intervening stroma is scant with absence of reticulin network. Mitoses are scant and these cells can be of acidophilic, basophilic or chromophobic. Cells with high mitoses and p53 expression have aggressive behaviour with invasion and recurrence and these are termed as **atypical adenomas.**

Anterior pituitary gland produces different hormones and clinical features depend upon the secretion of the hormones.

I. In prolactin-producing tumours, following are the clinical features.
  1. Amenorrhoea
  2. Galactorrhoea
  3. Loss of libido
  4. Infertility

II. Growth hormone producing tumours present with gigantism in children and acromegaly in adults. Gigantism has the following features:
  1. Epiphysis not closed
  2. Elevated GH levels
  3. Increase in body size
  4. Disproportionately long arms and legs.
  Acromegaly has the following features:
  1. Occurs after closer of epiphysis
  2. Elevated GH levels
  3. Bone density is increased and there is enlarged and broad jaw bones
  4. Feet and hands are large and fingers thickened
  5. Gonadal dysfunction, hypertension, CHF, and increased risk of GI cancer

III. ACTH producing adenomas (Cushing syndrome) have following features:
  1. Elevated levels of cortisol
  2. Hyperpigmentation

IV. Gonadotroph (LH and FSH) producing adenomas:
  1. Middle-aged females and males
  2. Neurological symptoms: Impaired vision, headache, diplopia
  3. Females present with amenorrhoea

V. TSH-producing adenomas presents with hyperthyroidism.

SELF-ASSESSMENT EXERCISE

1. **Increased thyroid antibodies with follicular destruction and granulomas are seen in:**
   A. Hashimoto thyroiditis
   B. Struma ovarii
   C. De Quervain's thyroiditis
   D. Hurthle cell disease

2. **Young male with hypertension, flushing, diarrhoea, with increased catacholamines:**
   A. Thyrotoxicosis
   B. Vipoma
   C. Insulinoma
   D. Phaeochromocytoma

3. **Phaeochromocytoma arises from:**
   A. Adrenal gland
   B. Mediastinum
   C. LN
   D. Liver

4. **All are true about Cushing syndrome *except*:**
   A. Adrenaline levels increased
   B. Oedema
   C. Violaceous cutaneous striae
   D. Polyuria

5. **For papillary carcinoma, all are true *except*:**
   A. Common thyroid carcinoma
   B. Psammoma bodies present
   C. Good prognosis
   D. Pleomorphic nuclei

6. **Most common cause for hypothyroidism is:**
   A. Graves
   B. Hashimoto's
   C. De Quervain's thyroiditis
   D. Iodine deficiency

7. **Which of the following is not seen in Cushing syndrome?**
   A. Central obesity
   B. Glucose intolerance
   C. Buffalo hump
   D. Hyperpigmentation

8. **Patients of diabetes mellitus have increased risk for the following *except*:**
   A. Infections
   B. Retinopathy
   C. Nephropathy
   D. Pancreatic carcinoma

9. **Patients of MENI can have the following:**
   A. Parathyroid tumour
   B. Abnormal proto-oncogene
   C. Marfanoid facies
   D. Develop medullary carcinoma

10. **Phaeochromocytoma can have the following:**
    A. Hypertension
    B. Aggressive malignant tumour
    C. Occurs only in adrenal gland
    D. Seconady to infection

Answers

1. C	2. D	3. A	4. A	5. D	6. D	7. D	8. D
9. A	10. A						

Diseases of Renal System

INTRODUCTION

The kidneys derive their nomenclature from the Latin term *renes,* which is related to the English word "reins", a synonym for the kidneys. Kidneys are commonly referred to as bean-shaped organs, having retroperitoneal location. The upper pole usually corresponds to the T12 vertebra and the lower pole to the body of L3 vertebra. The adult kidneys measure 11–12 cm in length, 5–7 cm wide and 2.5–3 cm thick depending on the gender, state of hydration and blood pressure. The weight of the kidney is nearly 13–44 grams in a newborn. In an adult male, it weighs 125–170 grams and 115–155 grams in females. William Bowman (1816–1892) was the first to describe the structural relationships between the glomerulus and the renal tubules, glomerular capillary tuft and its relations to the afferent and efferent arterioles.

The kidney is enveloped in Gerota's fascia and the external surface is brown in colour. Usually, the surface is smooth, however, normal fetal lobulations can be appreciated in some cases. The renal artery and renal vein usually form the blood supply of the kidney which enter the renal substance through the hilum. Hilum is located on the concave medial surface, and provides passage for renal artery, renal vein, lymphatics and nerve plexus. The hilum continues into cavity known as renal sinus. The cut surface of the kidney reveals a light-staining granular cortex because of the presence of glomeruli and convoluted tubules. Normally, it measures about 1–1.2 cm thick. Below the cortex is the darkstaining outer medulla. The inner medulla and papillae are less dense as compared to outer medulla (Fig. 39.1).

STRUCTURE AND FUNCTION OF NEPHRON

Nephrons are the functional unit of the kidney. Each kidney contains approximately one million of nephrons.

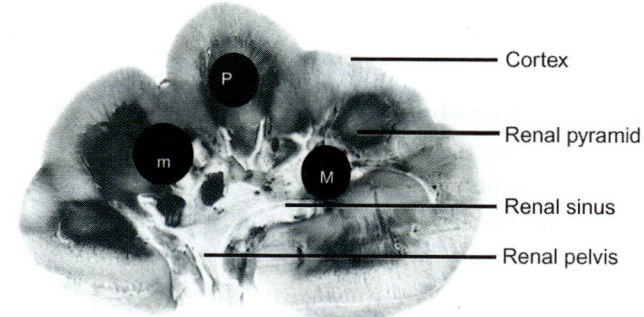

Fig. 39.1: Cut section of kidney reveals the pale staining cortex with darker medulla. Cut surface shows pyramids (P), the major calyces (M) and the minor calyces (m)

A nephron comprises a renal corpuscle known as glomerulus and complex tubular portion that drains into collecting duct. The renal corpuscle is the first segment of nephron which is involved in the formation of ultrafiltrate of blood. The human renal corpuscle measures about 150–240 μm in diameter. Renal corpuscle without parietal epithelial cells is known as glomerular tuft. The afferent arteriole enters renal corpuscle at the vascular pole, divides into several branches to form network of anastomosing capillaries which is called lobule. The supporting region of the lobule is the mesangium comprising of mesangial cells and matrix. The mesangial cells are involved in synthesis of the glomerular basement membrane (GBM) and phagocytosis. The capillaries further coalesce at the centre forming efferent arteriole which exits the glomerular tuft at the vascular pole forming a second capillary network around the tubules which are known as peritubular capillaries. The renal corpuscle consists of parietal epithelium, visceral epithelium (or podocytes), endothelial cells lining the capillaries, GBM and intraglomerular mesangial cells and matrix (Fig. 39.2).

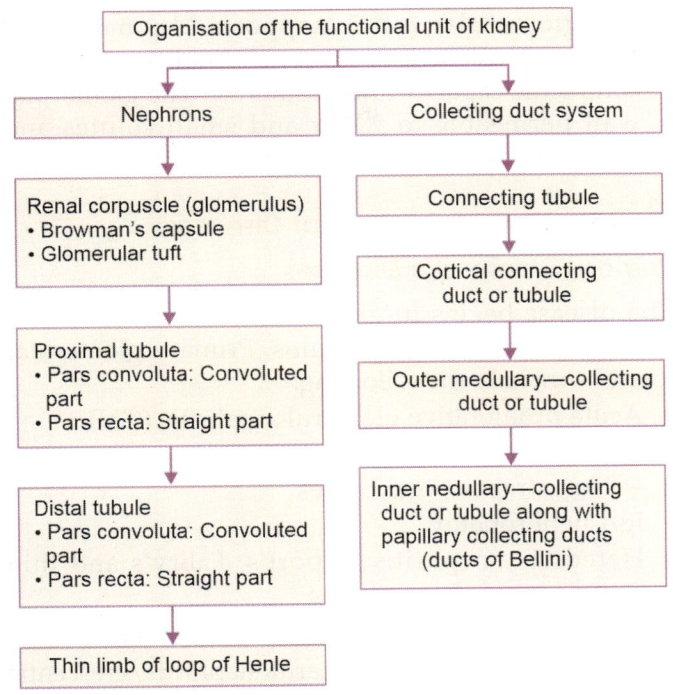

Fig. 39.2: The functional organization of the kidney

Symptoms in Glomerular Diseases

1. **Nephritic syndrome:** Syndrome characterised by glomerular haematuria and an active urine sediment having dysmorphic RBCs and RBC casts and often white blood cells and RBC casts. Patients usually have reduced glomerular filtration rate (GFR), variable degrees of hypertension, oliguria, azotemia, subnephrotic proteinuria and oedema.

2. **Nephrotic syndrome:** Syndrome characterised by heavy, albumin-dominant proteinuria (>3000 mg/day or spot urine protein/creatinine ratio of >3000 mg of protein/gram of creatinine), hypoalbuminaemia, oedema, hyperlipidaemia and lipiduria.

3. **Asymptomatic haematuria or proteinuria** or in combination of both is a manifestation of mild glomerular abnormalities.

4. **Rapidly progressive glomerulonephritis:** Important features are: Acute nephritis, proteinuria and acute renal failure. There is loss of renal function with microscopic haematuria, dysmorphic RBCs, RBC casts in the urine sediment and mild to moderate proteinuria.

5. **Acute renal failure** has oliguria or anuria, with recent onset of azotaemia. It can result from glomerular injury, interstitial injury, vascular injury or acute tubular necrosis.

6. **Chronic renal failure** is characterised by prolonged symptoms and signs of azotaemia followed by uraemia and this is the end result of different glomerular diseases.

7. **Haematuria:** Excretion of an abnormal number of red blood cells (RBCs) into the urine. The normal RBC excretion is about 1 million per day. Microscopic haematuria is defined as more than 3 RBC/HPF, but not enough RBCs to make the urine visibly red is known as microscopic haematuria. Asymptomatic haematuria is, if more than 3 RBC/HPF in at least two of three freshly voided, midstream, clean-catch urine specimen.

8. **Azotaemia:** Biochemical manifestation of acute and chronic kidney injury. There is elevated blood urea nitrogen and serum creatinine. This reflects reduced glomerular filtration.

Renal Biopsy

Indications of Kidney Biopsies

- Significant proteinuria (>1 g/day or protein to creatinine ratio >100 mg/mmol.
- Microscopic haematuria with any degree of proteinuria.
- Unexplained renal impairment (native or transplanted kidney).
- Renal manifestations of systemic disease (SLE, diabetes).
- To know the progression of disease.

Contraindications Associated with Renal Biopsy

- **Absolute contraindications:**
  - Uncontrolled hypertension
  - Bleeding diathesis
  - Widespread cystic disease
  - Hydronephrosis
  - Uncooperative patient
- **Relative contraindications:**
  - Individuals with single kidney
  - Patient who are on regular treatment with anti-platelet/clotting agents
  - Individuals having anatomical abnormalities
  - Patients with small kidneys
  - Patients having active infection
  - Obesity

Complications associated with renal biopsy:
- Macroscopic haematuria
- Bleeding that may require a blood transfusion.

GLOMERULAR DISEASES

The glomerulus consists of anastomosing network of capillaries invested by two layers of epithelium. The visceral epithelium (podocytes) is an inner layer which is in close proximity with capillary wall. The parietal layer lines the Bowman space (urinary space) and this is the space where the plasma ultrafiltrate first collects. The glomerular capillary wall is the filtration unit and consists of following structures as noticed under EM microscopy (Figs 39.3 to 39.5).

1. Inner most is a thin layer of endothelial cells which are fenestrated. The fenestrae are 70–100 nm in diameter.

2. The middle portion is glomerular basement membrane (GBM) which has central electron dense layer, inner lamina rara portion and outer lamina rara externa. The GBM has type IV collagen, laminin, proteoglycans, fibronectin and many other glyco-proteins.

3. The visceral epithelial cells, also called podocytes with their interdigitating foot processes, are adherent to the lamina rara externa of the basement membrane.

4. The glomerular tuft is supported by mesangial matrix. These are of mesenchymal origin, have contractile capacity and proliferate. The glomerular wall permeable to water and small solutes and impermeable to albumin of size 3.6 nm radius.

Classification of Glomerular Diseases

Primary Glomerular Diseases

The disease begins in glomerulus and causes direct damage only to the glomerulus. Primary glomerular diseases include the following:

- Acute proliferative glomerulonephritis (GN)
  - Post-streptococcal, and
  - Non-streptococcal causes
- IgA nephropathy
- Hereditary nephritis: Alport's, Fabry's and thin basement membrane lesion
- C3 glomerulopathy/dense deposit disease
- Rapidly progressive glomerulonephritis/crescentic glomerulonephritis:
  - Due to anti-GBM antibodies: Goodpasture syndrome
  - Due to immune complex deposition
- ANCA-associated glomerulonephritis
- Both anti-GBM disease and ANCAs-associated glomerulonephritis

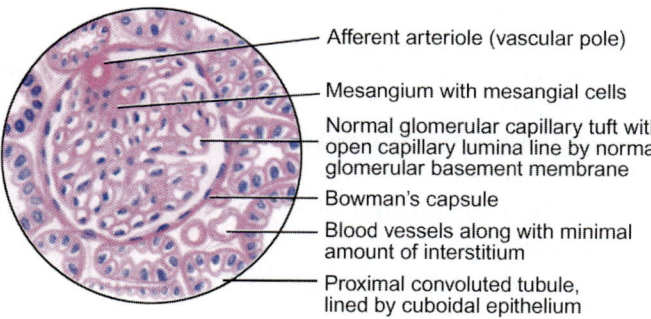

Afferent arteriole (vascular pole)

Mesangium with mesangial cells

Normal glomerular capillary tuft with open capillary lumina line by normal glomerular basement membrane

Bowman's capsule

Blood vessels along with minimal amount of interstitium

Proximal convoluted tubule, lined by cuboidal epithelium

Fig. 39.3: Normal histology of glomerulus (schematic)

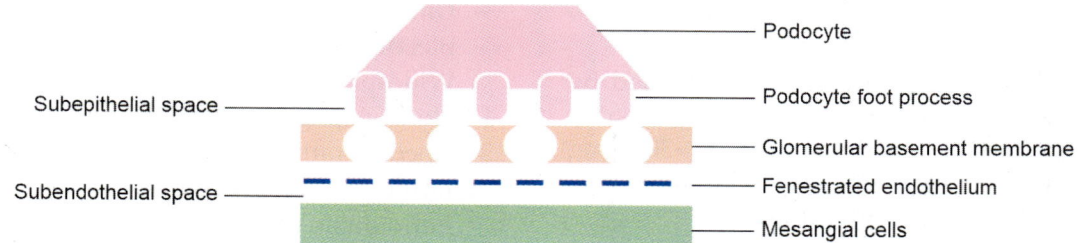

Podocyte

Subepithelial space

Podocyte foot process

Glomerular basement membrane

Subendothelial space

Fenestrated endothelium

Mesangial cells

Fig. 39.4: EM structure of glomerulus (schematic)

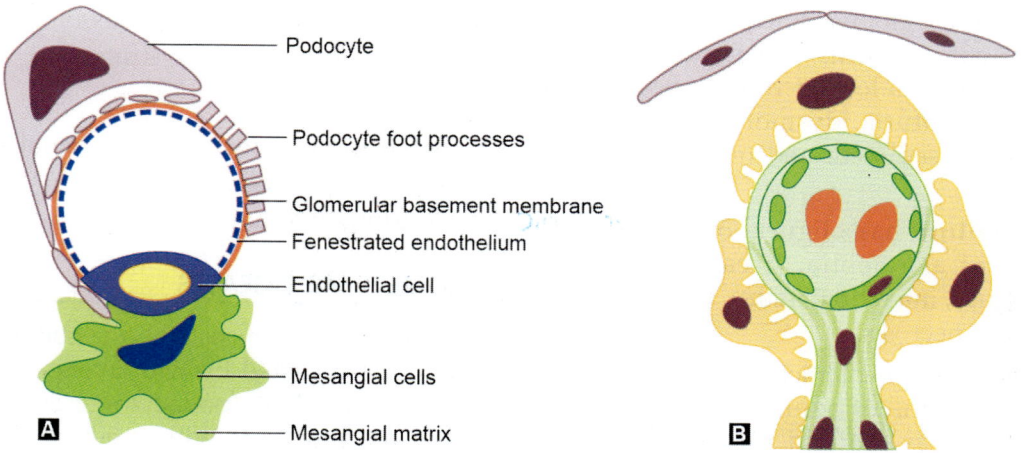

Podocyte

Podocyte foot processes

Glomerular basement membrane

Fenestrated endothelium

Endothelial cell

Mesangial cells

Mesangial matrix

A   B

Fig. 39.5: Details of EM structure of glomerulus (schematic)

- Minimal change disease
- Membranous glomerulopathy
- Focal and segmental glomerulosclerosis
- Membranoproliferative glomerulonephritis
- Chronic glomerulonephritis

Secondary Glomerular Diseases

Glomerular diseases that occur secondary to certain systemic diseases.

- Lupus nephritis
- Diabetic nephropathy
- Amyloidosis
- Cast nephropathy
- Goodpasture's syndrome
- Microscopic polyangiitis
- Wegener's granulomatosis
- Henoch-Schönlein purpura
- Bacterial endocarditis
- Microscopic polyarteritis/polyangiitis
- GN due to extrarenal infection
- Thrombotic microangiopathy

Pathogenesis of Glomerular Diseases

The immune mechanisms underline most types of primary glomerular diseases and many of the secondary glomerular diseases. GN is induced by antibodies, and glomerular deposits of immune complexes, and often along with various components of complements. Cell-mediated and humeral immune mechanisms and complement system also play role.

The important mechanisms established are:
1. **Antibody-mediated injury:**
   i. *In situ immune complex deposition:*
      - Antibodies directed against glomerular cell components
      - Antibodies against planted antigens
      - Heymann nephritis
   ii. *Circulating immune complex deposition:* Injury resulting from deposition of soluble circulating antigen-antibody immune complexes in the glomerulus
2. **Complement-mediated injury**
3. **Cell-mediated immune response**

Antibody-Mediated Injury

i. *In situ* **immune complex deposition-mediated glomerular injury:** This can be with following mechanisms:

- *Anti-GBM antibodies directed against normal components of the glomerular basement membrane:* The anti-GBM antibodies bind to intrinsic antigens

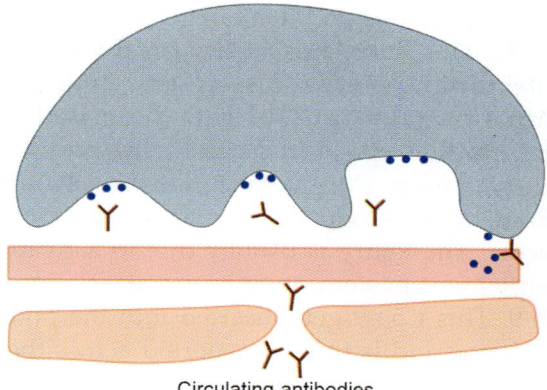
Circulating antibodies

Fig. 39.6: Anti-GBM antibodies directed against normal components of the glomerular basement membrane

in the GBM, results in linear pattern of staining by immunofluorescence technique. The anti-GBM antibodies crossreact with basement membrane of other tissues especially of the lung alveoli causing simultaneous lung and kidney lesions. This is termed as **Goodpasture syndrome**. The antibodies are to the GBM component which is non-collagenous domain NC1 of the alpha 3 chain of type IV collagen (Fig. 39.6).

- *Antibodies against planted antigens:* In this type of nephritis, the antibodies react with planted antigens in the glomerulus which are normally not present. The planted antigens include cationic molecules which bind to anionic components of the glomerulus. These are DNA, nucleosome, and other nuclear proteins. Viruses, bacteria and parasitic products and drugs may also get planted. Antibodies to these planted antigens induce a discrete pattern of immunoglobulin deposition which is granular by immunofluorescence and indistinguishable from intrinsic antigens (Fig. 39.7).

- *The Heymann nephritis:* Human counterpart of **membranous nephropathy** which is well explained by Heymann nephritis model in the rats is mediated by Th2 response, which is observed by increase in

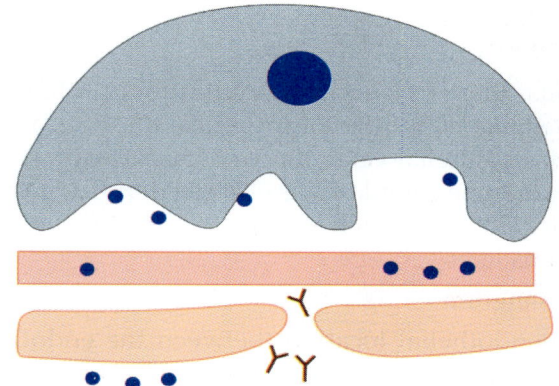

Fig. 39.7: Antibodies to the planted antigens in glomerulus (schematic)

percentage of IL-4 and IL-10 in the peripheral blood T cells. This correlates well with the amount of proteinuria. Once the disease sets in antibodies against megalin (gp330) gets deposited at the subepithelial space of glomerulus and trigger podocytes injury. Megalin in rats is present on brush border of proximal tubules and podocyte foot process. The injury is usually due to activation of complement system, membrane attack complex, C5b-9. This C5b-9 gets inserted into the podocyte membrane and is then transported across the cells into the urinary space.

It has been hypothesized that C5b-9 at cellular level generates hydrogen peroxide, triggers DNA damage and causes reversible damage of actin microfilaments, increased expression of TGF-β and its receptors leading to overproduction of extracellular matrix, thickening of the glomerular basement membrane and spike formation. C5b-9 also induces apoptosis in podocytes. No inflammatory response is accompanied as these deposits are at subepithelial location, which is inaccessible to circulating cells.

This model is difficult to explain in humans as megalin in human kidney is expressed in the proximal tubule and not at podocyte foot process. Secondly, the IgG4 which is the associated immunoglobulin with human membranous is incapable of activating the complement which is a major pathogenic factor in rat Heymann nephritis.

ii. Circulating immune complex deposition: Injury resulting from deposition of soluble circulating antigen-antibody immune complexes in the glomerulus. Here the antigen is not of glomerular origin. It is of endogenous origin as in SLE or exogenous as in streptococcal infection, hepatitis B viral infection, parasitic as in *Plasmodium falciparum* malaria and spirochete infection (*Treponema pallidum*). The antigen-antibody complexes are formed *in situ* or in the circulation and then they are trapped in the glomerulus. Here they produce injury, activate complement and recruit leucocytes (Fig. 39.8).

Thus, there is leucocytic infiltration, proliferation glomerular cells like endothelial, mesangeal, and parietal epithelial cells. Electron microscopy reveals these immune complexes as electron dense deposits or lumps/clumps which may lie at any of the three locations like:

1. Mesangium
2. Subendothelial location (between the endothelial cells and the GBM)
3. Subepithelial location (between the GBM and podocytes)

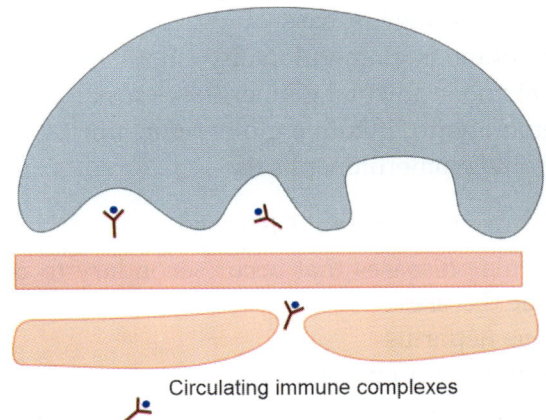

Circulating immune complexes

Fig. 39.8: Deposition of soluble circulating antigen-antibody immune complexes in the glomerulus (schematic)

The immunoglobulins and complement in these deposits can be demonstrated by immunofluorescence microscopy.

Mesangial deposits are usually observed in IgA nephropathy and class I and II of lupus nephritis. These deposits lead to activation of mesangial cells which initiate activation of the complement, coagulation and release of cytokines and growth factors. The C5b-9 mediated mechanism has been implicated in the pathogenesis of mesangial deposits as well. Following this the glomerular mesangial cells undergo a dysregulated process of proliferation and expansion leading to glomerular hypercellularity.

Subendothelial deposits in type 1 MPGN and class III and IV of lupus nephritis. These immune complexes recruit circulating inflammatory cells like neutrophils, lymphocytes, macrophages and platelets activate effector cells and cause injury. C5a and IL-8 recruit neutrophils at the site of injury, phagocytose immune complex aggregates get activated and generate reactive oxygen species following respiratory burst. RANTES and macrophage chemoattractant protein-1 (MCP-1) interact with deposited immunoglobulins and recruit macrophages. ICAM-1, VCAM-1 and MIF trigger macrophage migration leading to release of tissue factors and TGF-β which facilitates extracellular matrix accumulation causing glomerular sclerosis.

Subepithelial deposits are characteristic as in AGN (humps) and MGN with formation of spike-like deposits.

Complement-Mediated Injury

The major pathway for antibody initiated injury is complement leucocyte mediated. There is generation of complement components which are chemotactic mainly C5a. There is recruiting of neutrophils and monocytes. The neutrophils release proteases which damage and degrade the GBM. Oxygen-derived free radicals cause cell damage. In some cases, the C5–C9 membrane attack complexes cause damage to epithelial cells and detachment. Components of complement stimulate mesangeal and epithelial cells to secrete various mediators of cell injury. There is increased TGF-β which stimulates synthesis of extracellular matrix and altered GBM composition and thickening.

In complement-mediated injury, there is persistent activation of alternate complement pathway by following mechanisms.

Autoantibodies:

- *C3 nephritic factor (C3Nef):* This is an autoantibody to the alternate complement pathway's C3 convertase.
- *Autoantibodies to the complement alternative pathway regulatory proteins:* Complement factor H(CFH) and factor B.

Genetic abnormalities of complement component genes:

- C3 mutation
- Factor H mutation
- Allelic variants of complement factor I (CFI), CFH, C3

Complement may have a beneficial or harmful role on kidneys. Various renal diseases exhibit deposition of complement in the glomeruli like dense deposit disease, C3 glomerulopathy and C1q nephropathy. Certain renal diseases also show presence of immunoglobulins along with complement deposition like postinfectious glomerulonephritis, membranous nephropathy, IgA nephropathy and lupus nephritis.

Cell-Mediated Immune Response

The sensitized T cells formed during cell-mediated immune reaction can cause glomerular injury. In this type of injury, there no deposits of antibodies or immune complexes or the deposits do not correlate with severity of injury.

Role of T cells: Lymphocytes play an important role in pathogenesis of immune-mediated glomerular disease. The most important of all are the CD4 expressing T helper cells. These cells are involved in immunoglobulin production and also direct cellular immune mechanisms by activation of effector cells. It has been postulated that majority of the T cells are naïve which when stimulated by antigen-presenting cells, differentiate into either T helper 1 (Th1) or T helper 2 (Th2) cells. Th1 differentiation is facilitated via toll-like receptors, by secretion of IL-12 whereas IL-4 mediates Th2 differentiation. These activated Th1 cells are responsible for cell-mediated immunity through production of interferon γ (IFN-γ), interleukin 2 (IL-2)

and tumour necrosis factor α (TNF-α); leading to macrophage activation, induction of delayed-type hypersensitivity response, stimulate B-cells to produce complement-fixing antibody isotypes which mediate phagocytosis following opsonization. Th2 cells on the other hand produce IL-4, IL-5, IL-10 and IL-13, promoting production of non-complement-fixing IgG isotypes and IgE. Thus Th2 cells are involved in B cell-mediated response. The Th1-mediated responses in kidney are implicated by infiltration of circulating mononuclear cells and crescent formation. The Th2-mediated response is characterised by formation of immune complexes, deposition of these complexes in the glomerulus which further leads to activation of the complement system. Both the Th1 and Th2 responses bring about functional and structural changes in the glomerulus.

The T cell-mediated immune response and their role in various glomerulopathies: The cell-mediated immune responses are implicated in pathogenesis of minimal change disease, focal and segmental glomerulosclerosis (FSGS), pauci-immune crescentic glomerulonephritis and Class IV lupus nephritis. The lymphocytes and macrophages recruited at the glomerulus usually release tissue factors and TGF-β that initiate fibrin deposition as well as extracellular matrix deposition. It has also been postulated that T cells may be source of permeability factors that cause proteinuria and non-inflammatory glomerular disease especially in individuals with MCD and FSGS. The crescentic GN is predominantly thought to be of Th1-mediated response. T cells lead to delayed hypersensitivity reaction leading to cellular reaction and local fibrin deposition. Macrophages release ROS and inflammatory cytokines causing Bowman capsule injury, mediating formation of crescents and influx of inflammatory cells.

The humoral immune responses and their role in various glomerulopathies: Many glomerulonephritis are resultant of an autoimmune process. Loss of self-tolerance and exposure to etiological agents lead to immune complex formation, mostly by the mechanism of molecular mimicry and epitope spreading. Some antigens that are implicated are listed below:

Non-collagenous domain of the alpha-III chain of type IV collagen	Goodpasteur's syndrome
DNA-nucleosome complex	Lupus nephritis (non-renal self-antigens)
HCV antigen-containing cryoglobulins	HCV associated MPGN

NEPHRITIC SYNDROME

Nephritic syndrome is characterised by:

- Haematuria
- Urine sediment: Manifested by dysmorphic RBCs and RBC casts and often white blood cells.
- Reduced glomerular filtration rate (GFR)
- High serum creatinine and blood urea nitrogen levels
- Variable degree of hypertension
- Oliguria
- Oedema.

The primary glomerular diseases which fall under nephritic syndrome are:

1. Acute post-infectious glomerulonephritis
2. IgA nephropathy (Berger's disease)
3. Hereditary nephritis
4. C3 glomerulonephritis and dense deposit disease

Acute Postinfectious Glomerulonephritis

This can be due to following causes:

1. Streptococcal infection
2. Other causes:
    a. Bacterial infections (staphylococci, endocarditis, pneumococci, meningococcal infection)
    b. Viral (HBV, HCV, mumps, HIV, varicella and infectious mononucleosis)
    c. Parasitic (malaria and toxoplasma)

Postinfectious Streptococcal GN/Post-streptococcal GN

Acute post-infectious glomerulonephritis (PIGN), also known as acute post-streptococcal diffuse proliferative and exudative glomerulonephritis or formerly known as acute hemorrhagic Bright's disease, is acute glomerulonephritis related to recent streptococcal infection.

Clinical features and course of the disease:

1. Acute PIGN is usually disease of paediatric age group.
2. The incidence of this disease is less in developed countries due to better hygiene as compared to developing nations.
3. Nearly 1:1,000 develop PIGN post-streptococcal pharyngitis.
4. Beta haemolytic streptococci (types 12, 4 and 1) are responsible.
5. The peak age of presentation is between 6 and 8 years of life with a male to female ratio of 2:1.
6. The disease usually presents 1–4 weeks after infection by streptococci.
7. Haematuria is the most common symptom. The urine of these patients is typically described as "smoky", "Coca-Cola", and "tea" or "coffee" coloured.
8. Hypocomplementaemia, reduced serum C3 as well as C4 can be noted.
9. Demonstration of antistreptolysin O (ASO) titer is more specific for pharyngitis whereas anti-DNase-B for pyoderma.

Gross features: The kidneys are symmetrically enlarged to approximately 25–50% of normal and appear pale. The cut surfaces may have tiny red speckles caused by red blood cells in the lumen of the Bowman space and tubules.

Light microscopic features

Glomeruli (Figs 39.9 and 39.10):

- Appear hypercellular and are enlarged, reveal lobular accentuation.
- The hypercellularity is because of:
    1. Infiltration of leucocytes: Neutrophils, monocytes, eosinophils and plasma cells
    2. Proliferation of endothelial and mesangial cells (endocapillary proliferation) and migrant inflammatory cells, which include neutrophils, eosinophils, monocytes and plasma cells.
- The capillary lumina of glomeruli are narrowed.
- Diffuse and global changes: All lobules of all glomeruli involved.
- Interstitial areas show oedema and infiltration with polymorphonuclear leucocytes and mononuclear cells. Tubules may show neutrophilic casts.
- The arteries and arterioles are normal.

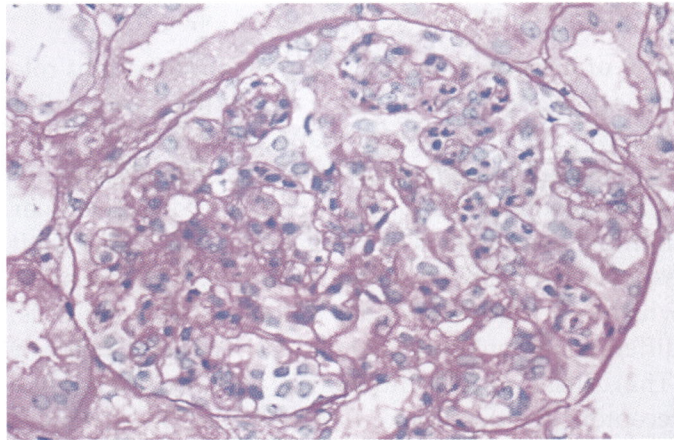

Fig. 39.9: Enlarged glomerulus with increase in number of nuclei in the glomerulus, the glomerular basement membrane is unremarkable. (PAS, ×400)

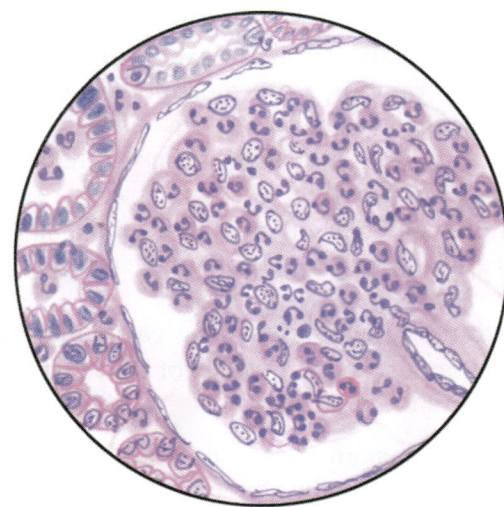

Fig. 39.10: Microscopy AGN (schematic)

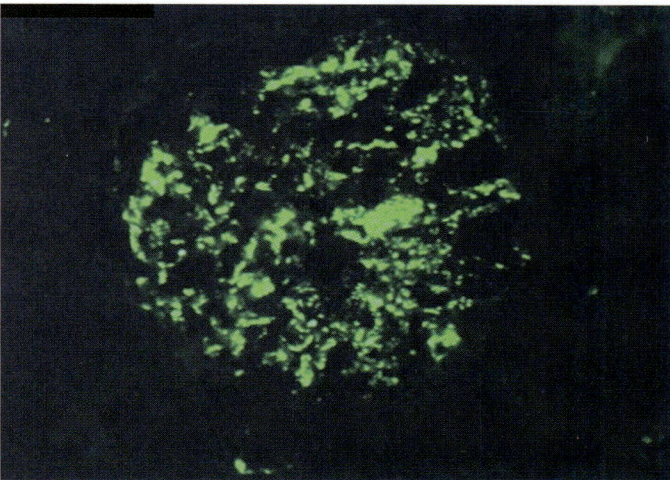

Fig. 39.13: Starry sky pattern: Irregular, fine, granular deposits that are present along the capillary wall large, post-infectious type deposit (humps) (anti-IgG, 400×)

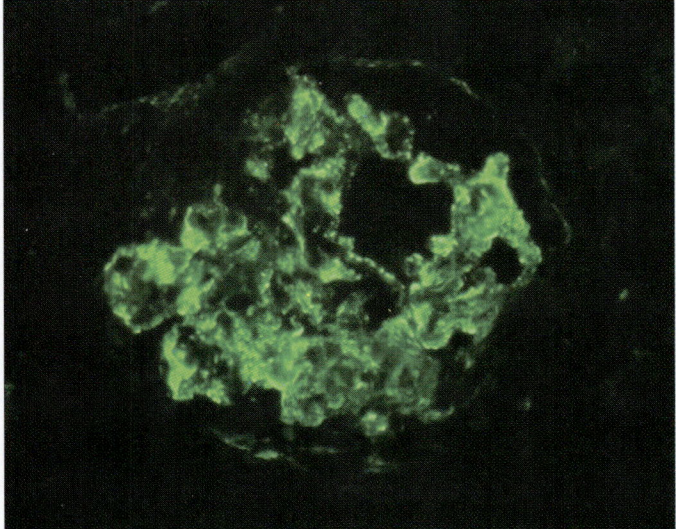

Fig. 39.11: IF Garland pattern: Intense, confluent and heavy deposits of anti-IgG are present along the glomerular basement membrane as well as mesangium (400×)

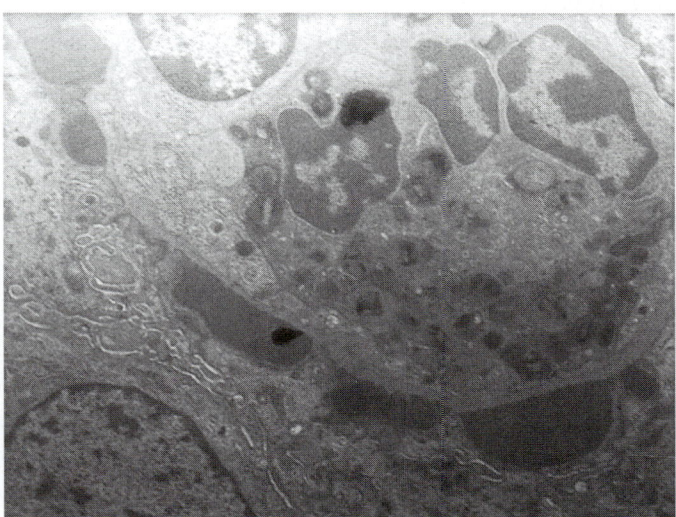

Fig. 39.14: EM structure subepithelial electron-dense immune deposits, AGN

Immunofluorescence: Immune deposits of immunoglobulin G and C3 in a **diffuse granular pattern** are present along the glomerular capillary wall and mesangium. Three different patterns of immunofluorescence are seen in cases of PIGN, namely the garland pattern, the starry sky pattern, and the mesangial pattern (Figs 39.11 to 39.13).

Electron microscopy findings: The most consistent and classic diagnostic finding is the presence of glomerular subepithelial electron-dense immune deposits (humps) on electron microscopy (Fig. 39.14).

Clinical course: A classical case is highlighted below.

1. A child of 5 to 6 years of age abruptly develops fever, malaise, nausea, oliguria, haematuria (smoky or cola-coloured urine) and generalized oedema.

2. This usually follows 1 to 2 weeks after recovery from sore throat.

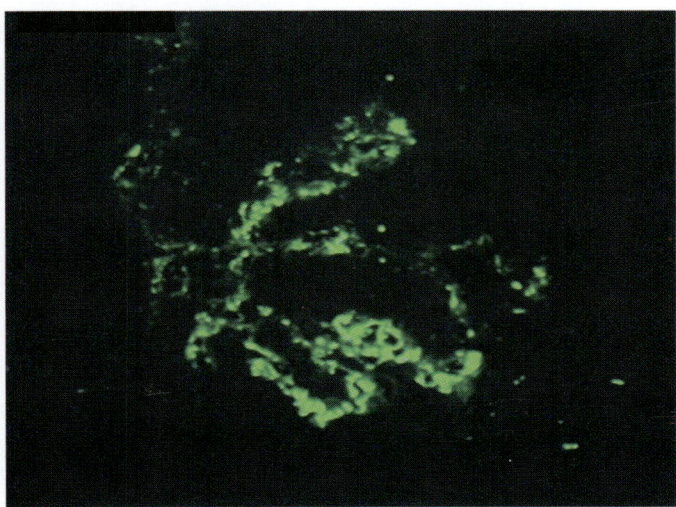

Fig. 39.12: IF mesangial pattern: Coarse deposits present in the mesangium (anti-IgG, 400×)

3. Patients have dysmorphic RBCs, red cells and red cell casts in urine and mild proteinuria of less than 1 g/day
4. Children have mild to moderate hypertension
5. In adults, the onset is atypical.

More than 95% of the children recover renal function with conservative therapy and less than 1% of the children develop RPGN.

IgA Nephropathy (Berger's Disease)

IgA nephropathy was first described by a French pathologist "Jene Berger" and "Nicole Hinglais" in cohort of patients presenting with persistent microscopic haematuria or episodes of macroscopic haematuria.

Primary idiopathic immunoglobulin A (IgA) nephropathy is a progressive glomerular disease with infrequent reversal and is characterised:

- Clinically by microscopic/episodic macroscopic hematuria and proteinuria
- Predominant IgA deposits (+2 or more intensity) in the mesangium of the glomeruli (normally 5–15 % of normal individuals may demonstrate IgA deposits in the mesangium); and
- Absence of systemic or other non-renal disease.

Nearly 20–30% patients develop renal failure within 10–20 years.

Clinical Features

IgA is one of the most common forms of primary glomerulitis in the world. IgA nephropathy mainly affects the young adults with a mean age of 30 years and paediatric population (older children).

1. Males are more commonly affected with M:F ratio of 2:1.
2. The most common presenting symptom is episodic haematuria, which is usually with a period of clinical quiescence and recurrence, associated with a URT (known as synpharyngitic haematuria).

Pathogenesis of IgA Nephropathy

1. The central pathogenesis of IgA nephropathy is abnormal glycosylation of the IgA1 molecule, which gets deposited in the mesangium and initiates the pathological process.
2. Patients with IgA nephropathy have IgA1 which is deficient in galactose. Autoantibodies to galactose-deficient IgA1 are produced which bind to GalNAc (N-acetylgalactosamine neoepitopes) on abnormally glycated IgA1.
3. Also, the galactose deficient IgA1 may bind to the mesangium.

Light microscopy findings: The glomeruli in IgA nephropathy exhibit a wide range of pathological morphology ranging from morphology of minimal change disease to globally sclerotic lesions.

1. Mesangial hypercellularity and accentuation of the mesangial matrix (Fig. 39.15).
2. Focal or segmental inflammation of the glomeruli, endocapillary hypercellularity, necrotizing lesions and crescents.
3. Interstitium shows variable degree of inflammation.
4. Tubules are packed with RBCs or RBC casts. Vessels usually are unremarkable.

Immunofluorescence microscopy findings: On immunofluorescence, the glomerular mesangial regions reveal IgA deposits along with C3 and properdin characteristically described as "Branches of a tree in winter, devoid of leaves" (Fig. 39.16).

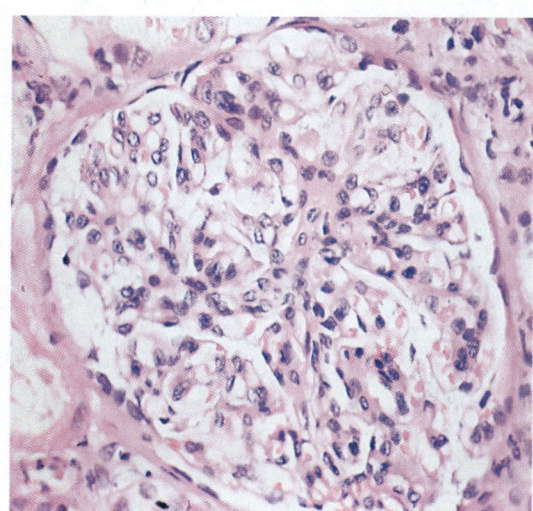

Fig. 39.15: IgA nephropathy with increase in the mesangial cellularity and mesangial matrix accentuation (400x)

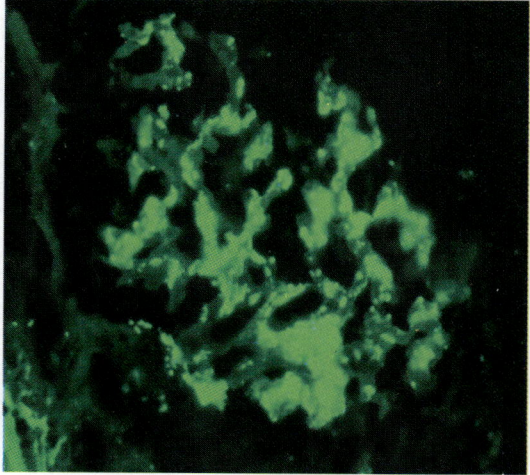

Fig. 39.16: IF deposits of IgA, which are mainly located in the mesangial region (anti-IgA, magnification x400)

Hereditary Nephritis (Alport's Syndrome and Thin Basement Membrane Nephropathy)

Alport's syndrome is characterised by renal, cochlear, and ocular involvement, usually in males with X-linked, and autosomal recessive (AR) can occur in males and females. The disease is usually caused by mutation of the type IV collagen genes *COL4A3*, *COL4A4*, and *COL4A5*. Grossly and microscopically, there are no structural alterations noted and glomeruli reveal unremarkable morphology.

Clinical Features

- Haematuria is the initial presentation in childhood along with proteinuria. 30 to 40% of the severe cases may develop nephrotic syndrome.
- Progressive sensory and neural hearing loss in late childhood or early adolescence.
- Ocular findings: Anterior lenticonus, maculopathy (whitish or yellowish flecks or granulations in the perimacular region), corneal endothelial vesicles (posterior polymorphous dystrophy), and recurrent corneal erosion.

Thin basement membrane nephropathy (Fig. 39.17) is characterised by persistent microscopic haematuria (benign familial haematuria). The affected individuals have benign course. However, some percentage of these cases may have renal insufficiency. Light microscopy has no specific lesions. EM shows marked thinning of lamina densa of GBM. Mutations of the type IV collagen genes *COL4A3* and *COL4A4* are detected.

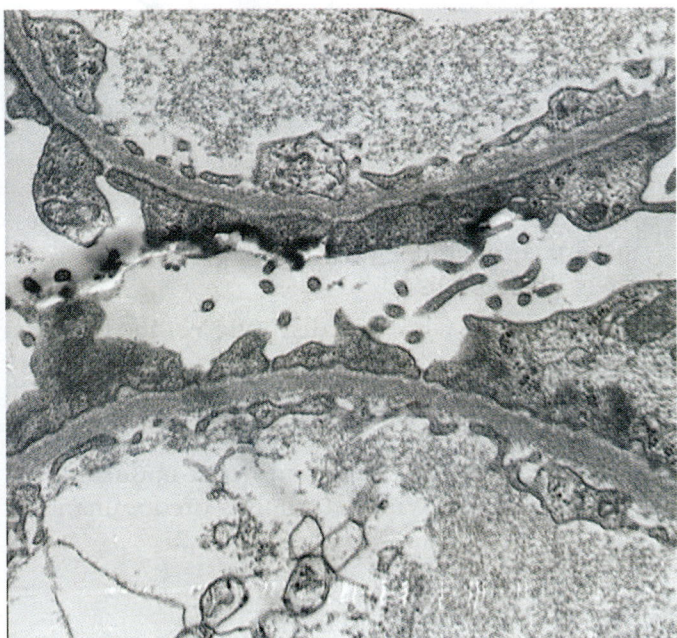

Fig. 39.17: Thinned out basement membrane (150 nm) at 2000× magnification

Electron microscopy:

- Splitting of the lamina densa into multiple interlacing strands of electron-dense material, resembling basket-weaving.
- Lacunae between these strands are occupied by round, electron-dense bodies.
- Diffuse thickening of the glomerular capillary wall with scalloping of the epithelial aspect.

C3 Glomerulonephritis and Dense Deposit Disease

C3 glomerulonephritis (C3GN) and dense deposit disease (DDD) are grouped under C3 glomerulopathy. DDD was earlier classified under MPGN type II, but now reclassified as complement-mediated glomerular disease. 'C3 glomerulopathy' the term has been used to encompass all glomerular lesions with predominant C3 accumulation and the term dense deposit disease reflects the linear appearing electron dense material in glomerular basement membrane.

DDD has electron dense material in the lamina densa of the GBM. IF shows C3 deposits along the capillary wall and mesangium. Immunoglobulin is not usually detected indicating that the disease not of classic antigen–antibody immune mechanism. There is dysregulation and activation of alternate complement pathway in these patients. Kidney biopsy shows MPGN histology.

The patients of DDD are children or adults, present with haematuria and features of chronic renal failure. They have decreased serum C3, but normal C1 and C4 levels. Circulating autoantibody to C3 nephritic factor (C3NeF) binds to C3 convertase and activates it. Mutations of Factor H have been associated with DDD.

C3GN has features similar to DDD. However, affects all age groups and both genders are equally affected. Oliguria and hypertension are common presenting features. Haematuria and proteinuria are the common urinary findings.[44] DDD may also present with nephrotic syndrome features.

CRESCENTIC GLOMERULONEPHRITIS/RAPIDLY PROGRESSIVE GLOMERULONEPHRITIS

Rapidly progressive glomerulonephritis (RPGN) is a disease of the kidney, characterised clinically by a rapid decrease in the glomerular filtration rate (GFR) to at least 50% over a short period, ranging from a few days to 3 months with features of nephritic syndrome. The onset is characterised by oliguria, advancing azotaemia, proteinuria, haematuria with cellular casts and hypertension.

Crescentic glomerulonephritis or proliferative extra-capillary or rapidly progressive glomerulonephritis (RPGN) is a histologic manifestation of severe glomerular damage with proliferation of parietal epithelial cells forming ≥2 layers occupying ≥25% of the Bowman's space. The patients usually present with rapidly progressive renal failure.

- At least 50% glomeruli should be displaying crescents.
- Cellular crescent: Predominant component is cellular.
- Fibrous crescent: >90% of the crescent component is fibrous.
- Fibrocellular crescent: Crescent with mixture of cellular and fibrous components.

The immunopathological classification of crescentic glomerulonephritis: According to immunopathological mechanisms involved, crescentic glomerulonephritis is classified as:

Type I: Produced by anti-glomerular basement membrane (GBM) antibodies.
- Idiopathic
- Goodpasture syndrome

Type II: Due to immune complexes deposited in glomeruli.
- Idiopathic
- Post-infectious GN
- SLE
- Henoch-Schönlein purpura
- IgA nephropathy

Type III: Pauci-immune and ANCA associated
- Idiopathic
- Wegener's
- Microscopic angiitis

Pathology in RPGN

Gross Features

The kidneys are usually normal sized; however, a few cases may show slightly enlarged kidneys. Kidneys on cut surface reveal multiple red dots on the cortical surface, typically described as *"flea-bitten"* appearance. These red hemorrhagic spots correspond to presence of blood in the tubular lumina or Bowman's capsule (Fig. 39.18).

Light Microscopy Findings (Fig. 39.19)

1. Characteristic histological lesion is the formation of cellular crescents with or without segmental fibrinoid necrosis in most of the glomeruli. The crescents are formed by proliferation of parietal cells and by migration of inflammatory cells like monocytes, and

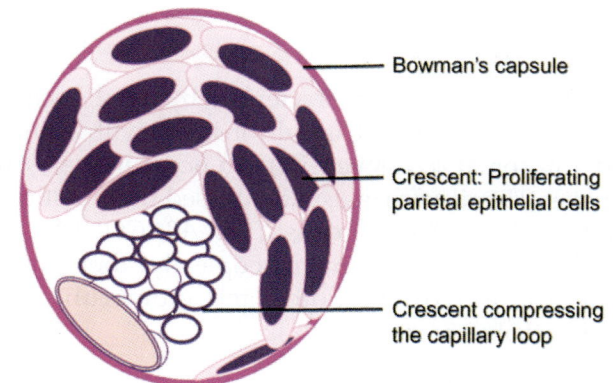

Fig. 39.18: A crescent which is formed due to proliferation of parietal epithelial cells.

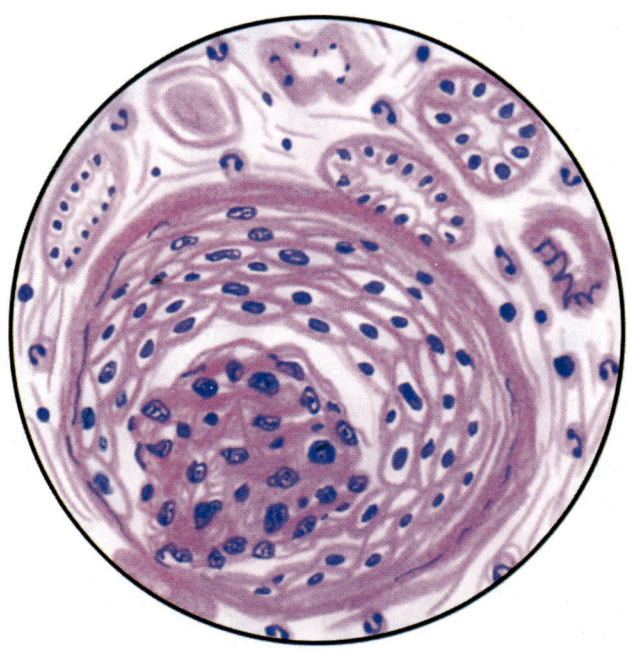

Fig. 39.19: Microscopy RPGN (schematic)

macrophages into the urinary space. Neutrophils and lymphocytes may be present. These may compress the glomerular tuft. Fibrin may be present in between the epithelial cells.

2. Rupture of the GBM and disruption of the Bowman capsule that elicits a periglomerular inflammatory reaction sometimes accompanied with giant cell reaction.

3. Capillary lumina reveal significant endocapillary hypercellularity, with neutrophils predominantly.

4. Tubular lumina as well as Bowman's space may show RBCs.

5. RBC casts are present in the tubules.

6. Interstitium is infiltrated by plasma cells, lymphocytes, neutrophils and macrophages.

Immunofluorescence

1. The characteristic strong, linear ribbon-like IgG staining of the GBM is diagnostic of anti-GBM disease.
2. Immune complex mediated cases show granular immune deposits, and
3. Pauci-immune cases have little or no immune deposits.

Diagnosis

Anti-GBM antibodies, antinuclear antibodies and ANCAs are helpful in diagnosis of Goodpasture syndrome. Plasmapheresis along with steroids and cytotoxic drugs can reverse lung and kidney changes. Despite therapy, patients may require chronic dialysis or transplacentation.

Anti-GBM Disease/Goodpasture Syndrome

Antiglomerular basement membrane disease (anti-GBM) is defined by the presence of autoantibodies directed at specific antigenic targets within the glomerular and/or pulmonary basement membrane. These antibodies bind to the α3 chain of type IV collagen. Ernest Goodpasture was the first to describe this disease in the year 1919. The antibodies cause inflammatory destruction of the basement membrane of glomeruli and pulmonary alveoli. There is rapidly progressive GN and necrotizing haemorrhagic interstitial pneumonitis.

Pathogenesis

The trigger that causes production of anti-GBM antibodies is not exactly known, but it is presumed that the cryptic antigens of the type IV collagen of BM are exposed, by the environmental insult such as viral infection, hydrocarbon solvents, smoking, etc.

Pathology

The lungs are heavy, red brown consolidation. Microscopy shows focal fibrinoid necrosis, hemosiderin-laden macrophages, late stages fibrosis of septa, hyperplasia and hypertrophy of type II pneumocytes.

Kidney shows features of proliferative GN of RPGN. There is fibrinoid necrosis and rupture of basement membrane and periglomerular inflammatory infiltration.

IF shows linear deposits of immunoglobulins along the BM of septal walls (Fig. 39.20).

Clinical Features of Goodpasture Syndrome

1. It can occur across all racial groups and at all age groups.

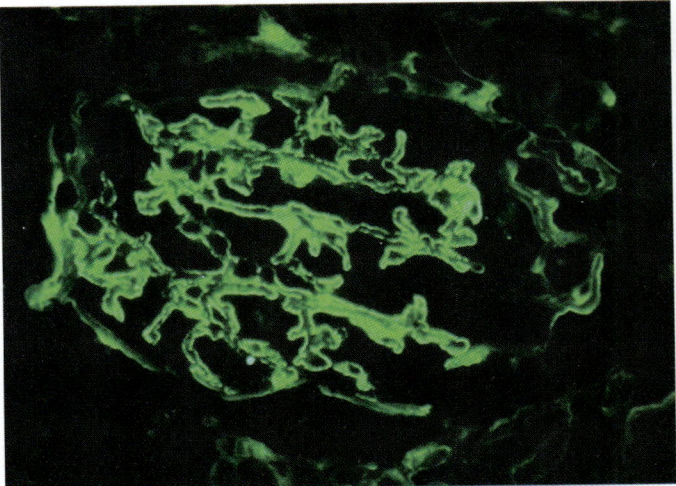

Fig. 39.20: IF showing linear deposits, Goodpasture syndrome

2. The disease has a typical bimodal presentation with a first peak incidence in the third decade and second peak in the sixth and seventh decades.
3. The disease affects men predominantly. Majority are smokers.
4. Flu-like illness may precede the onset of Goodpasture syndrome.
5. The patients may present with pulmonary and renal symptoms.
6. **Haemoptysis and dyspnoea** are the common symptoms.
7. **Haematuria** is the most common finding in patients with anti-GBM disease.

Treatment

Treatment includes plasmapheresis, immunosuppression and possible prevention of antibody formation.

NEPHROTIC SYNDROME

The primary and secondary to glomerular diseases which fall under nephrotic syndrome are:

Primary glomerular diseases:

1. Minimal change disease
2. Focal segmental glomerulosclerosis
3. Membranous glomerulonephritis
4. Membranoproliferative glomerulonephritis
5. IgA nephropathy

Secondary glomerular diseases:

1. Lupus nephritis
2. Diabetic nephropathy
3. Amyloidosis
4. Cast nephropathy
5. Goodpasture's syndrome
6. Microscopic polyangiitis
7. Wegener's granulomatosis

8. Henoch-Schönlein purpura
9. Bacterial endocarditis
10. Microscopic polyarteritis/polyangiitis
11. GN due to extrarenal infection
12. Thrombotic microangiopathy

The classical features are:

1. Heavy, albumin-dominant proteinuria (>3000 mg/day or spot urine protein/creatinine ratio of >3000 mg of protein/gram of creatinine)
2. Hypoalbuminaemia
3. Oedema
4. Hyperlipidaemia
5. Lipiduria.

Minimal Change Disease (Lipoid Nephrosis)

Minimal change disease (MCD) also known as nil disease or lipoid nephrosis is an idiopathic glomerular disease, usually presenting as nephrotic syndrome, commonly in paediatric age group. As most of the children with minimal change disease respond to steroid treatment, the disease is termed as steroid sensitive nephrotic syndrome".

The pathogenesis of primary MCD is attributed to effacement of the podocyte foot process due to negatively charged glycocalyx. The damage to podocytes is attributed to T cell-derived factor, however, still not established in humans.

Clinical Features

1. Most common cause of paediatric nephrotic syndrome and accounting for 70–90%.
2. Patients have nephrotic range proteinuria and most of the patients respond to steroid treatment.

Gross findings: The kidneys usually appear enlarged. The cut section has a typical waxy appearance. The cortex is usually yellow due to accumulation of lipids in the proximal tubules.

Light microscopic findings (Fig. 39.21):
1. The glomerular architecture is usually unremarkable on light microscopy.
2. The tubular cells reveal protein droplets, also known as "hyaline droplets" and lipid droplets.
3. The interstitium may show presence of foam cells.

Immunofluorescence: There is no immunological involvement noted on immunofluorescence studies.

Electron microscopy findings: The electron microscopic findings are characteristic and reveal (Fig. 39.22A and B):
1. Podocyte foot process effacement which is usually diffuse.

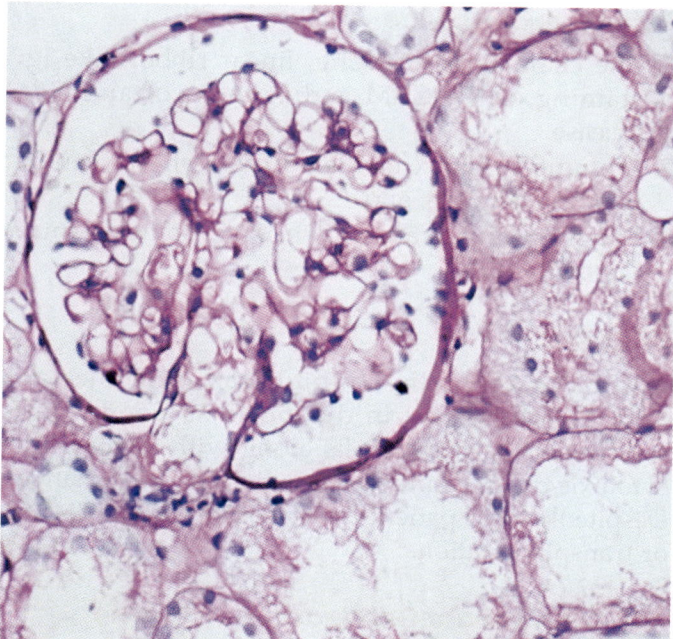

Fig. 39.21: Minimal change disease, glomeruli appear normal with patent lumina (HE, 200×)

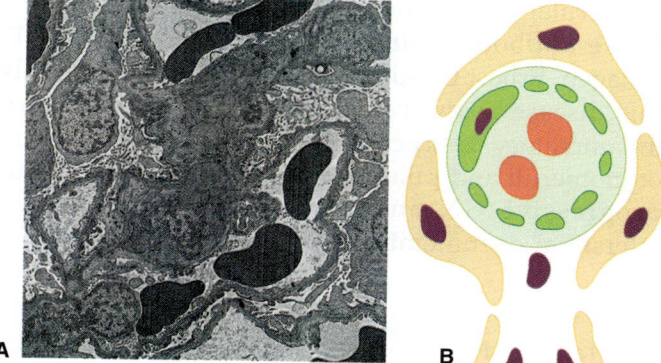

Fig. 39.22: (A) EM picture (B) with effacement of foot processes (schematic)

2. Swelling of the podocytes may show vacuolization and microvillus transformation.
3. Electron-dense resorption droplets are variably present in the tubules.

Focal Segmental Glomerulosclerosis

In focal segmental glomerulosclerosis (FSGS), there is focal (some glomeruli and not all) involvement of glomeruli and only segments of glomeruli are involved.

Etiology

Idiopathic and secondary causes like HIV infection, heroin addiction, sickle cell disease and massive obesity.

Pathogenesis

The pathogenesis of FSGS is unknown. As with MCD, permeability increasing factors produced by lymphocytes is blamed. There is entrapment of plasma proteins and lipids at the site of injury.

Pathology

Microscopy shows the glomerular lesion is focal, some but not all glomeruli are involved in FSGS with following features (Fig. 39.23).

1. A segment of glomerular capillary tuft [lobule(s)] is involved.
2. There is adhesion of glomerular tuft to Bowman's capsule, called synechiae, is often seen early in the process of sclerosis.
3. The glomeruli show sclerosis. There is an increased collagenous extracellular matrix expanding the mesangium with resultant obliteration of capillary lumina.
4. The affected glomeruli show hyalinosis with increased mesangial matrix with accumulation of glycoproteins, proteins and lipids.
5. The hypercellularity of segmental lesion is caused by proliferation of mesangial cells, epithelial cells and sometimes is accompanied with leucocytic infiltration.

IF: There is no deposition of immune complexes, but focal and segmental deposition of IgM and C3 in the sclerosed areas and mesangial expansion is present. Sometimes, less intense staining of IgA, IgG and albumin is also noted.

EM: There is effacement of foot processes, accompanied by podocyte alterations that include hyperplasia, hypertrophy and focal microvillous transformation.

Clinical Course

The clinical course is variable in FSGS. Spontaneous remission is less often and around 20% of the patients follow a rapid course and renal failure with 2 years.

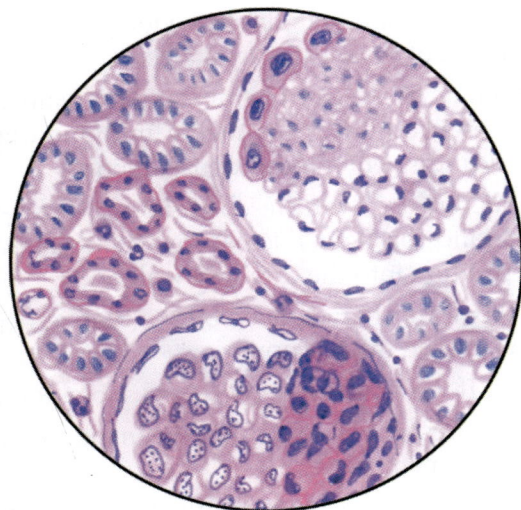

Fig. 39.23: Glomerulus in focal segmental glomerulosclerosis

Membranous Glomerulonephritis

Membranous nephropathy, known as membranous glomerulonephritis (MGN) or epimembranous nephropathy, is an idiopathic chronic glomerular disease characterised by deposition of diffuse subepithelial immune complexes with intervening formation of matrix (spikes) and clinically presents as nephrotic syndrome. The disease usually occurs in primary and secondary forms. Primary MGN is common and accounts for 75% of the cases. The secondary form is associated with the following causes:

1. Drugs: Pencillamine, non-steroidal anti-inflammatory drugs, gold, etc.
2. Malignant tumours: Carcinomas of lung and colon, melanomas, etc.
3. SLE: 10 to 15% of GN in SLE is MGN.
4. Infections: HBV, HCV, syphilis, schistosomiasis and malaria.
5. Other autoimmune disorders such as thyroiditis.

Clinical Features

Patients with nephrotic syndrome usually present with nephrotic range proteinuria. Haematuria is rare and if associated should raise a suspicion of renal vein thrombosis.

Pathology

Gross: Grossly the kidneys are symmetrically enlarged and appear pale.

Light microscopy: The microscopic changes can be studied under following headings:

1. **Glomerulus:** The hallmark is thickening of the glomerular basement membrane with no or minimal mesangial hypercellularity (Fig. 39.24). The PAS and silver stains usually reveal subepithelial deposits visible as "subepithelial spikes" (Fig. 39.25). The capillary lumina are fairly open. Presence of RBCs or leucocytes raises the possibility of renal vein thrombosis.

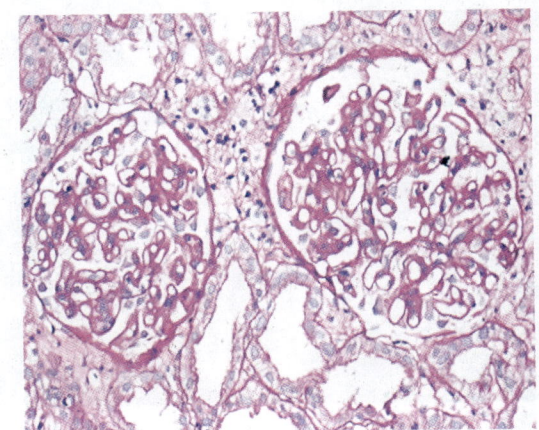

Fig. 39.24: Membranous nephropathy (PAS, 100×)

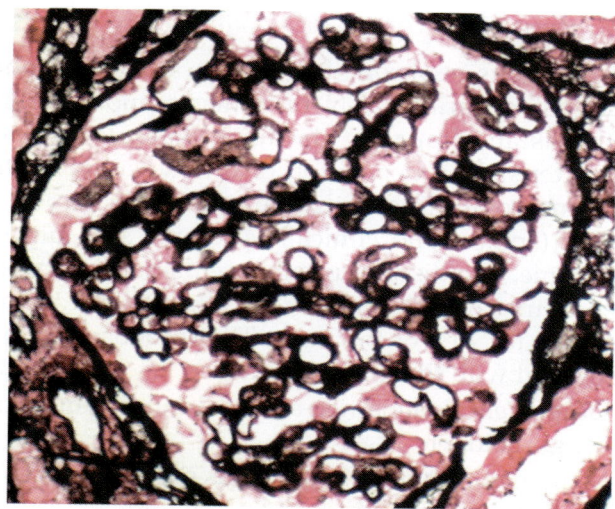

Fig. 39.25: Jones methenamine silver (400x)

2. **Tubules:** Tubules usually show presence of protein resorption droplets. Presence of tubular atrophy usually indicates a chronic phase or secondary nature of the disease.

3. **Interstitium:** Interstitial foam cells are quiet often identified and interstitial fibrosis is usually seen in advanced cases.

4. **Vessels:** Usually demonstrate arteriosclerosis.

Immunofluorescence (Figs 39.26 and 39.27): The hallmark of MGN is diffuse, global staining with fine deposits of IgG along the GBM, usually the IgG4 subclass predominates in subepithelial region. Complement deposits (usually C3) are also noticed but of lesser intensity when compared to IgG. Kappa and lambda light chain deposits are also seen.

Electron microscopy: The electron microscopy usually reveals presence of electron-dense deposits in the subepithelial region with effacement of podocyte foot processes. Usually four stages have been described by Ehrenreich and Churg. The stage I is characterised by

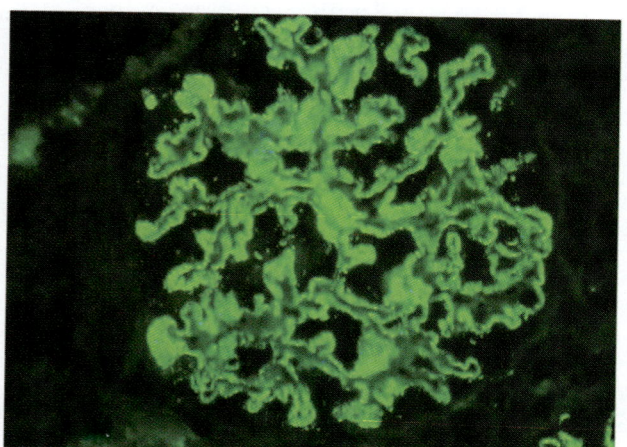

Fig. 39.26: IF with fine granularity in the peripheral capillary loops (400x)

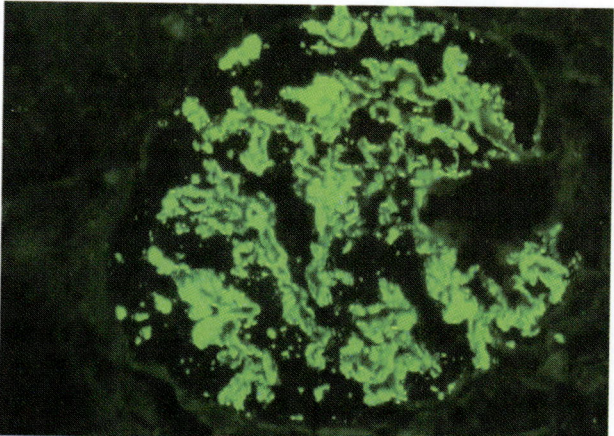

Fig. 39.27: IF with coarse granularity in the peripheral capillary loops (400x), late phase

presence of subepithelial deposits without significant basement membrane reaction between deposits. The stage II is where there is presence of basement membrane material ("spikes") between the deposits. Stage III is characterised by presence of subepithelial to intramembranous deposits and stage IV usually reveals electron-lucent deposits, which represent resorption of the previously formed subepithelial deposits.

Management

First, rule out the secondary causes which may reverse the injury. The course of the disease is variable and often indolent. Immunosuppressive drugs are used.

Membranoproliferative Glomerulonephritis

In membranoproliferative GN (MPGN), there are abnormalities of the complement (usually C3) and leads to an uncommon cause of chronic nephritis that occurs primarily in children and young adults. This pattern of glomerular injury has following three characteristic microscopic findings:

1. Proliferation of mesangial and endothelial cells and expansion of the mesangial matrix.

2. Thickening of the peripheral capillary walls due to the presence of subendothelial immune deposits and/or intramembranous dense deposits.

3. Characteristic double-contour or tram-track appearance on light microscopy due to mesangial interposition into the capillary wall.

The types are characterized on the type of deposits seen on electron microscopy:

- Type I: If the immune deposits are subendothelial.
- Type II: Presence of dense deposits in the glomerular basement membrane.
- Type III: Presence of subepithelial and subendothelial deposits.

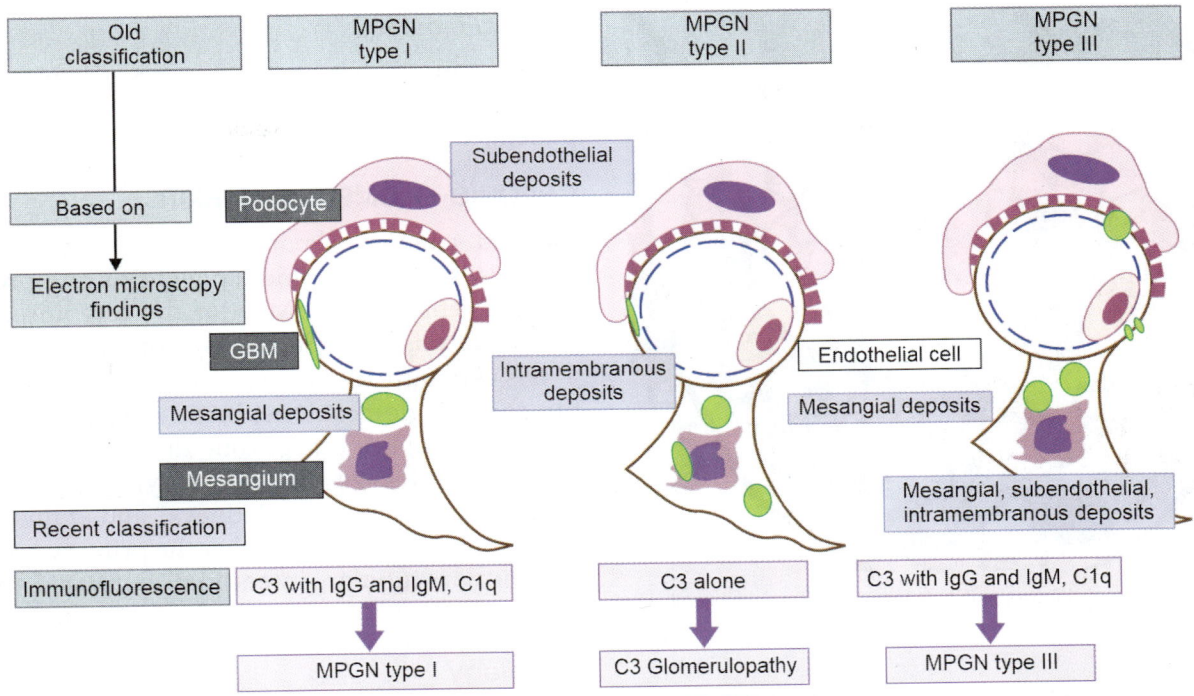

Fig. 39.28: Pathogenesis of MPGN I, II and III

Pathogenesis (Fig. 39.28)

Type I MPGN is caused by circulating immune complexes similar to serum sickness and this occurs in association with hepatitis B, and C infection and SLE, the immune complexes are deposited in subendothelial location.

Type II MPGN is due to dense deposit disease due to excess complement activation, C3 gets deposited in the basement membrane, mesangium, Bowman's capsule and tubular basememt membrane.

Type III MPGN: This is very rare.

Causes for MPGN can be primary or secondary: The secondary causes include: SLE, HBV, HCV, HIV, schistosomiasis, endocarditis, chronic visceral abscesses, malignancies (CLL, lymphomas), hereditary deficiency of complement regulatory proteins.

Morphology

Following are the classical features (Fig. 39.29).

1. The glomeruli are large with accentuated lobules.
2. There is proliferation of mesangial cells, endothelial cells, and leucocytes.
3. GBM is thickened, shows double contour or tram track appearance, evident in silver stains and periodic acid-Schiff (PAS) stain. This is due to splitting of the GBM by mesangial interposition, i.e. outward migration of mesangial cells, infiltrating mononuclear cells, margination of portions of

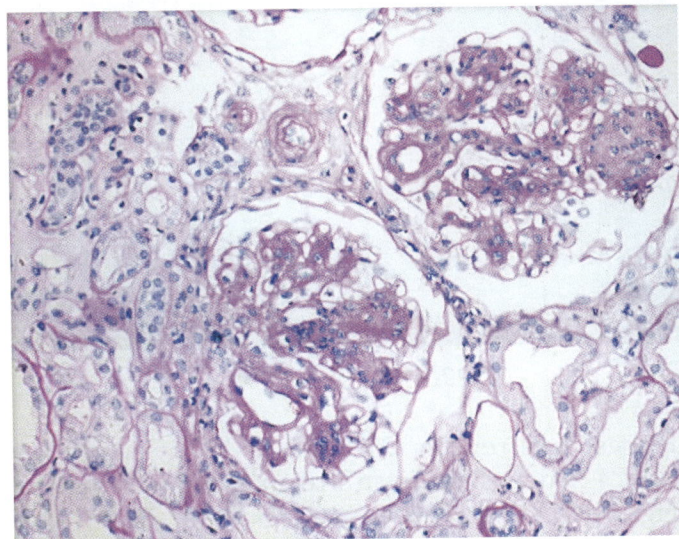

Fig. 39.29: MPGN, showing lobular accentuation, mesangial hypercellularity and thickened capillary walls (PAS, 200×)

endothelial cells along the inside of the capillary walls interposing themselves between endothelium and GBM (Fig. 39.30). This mesangial interposition can be circumferential or partially depending on whether the entire circumference or segment of capillary is involved. This corresponds to the subendothelial immune deposits present in between the duplicated GBMs.

Electron microscopy and immunofluorescence findings: With electron microscopy, Type I has subendothelial electron-dense deposits. Immuno-

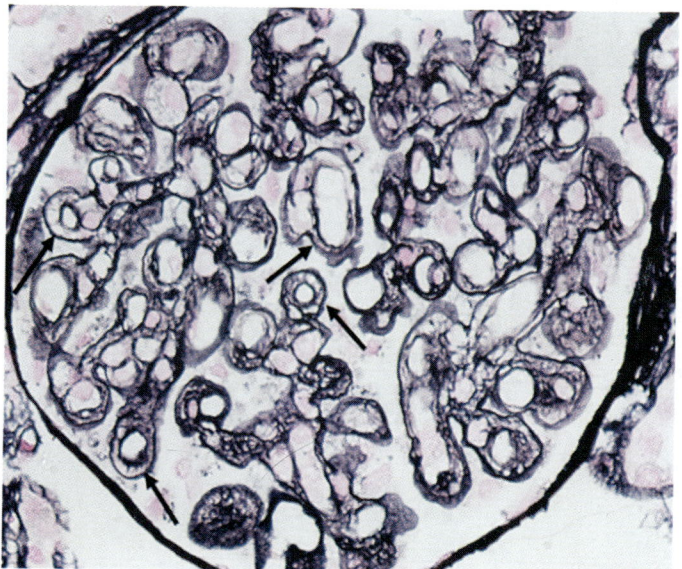

Fig. 39.30: Mesangial interposition (Jones methenamine silver, 400×)

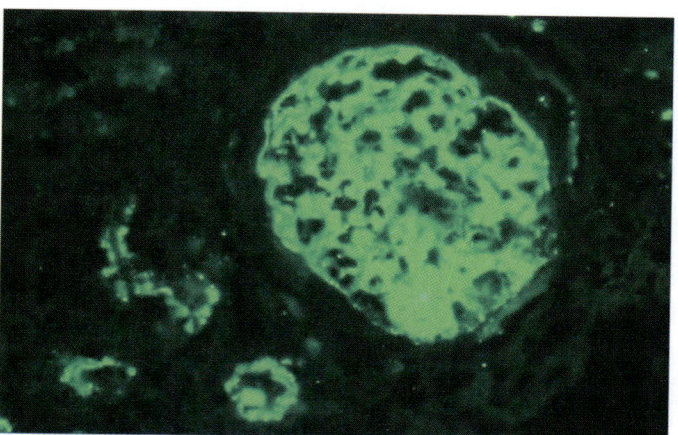

Fig. 39.31: IF in MPGN

fluorescence reveals C3 along with IgG and C1q and C4 is deposited in an irregular granular pattern (Fig. 39.31).

In type II, electron-dense ribbon-like material collects in GBM in lamina densa and subendothelial space. C3 is present in basement membrane and mesangiumin aggregates. IgG, C1q and C4 are absent.

Clinical Features

MPGN presents as nephrotic syndrome in most of the cases although it may begin as acute nephritis with mild proteinuria.

MPGN type I is usually disease of adults, rarely present in children. The disease usually presents as nephrotic syndrome along with recurrent episodes haematuria.

MPGN type II has hypocomplementaemia due to consumption of C3.

Clinical Course

Remissions occur in both types, disease slowly progresses, some may develop RPGN and 50% of the patients develop CRF.

CHRONIC GLOMERULONEPHRITIS

The end stage of primary and secondary glomerular diseases is chronic glomerulonephritis and present as chronic renal failure. Most of these require regular haemodialysis and renal transplantation.

It is very difficult to discern the original disease once the chronic glomerulonephritis sets in. Most of the diseases of nephritic, nephrotic and RPGN cases finally have this end stage. The markedly damaged kidneys are termed as "end stage kidneys" and at this stage, it is difficult to ascertain whether the primary lesion was glomerular, tubular, interstitial or related to blood vessel pathology.

Pathology

Gross: The kidneys are symmetrically contracted, surface red brown and diffusely finely granular.

Microscopy: The glomeruli show complete or partial sclerosis. There is interstitial fibrosis and atrophy of tubules. The vessels appear thick walled. The interstitial fibrous tissue is infiltrated by lymphocytes and plasma cells (Fig. 39.32).

Clinical Features

Patients have proteinuria, hypertension and azotaemia. Oedema may be present in some, if glomeruli are still functioning. Once the glomeruli are fully sclerosed, the proteinuria and oedema are less severe and disease is in advanced stage. Hypertension is common feature.

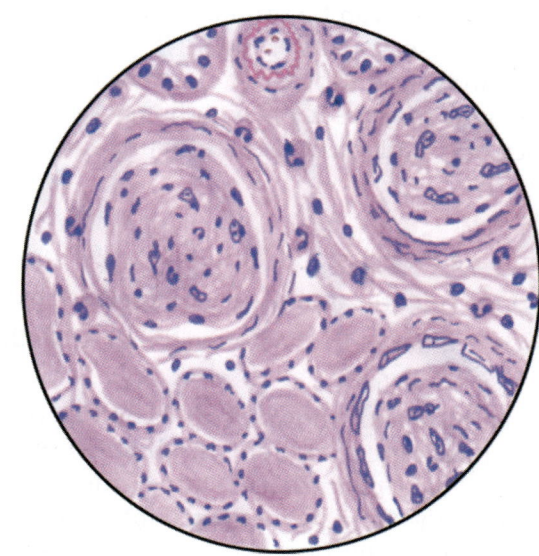

Fig. 39.32: Microscopy in GN (schematic)

TUBULOINTERSTITIAL NEPHRITIS

Tubulointerstitial nephritis (TIN) involves tubules and interstitium. The TIN diseases include:

1. Acute pyelonephritis
2. Pyonephrosis
3. Chronic pyelonephritis
4. Xanthogranulomatous pyelonephritis
5. Malakoplakia
6. Drug-induced interstial nephritis including analgesic nephropathy

The commonly occurring important lesions are discussed below.

ACUTE PYELONEPHRITIS

Acute pyelonephritis is a common acute inflammation of the kidney and renal pelvis. The organisms include the following.

1. Gram-negative organisms
   a. *E. coli* is the commonest organism.
   b. The other Gram-negative organisms:
      i. *Proteus*
      ii. *Klebsiella*
      iii. *Enterobacter*
      iv. *Pseudomonas*
2. Gram-positive organisms:
   a. Streptococci
   b. Staphylococci

It may be ascending infection or through haematogenous spread. The common causes include:

a. Urinary tract obstruction:
   i. Congenital or
   ii. Aquired
b. Instrumentation of UT
c. Indwelling catheters
d. Female sex
e. Vesicoureteric reflux
f. Pregnancy
g. Diabetes mellitus
h. Immunodeficiency syndromes
i. Immunosuppression

Gross findings: One or both kidneys are affected. The kidney size may be normal or enlarged. The kidney surface shows yellow discrete abscesses of 2 mm size surrounded by zone of hyperaemia. These coalesce to form big areas containing exudate. When obstruction is present, the exudate may fill the renal pelvis, calyces, and ureter producing pyonephrosis. Sometimes the renal papillae may show papillary necrosis.

Microscopic findings: There is suppurative necrosis and abscess formation within the renal parenchyma. The interstitium and tubules show collection of polymorphs.

Urine examination shows polymorphs and WBC casts.

Clinical Features

Fever and loin pain are the common clinical manifestations.

Complications of Acute Pyelonephritis

The complications include (Fig. 39.33):

1. Recurrent infection, pyonephrosis and perinephric abscess
2. Papillary necrosis
3. Chronic pyelonephritis and renal failure

CHRONIC PYELONEPHRITIS (PN) AND REFLUX NEPHROPATHY

Chronic pyelonephritis is a disorder in which *chronic tubulointerstitial inflammation and renal scarring are associated with pathologic involvement of the calyces and pelvis.* Chronic pyelonephritis is an important cause of end-stage kidney disease. It is sequelae of recurrent and persistent episodes of bacterial infection of the kidney.

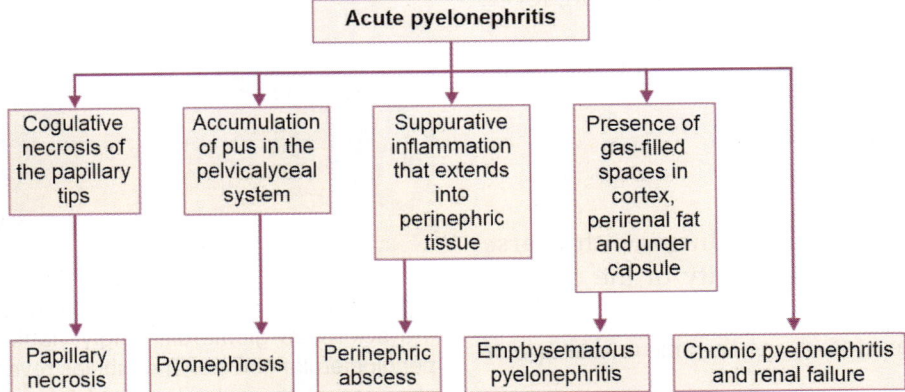

Fig. 39.35: Complications of acute pyelonephritis

Chronic pyelonephritis (PN) can be divided into two forms:

1. Chronic reflux-associated (chronic non-obstructive) pyelonephritis
2. Chronic obstructive pyelonephritis

Chronic Reflux-Associated Pyelonephritis (Reflux Nephropathy)

- Vesicoureteral reflux is a congenital disorder with regurgitation of urine from bladder into ureter. This is possibly due to inadequate development of muscle coat or due to short length of submucosa. This is often familial.
- There is superimposition of a urinary infection on congenital vesicoureteral reflux and intrarenal reflux.
- Occurs early in childhood with recurrent infection.
- It may cause scarring and atrophy of one kidney or involve both, leading to chronic renal insufficiency.
- The scars are usually placed at the upper or lower poles of kidney and associated with blunted calyces underneath in chronic reflux-associated pyelonephritis.

Chronic Obstructive Pyelonephritis

- Obstruction predisposes the kidney to infection.
- Obstruction causes can be: Posterior urethral valves, calculi, benign or malignat tumours).
- Recurrent infections superimposed on diffuse or localized obstructive lesions lead to recurrent bouts of renal inflammation and scarring.
- Parenchymal atrophy
- Both kidneys or one kidney can be affected depending on level of obstruction.
- When both kidneys are affected severe renal insufficiency occurs.

Clinical Features

- Insidious in onset or presents with back pain, fever, frequent pyuria, and bacteriuria.
- Polyuria and nocturia (because kidney looses its abitility to concentrate urine).
- May develop hypertension.

Radiological Findings

- Asymmetrically contracted kidneys with coarse scars and blunting and deformity of the calyceal system.
- Ultrasonograpy can determine the size and shape of the kidneys.
- Pyelogram is characteristic.

Other investigation findings:

- Significant bacteriuria may be present, but it is absent in the late stages.
- Proteinuria is mild

Pathology

Gross: Chronic pyelonephritis has deep 'U' shaped scars involving pelvis and calyces with papillary blunting and calyceal deformities (Figs 39.34 and 39.35).

- Kidneys are small, irregularly and asymmetrically scarred.
- Calyces are dilated, blunted, or deformed with flattening of the papillae.
- The uneven asymmetric scarring differentiates chronic pyelonephritis from symmetrically contracted kidneys of benign nephrosclerosis and chronic glomerulonephritis.

Microscopy (Figs 39.36 and 39.37):

- Involve predominantly tubules and interstitium.
- The tubules are atrophied.

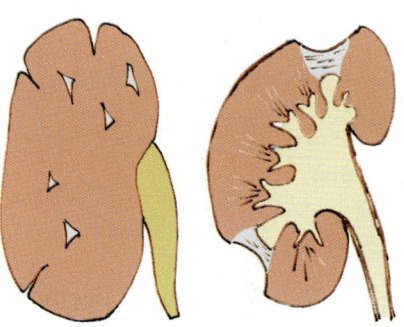 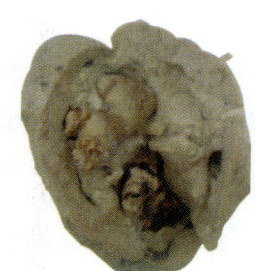

Figs 39.34A and B: Chronic PN with scars (schematic)

Fig. 39.35: Chronic PN with renal calculi (gross pictures)

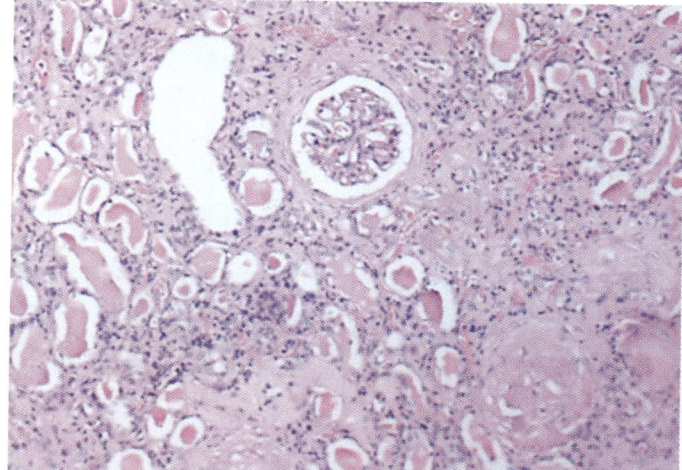

Fig. 39.36: Section from kidney with chronic pyelonephritis. Note the sclerosed glomeruli, singly viable glomerulus showing periglomerular fibrosis. The tubules reveal marked atrophy with changes of thyroidization and interstitium shows fibrosis. (haematoxylin and eosin, magnification ×200)

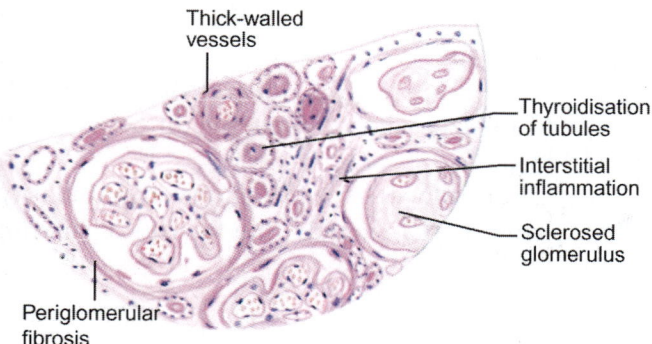

Fig. 39.37: Microscopy in chronic pyelonephritis

- Dilated tubules with flattened epithelium may be filled with colloid-like protein casts (thyroidization).
- Chronic interstitial inflammation and fibrosis in the cortex and medulla.
- Arcuate and interlobular vessels show obliterative intimal sclerosis.
- Glomeruli have periglomerular fibrosis.

DRUG-INDUCED INTERSTITIAL NEPHRITIS

This occurs with:
  i. Synthetic pencillins
 ii. Synthetic antibiotics (rifampicin)
iii. Diuretics
 iv. Non-steroidal anti-inflammatory drugs (NSAIDs)

Pathogenesis

- Immune mechanism plays role.
- It may be type I or type IV hypersensitivity.
- Drug acts as hapten and becomes immunogenic.

Pathology (Fig. 39.38)

- There is gross oedema.
- There is infiltration by mononuclear cells (lymphocytes and macrophages), eosinophils and neutrophils.

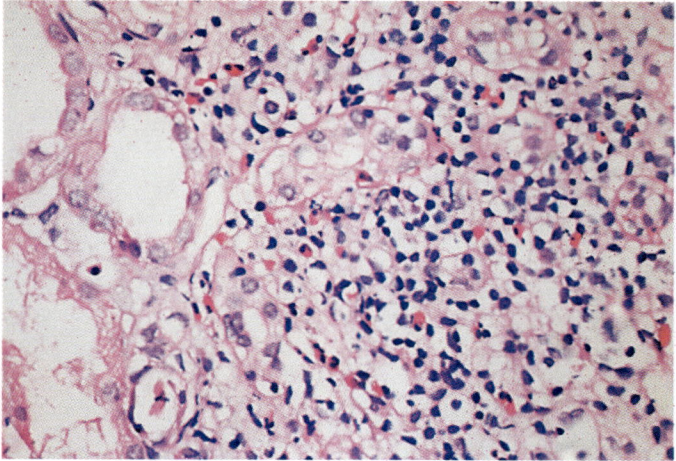

Fig. 39.38: Drug-induced interstitial nephritis

- With some drugs, non-caseating granulomas develop.
- There can be effacement of podocyte foot processes.

ANALGESIC NEPHROPATHY

This occurs with consumption of large amounts of analgesics (phenacetin, aspirin and acitaminophen) for long duration. This may result in renal papillary necrosis, acute interstitial nephritis and progessive renal failure.

Pathogenesis

There is co-valent binding and oxidative damage. The drugs predispose the renal papilla to ischaemia.

Pathology

Gross: The necrotic papillae appear yellow brown and later sloughed off.

Microscopy: Shows coagulative necrosis, tubular atrophy, interstitial scarring and inflammation.

ACUTE TUBULAR NECROSIS

Acute tubular necrosis (ATN), also called acute tubular injury (ATI), is a pathological process which manifests as acute renal failure. ATN is due to two mechanisms: (1) Ischaemia or (2) Toxin induced.

The ischaemic ATN follows hypotension or hypovolaemia. The underlying causes can be diseases involving vessels (hypertension, microangiopathies, etc.), haemolytic-uraemic syndrome (HUS), thrombotic thrombocytopenic purpura (TTP), disseminated intravascular coagulation or the causes of hypovolaemic shock.

In ischaemic ATN, both proximal and distal tubules are affected. The proximal tubules are dilated, lining cells are flattened and brush border is reduced. Distal tubules and ascending loop of Henle are also may be dilated and lined by flattened cells. There may be cell loss and basement membrane disruption. The spillage of the contents may induce localized inflammation with sometimes granulomas. Tamm-Horsefall protein casts may be present. Interstitium is oedematous and may be infiltrated by lymphocytes and monocytes. Overt necrosis may be seen.

Toxic ATN is dose related and tubular damage is mainly to proximal tubules, although distal tubules also can be affected and uniformly all nephrons are affected. Toxic injury can be due to heavy metals like mercury, drugs, radiocontrast dyes haemoglobin, myoglobin or monoclonal light chains, bilirubin and bile.

In toxic ATN, initially (3 days) there is extensive necrosis of the cells of proximal convoluted tubules (Fig. 39.39). The lining cells are desquamated and fill

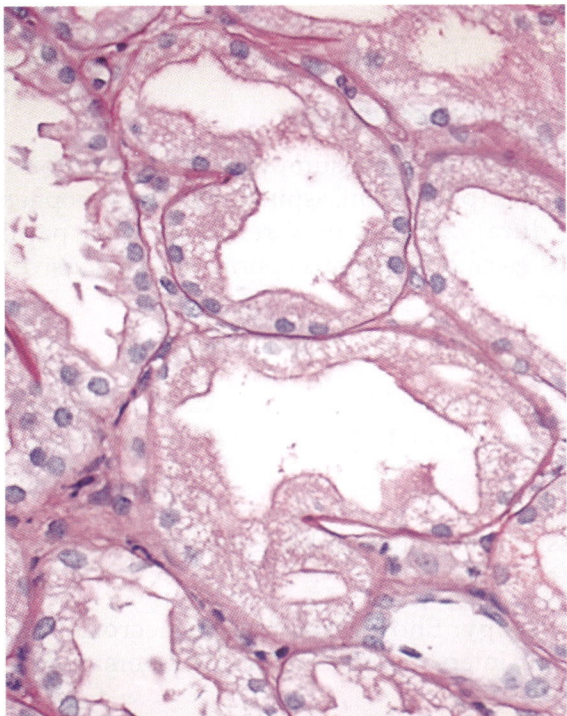

Fig. 39.39: Kidney in acute tubular necrosis

the lumen. Focal calcification may be present. After a few days (7 to 9 days), contents are not present and proximal tubules are dilated and are lined flattened cells. The epithelium regenerates and may show atypical nuclei. The mechanism may be (1) due to ischaemic injury, (2) due to mitochondrial dysfunction, or (3) due to development of thrombotic microangiopathy.

DISEASES INVOLVING BLOOD VESSELS

BENIGN NEPHROSCLEROSIS

Benign nephrosclerosis (NS) is associated with sclerosis of renal arterioles and small arteries resulting in ischaemia of parenchyma.

Pathogenesis

Two processes participate in the arterial lesions:

1. Medial and intimal thickening, as a response to haemodynamic changes, aging or genetic defects.
2. Hyaline deposition in arterioles.

Three groups of hypertensive patients with benign nephrosclerosis are at increased risk of developing renal failure: People of African descent, people with more severe blood pressure elevations, and persons with a second underlying disease, especially diabetes.

Clinical Features

- Uraemia
- Mild proteinuria

Morphology of Kidneys in Benign Nephrosclerosis

Gross (Fig. 39.40):

- The kidneys are either normal or moderately reduced in size, with average weight between 110 and 130 g.
- The cortical surfaces have fine and even granularity.
- The loss of mass is mainly due to cortical scarring and shrinking.

Microscopy (Fig. 39.41):

- There is narrowing of the lumens of arterioles and small arteries, caused by thickening and hyalinization of the vessel wall **(hyaline arteriolosclerosis).**
- Fine surface granulations are microscopic subcapsular scars with sclerotic glomeruli and tubular dropout.

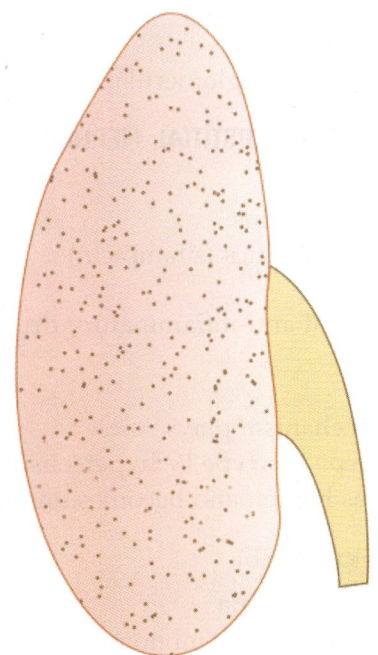

Fig. 39.40: Granular contracted kidney in benign nephrosclerosis

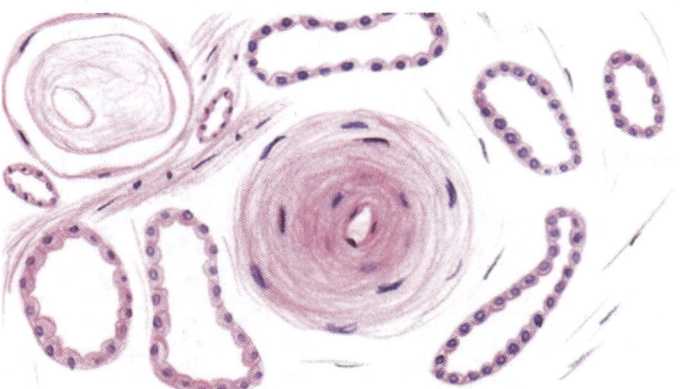

Fig. 39.41: Microscopy, benign nephrosclerosis (schematic)

- The interlobular and arcuate arteries show medial hypertrophy, reduplication of the elastic lamina, and increased myofibroblastic tissue in the intima, which narrow the lumen. This change is called **fibroelastic hyperplasia.**
- There is patchy ischaemic atrophy which consists of
  1. Foci of tubular atrophy and interstitial fibrosis, and
  2. A variety of glomerular alterations—collapse of the GBM, deposition of collagen within the Bowman space, periglomerular fibrosis, and total sclerosis of glomeruli.

MALIGNANT NEPHROSCLEROSIS

Malignant hypertension is less common than benign hypertension and accounts for only 5% of the individuals with raised blood pressure. The blood pressure is usually more than 180/120 mm Hg. It may occur *de novo* without pre-existing hypertension or may appear suddenly in a person who had mild hypertension.

The pathogenesis is not clear, but there is long standing benign hypertension with vascular wall damage especially of the kidneys.

Gross: The kidneys are normal or slightly reduced in size and surface shows pinpoint haemorrhagic lesions giving the flea bitten appearance (Fig. 39.42).

Microscopy: The vessels show necrotizing arteriolitis, fibrinoid necrosis, there is proliferation of intimal smooth muscle cells with onion skin concentric lamellated thickening of the arterioles with progressive narrowing. This is called hyperplastic arteriolosclerosis.

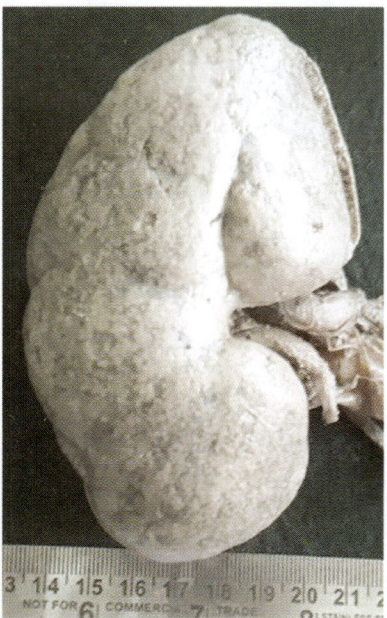

Fig. 39.42: Kidney in malignant hypertension

Prognosis

The rapid progression of kidneys is end organ damage with renal failure, hypertensive encephalopathy, left ventricular failure, retinal haemorrhages, exudates and papilloedema. Death is mostly due to uraemia and in small percentage of individuals due to cerebral haemorrhage and cardiac failure.

CYSTIC DISEASES OF KIDNEY

These can be:

1. Simple cysts
2. Polycystic kidney (AD and AR)
3. Medullary cystic kidney

   Some of these are described below.

POLYCYSTIC KIDNEY

This can be of autosomal dominant or autosomal recessive inheritance.

Polycystic Kidney: Autosomal Dominant

Multiple cysts of both kidneys. 1:500 to 1000. 10% of chronic renal failure (CRF). Mutations in PKD 1 gene on chromosome 16 and PKD2 on chromosome 4 are responsible for this condition.

Clinical features: Asymptomatic in one-third cases. May not produce symptoms until 4th decade.

Flank pain, heavy and dragging pain, haematuria, hypertension, chronic inflammation. End stage renal disease occurs by 50 yrs.

Gross: Varies from small to enormous in size. Weight may reach 4 kg. Cysts are 3–4 cm in diameter. Cysts are filled with fluid which is clear and turbid or hemorrhagic.

Microscopy: Cyst formation may involve any portion of nephron from tubule to collecting duct. Cyst compress the vasculature.

Polycystic Kidney: Autosomal Recessive

Autosomal recessive polycystic kidney (ARPCK) occurs in childhood, in 1:20000 live births. This is due to mutation in gene PKHD.

Clinical features: Serious manifestations are present at birth and death due to renal failure.

Gross: Numerous small cysts in the cortex and medulla forming sponge-like appearance. It is bilateral.

Microscopy: The cysts have cuboidal lining epithelium.

MEDULLARY CYSTIC KIDNEY

This disease presents with renal failure in children and young adults. The disease has mutations of several genes encoding epithelial cell proteins.

Gross: Kidneys are contracted and contain small cysts typically at corticomedullary junction.

Microscopy: Cysts lined by flattened or cuboidal epithelium.

URINARY TRACT OBSTRUCTION

There can be blockage to the flow of urine through its normal path. The obstruction can be at any level including kidneys, ureters, bladder and urethra. The blockage can lead to infection, kidney stones, hydro-nephosis and kidney damage.

KIDNEY STONES

Stones may be formed at any level in the urinary tract, but most commonly they arise in the kidney.

M: F ratio is 4:1. Common age of onset is 3–5 decades.

Clinical Features

- Pain and haematuria
- Pain is severe and abrupt.

Causes and Pathogenesis

The common stones are (Fig. 39.43):
1. **Calcium-containing stones (70%):** Calcium oxalate, calcium phosphate or mixture of these two.
2. **Triple phosphate stones (15%):** Comprised of magnesium, ammonium, phosphate and calcium carbonate
3. Uric acid stones (5–10%)
4. Cystine (1–2%)

There are many causes for initiation and propagation of stone formation, most important is an increased urinary concentration of stone constituents that exceeds their solubility in urine, i.e. **supersaturation.**

A low urine volume also may favour super-saturation.

Calcium phosphate stones:
1. These are formed in alkaline urine.
2. In conditions like renal tubular acidosis and hyper-parathyroidism.
3. These may be large in size.
4. These have smooth surface.

Calcium oxalate stones:
1. These are formed in acidic urine.
2. They are associated with hypercalcaemia and hyper-calciuria.

3. They are also associated with increased uric acid secretion.
4. These have spiky surface.
5. These cause acute pain and haematuria.

Triple phosphate stone:
1. These are associated with infections of urea splitting oraganisms (*Proteus* and some staphylococci) which convert urea to ammonia. The resultant alkaline urine causes precipitation of magnesium, ammonium phosphate salts.
2. Staghorn calculi belong to this category.
3. These are big in size and can damage the kidney.

Uric acid stones:
1. These are formed in acidic urine.
2. These are found in patients with hyperuricaemia such as gout and diseases with rapid turnover like leukaemias.
3. Uric acid stones are radiolucent.

Cystine stones:
1. They are formed in acidic urine.
2. They are caused by genetic defects in renal re-absorption of amino acids along with cystine leading to cystinuria.
3. The cystine crystals are flat hexagons in urine.

Complications

These can cause parenchymal changes like infection and obstruction leading to:
1. Pyelonephritis
2. Hydronephrosis and
3. Renal failure

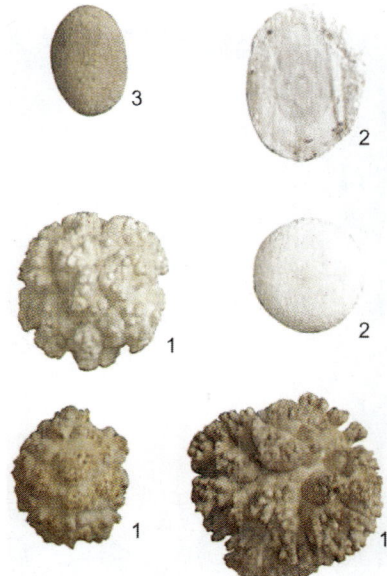

Fig. 39.43: Renal stones, note calcium oxalate stones with spikes (1), smooth surfaced calcium phosphate stones (2) and yellowish brown cystine stone (3) (gross pictures)

HYDRONEPHROSIS

Hydronephrosis (HN) is dilatation of renal pelvis and calyces with atrophy of renal parenchyma.

This may be due to obstruction to outflow of urine. Obstruction may be sudden or insidious.

Obstruction can be at any level from urethra to renal pelvis. Causes include the following.

1. **Congenital causes:** Atresia of urethra, posterior urethral valves, pyeloureteral junction stenosis and ureteral valves, aberrant renal artery compressing ureter (aberrant renal artery to the inferior pole cross anteriorly to the ureter) and kinking of ureter.

2. **Aquired causes:**
   - *Foreign bodies:* Calculi and necrotic papillae
   - *Tumours:* Nodular hyperplasia of prostate, prostatic carcinoma, bladder tumours, retroperitoneal tumours, carcinoma cervix and uterus
   - *Infections:* Prostatitis, urethritis, ureteritis, retroperitoneal fibrosis
   - *Neurogenic:* Spinal cord damage with neurogenic bladder
   - *Pregnancy*

Pathogenesis

With obstruction, there is back pressure on pelvicalyceal system with dilatation and gradually causing pressure atrophy of renal parenchyma. The high pressure also compresses vasculature causing arterial insufficiency and venous stasis. The tubules loose concentrating capacity and later stages eventually glomerular filtration is reduced.

Pathology

- It can be unilateral or bilateral.
- Bilateral obstruction occurs when obstruction is below the ureters.
- Unilateral obstruction occurs with obstruction to ureter.

Gross: One or both kidneys massively enlarged depending on level and nature of obstruction. Pelvicalyceal system is dilated. Renal parenchyma is compressed and atrophied with obliteration of papillae and flattening of pyramids (Fig. 39.44).

Microscopy: Tubules dilated. Atrophy and fibrosis replace tubules with relative sparing of glomeruli. In severe cases, glomeruli show atrophy and disappear with loss of reduced kidney parenchyma and renal papillae may show necrosis. Obstruction may cause infection causing pyelonephritis.

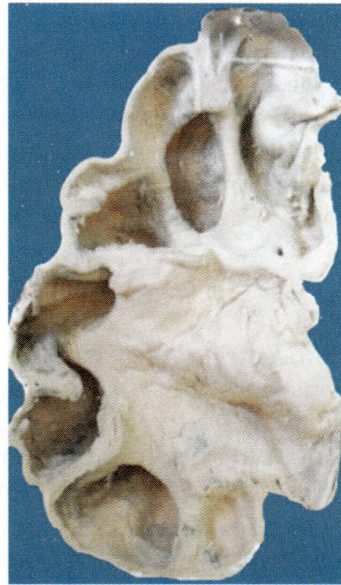

Fig. 39.47: Hydronephrosis (gross picture)

Clinical Features

- Anuria
- With incomplete obstruction: Polyuria and defects in glomerular filtration
- Unilateral may remain silent.

TUMOURS OF KIDNEY

Benign and malignant tumours occur in kidney. Malignant tumours are of great importance clinically. Renal cell carcinoma is a common tumour which occurs in adults followed by Wilms tumour which occurs in childhood. Urothelial carcinoma of calyces and pelvis also can occur. The common benign tumours of kidney are: Angiomyolipoma, renal papillary adenoma and oncocytoma.

BENIGN TUMOURS

Angiomyolipoma, renal papillary adenoma and oncocytoma are the common benign tumours.

Angiomyolipoma

It is a benign tumour of kidney. It is composed of vessels, smooth muscle and fat tissue originating from perivascular epithelioid cells. In patients of tuberous sclerosis with mutations of TSC1 and TSC2 genes, angiomyolipoma is commonly encountered. The clinical importance of this tumour is that it often leads to haemorrhage and usually retroperitoneal.

Renal Papillary Adenoma

These tumours arise from renal tubular epithelium. They are small, discrete, nodular, grey yellow tumours, present in the cortex and usually less than 0–5 cm. They are often called papillary adenomas because of their papillary morphology. Microscopy shows cells arranged in complex papillae, tubules, cords and sheets. The cells are cuboidal to polygonal with regular central nuclei. These tumours are potentially malignant and do not differ much from low grade papillary renal cell carcinoma and may metastasize even though smaller in size.

Oncocytoma

Familial are multicentric rather than being solitary in nature. This neoplasm is composed of large eosinophilic epithelial cells having small round benign appearing nuclei. It is thought to arise from intercalated cells of collecting ducts. These cells have numerous mito-chondria.

Grossly, they are tan to brown coloured homo-genous, and well capsulated. In one-third of the cases, there is a central scar. They may achieve large size.

MALIGNANT TUMOURS

The commonest malignant tumours are listed below.

- **Renal cell carcinoma**
  - Clear cell carcinoma
  - Papillary carcinoma
  - Chromophobe carcinoma
  - Xp11 translocation carcinoma
  - Collecting duct carcinoma
- **Wilms tumour**
- **Urothelial carcinoma**

Renal Cell Carcinoma

Renal cell carcinoma (RCC), also called hypernephroma, is the most common type of renal carcinoma in adults. It accounts for approximately 3% of adult malignancies and 90–95% of neoplasms arising from the kidney. Renal cell carcinoma is more common in people of Northern European ancestry and North Americans than in those of Asian or African descent. In United States, its incidence is slightly higher among black persons than among white individuals. Incidence is slightly higher in men than in women (M:F ratio – 1.6:1). Usually age of occurrence in 5th–6th decades of life, but may occur at earlier age.

Etiology

A number of environmental and genetic factors have been studied as possible causes for renal cell carcinoma (RCC), such as the following:

1. Cigarette smoking doubles the risk of renal cell carcinoma and contributes to as many as one-third of all cases.
2. Obesity is another risk factor, particularly in women.
3. Hypertension may be associated with an increased incidence of renal cell carcinoma.
4. In patients undergoing long-term renal dialysis, there is an increased incidence of acquired cystic disease of the kidney, which predisposes to renal cell cancer.
5. Tuberous sclerosis appears to be associated with renal cell carcinoma, although the exact nature of this is unclear.
6. In renal transplant recipients, acquired renal cystic disease of the native kidney also predisposes to renal cell cancer.
7. Hereditary and familial cause.

Pathogenesis

RCC originates from the proximal convoluted tubular epithelium. It occurs in a sporadic (non-hereditary) and a hereditary form, and both forms are associated with structural alterations of the short arm of chromosome 3(3p). Mutations of tumour suppressor genes (VHL, TSC) or oncogenes (MET) are also noticed in families with high risk of renal cancer.

Hereditary syndromes associated with renal cell carcinoma are:

- von Hippel-Lindau (VHL) syndrome
- Hereditary papillary renal carcinoma (HPRC)
- Familial renal oncocytoma (FRO) associated with Birt-Hogg-Dube syndrome (BHDS)
- Hereditary renal carcinoma (HRC)
- Hereditary leiomyomatosis and renal cell carcinoma syndromes: It is an autosomal dominant disease with mutation of fumarate hydratase (FH) gene, has cutaneous and uterine leiomyomas and aggressive papillary RCC with metastasis.

Pathology

Gross (Fig. 39.45): Clear cell renal cell carcinoma is typically a solitary tumour. Tumour size usually ranges from 0.3–30 cm in maximal diameter, with a mean of 6–7 cm. The tumour may be multifocal and bilateral in some cases.

The tumour is bosselated, well-circumscribed mass with a capsule or pseudocapsule and a pushing margin. Occasionally, an infiltrative margin is seen. On cut section, is typically yellow to golden colour because of the accumulation of lipid in the malignant cells, while areas of haemorrhage (brown), fibrosis (gray), necrosis, and cystic degeneration often give a variegated appearance.

Microscopy (Fig. 39.46): Typical clear cell renal cell carcinoma is characterized by epithelial cells with clear cytoplasm and a well-defined cell membrane, inter-spersed within a highly vascularized stroma. The

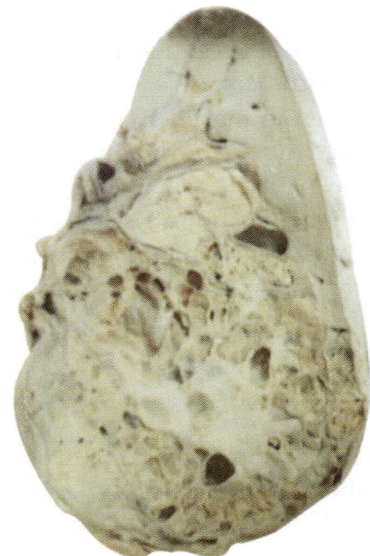

Fig. 39.45: Renal cell carcinoma (gross picture)

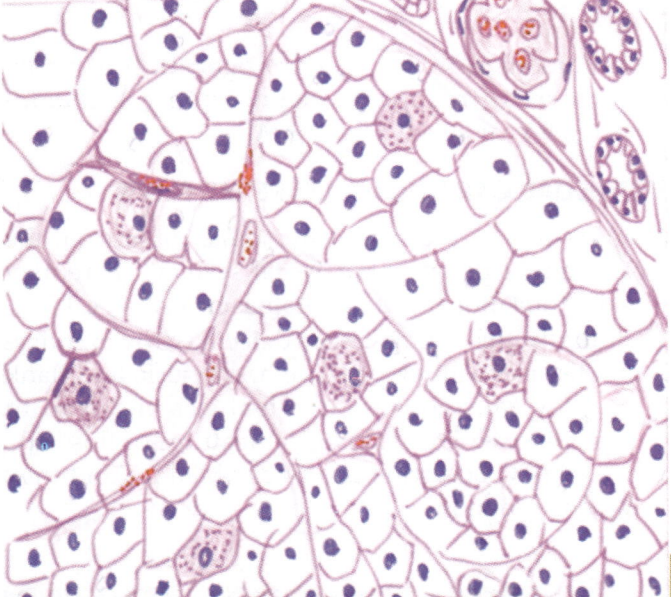

Fig. 39.46: Microscopy of renal cell carcinoma (clear cell RCC) (schematic)

transparency of the cytoplasm results from accumulated droplets of glycogen, phospholipids, and neutral lipids—in particular, cholesterol ester. Glycogen can be demonstrated by periodic acid-Schiff (PAS) stain, whereas neutral lipids can be identified using the Oil red O stain on unfixed tissue but are dissolved by histological processing. Clear cell variety may contain a variable proportion of cells with granular eosinophilic cytoplasm. Rarely, these granular cells are predominant or even the only cell type.

Architectural patterns like solid, alveolar, acinar, cystic growth patterns of cells with clear or ceosinophilic cytoplasm may be associated in clear cell RCC.

The other histological variants like papillary carcinoma, chromophobe carcinoma, Xp11 translocation carcinoma and collecting duct carcinoma are briefly described at the end of the topic.

Clinical Features

The most common presentations include haematuria (40%), flank pain (40%), and a palpable mass in the flank or abdomen (25%). Other signs and symptoms include weight loss (33%), fever (20%), hypertension (20%), hypercalcaemia (5%), night sweats, malaise and a varicocele usually left-sided due to obstruction of the testicular vein (2% of males).

Renal cell carcinoma is a unique and challenging tumour because of the frequent occurrence of paraneoplastic syndromes, including hypercalcaemia, erythrocytosis, and non-metastatic hepatic dysfunction (Stauffer syndrome). Polyneuromyopathy, amyloidosis, anaemia, fever, cachexia, weight loss, dermatomyositis, increased erythrocyte sedimentation rate (ESR), and hypertension are also associated with renal cell carcinoma.

Other clinical features associated may include:

1. Faminisation: Estrogen production
2. Musculinisation: Androgen production
3. Cushing syndrome
4. Eosinophilia
5. Leukaemoid reactions

Prognosis

The five-year survival rate is around 90–95% for tumours less than 4 cm. For larger tumours confined to the kidney without venous invasion, survival is still relatively good. For tumours that extend through the renal capsule and out of the local fascial investments, the survival reduces to near 60%. If it has metastasized to the lymph nodes, the 5-year survival is around 5 to 15%. If it has spread metastatically to other organs, the 5-year survival rate is less than 5%.

Wilms' Tumour

Wilms' tumour (also known as nephroblastoma) is a rare malignant tumour of the kidney that primarily affects children. It is the most common tumour of the kidney in children and accounts for 6% of all paediatric tumours. Wilms' tumour most often affects children at peak ages 2–4 years, 90% are less than 10 years old. Wilms tumour most commonly affects one kidney and is bilateral in 5% of the cases. A minority of these are associated with syndromes or congenital anomalies.

Etiopathogenesis

Genetic mutations of nephrogenic rests (benign foci of embryonal kidney cells that persist abnormally into postnatal life) and frequently associated with deletions or mutations of WT1.

Gross: Solitary/multiple cystic mass, soft, bulging, grey-white with focal haemorrhage and necrosis.

Microscopy (Fig. 30.47): Wilms' tumour is a triphasic malignant tumour containing three elements—metanephric blastemal, stromal and epithelial derivatives.

- Blastemal components in the form of sheets of small blue cells without differentiation.

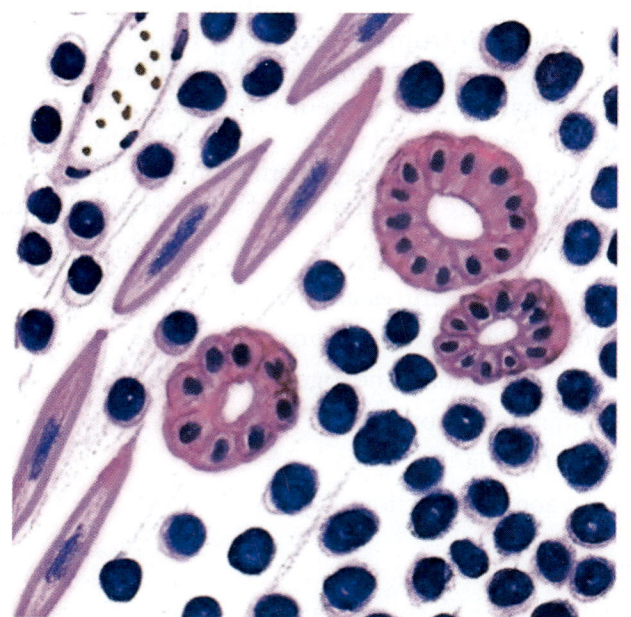

Fig. 39.47: Microscopy of Wilms' tumour. Note triphasic pattern (schematic)

- Characteristic is the presence of abortive tubules and glomeruli (epithelial components) surrounded by a spindled cell stroma.
- The stroma or the mesenchymal component may include striated muscle, cartilage, bone, fat tissue and fibrous tissue.

The tumour usually compresses the normal kidney parenchyma. The mesenchymal component may include cells showing rhabdomyoid (skeletal muscle) differentiation. The rhabdomyoid component may itself show features of malignancy (rhabdomyosarcomatous Wilms).

Clinical Manifestations

- In an isolated case may present with asymptomatic/palpable abdominal mass, hypertension (25%), haematuria (25%), fever (25%), pain and intestinal obstruction.
- It may present with any of the syndromes mentioned with a renal mass.

Prognosis

It is a tumour with very good prognosis. It is highly responsive to treatment, (nephrectomy + chemotherapy). 5-year survival rate is 90%.

UROTHELIAL CARCINOMA OF RENAL PELVIS

About 5–10% of the renal carcinomas arise from the urothelium of pelvis and calyceal system. There may be renal transitional cell papillomas or invasive TCC.

Clinically, these tumours are detected early in course of the diseases as they produce haematuria and flank pain. They cause obstructive features and lead to hydronephrosis. The histological features of this TCC resemble TCC occurring in urinary bladder and they have poor prognosis.

NICE TO KNOW

SYNDROMES ASSOCIATED WITH RCC

Von Hippel-Lindau Syndrome

von Hippel-Lindau disease is an autosomal dominant syndrome that confers predisposition to a variety of neoplasms, including the following:

1. Renal cell carcinoma with clear cell histologic features
2. Pheochromocytoma
3. Pancreatic cysts and islet cell tumours
4. Retinal angiomas
5. Central nervous system (CNS) haemangioblastomas
6. Epididymal cystadenomas

Renal cell carcinoma develops in nearly 40% of patients with von Hippel-Lindau disease and is a major cause of death among these patients.

Deletions of 3p occur commonly in renal cell carcinoma associated with von Hippel-Lindau disease. The *VHL* gene (located on 3p25.3) is mutated in a high percentage of tumours and cell lines from patients with sporadic (nonhereditary) and hereditary clear cell renal carcinoma.

Mutations of the *VHL* gene result in the accumulation of hypoxia inducible factors (HIFs) that stimulate angiogenesis through vascular endothelial growth factor (VEGF) and its receptor (VEGFR). VEGF and VEGFR are important new therapeutic targets.

Hereditary Papillary Renal Carcinoma

Hereditary papillary renal carcinoma is an inherited disorder with an autosomal dominant inheritance pattern; affected individuals develop bilateral, multifocal papillary renal carcinoma. Germline mutations in the tyrosine kinase domain of the MET gene have been identified.

Familial Renal Oncocytoma and Birt-Hogg-Dube Syndrome

Individuals affected with familial renal oncocytoma can develop bilateral, multifocal oncocytoma or oncocytic neoplasms in the kidney. Patients with Birt-Hogg-Dube syndrome have a dominantly inherited predisposition to develop benign tumours of the hair follicle (i.e. fibrofolliculomas), predominantly on the face, neck, and upper trunk, and these individuals are at risk of developing renal tumours, colonic polyps or tumours, and pulmonary cysts.

Hereditary Renal Carcinoma

Affected individuals with this inherited condition have an increased tendency to develop oncocytomas, benign renal tumours that have a low malignant potential.

Other Histological Variants of RCC: Papillary Carcinoma

This variant accounts for 10 to 15% of the renal cell carcinomas. It has both familial and sporadic forms. These are not associated with 3p deletions. The genetic abnormalities seen are: Trisomy 7, trisomy 17 and loss of Y in male patients in sporadic form and trisomy 7 in familial form. MET proto-oncogene is present on chromosome which is mutated in these tumours. MET encodes hepatocyte growth factor which mediates growth, mobility and differentiation. Papillary renal cell carcinoma are categorized as type I and type II. Nuclear grade of 2 or less is encountered in type I, whereas type II has grade 3 and above. Type II is believed to have worse prognosis than the type I. Grossly, these are multifocal in origin and microscopically has papillary morphology.

Chromophobe Carcinoma

These represent 5% of the RCC. These are thought to arise from intercalated cells of collecting ducts and have good prognosis, when compared to clear cell RCC and papillary variant of RCC. These have multiple chromosomal abnormalities.

Microscopically, the cell outlines are very distinct, have pale eosinophilic cytoplasm with clear halo around the nucleus and nuclei appear pleomorphic. Ferman grading is not applied to these tumours.

Xp11 Translocation Carcinoma

This occurs in young people, with translocation of TFE3 gene located on Xp11.2 region. The translocation overexpresses TFE3 transcription factor. The neoplastic cells have clear cytoplasm but have papillary architecture.

Collecting (Bellini) Duct Carcinoma

These represent less than 1% of the renal cell tumours. It affects young patients. They arise from collecting duct cells in the medulla. It is associated with aggressive local invasion and distant spread with poor prognosis. Microscopy of these tumours shows glands and irregular channels with dense stroma. The epithelium lining cells shows atypia of high grade morphology with hobnail pattern.

SYNDROMES ASSOCIATED WITH WILMS TUMOUR

Beckwith-Wiedemann Syndrome

- Hemihypertrophy
- Organomegaly
- High birth weight
- Omphalocele
- Neonatal hypoglycaemia
- Wilms tumour, hepatoblastoma (5%)
- 11p15 Loss of imprinting IGF2/H19 genes

WAGR Syndrome

- Wilms tumour
- Aniridia
- Genitourinary malformations
- Hypospadias
- Undescended testes
- Mental retardation
- 30% chance of Wilms
- 11p13 deletions
- Germline mutations of WT1

Denys-Drash Syndrome

- Gonadal dysgenesis (male pseudohermaphroditism)
- Nephropathy—renal failure
- Germline anomalies of WT1 (renal and gonadal development)
- Gonadoblastoma

TUMOURS OF KIDNEY

Classification of kidney tumours[45]

- Renal cell tumours
  - Clear cell renal cell carcinoma
  - Multilocular cystic renal neoplasm of low malignant potential
  - Papillary cell renal cell carcinoma
  - Clear cell papillary carcinoma
  - Chromophobe cell renal cell carcinoma
  - Collecting duct carcinoma
  - Renal medullary carcinoma
  - Renal cell carcinoma unclassified
  - Hereditary leiomyomatosis and renal cell carcinoma
  - Succinate dehydrogenase deficient renal cell carcinoma
  - Mucinous, tubular and spindle cell carcinoma
- Tubulocystic renal cell carcinoma
  - Acquired cystic disease associated renal cell carcinoma
  - Oncocytoma
  - Papillary adenoma
- Metanephric tumours
- Nephroblastic and cystic tumours
  - Nephrogenic rests
  - Nephroblastoma
  - Cystic partially differentiated nephroblastoma
- Paediatric cystic nephroma
- Mesenchymal tumours
  - Mesenchymal tumours in children
  - Clear cell sarcoma
  - Rhabdoid tumour
- Congenital mesoblastic nephroma
- Ossifying renal tumour of infancy
  - Mesenchymal tumours in adults

- Mixed epithelial and stromal tumours
  - Cystic nephroma
  - Mixed epithelial and stromal tumour
- Neuroendocrine tumours
- Miscellaneous tumours
- Metastatic tumours

Note: WHO 2016 Classification with slight modification

WHO/International Society for Urological Pathology grading system for renal cell carcinoma and other prognostic parameters[46]

Grade	Description
Grade I	Nucleoli absent, or inconspicuous and basophilic at 400 magnification
Grade II	Nucleoli conspicuous and eosinophilic at 400 magnification
Grade III	Nucleoli conspicuous and eosinophilic at 100 magnification
Grade IV	Extreme pleomorphism, multinucleate giant cells, rhabdoid and sarcomatoid differentiation

Fuhrman grading system **(WHO/International Society for Urological Pathology grading system for renal cell carcinoma and other prognostic parameters):**

Grade 1: Nuclei uniform, 10 mm, absent/inconspicuous nucleoli.

Grade 2: Nuclei irregular, 15 mm, and small nucleoli

Grade 3: Nuclei irregular, 20 mm, and nucleoli prominent.

Grade 4: Nuclei irregular/bizarre/multilobed, more or equal to 20 mm, nucleoli prominent/heavy chromatin clumps.

LOWER URINARY TRACT

The lower urinary tract lesions include anomalies, inflammation neoplasms arising from ureters, urinary bladder and urethra. These are lined by urothelium which is transitional epithelium.

Congenital anomalies of urethra include: Double and bifid ureters, ureteropelvic junction obstruction, and diverticula.

Inflammation of ureters: These may be ureteritis follicularis or ureteritis cystica.

Obstructive lesions of ureters: These may be intrinsic or extrinsic origin and are listed in Table 39.1. These cause not just ureteral obstruction followed by dilatation but also cause back pressure on kidneys leading to hydronephrosis.

Table 39.1	Causes of ureteral obstruction
Duplication	Ureteropelvic junction anomalies
Ureterocele	Stones
Retroperitoneal fibrosis	Vesicoureteric reflux
Ureteral stricture	Factors compressing from outside

URINARY BLADDER

Vesicoureteric reflux, congenital or acquired diverticula, congenital abnormalities, endometriosis, metaplasia, inflammations and neoplasms are encountered in urinary bladder. Often bladder lesions are of clinical importance and disabling and sometimes are lethal. The bladder tumours can cause morbidity and mortality.

Vesicoureteric Reflux

This is the most common anomaly and can cause infection and scarring.

Diverticulosis

Diverticula

These are pouch-like extension of the bladder of 1 to 10 cm diameter. These may be congenital or acquired.

Congenital diverticula: This occurs in absence of obstructive factors and is related to deficient detrusor layer.

Aquired diverticula: Most of these are acquired because of obstruction in the urethra or bladder neck. These are most often seen with posterior urethral valves, neurogenic bladder, benign prostatic hyperplasia or neoplasia producing obstruction to the urinary flow. There is increased vesical pressure which causes out pouching of the bladder wall. They are usually small and asymptomatic. These are sites of stasis and source of infection. They can be source of calculi formation also.

Congenital Abnormalities

Urachal Lesions

Urachus in fetal life connects the urinary bladder with allantois. At birth, it retaracts from bladder lumen but may persist with bladder wall. Anomalies like patent urachus, blind sinus, abscess or granuloma may be encountered with urachus.

Exstrophy

There is absence of lower abdominal wall and bladder is exposed.

Endometriosis

Endometriosis of bladder occurs due to previous operation of the area and patient has symptoms related to female genital tract.

Metaplasia

Von Brunn's nests are present as solid areas below the transitional epithelium. Cystic dilation of these nests with transitional epithelium is cystitis cystica. When there is metaplasia to colonic/glandular epithelium, it is cystitis glandularis.

Squamous metaplasia: This is also called leukoplakia of bladder which develops with chronic irritation.

Inflammation of Urinary Bladder

Cystitis presents with lower abdominal/suprapubic/perineal pain and urinary frequency. This can be of different histological types as mentioned below:
1. Eosinophilic cystitis
2. Polypoidal cystitis
3. Emphysematous cystitis
4. Tuberculous cystitis
5. Malakoplakia

Malakoplakia

It is chronic inflammation of urinary tract which can involve many other organs. There is acquired condition with defect in bactericidal activity of macrophages.

Gross: It presents with multiple nodular thickening of mucosa and submucosa usually in the region of trigone and mistaken for carcinoma.

Microscopy: This has collection of histiocytes with granular acidophilic cytoplasm. Some cells have intra-cytoplasmic concentric basophilic layered inclusions called Michaelis-Gutmann bodies or calco-spherites which are PAS positive. These stain for iron and calcium. These cells are present beneath the surface epithelium.

Neoplasia

Inverted Papilloma

This occurs in adults/elderly males, common in the region of trigone of bladder, neck or prostatic urethra. Microscopy shows invagination of transitional epithelium. Papillae are absent. Connective tissue is scanty and has no atypia.

TUMOURS OF URINARY BLADDER

Urinary bladder cancer accounts for 2 to 6% of all malignancies in United States. It ranks fourth most common malignancy. About 95% are epithelial in origin and rest being mesenchymal tumours. The most common epithelial tumour includes the one arising from transitional epithelium but squamous cell carci-noma and adenocarcinoma also can occur (Table 39.2).

These are more common in men than women with ratio 3:1. The disease is common in Whites than Blacks.

UROTHELIAL CARCINOMA

About 95% of the bladder carcinomas are transitional cell carcinoma (TCC).

Etiology

Following are the common risk factors:
1. Major cause is smoking: Four times higher risk in smokers, risk depends upon duration and amount of smoking.
2. Analgesic abuse: Phenacetin
3. Other drugs: Cyclophosphamide, piaglutazole
4. Urinary tract inflammation and stones
5. Persons working in rubber, leather, textile, paint and dye industries have risk of bladder carcinoma.

Table 39.2   Urinary bladder tumours

Non-invasive urothelial neoplasms
1. Urothelial carcinoma *in situ*
2. Non-invasive papillary urothelial carcinoma, low grade
3. Papillary urothelial neoplasm of low malignant potential
4. Urothelial papilloma
5. Inverted urothelial papilloma
6. Urothelial proliferation of uncertain malignant potential
7. Urothelial dysplasia

Infiltrating urothelial carcinoma, usual type (TCC)

Infiltrating urothelial carcinoma with divergent differentiation
1. Nested, including large nested
2. Microcystic
3. Micropapillary lymphoepithelial like
4. Plasmacytoid/signet ring/diffuse
5. Sarcomatoid
6. Giant cell
7. Poorly differentiated
8. Lipid rich
9. Clear cell

Squamous cell neoplasms
1. Pure squamous cell carcinoma
2. Verrucous carcinoma
3. Squamous cell papilloma

Glandular neoplasms
1. Adenocarcinoma—NOS
2. Villous adenoma

Urachal carcinoma

Tumours of Mullarian type

Neuroendocrine tumours

Melanocytic tumours

Mesenchymal tumours

Miscellaneous tumours

(**Note:** Modified from WHO 2016 classification of urinary system and male genital organs)

6. Occupational exposure to chemicals like aniline dyes and aromatic dyes such as beta naphthylamines (2 naphthylamine, benzidine and 4-aminobiphenyl)
7. Arsenic in drinking water
8. Genetics: Families with Lynch syndrome, PTEN mutations as in Cowden syndrome, mutations of retinoblastoma gene have higher risk.
9. *Schistosoma haematobium* infections in endemic areas (e.g. Egypt, Sudan)
10. Irradiation has high risk cancer.

Clinical Features

Majority of the patients present with gross or microscopic haematuria. Urgency, frequency and dysuria can be other symptoms.

Investigations

1. Cystoscopy
2. Biopsy of larger suspected lesions resected as completely as possible transurethrally, if possible, should include muscle layer and smaller and flat lesions by cold cup biopsy forceps.

Pathology

Gross: Most tumours have single, solid, polypoid mass with or without ulceration. The mass may sessile or even may infiltrate the bladder wall.

Microscopy: The epithelium may show ulceration with increased number of layers. The cells have moderate to abundant amphophilic cytoplasm, large hyperchromatic nuclei which are hyperchromatic having irregular contours. Nucleoli are present. Mitoses are common. Invasion beyond the basement membrane with cells arranged in sheets, cords, trabaculae and small clusters and are often separated by desmoplastic stroma. Squamous or glandular differentiation can be present.

Histological grading of the cells (grade 1/2/3) to be mentioned. Invasion is common in high grade tumours. The invading fronts have irregular contour with irregularly shaped nests of tumour cells or individual tumour cells invading the stroma. The lamina propria shows dense inflammatory cells.

The variants like inverted, papillary, microcystic, lymphoepithelioma like, lymphoma/plasmacytoma like, lipoid cell, clear cell (glycogen rich), TCC with syncytiotrophoblastic giant cells, sarcomatoid, TCC with rhabdoid features, small cell carcinoma, large cell undifferentiated carcinoma can be encountered.

Following are the cell features in different histological types:

Grade 1. Urothelial carcinoma: Has following features:
1. Well-formed papillae—present
2. Layers—more than 7 layers
3. Superficial umbrella cells—usually present
4. Cytological variations—mild
5. Nuclear enlargement—slight to moderate
6. Nuclear hyperchromasia—slight
7. Chromatic: Slightly coarse or granular
8. Nucleoli may be present
9. Mitoses: Rare, basally present
10. Stromal invasion—uncommon.

Grade 2. Urothelial carcinoma: The histological features lie in between the grade 1 and grade 3 features.

Grade 3. Urothelial carcinoma: Has following features:
1. Marked loss polarity
2. Loss of normal architecture
3. Superficial cell layer: Absent

4. Cellular dyscohesion: Present
5. Cellular anaplasia: Marked cellularity, nuclear crowding, nuclear pleomorphism, variation in size and shape of cells, coarse chromatin and occasional tumour giant cells.
6. Atypical mitoses: Plenty.

Papillary Urothelial Neoplasm of Low Malignant Potential

In WHO 2004 classification, this lesion is similar to exophytic transitional cell papilloma. This lesion is with increased number of layers, cytological atypia is minimal or absent, architectural abnormalities are minimal with preserved polarity. Mitoses are minimal and limited to basal layer. These have male pre-pondarance with M: F ratio of 3:1. Occur around mean age of 65 years. These are 1–2 cm in diameter, located on the lateral wall or near the ureteric orifices and described as seaweed in the ocean. Thes are commonly encountered while investigating for haematuria.

Low grade urothelial carcinoma: The low grade papillary urothelial neoplasms show slender papillae, with frequent branching, nuclear enlargement and irregularity, nuclei vesicular, nucleoli often present with variation in polarity. Grade 1 of WHO 1973 classification fall into this group.

High grade urothelial carcinoma: High grade papillary urothelial carcinoma has disorederly arrangement of cells with cytological atypia. The nuclei are pleomorphic with prominent nucleoli with loss of polarity. Mitoses are frequent. With endoscopy, mass appears as papillary to nodular or solid growth. Grade 3 and grade 2 of WHO 1973 classification fall into this group.

Adenocarcinoma/Adenocarcinoma—NOS of Urinary Bladder

This accounts for 0.5 to 2% of the malignant bladder tumours. Metaplasia to glandular epithelium is thought to be precursor lesion for adenocarcinoma. This occurs frequently in males than females. Peak incidence is 65 years. This may arise from bladder proper or urachus. The cells are arranged in glandular pattern with different variants like NOS, colonic, hepatoid, signet ring cell and clear cell variant.

Squamous Cell Carcinoma/Pure Squamous Cell Carcinoma

When pure squamous component is present, it sis labelled as squamous cell carcinoma. In association with TCC, it is labelled as TCC with squamous differntiation.

The risk factors are:
1. Smoking
2. Chronic urinary tract infection
3. Schistosomiasis

These tumours are often bulky and exophytic and microscopy is similar to squamous cell carcinoma found in other location.

Neuroendocrine Tumour/Small Cell Carcinoma

This is malignant neuroendocrine neoplasm of the urothelium. It is extremely rare and accounts for less than 1% of the bladder tumours. Majority of the patients are male, history of smoking present, and occasionally can have paraneoplastic syndromes with hyper-calcaemia, hypophosphataemia, ectopic secretion of adrenocorticotrophic hormone.

SELF-ASSESSMENT EXERCISE

1. **Renin-secreting cells are mainly confined to:**
   A. Afferent arteriole   B. Efferent arteriole
   C. Glomerulus   D. Bowman's capsule

2. **A 5-year-old child with acute onset of haematuria, mild proteinuria, azotaemia, and hypertension indicates:**
   A. Nephrotic syndrome   B. Nephritic syndrome
   C. Pyelonephritis   D. Renal failure

3. **In Berger's disease, there is change in the form of:**
   A. Podocyte fusion
   B. Tubular necrosis
   C. Mesangial deposition of IgA and C3
   D. Mesangial deposition of IgG and C3

4. **The defective gene of adult polycystic kidney PKD1 is on the following location:**
   A. Short arm of chromosome 16
   B. Short arm of chromosome 15
   C. Short arm of chromosome 20
   D. Short arm of chromosome 21

5. **An adult male has generalized oedema and sub-nephrotic proteinuria and microscopic haematuria, serum complement reduced and positive anti-HBC antibodies. The most likely diagnosis is:**
   A. Rapidly progressive GN
   B. Mesangioproliferative GN
   C. Focal segmental glomerulosclerosis
   D. Post-streptococcal GN

6. **Loss of foot process of podocytes is observed in:**
   A. Minimal change GN
   B. Nephritic syndrome
   C. RPGN
   D. Alport's syndrome

7. **Beckwith-Wiedeman syndrome is associated with:**
   A. Ewing's sarcoma   B. Wilms tumour
   C. Neuroblastoma   D. Teratoma

8. **Multicentric and recurrent RCC seen in:**
   A. NF1
   B. NF2
   C. Sipple's syndrome
   D. Von Hippel-Lindau disease

9. **Renal vein thrombosis, most frequent cause is:**
   A. Loss of antithrombin III
   B. Decreased fibrinogen
   C. Decreased vitamin K
   D. Reduced vitamin C

10. **Mutation in gene alpha 3 chains of type IV collagen is associated with:**
    A. Alport's syndrome
    B. Benign familial haematuria
    C. Down syndrome
    D. Goodpasture syndrome

11. **Mutations of gene encoding alpha 4 chain of type IV collagen is associated with:**
    A. Down's syndrome
    B. Alport's syndrome
    C. Benign familial haematuria
    D. Goodpasture syndrome

12. **Autosomal recessive PCKD is associated with:**
    A. Chromosome 6   B. Chromosome 2
    C. Chromosome 5   D. Chromosome 7

13. **Autosoma dominant PCKD is associated with:**
    A. ADPKD1 on chromosome 4 and ADPKD2 on chromosome 16
    B. ADPKD1 on chromosome 6 and ADPKD2 on chromosome 14
    C. ADPKD1 on chromosome 4 and ADPKD2 on chromosome 4
    D. ADPKD1 on chromosome 16 and ADPKD2 on chromosome 4

Answers

1. A	2. B	3. C	4. A	5. B	6. A	7. B	8. D
9. A	10. D	11. C	12. A	13. D			

Bone Lesions

NORMAL STRUCTURE OF BONE

Adult human body has 206 bones which account for about 12% of the body weight. Bones have structural, protective and metabolic functions. Bone formation is a dynamic process. Extracellular matrix, specialized cells for production and maintenance of matrix constitute a bone. Characteristic feature of bone is its hard matrix which is composed of matrix protein and minerals.

In human body, two types of bones are noted:
1. Compact bone (cortical bone)
2. Spongy bone (trabecular bone/cancellous bone)

Bone is a specialized connective tissue and has following cells:
- Osteoblasts
- Osteocytes
- Osteoclasts

Osteoblasts: Osteoblasts play an important role in synthesis of the bone matrix. Serum alkaline phosphatase is a biomarker for osteoblastic activity as they contain alkaline phosphatase in their cytoplasm.

Osteocytes: Osteocytes help to control microenvironment of bone by controlling calcium and phosphate levels.

Osteoclasts: Osteoclasts are multinucleated giant cells (macrophages) which play an important role in bone resorption. Osteoclasts and osteoblasts act in co-ordination to control bone growth and metabolism through the bone remodelling cycle.

Cortical bone forms diaphysis of long bone and outer surface of trabecular bone as it has structural load-bearing function. Trabecular bone (cancellous bone) predominantly contributes to the metabolic functions of the bone. Since it is metabolically more active, it is more prone to diseases such as postmenopausal osteoporosis and metastatic deposits from malignancies.

OSTEOMYELITIS

- Infection of bone followed by inflammation is termed as osteomyelitis.
- It may be caused by direct inoculation of the causative organism (most commonly bacteria) or spread from systemic infectious disease.
- Two most common forms are:
  1. Pyogenic osteomyelitis
  2. Tuberculous osteomyelitis.
  Other organisms causing osteomyelitis include:
  Fungi: *Coccidioides immitis, Histoplasma* (*capsulatum* and *duboisii*), *Cryptococcus neoformans, Blastomyces dermatitidis, Actinomyces israelii.*
  Parasites: Hydatid cyst (echinococcus).

PYOGENIC OSTEOMYELITIS

- Long bones most commonly affected.
- Bacterial infection is the most common cause of osteomyelitis.
- *Staphylococcus* is the most common organism. Other organisms include streptococci, gram-negative bacilli and *Brucella* organisms.
- *Pseudomonas aeruginosa* is the most common cause in IV drug abusers. *Salmonella* is frequent in patients with sickle cell disease.
- In infants and young children, haematogenous spread occurs in long bones.
- It may also occur as a complication of fractures, surgical procedures, immunosuppression, gangrene of limbs, etc.

Pathogenesis and Pathology

- Organisms cause acute inflammatory reaction at the metaphyseal end of the bone leading to oedema, exudative inflammatory infiltrate (predominantly neutrophils) and congestion.
- Marrow cavity pressure rises.
- Spread of infection to periosteum leading to periostitis.
- Compression and decreased blood supply leads to erosion of cortical bone, thinning and necrosis. Infarcted bone is called "sequestrum".
- With the passage of time, new bone is formed beneath the periosteum. This new bone forms a sheath around necrosed bone. This is called "involucrum".
- Encapsulated osteomyelitis forming a well demarcated abscess is called Brodie's abscess.

Gross: Sequestrum—the dead necrotic bone and involucrum—the reactive bone are the features. There can be sinus tracts extending from bone, passing through soft tissues and extending up to skin surface. Exudate and necrotic bony spicules may come out of the opening of sinus tracts (Fig. 40.1).

Microscopy: Mixed inflammatory cells (predominantly neutrophils) along with chronic inflammatory cells, congestion, oedema and necrotic bony spicules are common features (Fig. 40.2).

Complications

- Septicaemia
- Acute bacterial arthritis

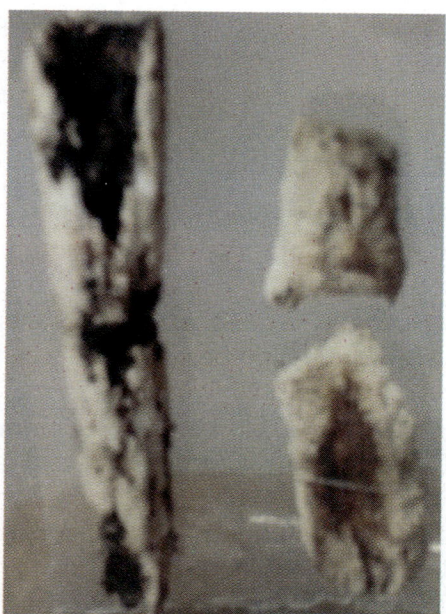

Fig. 40.1: Osteomyelitis, note dead bone sequestrum (gross picture)

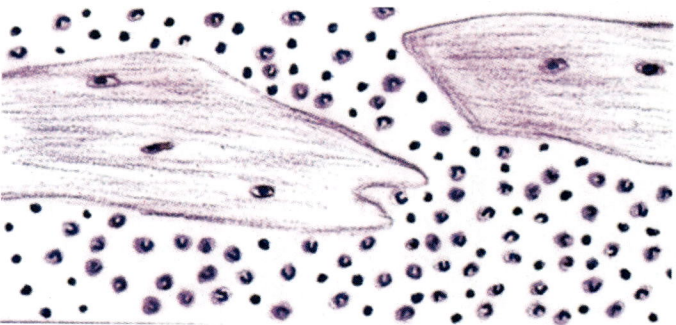

Fig. 40.2: Microscopy of osteomyelitis (schematic)

- Endocarditis
- Pathological fracture
- Squamous cell carcinoma or sarcoma in long standing cases
- Fusion of joint spaces
- Shortning of limbs in children
- Amyloidosis—secondary (AA type)

Clinical Features

- Pain
- Fever
- Leucocytosis
- Malaise

GRANULOMATOUS OSTEOMYELITIS (Mycobacterial Osteomyelitis/Tuberculous Osteomyelitis)

The common cause for granulomatous osteomyelitis is tubercolosis. It is rare in developed countries but common in developing countries. Following are the features:

- Haematogenous dissemination of *Mycobacterium tuberculosis* from primary site of infection into the bone or sometimes direct extension from pulmonary or GI tuberculosis.
- Most commonly affected site is spine (lower thoracic and lumbar vertebrae), tibia and fibula. Spine is affected in 50% of the tuberculous osteomyelitis cases. Affected bone is eroded by the granulomatous inflammation caused by bacilli, also the intervertebral disc is affected. Collapse of the eroded vertebrae causes symptoms of nerve compression.
- Pus from the lesion spreads into the surrounding areas, sheaths of psoas muscle producing psoas abscess or lumbar cold abscess.
- On microscopic examination, the lesion shows the same general histological features noted in tuberculosis in other organs such as caseous necrosis surrounded by epithelioid cells, giant cells, fibroblasts and lymphocytes. Along with the above mentioned features, fragments of necrotic bone are also noted.

- The cold abscess, if not treated, may lead to formation of sinuses
- Long-standing cases may develop amyloidosis.

DEVELOPMENTAL ABNORMALITIES

Inherited mutations frequently result in developmental abnormalities of the skeleton. These abnormalities manifest during the early life when bone formation takes place. Problems in the migration and condensation of mesenchyme or global disorganization of bone and/or cartilage can result in developmental anomalies.

ACHONDROPLASIA

Achondroplasia is the most common skeletal dysplasia. It is one of the major causes of dwarfism.

It is an autosomal dominant disorder having reduced cartilage formation. Affected individuals have short limbs with macrocephaly. Intelligence and reproductive function is not affected.

OSTEOGENESIS IMPERFECTA (Brittle Bone Disease)

Osteogenesis imperfecta is the most common inherited disorder of the connective tissue. It is caused by the deficiency in the synthesis of type 1 collagen. Apart from bone, it also affects other sites which are rich in type 1 collagen, viz. joints, eyes, ears, skin and teeth.

Following are characteristic features:
- There is extreme skeletal fragility due to too little bone.
- Findings noted in osteogenesis imperfecta include— blue sclera, hearing loss, dental abnormalities (small, blue–yellow teeth).
- Four clinical subtypes are noted based on the location of mutation within the protein.
- Subtype include following:
  - Type I: Autosomal dominant—compatible with life.
  - Type II: Most autosomal recessive—perinatal death. Some autosomal dominant
  - Type III: Autosomal dominant (75%)—progressive with deformity. Autosomal recessive (25%)
  - Type IV: Autosomal dominant—compatible with life. (Genetically differs with type I)
- Type II is fatal variant characterised by extraordinary bone fragility with multiple intrauterine fractures; whereas individuals with type I variant lead a normal life but experience fractures during childhood which decreases in frequency after puberty.

OSTEOPETROSIS

Osteopetrosis is also known as marble bone disease or Albers–Schonberg disease. It is a genetic disease characterised by reduced bone resorption and diffuse symmetric skeletal sclerosis due to impaired formation or function of osteoclasts. The bones are brittle and prone to fracture. Genetic mutation interferes with the acidification of osteoclast resorption pit, which is essential for dissolution of calcium hydroxyapatite in the matrix. Bones involved by osteopetrosis lack medullary canal due to deficient osteoclast activity which makes the ends of long bones bulbous (Erlenmeyer flask deformity).

It has following characteristic features and presentations:
- The neural foramina are small and compress exiting nerves.
- The medullary cavity is filled with primary spongiosa leaving no room for haematopoietic marrow.
- Severe infantile osteopetrosis is an autosomal recessive disorder. It manifests *in utero* or soon after birth. It is characterised by fractures, anaemia and hydrocephaly leading to postpartum mortality.
- If a child survives to infancy, it manifests as cranial nerve defect, repeated infections due to leukopenia and prominent hepatosplenomegaly due to extramedullary haematopoiesis.
- Autosomal dominant form of osteopetrosis may go unnoticed until adolescence. Individual presents with history of repeated fracture, mild cranial nerve defects and anaemia.
- Osteopetrosis was the first genetic disease treated with haematopoietic stem cell transplantation.

OSTEOPOROSIS

Osteoporosis is a disease characterized by reduction in bone mass in the presence of normal mineralization. Radiographically bone mass is 2.5 standard deviation below the mean value for young adult of same sex. Characteristic findings are as shown below.
- It may be localized or may involve entire skeleton.
- The most common forms of osteoporosis are the senile and postmenopausal type.
- Hereditary factors, physical activity, muscle strength, diet and hormonal state play an important role in formation of peak bone mass.
- Average bone loss is 0.7% per year which is normal biologic phenomenon. Osteoblastic activity in older individual is on the lower side as compared to that in younger individuals resulting in reduced capacity to make bone. This form of osteoporosis is known as senile osteoporosis.

Mechanical forces are known to play an important role in bone remodelling. Reduced physical activity increases the rate of bone loss. Decreased physical activity in the elderly contributes to senile osteoporosis.

Genetic makeup of an individual plays a role in peak bone density (gene encoding regulation of osteoclasts, estrogene receptor gene and HLA focus). Calcium plays an important role in peak bone mass. Calcium-deficient diet during the period of rapid bone growth restricts the bone mass thus increasing the risk of osteoporosis. Calcium deficiency, increased parathyroid hormone and decreased vitamin D concentration may lead to development of senile osteoporosis.

- Estrogen levels play an important role in bone remodelling. Postmenopausal estrogen deficiency increases bone resorption and bone formation but bone resorption is more as compared to bone formation leading to osteoporosis. Bone loss is around 35% of the cortical bone and 50% of cancellous bone by 30–40 years after menopause.

Decreased estrogen increases secretion of inflammatory cytokines which in turn stimulates osteoclastic activity and preventing osteoclast apoptosis.

In postmenopausal osteoporosis, the bones with increased surface areas are affected such as vertebrae. The trabeculae become perforated, thinned leading to microfractures and eventually vertebral collapse. Vertebral fractures that frequently affect thoracic and lumbar regions are painful and cause various deformities, if there is significant damage.

Diagnosis

1. Osteoporosis is detected on radiography only when 30 to 40% of bone mass is lost.
2. Blood levels of calcium, phosphorus and alkaline phosphatase are non-diagnostic.
3. The best mode of diagnosis is measurement of bone density using specialized radioimaging techniques.
4. Trabaculae bone, trabaculae are thinner and widely separated than normal.

PAGET'S DISEASE OF BONE (Osteitis Deformans)

Paget's disease is a disorder of increase but disordered and structurally unsound bone mass.

There are three phases:
1. Initial osteolytic stage
2. Mixed osteoclastic–osteoblastic stage
3. Osteosclerotic stage

Paget's disease is a disease of adulthood, with variation in incidence all over the world. Some areas with high incidence whereas some areas with hardly few cases.

Paget's disease is a disease of unknown etiology with some evidence suggesting contribution of genetic and environmental factors. Mutation in RANK (receptor activator of nuclear factor kappa B) and OPG (osteoprotegerin) account for a few cases of juvenile Paget's disease of bone.[47] A few studies have shown the role of measles virus, respiratory syncytial virus or canine distemper virus in the pathogenesis of Paget's disease with the presence of viral inclusion in osteoclasts.[48] Following are the features in Paget's disease of bone:

- The hallmark is mosaic pattern of lamellar bone, noted in sclerotic phase.
- The osteoclasts are large with increased number of nuclei (around 100 nuclei) during the initial lytic phase.
- During mixed phase, bone surfaces are lined by osteoblasts. Adjacent marrow is replaced by loose connective tissue.
- As the mosaic pattern unfolds, the periosseous fibrovascular tissue recedes and is replaced by normal marrow.
- In the end, bone formed has thickened trabeculae and soft and porous cortex that lacks stability, making it vulnerable for fracture.
- Paget's disease generally affects multiple bones. Axial skeleton or proximal femur is involved in about 80% of cases.
- Enlargement of craniofacial skeleton may give appearance of lion face (leantiasis ossea), making it difficult for individual to hold the head erect due to heaviness.
- Weight-bearing causes bowing of femurs and tibia leading to secondary osteoarthritis.
- Chalk stick fractures are known complication in long bones.
- Variety of secondary lesions are encountered in bones affected with Paget's disease such as giant cell tumour, giant cell reparative granuloma and sarcoma (osteosarcoma or fibrosarcoma).
- Radioimaging plays an important role in diagnosis of Paget's disease of bone.

RICKETS AND OSTEOMALACIA

Vitamin D plays an important role in mineralization of epiphyseal cartilage and osteoid matrix. In collaboration with parathyroid hormone, it maintains the normal blood level of calcium and phosphorus. Deficiency of vitamin D manifests in three forms:

1. Rickets in childhood
2. Osteomalacia in adults
3. Hypocalcaemic tetani

Deficiency of vitamin D can be due to following causes:
1. Dietary deficiency
2. Inadequate exposure to sunlight
3. Reduced synthesis
4. Derangement of vitamin D metabolism
5. Defective fat absorption leading to calcium deficiency
6. Resistance of end organ to respond to vitamin D

Rickets

It is a disease of childhood caused either by deficiency of vitamin D or resistance to its action. Primary defects in rickets are:
1. Interference with mineralization of bone
2. Deranged bone growth.

Clinical Features

Age group—6 months to 2 years, listless and irritable child.

Skeletal changes:
1. Craniotabes—box-like skull due to unossified areas.
2. Rickety rosary—swelling of costochondral junctions of ribs.
3. Pigeon chest/funnel chest—anterior protrusion of sternum.
4. Bow legs—bending of the weak long bones.
5. Knock knee.
6. Delayed eruption of teeth.
7. Muscular weakness.

Biochemical findings:
- Serum calcium and serum phosphorus levels are lower than normal for age.
- Serum alkaline phosphatase levels are raised due to osteoblastic activity.

Pathogenesis
- Vitamin D deficiency reduces absorption of calcium from intestine and mobilization of calcium from bones.
- Calcium levels fall leading to secretion of PTH (parathyroid hormone) thus increasing resorption of calcium in kidney but at the cost of phosphate leading to hypophosphataemia.
- Due to hypophosphataemia, mineralization of bone stops.

Osteomalacia

This is an adult counterpart of rickets due to failure in mineralization of osteoid matrix. This has following features:

- First affects vertebrae, pelvis and other bones of trunk.
- Long bones are last affected and with low severity.
- New bone formed has thin core of ossified bone surrounded by unossified osteoid.
- Cortex of the affected bone is thinned out and Haversion canals enlarge.
- Serum calcium and phosphorus levels are low whereas alkaline phosphatase levels are raised.
- Severe form can lead to fracture.
- Compression fractures of vertebrae and long bones are common.

Clinical Features
- Mascular weakness
- Vague bony pains
- Pathological fractures (greenstick fracture)
- Looser's zone or pseudo-fractures at weak places in bones.

RENAL OSTEODYSTROPHY

The skeletal changes that occur in chronic renal disease including those associated with dialysis are collectively called renal osteodystrophy.

The histologic bone changes in individuals with end stage renal failure can be divided into three types:
1. High turnover dystrophy—increased bone resorption and formation but resorption is more.
2. Low turnover or aplastic disease—decreased osteoblastic and osteoclastic activity.
3. Mixed pattern—areas of high and low turnovers.

Skeletal abnormalities are caused through three mechanisms:
1. Tubular dysfunction—low pH associated with renal tubular acidosis dissolves hydroxyapatite leading to demineralization and osteomalacia.
2. Generalized renal failure—it reduces excretion of phosphate, thus causing hyperphosphataemia and hypocalcaemia. Thereby leading to secondary hyperparathyroidism.
3. Decreased production of secreted factors—kidney plays an important role in formation of vitamin D_3 and regulation of calcium and phosphate levels by converting vitamin D and secreting BMP-7, FGF-23 and membrane proteins Klotho. Decreased synthesis of vitamin D_3 results in hypocalcaemia thus contributing to secondary hyperparathyroidism. The reduced signals for secretions of proteins with chronic renal failure thus resulting in osteopenia and osteomalacia.

Alternate areas of thickened bone and osteoporosis are noted in the cases with long-standing disordered bone remodelling due to combination of secondary hyperparathyroidism and osteomalacia. This characteristic appearance is known as "rugger jersey spine".

BROWN TUMOUR

Brown tumour also called **osteitis fibrosa cystica** is a localized bone lesion which occurs in hyperparathyroidism due to excessive osteoclast activity. It is not a true neoplasm. The bones have cystic and fibrotic areas.

It occurs due to primary or secondary hyperparathyroidism. 2% of the patients suffering from hyperparathyroidism develop brown tumour.

Excessive urinary excretion of calcium leads to reduced serum levels which stimulates parathyroid to secrete PTH. This mobilizes calcium from bones through osteoclast activity to maintain normal serum calcium levels.

Clinical Features

Brown tumour may cause swelling, pathological fracture and bone pain.

X-ray: Lytic expansile lesion with thinned cortex, may have fractures.

Gross: Bones have lytic lesions, with haemorrhage and reparative granulation tissue which may relpace bone marrow with fibrosis. The cortex is thinned and expanded. The colour is brown due haemorrhage and hemosiderin deposition.

BONE TUMOURS

Primary bone tumours are rare. As compared to primary tumours, metastatic and haematopoietic tumours are more common in bones. Bone tumours have the following features:

- Bone tumours have predilection for long bones of the extremities.
- Involved site and age group gives a clue towards the specific type of tumour.
- Radiological investigations play an important role in diagnosing these tumours. Definitive diagnosis needs histopathological study of the biopsy.
- Diagnosis of bone tumours is a team work involving clinicians, radiologist and pathologist.

CLASSIFICATION OF BONE TUMOURS

Table 40.1 describes classification of bone tumours.

BONE-FORMING TUMOURS

Osteoid Osteoma and Osteoblastoma

These two tumours are with identical histologic feature but difference in size, site and clinical features. Differences between the two are given in Table 40.2.

Table 40.1	Classification of bone tumours[49]	
Category	**Benign**	**Malignant**
Bone forming	Osteoma Osteoid osteoma Osteoblastoma	Osteosarcoma
Cartilage forming	Osteochondroma Chondroma Chondroblastoma Chondromyxoid fibroma	Chondrosarcoma
Uncetrain origin	Giant cell tumour	Malignant giant cell tumour Ewing's sarcoma
Metastatic		Malignant
Tumour-like lesions	Aneurysmal bone cyst, fibrous cortical defect, fibrous dysplasia, nonossifying fibroma	

Note: Simplified 2013 WHO classification of bone tumours

Table 40.2	Differences between osteoid osteoma and osteoblastoma
Osteoid osteoma	**Osteoblastoma**
1. Less than 2 cm	More than 2 cm
2. Predilection to appendicular skeleton (femur or tibia)	Posterior spine (laminae and pedicles)
3. Thick reactive cortical bone	Bony reaction not marked
4. Pain responds to aspirin	Does not respond to aspirin
5. Treated by radiofrequency ablation	Curettage or en block excision

Gross: Both are round to oval, hemorrhagic and tan-coloured, rim or sclerotic bone present at the edge which is more pronounced in osteoid osteoma.

Microscopy:

- Well circumscribed, randomly interconnecting trabeculae of woven bone rimmed by single layer of osteoblasts.
- Surrounding stroma contains loose connective tissue with giant cells and dilated congested capillaries.
- Small size, well-defined margins and benign cytologic features distinguishes these tumours from osteosarcoma.

Osteosarcoma

Osteosarcoma is a malignant mesenchymal tumour characterised by production of osteoid matrix or mineralized bone by malignant tumour cells. It is a most common primary bone tumour after myeloma and lymphoma.

Genetic abnormalities play an important role in pathogenesis of osteosarcoma. Mutation in tumour suppressor gene; commonly affected genes are RB gene, TP53 gene mutation, INK4a, MDM2 and CDK4.

It has following features:
- Bimodal age distribution
  I. Younger age (<20 years)—primary
  II. Older adults (secondary to other bone disorders, viz. Paget's disease of bone, bone infarcts, prior irradiation, fibrous dysplasia.)
- Metaphyseal region of long bone is involved.
- 50% cases occur commonly around knee (distal femur, proximal tibia or proximal humerus).
- Painful, progressive mass. Sometimes presented with fracture.
- Radiograph shows mixed bulky destructive lesion with cystic areas and Codman's triangle.
- **Codman's** triangle—tumour lifts the periosteum, breaking through cortex. The shadow between the cortex and raised end of periosteum is radiologically called Codman's triangle.
- **Sunburst appearance:** Appearance of rays of sun produced due to parallel lines of mineral deposition by tumour cells in the periosteal region.

Gross: These tumours are bulky masses, gritty, grey-white in colour and have areas of haemorrhage and cystic degeneration. They can destroy the cortex and produce soft tissue masses (Fig. 40.3).

Microscopy: The tumour cells vary in size and shape. They have large hyperchromatic nuclei (Fig. 40.4).

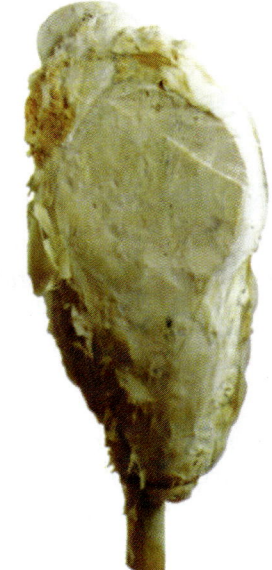

Fig. 40.3: Osteosarcoma (gross picture)

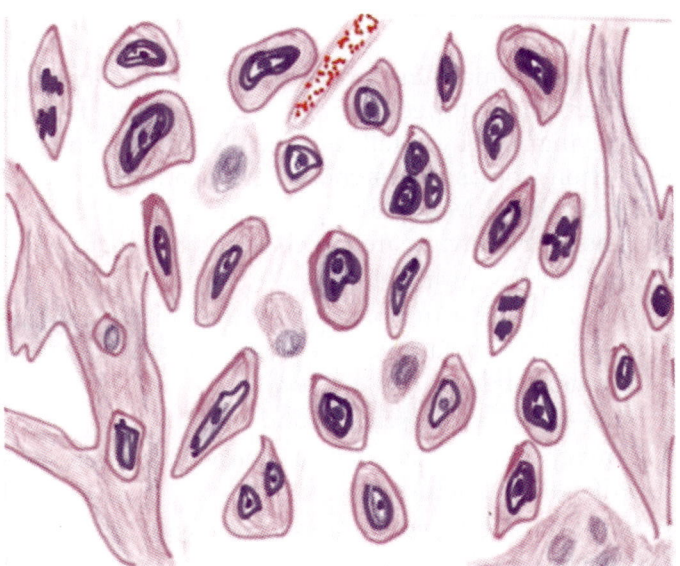

Fig. 40.4: Microscopy of osteosarcoma (schematic)

Bizarre tumour, and giant cells along with mitosis (some abnormal) are noted. Formation of new bone by tumour cells is diagnostic feature. Newly formed neoplastic bone has fine lace-like architecture. Areas of haemorrhage and cystic change are present. Vascular invasion is common and also extensive necrosis is prominent.

Destruction of surrounding cortices with extension into medullary cavity and replacing haematopoietic cells and also extends into soft tissues.

Histological variants of osteosarcoma: The different histological variants of osteosarcoma are:

1. Conventional osteosarcoma
2. Fibroblastic

3. Chondroblastic
4. Telangiectatic
5. Small cell
6. Fibrohistiocytic
7. Anaplastic
8. Well-differentiated intramedullary osteosarcomas.

If invasion occurs, tumour spreads along with tendo-ligamentous structures. By haematogenous route, spread to the lungs. Also, can metastasize to other bones, brains, etc.

Clinical Course

Osteosarcoma is treated with neoadjuvant chemotherapy followed by surgery. If metastasis occurs, lung is the organ involved. At the time of diagnosis, 10–20% of patients have evidence of pulmonary metastasis. Prognosis is poor in patients with metastasis.

CARTILAGE-FORMING TUMOURS

Osteochondroma (Exostosis)

Osteochondroma is the most common benign tumour. It is cartilage-capped tumour which is attached to underlying bone by a stalk and usually solitary. Solitary osteochondromas are diagnosed in late adolescent and early adulthood. Multiple osteochondroma noted during childhood. Following are the characteristic features:

- Predilection for male.
- Develops only in bones of endochondral origin, arises from metaphysis near growth plate of long tubular bones.
- Site—knee, pelvis, scapula and ribs.
- Slow growing mass, painful if nerve is compressed or if stalk is fractured.
- EXT 1 or EXT 2 genes are associated with hereditary exostosis.
- Osteochondromas may be sessile or pedunculated with size ranging from 1 to 20 cm.
- Cap is composed of benign hyaline cartilage of varying thickness.
- Cartilage has appearance of disorganized growth plate which undergoes ossification. The ossified bone forms head and stalk.
- Cortex of stalk and host bone merge so medullary cavity is in continuity.

Chondroma

This is benign cartilaginous tumour composed of lobules of mature hyaline cartilage. This is also called enchondroma when occurs in medullary cavity and called perosteal or juxtacortical chondroma when occurs on the surface. Most of the enchondromas occur in small bones of hands and feet. Next common site is long bones. It is rare in flat bones.

There are syndromes associated with chondromas.
1. Ollier's syndrome: Multiple enchondromsa, skeletal dysplasia.
2. Maffucci's syndrome: Multiple enchondromas, haemangiomas of skin, with risk for ovarian and liver malignancy.

Chondrosarcoma

Chondrosarcoma is a cartilage producing malignant tumour. It is subclassified as:
I. Conventional (produces hyaline cartilage)
II. Clear cell
III. Dedifferentiated
IV. Mesenchymal

Conventional chondrosarcoma is the most common variant. Chondrosarcoma is next to osteogenic sarcoma in its occurrence as malignant matrix producing bone tumour. Age of onset is 5th decade or above.

Clear cell and mesenchymal variants occur in teens and young adults. Males are more commonly affected than females. Axial skeleton is involved (pelvis, shoulder, ribs) more commonly. Low grade tumour causes thickening of cortex whereas high grade tumour destroys the cortex forming a soft tissue mass.

Clear cell variant is noted at epiphysis of long bone. 15% of chondrosarcoma arises from pre-existing benign cartilage producing tumours (enchondroma or osteochondroma).

Mutations in EXT, IDH1 and IDH2 genes are associated with chondrosarcomas and usually present as painful, progressively enlarging masses.

Morphology

Gross findings:
- Large, bulky, nodular tumours with glistening grey white translucent cartilage. Matrix is often gelatinous or myxoid.
- Cystic change may be noted due to necrosis.
- Calcification usually present.

Microscopic findings:
- Tumour varies in cellularity and cellular features (atypia and mitosis).
- Grade I: Mild hypercellular with chondrocytes having plump, vesicular nuclei and small nucleoli. Mitotic figure is rare. Cartilage may undergo endochondral ossification.
- Grade III: Marked hypercellularity, highly pleomorphic cells with bizarre tumour, giant cells and mitosis.

EWING SARCOMA FAMILY TUMOUR (ESFT)[50]

ESFTs are highly aggressive malignancies. Ewing sarcoma is malignant tumour composed of primitive round cells without differentiation.

Earlier Ewing sarcoma and primitive neuro-ectodermal tumour (PNET) were two different entities but recently these have been included in single category of Ewing sarcoma family tumour (ESFT) due to similar clinical, morphological, biochemical and molecular features. It constitutes 6 to 10% of primary malignant bone tumours. These are 2nd most common bone sarcomas in children after osteosarcomas and show a slight predilection for males.

It is characterised by recurrent chromosomal translocations [t(11;22) EWSR1-FLI1 or t(21;22) EWSR1-ERG] and membranous MIC2/CD99 over expression.

Following are some characteristic features:
- About 80% of cases are younger than 20 years.
- Predilection for boys and Whites.
- Ewing's sarcoma usually arises from diaphysis or metadiaphyseal region of long bones, pelvic bones and ribs.
- The rare locations are the skull bones, vertebra, scapula, and the small bones of hands and feet. Any soft tissue site can be affected. Ewing's sarcoma shows a permeative pattern with periosteal reaction.

Clinical Features

- Painful enlarging mass with raised local temperature.
- Fever, elevated ESR, anaemia, leucocytosis.
- These clinical features mimic infection that is osteomyelitis.

Radiological Findings

The radiological findings are essential for histopathological diagnosis. They are:
1. Destructive, lytic tumour with deposition of reactive periosteal bone resembling 'onion skin'.
2. Widening of medullary canal.

Morphology

It arises in medullary cavity and invades cortex, periosteum and soft tissue. Grossly, the tumour is soft, tan white mass with areas of haemorrhage and necrosis.

Microscopy (Fig. 40.5): Ewing's sarcoma is a highly malignant small round blue cell tumour, histologically composed of sheets of small cells with high nuclear to cytoplasmic ratio. The cytoplasm is scant, eosinophilic, and usually contains glycogen, which is detected by periodic acid-Schiff stain and is diastase degradable.

The nuclei are round, with finely dispersed chromatin, and one or more tiny nucleoli. This tumour frequently

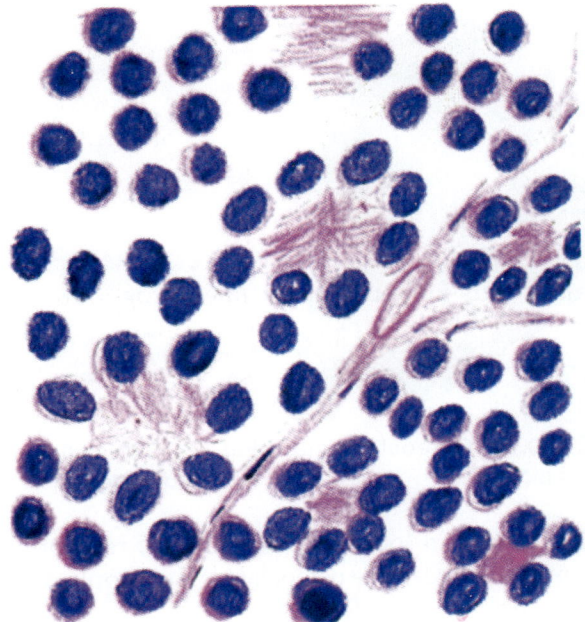

Fig. 40.5: Microscopy of Ewing's sarcoma, note rosettes (schematic)

undergoes necrosis and shows a "peritheliomatous" or a perivascular distribution. Homer–Wright rosettes, cells arranged in a circle around a central fibrillary structure is indicative of a neural differentiation.

GIANT CELL TUMOUR

Recent WHO classification categorizes giant cell tumour (GCT) as intermediate grade neoplasm. Rarely, it can metastasize to lungs. Giant cell tumours are characterised by presence of multinucleated osteoclasts like giant cells (synonym—osteoclastoma). It is believed to arise from monocyte–macrophage lineage. Following are characteristic features:

- It is locally aggressive tumour and rate of recurrence is very high (>50%).
- Commonly occurs in individuals in the age group of 20–40 years.
- Tumour arises in the epiphysis and may extend in metaphysis.
- It occurs most commonly around the knee and lower end of the radius; but any bone may be involved.
- It is associated with pathological fracture.

Pathogenesis

Primitive osteoblast precursors (mononuclear cells) are the neoplastic cells (minor component).

Major component of GCT is non-neoplastic osteoclasts and their precursors. The neoplastic cells stimulate proliferation of osteoclast precursors which later differentiate into mature osteoclasts.

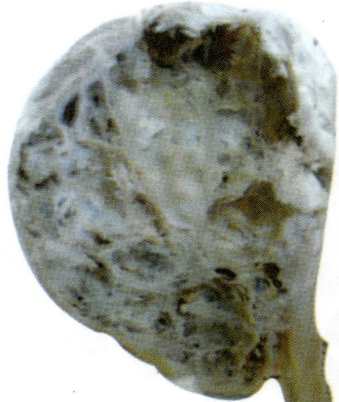

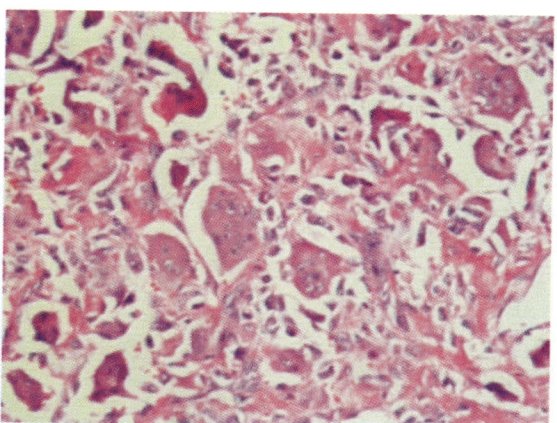

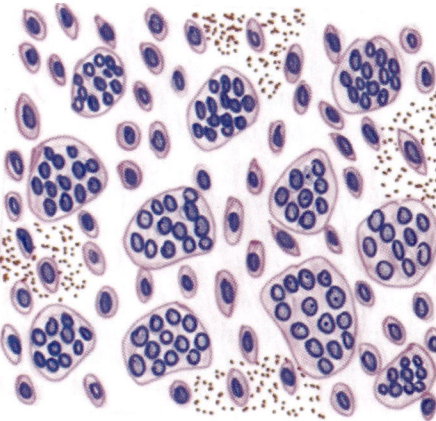

Fig. 40.6: Osteoclastoma (gross picture)

Fig. 40.7: Microphotograph of osteoclastoma, note numerous osteoclasts

Fig. 40.8: Microscopy of osteoclastoma (schematic)

This results in localized, destructive, resorption of bone matrix by reactive osteoclasts. The neoplastic cells express high levels of RANKL.

Radiology

X-ray shows lytic lesion with multiple cystic areas surrounded by thin bony shell gives "soap bubble" appearance.

Morphology

Grossly has a bulging soft tissue mass with club-shaped deformity lined by thin shell of reactive bone. The cut section shows red-brown solid areas and cystic areas containing haemorrhage (Fig. 40.6).

Microscopy: There are sheets of oval mononuclear cells and numerous multinucleated osteoclasts like giant cells with 100 or more nuclei. The nuclear feature of mononuclear cells decides the biological behaviour of tumour. Necrosis, haemorrhage and haemosiderin deposition are common features (Figs 40.7 and 40.8).

No bone or cartilage is synthesized by the tumour cells.

Clinical Features

- 40–60% recur locally after curettage.
- 4% metastasize to lung, with each recurrence chances of metastasis increases.
- Nature of stromal cells (neoplastic cells) decides the biological behaviour of the giant cell tumour of bone.
- At the time of initial diagnosis, a baseline X-ray chest is advised. This can be used in future lung metastasis for comparison.

AMELOBLASTOMA

This is an odontogenic bone tumour, frequently occurring in mandible (jaws) and has aggressive behaviour. Exact origin is not known, thought to arise from cell rests of the enamel organ or epithelium lining the dentigerous cysts.

Gross: The tumour is grey-white with solid to cystic areas expanding the affected bone.

Microscopy: There are different histological patterns such as follicular, plexiform, acanthomatous and granular cell pattern. The follicular pattern is more common. There is central area of stellate cells resembling stellate reticulum and peripheral layer of cuboidal to columnar epithelium with polarization of the nuclei away from the basement membrane (Fig. 40.9).

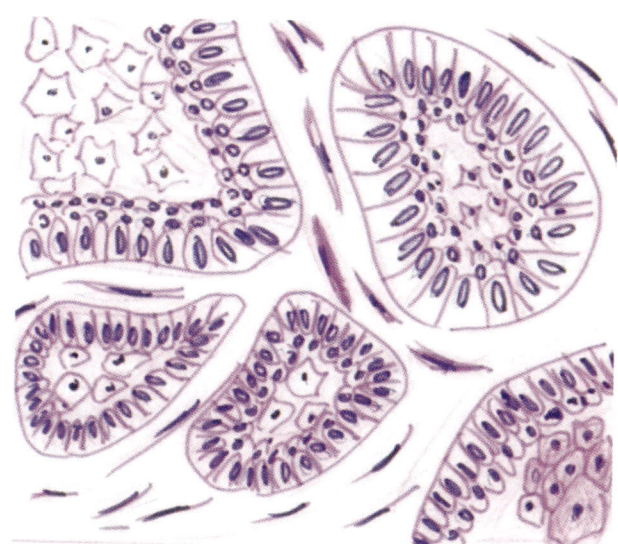

Fig. 40.9: Microscopy of ameloblastoma (schematic)

SELF-ASSESSMENT EXERCISE

1. **Osteoid osteoma originates from:**
   A. Cortex
   B. Periosteum
   C. Medullary cavity
   D. All of the above

2. **Sunray appearance in osteosarcoma is due to:**
   A. Perosteal reaction
   B. Osteonecrosis
   C. Formation of osteoid along vessels
   D. Calcification

3. **Bone metastasis is common due to tumour of:**
   A. Prostate
   B. Kidney
   C. Thyroid
   D. All of the above

4. **Synonym for Paget's disease is:**
   A. Osteitis deformans
   B. Osteitis imperfecta
   C. Osteitis fibrosa
   D. None of the above

5. **Enzymes in osteoblasts:**
   A. Alkaline phosphatase
   B. Acid phosphatase
   C. Elastase
   D. Cytochrome oxidase

6. **Ewing's sarcoma has following appearance on X-ray:**
   A. Plaque
   B. Onion skin
   C. Cannon ball
   D. All of the above

7. **Dysfunction of osteoclasts leads to:**
   A. Osteopetrosis
   B. Osteogenesis imperfecta
   C. Osteomalacia
   D. All of the above

8. **Osteogenesis imperfecta following observed:**
   A. Defect in Type I collagen synthesis
   B. AD
   C. Sclera translucent
   D. All of the above

9. **Tumour with soap bubble appearance is located in:**
   A. Epiphysis
   B. Metaphysis
   C. Diaphysis
   D. All of the above

10. **Ewing's sarcoma is located in following site:**
    A. Epiphysis
    B. Metaphysis
    C. Diaphysis
    D. All of the above

11. **HLA-B27 is associated with:**
    A. Rheumatoid arthritis
    B. Psoriatic arthritis
    C. Enteropathy associated arthritis
    D. All of the above

12. **Ewing's has following genetic abnormality:**
    A. t(11:22) (q24:q12)
    B. 11p13 deletion
    C. 13q14
    D. N-myc amplification

13. **Mosaic pattern of lamellar bone is observed in following disease:**
    A. Osteoporosis
    B. Osteopetrosis
    C. Paget's disease of bone
    D. All of the above

14. **Pathogenesis of osteopetrosis is:**
    A. Poor osteoclast function
    B. Defective mineralization
    C. Imbalance between osteoclast and osteoblast activity
    D. None of the above

Answers

1. A	2. C	3. D	4. A	5. A	6. B	7. A	8. D
9. A	10. C	11. D	12. A	13. C	14. A		

Skeletal Muscle Lesions

SKELETAL MUSCLE ATROPHY

This develops due to varied muscle disorders mentioned below.

1. Disuse atrophy
2. Corticosteroids: Exogenous or endogenous (Cushing syndrome).

   The disuse and corticosteroids cause mainly type II fibre atrophy.
3. Neurogenic atrophy: Group atrophy.
4. Dermatomyositis: Perifascicular atrophy.

INFLAMMATORY MYOPATHIES

Types

1. Dermatoyositis
2. Polymyositis

Note: Refer to autoimmune diseases.

INHERITED DISORDERS

DUCHENNE MUSCULAR DYSTROPHY

This is the most common of all the inherited dystrophies and transmitted as X-linked recessive pattern of inheritance. This is due to dysfunction of protein dystrophin. Pelvic and shoulder girdle muscle are commonly affected.

Incidence: 1 in 3500 live male births.

Clinical Course

The children are normal at birth; however, mother notices the symptoms as the child grows. These are difficulty in walking, standing, frequent fall, difficulty in getting up from lying or sitting position, difficulty in running and jumping, muscle pain and stiffness.

There is waddling gait and children have learning disabilities. The disease is evident by 5 years; there is progressive weakness and children become wheelchair bound by 15 years and death by 20 years.

Pathogenesis

There is mutation of large gene on Xp21 which codes for dystrophin. It is 427 kd protein, localised on the inner surface of the sarcolemma. Dystrophin acts as link between sub-sarcolemmal cytoskeletal contractile apparatus and extracellular matrix to maintain muscle integrity.

Pathology

Following are the features (Fig. 41.1):
- There is degeneration of muscle fibres including fibre splitting, necrosis.
- Muscle fibre regeneration and atrophic fibres are seen.

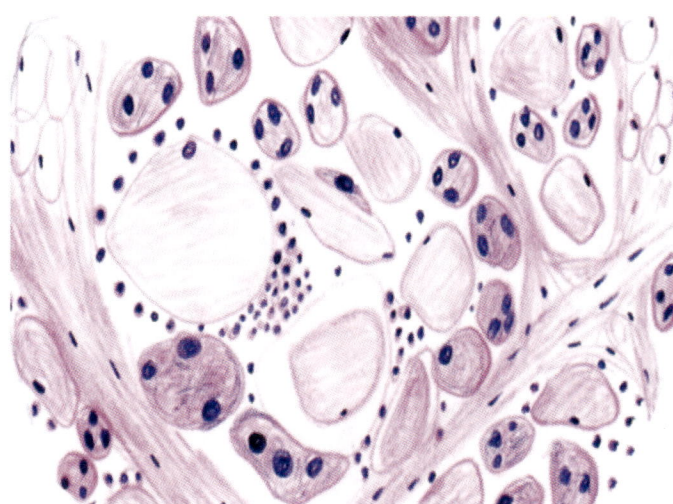

Fig. 41.1: Microscopy in Duchenne muscular dystrophy

- There is marked variation in fibre size with hypertrophy and atrophy.
- Fibrous and fatty replacement of muscle fibres (classical findings).
- Loss of membrane positivity for dystrophin protein on immunohistochemistry.

BECKER MUSCULAR DYSTROPHY

This is a milder form of Duchenne muscular dystrophy. All the findings described above are present in a milder form. There is partial loss of dystrophin protein on immunohistochemistry.

OTHER INHERITED MUSCLE DISORDERS

1. Myotonic dystrophy
2. Congenital myopathies
3. Emery-Dreifuss muscular dystrophy
4. Fascioscapulohumeral dystrophy
5. Limb-girdle muscular dystrophy
6. Mitochondrial myopathies
7. Spinal muscular atrophy

SELF-ASSESSMENT EXERCISE

1. Histological features of muscular dystrophy do not include:
   A. Degeneration, necrosis and phagocytosis
   B. Regeneration of muscle fibres
   C. Decreased number of internalised nuclei
   D. Proliferation of endomysial connective tissue

2. Most common inheritance of muscular dystrophy is:
   A. AR   B. AD
   C. X-linked recessive   D. Mitochondrial

3. Features of DMD are all *except*:
   A. Gower's sign
   B. Pseudohypertrophy of calf muscle

   C. Intact cognitive ability
   D. Elevated serum creatine kinase

4. Rash and calcinosis is seen in which of the following muscle disorders?
   A. Polymyositis
   B. Dermatomyositis
   C. Inclusion body myositis
   D. Becker muscular dystrophy

5. Which of the following statements is false?
   A. In DMD, there is no dystrophin
   B. In Becker's nevus, there is reduced dystrophin
   C. Perifascicular atrophy is seen in Becker's nevus
   D. DMD has X-linked inheritance

Answers

1. C   2. C   3. C   4. B   5. C

CNS Lesions

BERRY ANEURYSMS/SACCULAR ANEURYSMS

These are sac-like dilatations of the vascular wall. In aneurysms, the vascular wall is deficient of muscle layer and internal elastic lamina and composed of fibrous tissue at the neck and sac of the aneurysm.

They commonly occur at the following sites (Fig. 42.1):

1. Junction of anterior communicating artery and anterior cerebral artery (40%)
2. At branching of middle cerebral artery (34%)
3. Internal carotid artery and posterior communicating artery (20%)

Rupture usually occurs with straining during defaecation or during sexual orgasm. Rupture occurs at the apex with extravasation of blood into the subarachnoid space causing subarachnoid hemorrhage (SAH). This is the frequent cause of SAH.

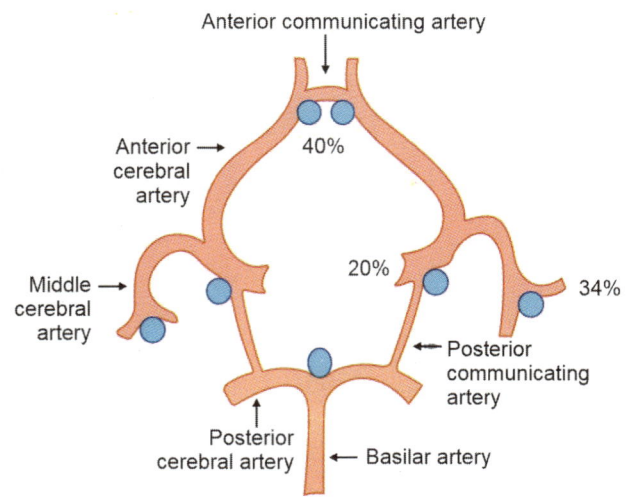

Fig. 42.1: Berry aneurysms

SUBARACHNOID HAEMORRHAGE

Haemorrhage into subarachnoid space is called sub-arachnoid haemorrhage (SAH).

Causes

Aneurysms:

- Rupture of the Berry aneurysm is the frequent cause;
- Other types of aneurysms are:
  i. Fusiform aneurysm (mostly due to atherosclerosis of basilar artery)
  ii. Mycotic aneurysm
  iii. Syphilitic aneurysm
  iv. Traumatic aneurysm
  v. Dissecting aneurysm

Other causes include:

1. Vascular malformation
2. Trauma (head injury)
3. Hypertension
4. Bleeding disorders
5. Anticoagulant therapy
6. Autosomal disorders: Marfan syndrome, polycystic kidney disease, neurofibromatosis type 1 and Ehlers-Danlos syndrome.

The patients experience following features:

1. Sudden excruciating headache, followed by
2. Rapid loss of consciousness.
3. About 25 to 50% of the patients die with first rupture.

CSF Findings in SAH

CSF in SAH will be mixed with the blood, the three bottle test is done to differentiate traumatic tap from SAH. In traumatic tap, only the first and second bottles will show blood and third bottle will be free of blood whereas in SAH all the bottles will show blood mixed CSF. Centrifuged sample in SAH shows yellowish discolouration of CSF (xanthochromia).

Brain in SAH

Brain shows cerebral oedema, subarachnoid and intracerebral haemorrhage with possible rupture of aneurysm of the circle of Willis, or atherosclerotic vessel or due to hypertensive changes of the vessel wall.

INTRACEREBRAL HAEMORRHAGE

In intracerebral haemorrhage (ICH), there is haemorrhage into the brain parenchyma.

Causes

- Hypertension: This accounts for 15% of the deaths.
- Cerebral amyloid angiopathy
- Local and systemic factors: Coagulation disorders, vasculitis, neoplasms, aneurysms, and vascular malformations.

Clinical Features

These depend upon the portion of the brain involved, large or small areas and which of the areas are involved. Large ICH may extend into ventricles. Hypertensive ICH commonly involves putamen, thalamus, pons and cerebellar hemisphere. The patients usually have neurological symptoms (stroke).

Gross and Microscopic Features

Recent haemorrhage: Shows clotted blood rimmed by brain tissue having anoxic neuronal cells and oedema.

Old haemorrhage: With resolution of haemorrhage, brain parenchyma can have cyst formation. There is rim of brownish discolouration. Brain oedema resolves over the time, hemosiderin pigment and lipid-laden macrophages appear. The adjacent parenchyma may show features of compression.

MENINGITIS

Meningitis is the inflammation of the meningeal layers of the brain and spinal cord. Pachymeningitis is the inflammation of dura mater and leptomeningitis is inflammation of the arachnoid and pia mater.

Types

Infectious: Due to bacterial, viral, fungal and parasite.

Non-infectious: It is rare and is due to drugs, autoimmune hypersensitivity reactions, neoplasms and chemical agents.

INFECTIVE MENINGITIS

Meningitis most commonly occurs due to the viruses and bacteria. It is rarely due to fungi and parasites.

Mode of Spread

1. Contagious spread: From the infections in the neighbouring sites like ear and orbit.
2. Haematogenous spread from the infections in other sites like gastrointestinal, genitourinary, respiratory tracts, etc.
3. Direct entry following a neurosurgical procedure.
4. Along the nerves as in viral meningitis.

Classification of Infective Meningitis

Based on the organisms, meningitis can be:
1. Bacterial
2. Viral
3. Fungal
4. Parasitic

Bacterial Meningitis

Most common in the age group of less than 5 yrs, but can occur in any age group.

Following are the different organisms responsible in various age groups.
1. **In neonates:** *E. coli* and group B streptococci
2. **Infants and children:** *H. influenzae*
3. **Adolescents and young adults:** *N. meningitidis*
4. **Elderly:** *Streptococcus pneumoniae* and *Listeria monocytogenes*

Clinical Features

Headache, neck stiffness, photophobia, fever and altered sensorium.

Pathology

Depending on duration, meningitis can be (Table 42.1):
1. Hyperacute: Within 24 hours
2. Acute: 2–7 days
3. Subacute: >7 days

Gross: Meningeal vessels are engorged. There is exudate in the subarachnoid space; in *H. influenzae* meningitis, exudate is predominantly at the base of brain and in *N. meningitidis* infection over the cerebral convexities. Exudate is present along the vessels in early stages (Fig. 42.1).

It may be seen in the ventricles also. Later stages, exudate fills the SA space.

Microscopy: Neutrophils fill the subarachnoid space. The vessels are congested. Cerebritis may be present.

Table 42.1	Findings in pyogenic meningitis		
Hyperacute	**Acute**	**Subacute**
Death within 24 hours Adrenal haemorrhage, centrilobular necrosis of liver are common features DIC Exudate scant Organisms numerous Mimics SAH	2–7 days **On early second day:** Grossly difficult to make out Microscopy and culture are useful for diagnosis Pus in the basal cisterns **Between 3 and 7 days:** Pus all over Fibrin + Bacteria + Neutrophils numerous Neurons hypoxic Brain oedematous	More than 7 days Neutrophils reduced Lymphocytes, plasma cells and macrophages present Fibrin + Vessels show fibrinoid necrosis with infarcts of cortical zones

Phlebitis may lead to venous obstruction and subsequent infarction of brain parenchyma (Figs 42.2 to 42.4).

Complications

If not treated, fibrous adhesion with hydrocephalus is known to occur.

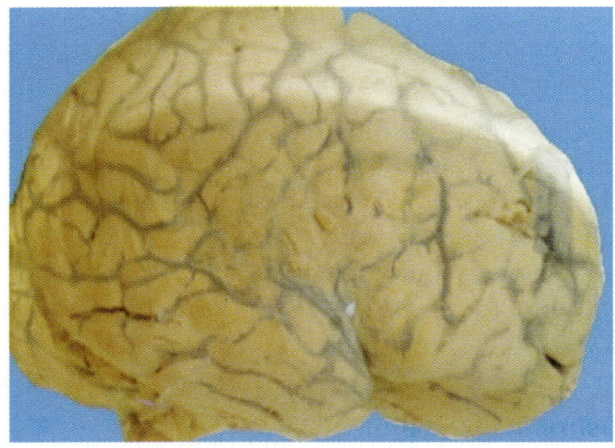

Fig. 42.2: Pyogenic meningitis (gross picture)

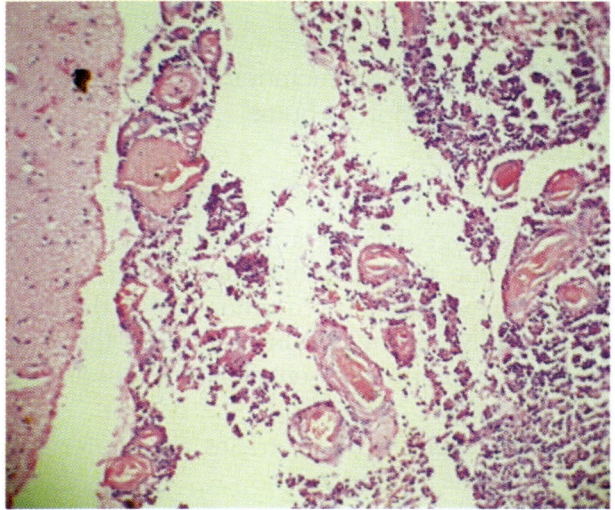

Fig. 42.3: Microphotograph of pyogenic meningitis, note exudate in subarachnoid space

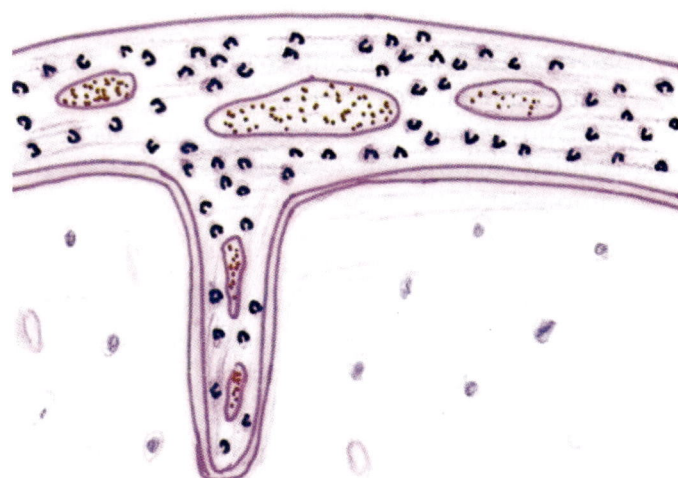

Fig. 42.4: Microscopy in pyogenic meningitis (schematic)

Laboratory Diagnosis

- By CSF examination
- Blood culture (gold standard)

The disease is associated with high morbidity and mortality especially in children with seizures and permanent neurological deficits.

Viral Meningitis

This is a condition, where the patient will have all the clinical signs of meningitis with CSF pleocytosis and absence of organisms in culture.

In majority of cases, the causative organism is not identifiable. Amongst the organisms identified, enterovirus is common, followed by mumps virus, HIV and HSV. Laboratory diagnosis is made by the examination of the CSF pleocytosis with elevation of protein and normal to decreased sugar. Molecular technique like PCR is required to establish the etiological agents.

Fungal and Parasitic Meningitis

Fungal and parasitic meningitis are rare and observed in immunocompromised hosts. *Cryptococcus neoformans*, *Aspergillus* and *Mucormycosis* species are common. Parasites like *Neisseria flowri* and *Acanthamoeba* species are the organisms causing meningitis. Fungal and parasitic meningitis mimic like chronic tubercular meningitis clinically.

TUBERCULOSIS OF CENTRAL NERVOUS SYSTEM

Central nervous system tuberculosis occurs in three different forms:
1. Tubercular (TB) meningitis
2. Tuberculoma
3. Tubercular abscess.

Brain is the target organ for TB bacilli next to lungs. They reach the brain through haematogenous route. In an immunocompetent host, initially they form Rich's foci in the meningeal layer and remain dormant. When immunity is lowered, bacilli proliferate producing the disease.

In TB meningitis, there will be a thick exudate formed in the basal region of the brain, which extends along the Sylvian fissure, it also surrounds the arteries causing end-arteritis and infarction. If untreated, the exudate can get organized and can block CSF flow causing hydrocephalus.

If the bacilli enter within the parenchyma, it leads to tuberculoma. Tuberculoma is a well-circumscribed intraparenchymal mass measuring 2 to 10 cm clinically mimics like a glioma.

Microscopically, they show central areas of caseous necrosis surrounded by granuloma. Acid-fast bacilli can be demonstrated.

Tuberculous abscess resembles clinically like a pyogenic abscess but microscopically shows caseous necrosis and acid-fast bacilli can be demonstrated.

CENTRAL NERVOUS SYSTEM TUMOURS

Central nervous system (CNS) constitutes 2% of all the cancers and in paediatric population, it accounts for 20% of all childhood tumours. About 70% of the childhood tumours occur in the posterior fossa whereas most of the adult CNS tumours occur within the cerebral hemispheres. Metastatic tumours are more common than the primary tumours.

The CNS tumours need special attention due to the following reasons:
1. The clinical course of a patient with brain tumour is strongly influenced by patterns of growth and location. Even low grade tumours may have infiltrative margins, clinical deficits and poor outcome.
2. The tumour may not be amenable to surgical resection due to infiltrative margins.
3. Even benign tumours may compress vital organs, if the tumours are adjacent to the vital structures.
4. The tumours may spread through CSF pathway and implants can be present along brain and spinal cord in distant sites away from primary tumour.

CLASSIFICATION OF CNS TUMOURS

In the year 2007, WHO has classified the brain tumours on the basis of phenotype into grade I to IV, however, in the year 2016, WHO revised the classification of the CNS tumours based on molecular changes, i.e. genotypic and phenotypic classification which is target therapy based. The detailed classification is beyond the scope of this book.

Depending upon the cell of origin, the CNS tumours are named as below.
- Glioma: Arising from the glial cells
- Astrocytes: Astrocytoma
- Oligodendrocytes: Oligodendroglioma
- Ependymal cells: Ependymoma
- Choroid plexus: Choroid plexus papilloma
- Meningeal cells: Meningioma
- Ganglion cells and neural cells: Ganglioneuroma

The simplified **WHO 2016 classification of CNS** tumours is presented in Table 42.2.

ASTROCYTOMA

Different types of astrocytic tumours are recognized. These occur in the cerebral hemispheres and may also occur in the cerebellum, brainstem or spinal cord. They commonly occur during 4th–6th decades.

Astrocytomas can be:
1. Localised (grade I astrocytoma): Pilocytic astrocytoma and subependymal giant cell astrocytoma
2. Infiltrating (grade II to grade IV astrocytomas)

Clinical Features

The most common presenting signs and symptoms are seizures, headache, and focal neurologic deficits related to the anatomic site of involvement.

Pilocytic Astrocytoma

Pilocytic astrocytomas are Grade I astrocytomas, occur in children and young adults and these are relatively benign tumours. They are located in the cerebellum but may also appear in the floor and walls of the third ventricle, the optic nerve and occasionally cerebral hemispheres.

Table 42.2 Classification of CNS tumours[51]	
Astrocytic and oligodendroglial tumours	**Mixed glial and neuronal**
Astrocytoma	Ganglioneuroma
Diffuse astrocytoma IDH mutant	**Embryonal tumours**
Diffuse astrocytoma NOS	Medulloblastoma
Gemistocytic astrocytoma	• WNT activated
Anaplastic astrocytoma IDH mutant	• SHH activated and TP53 mutant
Glioblastoma IDH mutant and IDH wild type	• Non-WNT and Non-SHH activated
Glioblastoma NOS	• Classical
Oligodendroglioma NOS	• Desmoplastic
Oligodendrogliolma IDH mutant and 1p/19q codeleted	• Anaplastic
Oligoastrocytoma NOS	• NOS
Anaplastic oligodendroglioma IDH mutant and 1p/19q codeleted	Pineloblastoma
Other astrocytic tumours	Neuroblastoma
Pilocytic astrocytoma	Atypical teratoid rhobdoid tumour
Subependymal giant cell astrocytoma	**Nerve sheath tumours**
Pleomorphic xanthoastrocytoma	Neurofibroma
Anaplastic pleomorphic xanthoastrocytoma	Schwannoma
Ependymal	Malignant peripheral nerve sheath tumour (MPNST)
Subependymoma	**Meningiomas**
Ependymoma RELA fusion positive	Meningioma
Myxopapillary ependymoma	Atypical meningioma
Papillary ependymoma	Anaplastic meningioma
Clear cell ependymoma	**Tumours of sellar origin**
Anaplastic ependymoma	Pituitary adenoma
Choroid plexus	Craniophyaryngioma
Choroid plexus papilloma	**Miscellaneous**
Atypical choroid plexus papilloma	CNS lymphoma
Choroid plexus carcinoma	Germ cell tumour
Tumours of neural origin	Haemangioblastoma
Ganglioneuroma	Malignant melanoma
Neuroblastoma	**Metastatic tumours**

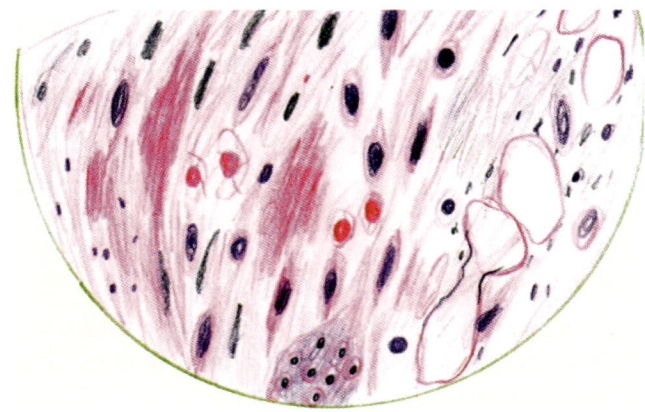

Fig. 42.5: Pilocytic astrocytoma (schematic)

Gross: Pilocytic astrocytoma is often cystic and if solid well circumscribed. They have localized growth.

Microscopy: The tumour is composed of bipolar cells with long, thin "hair-like" processes that are GFAP-positive and form dense fibrillary meshwork. Cystic areas, Rosenthal fibres and eosinophilic granular bodies are often present. Necrosis and mitoses are absent (Fig. 42.5).

Site: Cerebellum, spinal cord, optic nerve (neurofibromatosis 1).

Treatment and prognosis: Amenable to excision with good prognosis.

SUBEPENDYMAL GIANT CELL ASTROCYTOMA (SEGA)

This has benign course and grouped under WHO grade I. SEGA occurs exclusively in young patients and children. They may be symptomatic or asymptomatic tumours. They arise within the wall of the ventricles or may present as intraventricular mass producing obstructive features because of hydrocephalus.

These tumours can be seen in patients with tuberous sclerosis, who present with mental retardation and seizures. Earlier the onset of seizures, poor will be the intelluctual outcome of the patients.

Gross: SEGA presents as focal discrete and firm lesions. These are often calcified and showing cystic degeneration.

Microscopy: The tumour cells are having prominent nucleoli and abundant eosinophilic cytoplasm, consist of large pleomorphic giant cells. There is clustering of tumour cells and perivascular pseudopallisading is seen. Mast cells and calcification may be present.

Infiltrating astrocytoms can be:

1. Diffuse astrocytomas
2. Anaplastic astrocytoma
3. Glioblastoma

Diffuse Astrocytoma

This is WHO grade II and has following different histological types:

1. Pleomorphic xanthoastrocytoma
2. Gemistocytic astrocytoma

The protoplasmic astrocytoma and fibrillary astrocytoma have been taken out in WHO 2016 classification.

Site: Supratentorial region commonly frontal lobes.

Age: 20–30 yrs.

Gross: These tumours, as the name suggests, are having highly infiltrative type of growth, they diffusely involve the white matter of the brain. It extends to different parts of the brain and the borders cannot be determined. Cut section is firm or soft and gelatinous. Cystic degeneration may be seen.

Microscopy: The tumour is cellular and shows fibrillary background. There is variable degree of pleomorphism. Necrosis and mitoses indicate higher grade and aggressive course.

The cells having abundant eosinophilic glassy cytoplasm with eccentric nuclei and prominent nucleoli are called gemistocytic astrocytoma. The background of the tumour has fibrillary network and GFAP and Vimentin are positive.

Anaplastic Astrocytoma

This is of WHO grade III and have densely cellular and have greater degree of pleomorphism. The cells show increased mitotic activity.

Glioblastoma

This was previously called glioblastoma multiforme (GBM), corresponds to WHO grade IV.

Age: Above 40 yrs of age.

Types: *De novo*—primary.

Secondary: Develops from the pre-existing anaplastic astrocytoma.

Sites: This tumour can occur in any part of the brain but more common in the supratentorial region, rare in cerebellum and spinal cord.

Gross: GBM is having infiltrative type of growth; they have variegated appearance solid, cystic and soft areas represent necrosis and haemorrhage (Fig. 42.6).

Microscopy: The tumour cells are highly anaplastic with pleomorphic nuclei. The cells range from spindle to epithelial, bizarre giant cells sometimes round cells seen. Good numbers of mitotic figures are seen. The hallmark and diagnostic point is the presence of necrosis and vascular proliferation. Two types of necrosis noted: One is pseudopalisading wherein tumour cells surround the necrotic foci and another is foci of necrosis. A criterion for vascular endothelial proliferation is vessel having more than two endothelial layers. With marked vascular endothelial cell proliferation, the tuft forms a ball-like structure, called the glomeruloid body (Fig. 42.7).

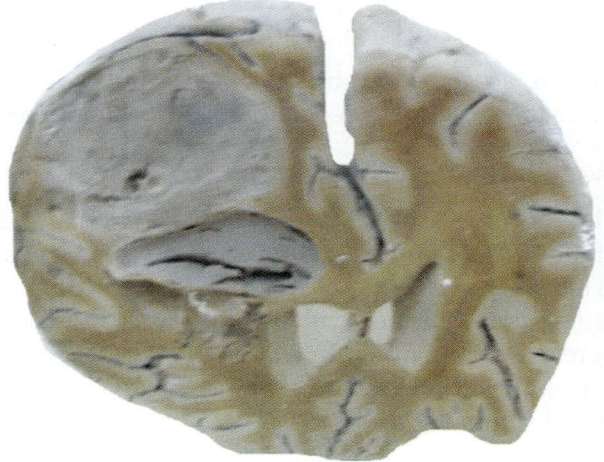

Fig. 42.6: Brain tumour (gross picture)

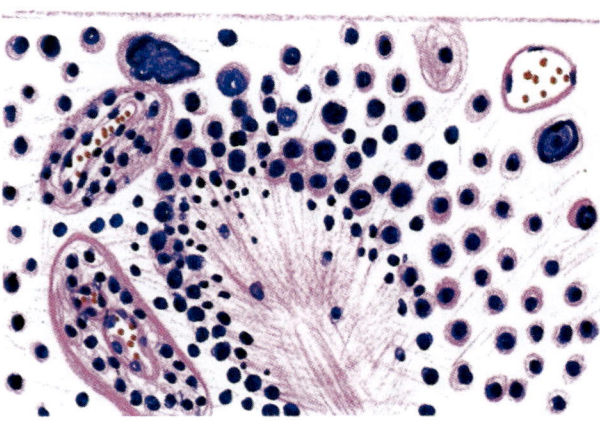

Fig. 42.7: Microscopy of glioblastoma (schematic)

Glioblastoma Cerebri

This is a diffuse glioma with extensive infiltration of multiple regions of brain, sometimes involving entire brain. This has aggressive course.

OLIGODENDROGLIOMA

- These account for 5–15% of gliomas.
- Occur in fourth and fifth decades.
- The lesions are found mostly in the cerebral hemispheres, with a predilection for white matter.

Morphology

Gross: Oligodendrogliomas are gelatinous, gray masses, often with cysts, focal haemorrhage and calcification.

Microscopy: The tumours are composed of sheets of regular cells with spherical nuclei containing finely granular chromatin and containing small nucleoli. Perinuclear halo is present giving **"fried egg"** appearance. The tumour typically contains a delicate network of anastomosing capillaries **(chicken wire network)**. Calcification is seen in 90% of the cases (Fig. 42.8).

Anaplastic Oligodendrogliomas

These are characterised by increased cellular density, nuclear anaplasia, increased mitotic activity and necrosis.

Molecular Markers in Gliomas[52–54]

Mutations of isocitrate dehydrogenase (IDH) 1 and 2 mutations and 1p/19q deletion are used as prognostic markers. The gliomas with these mutations and deletions are associated with overall good survival and progression free survival of the patient. IDH mutant forms have good prognosis and progession free survival compared to wild type.

Glioblastomas occur in two forms—primary and secondary. Primary glioblastomas are *de novo*, occur without the pre-existing tumours and associated with

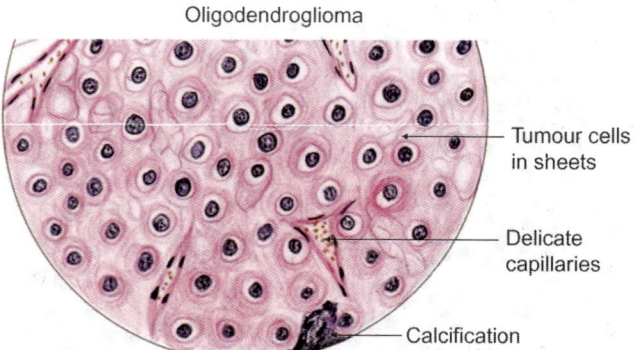

Oligodendroglioma

— Tumour cells in sheets

— Delicate capillaries

— Calcification

Fig. 42.8: Microscopy of oligodendroglioma (schematic)

mutation in PTEN, deletion of chromosome 10 and amplification of EGFR. Secondary glioblastomas arise from the anaplastic astrocytoma and are associated with mutation of IDH1 and IDH2, over expression of PDGFRA and P53 mutations.

NOS is applied when (1) genetic testing is not available, (2) genetic testing does not show diagnostic alterations, or (3) uncertainity of tumour architecture/cytological features or insufficient tissue.

KIAA 1549–BRAF15-9 fusions are common with midline pilocytic astrocytoma than within the cerebellum.

EPENDYMOMA

These tumours arise from the ependymal lining of the ventricle, hence they are common in lateral ventricle, fourth ventricle and in spinal cord. The tumours range from Grade I to Grade III. Grade I are subependymoma and myxopapillary ependymoma most frequently occur in adults whereas ependymomas (WHO grade II) and anaplastic ependymomas (WHO grade III) occur in children.

The tumour usually stains positive for glial fibrillary acidic protein, vimentin, and CD56. Supratentorial ependymomas with *RELA* fusion positive are associated with unfavourable prognosis. Group A posterior fossa ependymomas are enriched for the CpG island methylator phenotype and group B posterior fossa ependymomas are associated with extensive chromosomal abnormalities. Group B posterior fossa ependymomas are transcriptionally similar to spinal ependymomas and have a better prognosis than group A ependymomas.

Subependymoma

This is WHO grade I and arises from the subependymal glia, has indolent course and accidentally detected at autopsy. They occur in ventricles and spinal cord.

Gross: They appear as pedunculated masses.

Microscopy: Consists of tumour cells resembling subependymal glia with or without pleomorphism and anaplasia. These tumour cells are embedded in a fibrillary framework with areas of microcystic change and calcification. They have indolent course, but because of the site, they may present with obstructive hydrocephalus.

Myxopapillary Ependymoma

This tumour is WHO grade I and arises from the ependymal cells in the region of filum terminale and cauda equina. As the name suggests, these tumours will have myxoid and papillary structures. They have benign and indolent course.

Both subependymoma and myxopapillary ependymoma will have benign and indolent course and may pose to problem to the neurosurgeon due to their site.

Ependymoma Grade II

Cell of origin:
- Ventricle: Ependymal cells.
- Parenchyma: Stem cell with ependymal differentiation.

Age: 2nd–3rd decade.

Gross: They appear gray-white and localised lesions.

Microscopy: They show tumour cells arranged in true rosettes, pseudorosettes, and ependymal canals and in solid pattern. True rosette is the one where tumour cells surround the blood vessel without intervening fibrillary matrix. In pseudorosettes, the tumour cells surround the blood vessel but both are separated by intervening fibrous tissue. Mitotic activity is inconspicuous.

Anaplastic Ependymoma (WHO Grade III)

These are similar to Grade II but exhibit increased mitotic activity.

These are malignant gliomas with ependymal differentiation, hypercellularity, nuclear pleomorphism, high mitotic activity, microvascular proliferation, and pseudopalisading necrosis. As in grade II ependymomas, perivascular pseudorosettes are common. Areas of cytologic atypia, including increased nuclear-to-cytoplasmic ratio and cellular pleomorphism, may be seen.

CHOROIDAL PLEXUS TUMOURS

They are rare; they arise from the epithelium lining the choroid plexus. The tumour may arise in cerebellopontine angle from embryonic remnants of choroid plexus analage. These tumours occur in ventricles. These are commonly seen in children. These are graded by the WHO classification as choroid plexus papilloma (WHO grade I), atypical choroid plexus papilloma (WHO grade II), and choroid plexus carcinoma (WHO grade III).

Gross: These tumours have circumscribed cauliflower-like growth masses that are adhering to ventricular wall, but well delineated from the brain parenchyma.

Microscopy: Shows papillary-like pattern with delicate fibrovascular core, the papillae are lined by colllumnar cells with basally placed nuclei. Mitotic activity is very less.

EMBRYONAL/UNDIFFERENTIATED TUMOURS

MEDULLOBLASTOMA

Medulloblastoma is the most common of all the embryonal tumours, occurs in children and confined to the cerebellum. The tumour occurs in the midline of the cerebellum, well circumscribed and has variegated appearance having solid and cystic and soft areas.

Microscopy: Classical medulloblastoma shows small blue round cells, the tumour cells are carrot-shaped and undifferentiated, they have hyperchromatic, pleomorphic nuclei with anaplasia, the cytoplasm is scanty. Good number of mitotic figures are present. The tumour cells are arranged in solid pattern, sheets and in rosettes (Homer-Wright). At places, they show neuronal differentiation which appears as pale areas. The tumour cells exibit GFAP (glial) and synptophysin (neuronal) markers. Neuronal differentiation is associated with good prognosis.

Nodular desmoplastic variant is associated with more pronounced neuronal differentiation marked by synptophysin positivity.

Large Cell/Anaplastic Variant

In this, the tumour cells have more anaplasia and large cells and carries a bad prognosis.

NEWER MOLECULAR CLASSIFICATION OF EMBRYONAL/UNDIFFERENTIATED TUMOURS

1. WNT type: Classical medulloblastoma—good prognosis.
2. SHH type: Nodular medulloblastoma— intermediate prognosis.
3. MYC amplification—worst prognosis.
4. Isochromosome 17q—poor prognosis.

Tumours with similar morphology in children are also noted in pineal region and are termed as pineloblastoma and in cerebrum they are called CNS PNET.

ATYPICAL TERATOID/RHABDOID TUMOUR

This is a childhood tumour, highly malignant and occurs in cerebellum. The tumour cells are rhabdoid in morphology and resemble rhabdomyosarcoma. The tumour is characterised by loss of INI 1 mutation. This serves as molecular diagnostic marker. These tumours carry bad prognosis.

CNS LYMPHOMAS

Lymphomas of the CNS are rare tumours, constituting 4% of all intracranial neoplasm 4–6% of extranodal lymphoma.

Types

- Primary: No lymphoma else where.
- Secondary: Involvement of CNS lymphoma due to systemic lymphomas.

Primary CNS Lymphomas

They occur in two settings—in immunocompetent individuals and in immunodeficiency patients. In immunocompetent individuals, the tumour usually occurs after the age of 60 yrs. The etiology is not known and is not associated with EBV. Immunocompromised patient lymphoma occurs early and is EBV associated. The immunodeficiency conditions which can pre-dispose to lymphoma are AIDS, chemotherapy for cancer, transplant recipient, connective tissue disorder.

Gross: These tumours occur as a circumscribed localised lesion in the supratentorial region which mimics like a glioma. The lesion is periventricular in location. It will have variegated appearance having solid, cystic and areas of necrosis. They can also present as an infiltrative growth involving more than one lobe what is called lymphomatosis cerebri.

Microscopy: The tumour is similar to lymphoma else where, i.e. they are monomorphic population of lymphoid cells in sheets and in follicle formation, these tumours also surround the blood vessel (angiocentric). Immunohistochemistry helps in diagnosis.

Secondary Lymphoma

It commonly involves the subarachnoid space and shows CSF pleocytosis. CSF examination and flow cytometry is needed for diagnosis.

GERM CELL TUMOUR

Germ cell tumours are rare intracranial neoplasms. They occur in the central axial of the body in sellar and suprasellar regions. The similar to testicular counterpart of seminoma is called germinoma. Before making a diagnosis of primary germ cell tumour of CNS, meta-stasis from testis needs to be ruled out.

MENINGIOMA

Although histogenesis of meningioma is uncertain, it is thought to arise from arachnoid cells. These tumours usually occur in adults and in all locations including spinal cord. They compress the underlying parenchyma producing neurological deficits.

Like mesothelial cells, meningothelial cells are also having divergent differentiation hence it is having many variants.

Gross: These tumours are having well-circumscribed with a fibrous capsule. They may grow enplaque, the tumour spreads in sheet-like fashion along the surface of the dura. Grossly haemorrhage and necrosis are absent. They invade the skull and dura mater and compress the underlying brain parenchyma.

Microscopy: Varies different histological types. Following are the different variants:

1. *Meningothelial meningioma:* Meningeal cells show epithelial differentiation, consist of lobules of meningothelial cells separated by fibrous tissue.
2. *Fibrous meningioma:* Meningothelial cells show mesenchymal differentiation, consist of spindle cells intermingled with collagen fibres.
3. *Transitional meningioma:* Combination of mesen-chymal and fibrous meningioma.
4. *Psammomatous meningioma:* It is of the transitional type with good number of psammoma bodies commonly occur in vertebral column.
5. *Angiomatous meningioma:* A variant consisting pre-dominantly of hyalinised blood vessel surrounded by meningothelial cells.
6. *Microcystic meningioma:* Consists predominantly of microcystic areas.
7. *Secretory meningioma:* This variant will have PAS +ve, secretory granules in the cytoplasm.
8. *Lymphoplasmacyte rich meningioma:* Meningioma with lymphoplasmacytic differentiation.
9. *Metaplastic meningioma:* Here the stroma shows metaplstic tissues like cartilage, bone, etc.

The variant does not have prognostic significance. Most of the meningiomas are of WHO Grade I which are benign tumours with indolent course.

Atypical Meningioma

This meningioma is of WHO Grade-II. Any of the above mentioned meningioma exhibiting increased mitotic count >4/10 HPF or with brain parenchyma invasion. These tumours have clear cells or chrondroid morpho-logy.

Anaplastic/Malignant Meningioma

This is WHO grade III. Mitoses are high. Any of the above mentioned grade I meningiomas with mitotic activity >20/10 HPF. Papillary or rhabdoid morphology menin-gioma. Grade II and III meningiomas carry a high risk of recurrence hence patient needs to be followed.

CRANIOPHARYNGIOMA

It is a tumour arising from the Rathke cleft/remnants of the craniopharyngeal duct and situated in sellar and suprasellar regions. There are two types of cranio-pharyngioma. One is adamantinomatous and the other is papillary type. These tumours show islands of squmous epithelium surrounded by columnar epithelium with whorls of mature keratin. In papillary variant, papillae are seen.

PITUITARY ADENOMA

This tumour occurs in sellar or suprasellar region. Commonly presents with visual disturbances. They are classified based on the hormone which they elaborate.

METASTATIC TUMOURS

Metastatic tumours are most common neoplasm in adults and they constitute only 2% in case of paediatric neoplasm.

Cerebral hemisphere is the most common site of metastasis. These lesions are situated in watershed areas of the brain. The lesions may be single or multiple. Tumours reach the brain either by direct extension or through haematogenous route. Most of the time, they are singles or they may be multiple.

Table 42.3	Syndromes and CNS tumour association
Neurofibromatosis 1	Neurofibroma, meningioma, schwannoma
Neurofibromatosis 2	Schwannoma
VHL disease	Hamangioblastoma
Tuberous sclerosis	SEGA
Li-Fraumani syndrome	Glioblastoma, astrocytoma
Cowden syndrome	Dysplastic cerebellar gangalio-neuroma
Turcot syndrome	Glioma
Naevoid basal cell carcinoma	Medulloblastoma
Rhabdoid tumour	ATRT

Common tumours which can metastasis to brain are lung carcinoma, breast, melanoma and renal cell carcinoma. In paediatric age group, lymphoma and leukaemia are common. In the spinal cord, NHL, renal cell carcinoma, lung, breast and prostate are common (Table 42.3).

SELF-ASSESSMENT EXERCISE

1. **Child with abnormal gait is:**
   A. Acoustic neuroma   B. Medulloblastoma
   C. Craniopharyngioma D. Astrocytoma

2. **Hormone oxytocin is produced from following pituitary area:**
   A. Pars tuberalis   B. Pars anterior
   C. Posterior lobe   D. Paraventricular nucleus

3. **Fever, headache and Durck's granuloma most likely seen in:**
   A. Cerebral malaria   B. Encephalitis
   C. Neurocysticercosis D. Cerebral toxoplasmosis

4. **Flexner-Wintersteiner rosettes are seen in:**
   A. Hepatoblastoma   B. Retinoblastoma
   C. Nephroblastoma   D. Neuroblasttoma

5. **Most common CNS tumour in NF1 is:**
   A. Optic nerve glioma   B. Meningioma
   C. Astrocytoma   D. Schwannoma

6. **Rosenthal fibres are seen in following:**
   A. Glioblastoma multiforme
   B. Medulloblastoma
   C. Pilocytic astrocytoma
   D. PNET

7. **Meningioma arises from:**
   A. Meningael cells of arachnoid layer
   B. Neuronal cells

   C. Oligodendrocytes
   D. Astrocytes

8. **Pilocytic astrocytomas are:**
   A. WHO grade I tumours
   B. WHO grade II tumours
   C. WHO grade III tumours
   D. WHO grade IV tumours

9. **Vast majority of primary brain lymphomas are of:**
   A. B cell type   B. T cell type
   C. NK cell   D. Precursor B cell

10. **Most common CNS tumour in HIV patients is:**
    A. Non-Hodgkin lymphoma B cell
    B. Non-Hodgkin lymphoma T cell
    C. Non-Hodgkin lymphoma NK cell
    D. Hodgkin lymphoma

11. **Seizures, mental retardation, hemiplegia, facial naevus and angiomas are seen in:**
    A. Sturge-Weber syndrome
    B. Tuberous sclerosis
    C. VHL disease
    D. Von Recklinghausen disease

12. **Phagocytic cells of brain are:**
    A. Microglia   B. Neuronal cells
    C. Oligodendrocytes   D. Astrocytes

Answers

| 1. B | 2. C | 3. A | 4. B | 5. D | 6. C | 7. A | 8. A |
| 9. A | 10. A | 11. A | 12. A | | | | |

Skin Lesions

VIRAL INFECTIONS

These include infection by poxvirus (molluscum contagiosum), human papilloma virus and herpes group.

MOLLUSCUM CONTAGIOSUM

The virus belongs to poxvirus group which is a DNA virus. Mainly children, and persons with impaired cellular immunity are commonly affected.

IP period: 14 to 50 days.

Mode of spread: Skin-to-skin contact and auto-inoculation (Koebner phenomenon), contact with fomites and sexual contact.

Clinical findings: The lesions are firm; smooth-surfaced and dome-shaped pearly white papules. They are 3 to 5 mm in diameter. Central umbilication is characteristic. They are common on face, trunk and extremities.

Pathology: There is inverted cup-shaped lesion comprised of acanthotic squamous cells. There are eosinophilic intracytoplasmic inclusions (Handerson-Patterson bodies) and progressively enlarge until it fills the cell cytoplasm. These cells are finally extruded from the central crater like ostium.

Course: These resolve spontaneously in immuno-competent patients or may need immunomodulators, cryotherapy or electrodissection.

VIRAL WARTS

These are caused by human papilloma virus of papovavirus group.

Clinical findings: They may be flat (verruca plana), papule (verruca vulgaris) or filiform.

Verruca Vulgaris

These usually present as multiple papules on hands. Microscopy has hyperkeratosis, acanthosis, hypergranulosis, parakeratosis and elongation of rete pegs. The rete pegs curve inward and point towards the centre. Large cells called koilocytotic cells are seen in the upper epidermis. The cytoplasm of these cells is vacuolated, the nucleus is small, dark, hyperchromatic with irregular contours.

INFLAMMATORY DERMATOSIS

These can be acute or chronic. The acute can be urticaria, acute eczematous dermatitis and erythema multiforme. The chronic lesions include: Psoriasis, lichen planus and lichen simplex chronicus. The details of psoriasis and lichen planus are given below.

PSORIASIS

Psoriasis is a chronic disorder resulting from triggering factors like trauma, infection, medications, psychological stress, etc. The prevalence of psoriasis is around 2% of the world's population. It may be associated with arthritis, myopathy and enteropathy.

Pathogenesis: Psoriasis is a immunological disease. The inciting antigens are from self or environment. The sensitized CD4 and CD8 T cells accumulate in the epidermis.

Morphology: The characteristic lesion is a sharply demarcated erythematous plaque with silvery white scales.

Microscopy: The scaly red plaque is due to hyperkeratosis, parakeratosis, acanthosis with downward elongation of rete ridges. There is loss of stratum granulosum. Over the tips of the dermal papillae

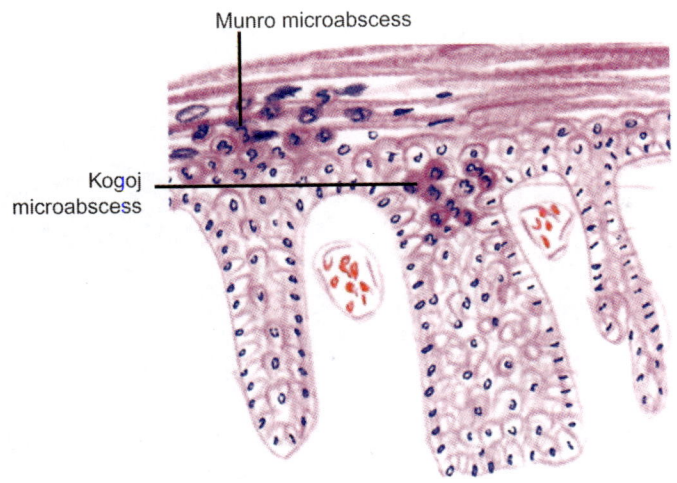

Fig. 43.1: Microscopy in psoriasis (schematic)

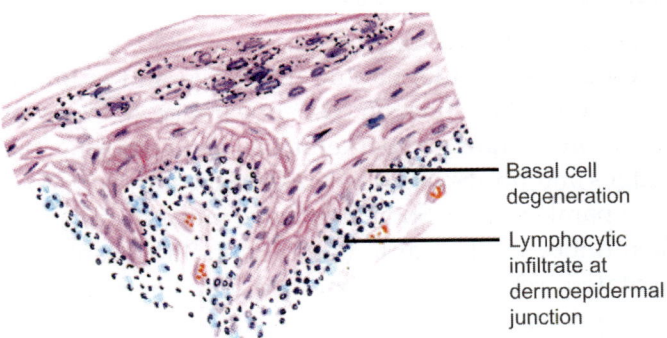

Fig. 43.2: Microscopy in lichen planus (schematic)

(suprapapillary), the epidermal cell layer is thinned out. The blood vessels within the papillae are dilated and tortuous. These vessels bleed easily when the scale is removed (Auspitz sign). Neutrophils form abscesses in parakeratotic layer (Munro microabscess) and in the spongiotic superficial epidermis (pustule of Kogoj) (Fig. 43.1).

Clinical features: Psoriasis affects most commonly skin of elbows, knees, scalp, lumbosacral areas intergluteal cleft and glans penis. The most common lesion is a well demarcated pink to salmon-coloured erythematous plaque covered with loosely adherent silvery white scale. Nail changes may occur in 30% of the cases.

LICHEN PLANUS

Lichen planus in a self-limited disorder which resolves within 1–2 years of onset.

Pathogenesis: The exact etiology is not known. There is expression of altered antigens at the basal layer of epidermis. D-E junction has CD8+ T cells. The altered antigen could be due to viral infection or due to drugs.

Morphology: Grossly, has pruritic violaceous flat-topped papules which coalesce and form plaques. Microscopically, has hyperkeratosis, no parakeratosis, focal increase in granular cell layer, irregular acanthosis with sawtoothed appearance of the rete pegs. There is basal cell degeneration of basal layer and band like lymphocytic infiltrate at dermo-epidermal junction. Colloid bodies (civatte, hyaline or cytoid) are apoptotic or dyskeratotic keratinocytes and are present in the epidermis. Vacuolar changes in the basal layer may show separation between epidermis and dermis

(Max-Joseph spaces). There is pigment incontinence and accumulation of dermal melanophages (Fig. 43.2).

Clinical features: Pruritic, purple, polygonal, planar papules and plaques are "Ps" of lichen planus. Mucosal lesions may be seen in 15% of the patients. The plaques may have white dots or lines called Wickham's striae. The lesions are multiple and these are symmetrically distributed. There may be hyperpigmentation of the lesions.

ADENEXAL TUMOURS

These can be classified as below:

1. **Tumours with follicular differentiation:**
   - *Benign:* Pilar sheath acanthoma, trichofolliculoma, infundibuloma, trichoblastoma and tricho-epithelioma, tricholemmoma and pilomatricoma.
   - *Malignant:* Basal call carcinoma, pilomatrix carcinoma.

2. **Tumours with eccrine differentiation:**
   - *Benign:* Eccrine adenoma, apocrine adenoma, hidradenoma papilliferum, syringoma, syringo-cystadenoma papilliferum, acrospiroma, spiradenoma, cylindroma, chondroid syringoma, myoepithelioma.
   - *Malignant:* Microcystic adenexal carcinoma (sweat duct adenocarcinoma), malignant poroma, hidradenocarcinoma, cribriform carcinoma, apocrine carcinoma (mucinous adenocarcinoma), extramammary Paget's diseases, sweat gland carcinoma, adenoid cystic carcinoma, malignant myoepithelioma and carcinosarcoma.

Basal cell carcinoma is described later in this chapter. The details of rest of the adnexal tumours are not in the purview of this book and can be referred from the dermatology textbooks.

TUMOURS ARISING FROM THE STRATIFIED EPITHELIUM

SEBORRHOEIC KERATOSIS

This is a benign tumour occurring in skin. Clinically, presents as macule, papule or plaque and is brown coloured. It has stuck on end appearance. Microscopy most often shows hyperkeratosis, anastomosing rete ridges and horn cysts. They may show papillomatosis and parakeratosis. Some may have melanocytes in the keratinocytes. The different variants like acanthotic, irritated, reticulated, pigmented, etc. have differing microscopic features.

SQUAMOUS CELL PAPILLOMA

This benign tumour arises from the stratified squamous epithelial surface. The epithelium proliferates and is thrown into papillary folds which become increasingly complex. The proliferation is accompanied by a corresponding growth of supportive connective tissue.

Etiology: Chronic irritation and infection with human papilloma virus (HPV) are two proposed etiologies. HPV 6 and HPV 11 have been implicated for squamous cell papilloma in different sites.

Gross: It is a warty growth with finger-like projections.

Microscopy: This benign neoplasm shows a papillomatous lesion lined by hyperplastic and hyperkeratotic stratified squamous epithelium. The thin core of the papillae has lymphatics and blood vessels, e.g. wart (Figs 43.3 and 43.4).

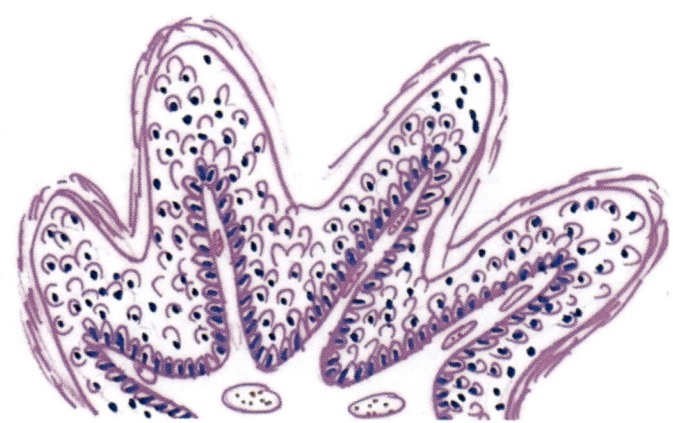

Fig. 43.4: Microscopy of sqamous cell papilloma (schematic)

SQUAMOUS CELL CARCINOMA

Predisposing factors for this malignant tumour are as follows: Exposure to UV light, chemicals (tars and oils), chronic ulcers such as Marjolin's ulcer, burn scars, osteomyelitis, radiation, tobacco and betel nut chewing, xeroderma pigmentosum and so on.

HPV 16 and 18 are associated with squamous cell carcinoma of skin as well as squamous cell carcinoma of genital system.

Gross: The tumour presents as a nodular cauliflower-like growth. It is prone to bleed and ulcerate (Fig. 43.5).

Microscopy: The epithelium shows atypical squamous cells. There is a breach in the basement membrane and the neoplastic cells invade the subepithelial tissue. The cells are polygonal with atypical pleomorphic nuclei, arranged in sheets and exhibit good amount of keratinisation (well-differentiated/keratinizing) to highly anaplastic cells with scanty or no keratinisation (poorly differentiated/non-keratinising) (Figs 43.6 and 43.7).

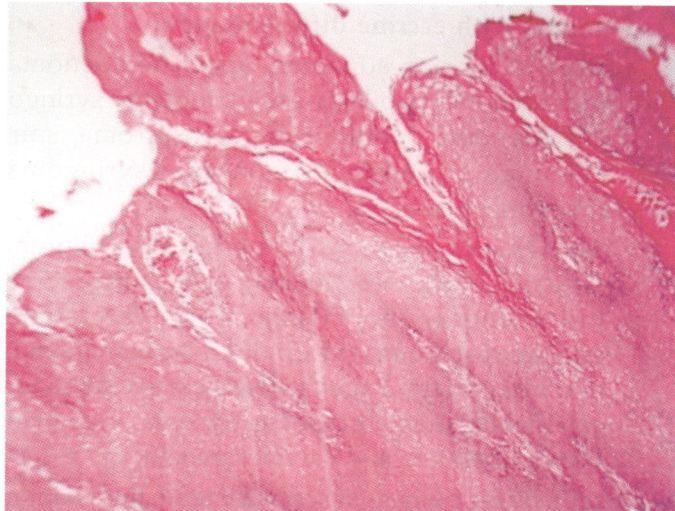

Fig. 43.3: Microphotograph of sqamous cell papilloma, note papillae lined by stratified squamous epithelium; shows hyperkeratosis

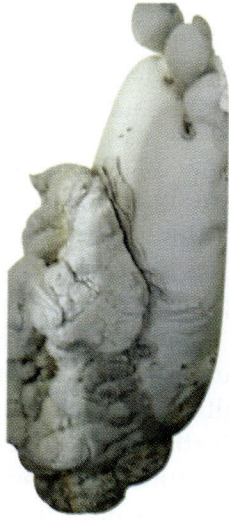

Fig. 43.5: Squamous cell carcinoma (gross picture)

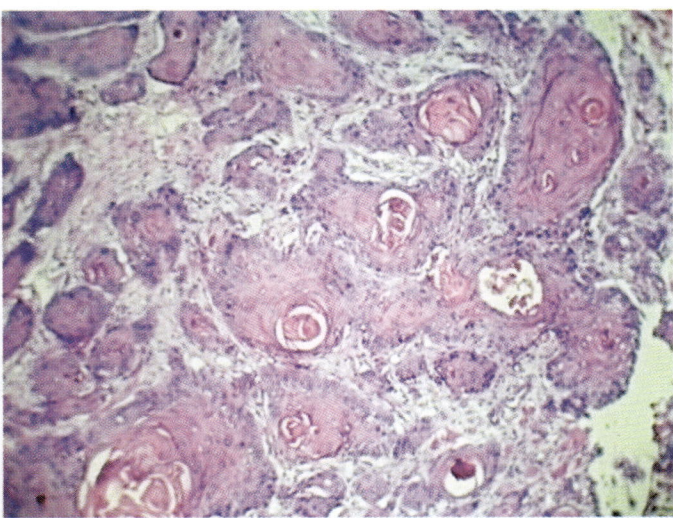

Fig. 43.6: Microphotograph, note malignant squamous cells with epithelial pearls

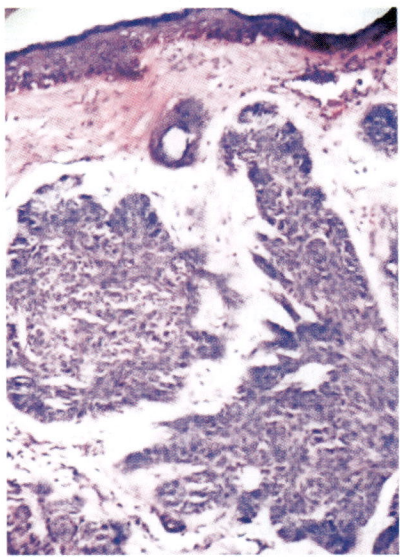

Fig. 43.8: Microphotograph of basal cell carcinoma, note islands of cells and peripheral cells showing palisaded nuclei

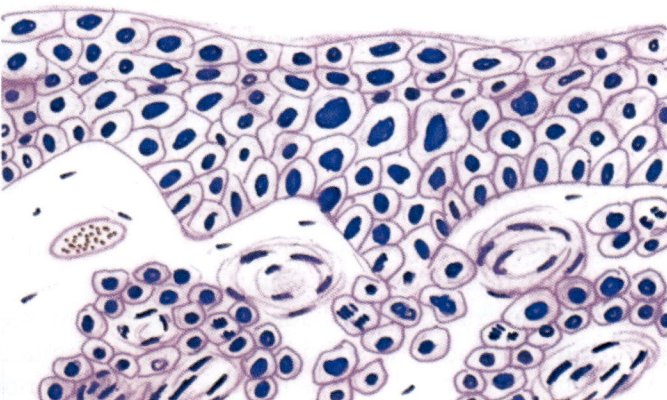

Fig. 43.7: Microscopy of sqamous cell carcinoma (schematic)

BASAL CELL CARCINOMA (BCC)

It is a slow growing, locally malignant tumour which rarely metastasizes.

Predisposing factors: Light pigmented people (Whites), immunosuppression and other predisposing factors similar to squamous cell carcinoma.

It occurs in elderly people. It arises from the basal epithelium or from the follicular epithelium.

Clinically, there are three types:

1. **Nodular BCC:** It is pearly white, firm nodule with ulceration and adjacent telangiectasia.

2. **Superficial BCC:** This presents as erythematous flat lesion having distinct pearly white raised border with adjacent telangiectasia.

3. **Morphoeic BCC:** It shows depressed white plaque with erythematous border.

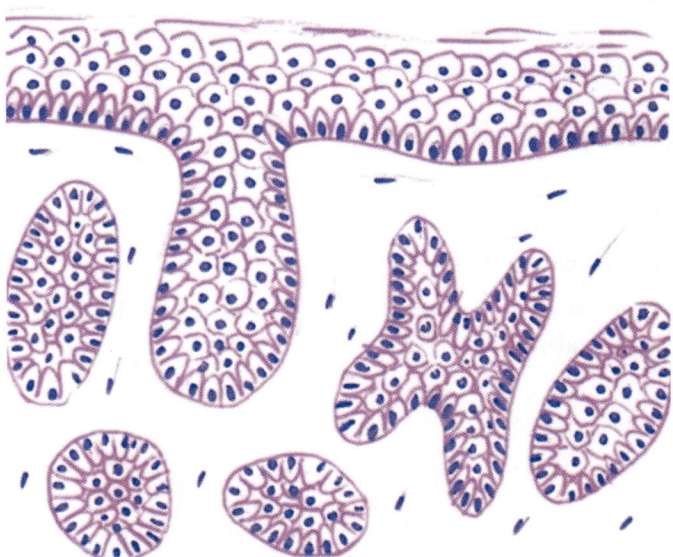

Fig. 43.9: Basal cell carcinoma (schematic)

Microscopy: The cells grow from basal epithelium downwards into the dermis as cords or islands. The neoplastic cells are basophilic with slight nuclear enlargement and hyperchromatic nuclei. The nuclei of the peripheral cells are arranged in palisading pattern (Figs 43.8 and 43.9).

MERKEL CELL CARCINOMA

This is also called neuroendocrine carcinoma of skin, presents as erythematous or violaceous papule or nodule. The cells are small to intermediate and sometimes large blue cells with scant cytoplasm with finely granular (salt and pepper) nuclei. Nuclear moulding is seen. Organoid pattern may be present. These express neuroendocrine markers, CK20 and other markers.

MELANOCYTIC LESIONS

NAEVUS

Mole or melanocytic naevus is generally used to designate localized benign lesion of melanocytes.

These are acquired or congenital.

Majority are located in the skin and mucous membranes.

These naevi can be categorised as:
- Junctional naevus
- Intradermal naevus
- Compound naevus

Junctional Naevus

- The melanocyte proliferation is restricted to the basal portion of the epithelium (junctional area).
- Naevi of palms and soles are of this type.
- **Grossly,** flat or slightly elevated, non-hairy.
- **Microscopically,** nests of melanocytes are seen on epithelial side of the dermoepidermal junction.
- Malignant melanoma can arise from these lesions.

Intradermal Naevus

The proliferated melanocytes are in the dermis. It may be flat, pedunculated or papillomatous.

Compound Naevus

Junctional and dermal components, melanin production is abundant (Figs 43.10A and B).

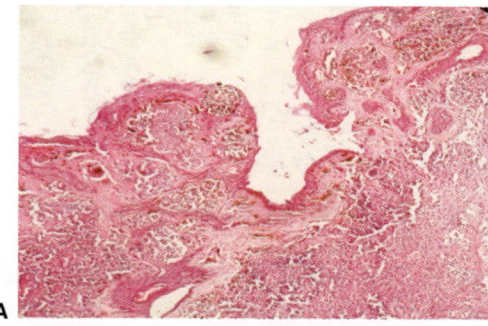

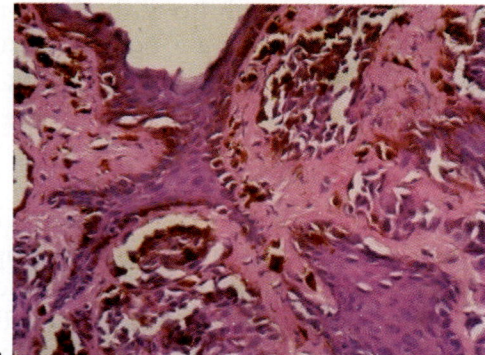

Fig. 43.10A and B: Microphotographs of naevus (compound naevus)

MALIGNANT MELANOMA

Majority of the melanomas arise from:
- Skin especially of head and neck area and lower extremities
- The other sites are:
  - Oral and anogenital mucous membranes
  - Palms and soles
  - Subungual region
  - Esophagus
  - Meninges
  - Eye: Uvea, choroid, ciliary body, conjunctiva, eyelid

Etiology and Predisposing Factors

- Sunlight plays important role.
- People who develop freckles after sun exposure are susceptible.
- Lightly pigmented individuals (Whites/fair-skinned) are more prone than the deeply pigmented individuals.
- Occurs in pre-existing dysplastic naevus.
- Mutations of B-raf oncogene, CMM1 gene on chromosome 1p36 and tumour suppressor gene mapped on 9p21 are found in some families.

Clinical Features

Malignant melanomas are usually asymptomatic. Itching or pain may be early sign.

Change in colour with shades of black, brown, red dark-blue, and grey is striking feature in malignant melanoma. Unlike benign neavi, the borders are not smooth, round and uniform.

The warning signs of malignant melanoma (ABCD rule) in naevus are:
1. **A**symmetry of shape
2. **B**order irregularity
3. **C**olour variation
4. **D**iameter more than 6 mm

Morphological Features in General—Malignant Melanoma

Gross: Malignant melanoma usually presents as ulcero-nodular friable mass. It is grey to black in colour. The naevus with malignant change shows irregular enlarging borders; it has itching and shows change of colours (Fig. 43.11).

Microscopy: There is junctional activity of melanocytes. The neoplastic cells may be epithelioid or spindle shaped. The cells may be extremely bizarre. The cytoplasm can be eosinophilic, basophilic, foamy or clear. Melanin pigment in the cytoplasm of these cells may be abundant, scant or absent. The nuclei are

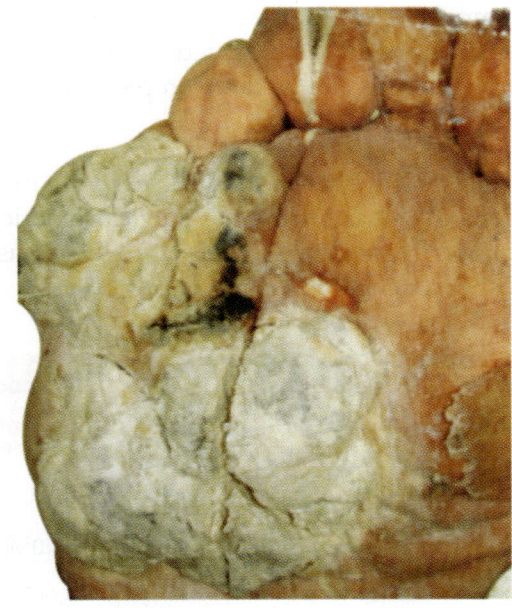

Fig. 43.11: Malignant melanoma (gross picture)

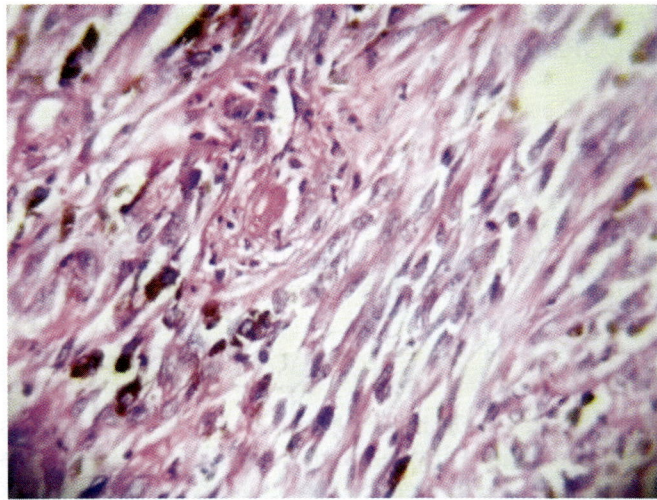

Fig. 43.12: Microphotograph of malignant melanoma

markedly atypical. The cells have vertical growth phase and radial growth phase (Figs 43.12 and 43.13).

Malignant melanoma cells are positive for vimentin, S-100, HMB-45, Melan-A (Mart-1), and tyrosinase. However, desmoplastic variety is positive for S-100; HMB-45 and Melan-A are negative.

The different types of malignant melanomas are:
1. Superficial spreading melanoma
2. Nodular melanoma
3. Acral (lentiginous) melanoma
4. Lentigo maligna (Hutchinson's freckle) melanoma

Superficial spreading melanoma:
1. This is the most common form. It has variegated appearance, has different shades of colours from blue admixed with tan, brown or black.
2. The surface is slightly elevated, margins are barely palpable.
3. May have white areas.
4. The borders are irregular and notched.
5. With deep invasion, there is appearance of elevated nodule on the surface.
6. Microscopically, shows proliferation of atypical melanocytes with nest formation along the basal layer of the epithelium.

Nodular melanoma:
1. It is an uncommon form, appears in short duration, in younger people.
2. Presents as a nodule covered with epithelium, or as an elevated blue black plaque, or as a polypoid ulcerated mass.
3. It has vertical growth.

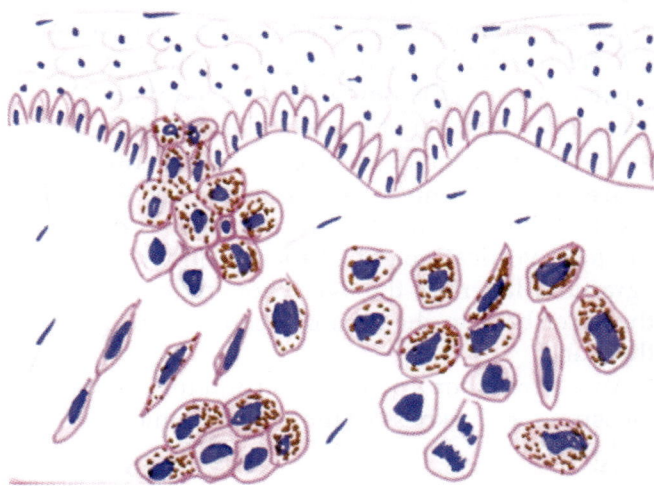

Fig. 43.13: Malignant melanoma microscopy (schematic)

Acral (lentiginous) melanoma:
1. Has intraepidermal radial and vertical growth.
2. Atypical melanocytes are present in dermo-epidermal junction with focal upward growth. In vertical growth phase, atypical melanocytes fill and expand the papillary dermis.

Lentigo maligna (Hutchinson's freckle) melanoma:
1. Typically seen in elderly
2. Sun-exposed areas
3. Fair-skinned people or Whites
4. Flat slowly growing lesion
5. Colour varying from tan to black
6. Microscopically, proliferation of atypical melano-cytes at the basal layer distributed individually and in nests. The cells are spindle shaped.
7. This has low degree of aggressiveness.

Most of the malignant melanomas produce melanin pigment; however, some may not and in such instances demonstration of presence of an enzyme thyrosinase by DOPA reaction can diagnose amelanotic melanomas.

DOPA Reaction

Melanin is produced from tyrosine by the action of an enzyme tyrosinase (DOPA oxidase). To know the presence of the enzyme, DOPA reaction test is done. If the enzyme is present in the tissue (as in amelanotic melanoma) acts on dihydroxyphenylalanine (DOPA)

and demonstrates the presence of an enzyme DOPA oxidase/tyrosinase which converts DOPA into melanin-like pigment. This can be done on paraffin sections or frozen sections.

Note: False positive results may be seen with mast cells. Mast cells can be confirmed by metachromatic stains. IHC for Mart-1, Melan-A, S-100 HMB-45 are usual for diagnosing amelanotic melanoma.

NICE TO KNOW

The Clark levels refer to how deep the tumour has penetrated into layers of the skin. This system was originally developed by WH Clark, in 1966. Clark levels are defined as follows:
- *Level I:* Confined to the epidermis (intraepidermal/ *in situ* melanoma).
- *Level II:* Invasion of the papillary (upper) dermis.
- *Level III:* Filling of the papillary dermis, but no extension into the reticular (lower) dermis.
- *Level IV:* Invasion of the reticular dermis.
- *Level V:* Invasion of the deep subcutaneous tissue.

Breslow thickness first reported by Alexander Breslow, in 1970, the Breslow thickness is defined as the total vertical height of the melanoma, from the **"granular layer"** of the overlying epidermis or from the ulcer base to the area of deepest penetration in the skin.[55]

An instrument "ocular micrometer" is used to measure the thickness of the excised tumour.

Risk assessment depending upon the depth of tumour

Risk	Depth of invasion
Low risk	Up to 0.76 mm
Intermediate risk	0.76 to 1.5 mm
High risk	More than 1.5 mm

Staging system for cutaneous melanoma of the American Joint Committee on Cancer[56]

Stage	Description
0	Melanoma *in situ*, Clark level I (pTisN0M0)
IA	Localized melanoma ≤0.75 mm thick or Clark level II (pT1N0M0)
IB	Localized melanoma 0.76–1.50 mm thick or Clark level III (pT2N0M0)
IIA	Localized melanoma 1.51–4.00 mm thick or Clark level IV (pT3N0M0)
IIB	Localized melanoma >4.00 mm thick or Clark level V (pT4N0M0)
IIIA	Regional lymph node(s) metastasis ≤3 cm in the greatest dimension (any pT, N1M0)
IIIB	Regional lymph node(s) metastasis >3 cm in greatest dimension and/or in-transit metastasis (any pT, N2M0)
IV	Distant metastasis (any pT, any N, M1)

pT: primary tumour; N: lymph node; M0: no distant metastasis; M1: distant metastasis

SELF-ASSESSMENT EXERCISE

1. **Recurrent pain and diarrhoea are seen in:**
   A. Dermatitis herpetiformis
   B. Bullous pemphigoid
   C. Herpes simplex infection
   D. Pemphigus vulgaris

2. **Red-coloured lesions on skin with diagnosis of Kaposi sarcoma: Causative agent is:**
   A. HHV8
   B. HPV
   C. HTLV1
   D. Candida

3. **Munro abscesses are seen in:**
   A. Psoriasis
   B. Lichen planus
   C. Mycosis fungoides
   D. Bullous pemphigoid

4. **Civatte bodies seen in:**
   A. Psoriasis
   B. Lichen planus
   C. Pemphigus vulgaris
   D. Inflammatory dermatosis

5. **Acantholytic cells in pemphigus vulgaris are from:**
   A. Stratum basalis
   B. Stratum spinosum
   C. Stratum granulosum
   D. Keratinous layer

6. **Mutation in malignant melanoma may be of:**
   A. BRCA   B. N-myc
   C. Rb   D. BRAF

7. **Marker of malignant melanoma is:**
   A. Cytokeratin   B. AFP
   C. CEA   D. HMB-45

8. **Antibodies to desmogleins, transmembrane desmosomal adhesion molecules seen in:**
   A. Pemphigus vulgaris
   B. Psoriasis
   C. Lichen planus
   D. Inflammatory dermatosis

9. **Mycosis fungoides is malignant disorder of following cells:**
   A. T cells   B. B cells
   C. NK cells   D. Null cells

Answers

1. A	2. A	3. A	4. B	5. B	6. D	7. D	8. A

9. A

Eye Lesions

In eye, following can be encountered:
- Conjunctivitis: Bacterial, viral, chlamydia, etc.
- Corneal ulcers
- Vitamin A deficiency features
- Inflammation of lacrimal duct

Other common lesions and tumourous conditions:
- *Conjunctival tumours:* Dermoid cyst, papilloma, adenoma, naevus, Bowen's disease and squamous cell carcinoma, basal cell carcinoma and malignant melanoma.
- *Lacrimal gland:* Benign mixed tumour, malignant mixed tumour, adenoid cystic carcinoma, muco-epidermoid carcinoma and adenocarcinoma.
- *Eyelid lesions:* Blepharitis (bacterial and parasitic), inflammation of meibomian glands, stye, chalazion, papilloma, xanthelasma, haemangioma, kerato-acanthoma, actinic keratosis, squamous cell carcinoma, basal cell carcinoma, sebaceous gland carcinoma or meibomian gland carcinoma and malignant melanoma.
- *Orbit:* Hypertensive retinopathy, retinitis pigmentosa, dermoid cyst, meningioma, lymphoproliferative lesions, retinoblastoma, malignant melanoma, mesenchymal tumours (vascular tumours, optic nerve glioma, etc.) and metastatic tumours (from breast, lung, prostate, kidney, thyroid, GIT, etc.)

The detailed description of all the entities of eye is out of reach of this book. Only some of the lesions are given below.

TRACHOMA

This is caused by *Chlamydia trachomatis.* This produces chronic keratoconjunctivitis with intracytoplasmic inclusions. The disease is more common in poor socio-economic group individuals and dry and dusty weather.

Direct spread, vector spread, or with use of common towels and handkerchiefs is known in this disease.

Clinical Features
- Foreign body sensation
- Stickiness of eyelids
- Scanty discharge
- With secondary infection: Mucopurulent discharge

On examination, the following findings may be noticed.
- Follicular conjunctivitis
- Intense inflammation of conjunctiva
- Trichiasis
- Corneal opacity
- Scarring

Diagnosis
- Conjunctival cytology: Plenty of neutrophils and plasma cells and Leber cells
- Detection of inclusion bodies with Giemsa stain
- ELISA for chlamydia antigens
- Isolation of organisms (yolk sac inoculation and tissue culture)
- Serotyping

Complications: Corneal opacity and blindness.

CHALAZION/TARSAL/MEIBOMIAN CYST

This is chronic granulomatous lesion of meibomian glands. The ducts are blocked and there is lipogranulomatous inflammation of the glands.

STYE/EXTERNAL HORDEOLUM

Definition: This is an acute inflammation of eyelash follicles and associated glands of Zeis or Moll. *Staphylococcus aureus* is the commonest organism causing this inflammation. One or multiple stye may be present.

Clinical features: Pain, swelling, watering and photophobia are the usual symptoms.

Pathology: There is stage of cellulitis or abscess formation.

INTERNAL HORDEOLUM

Definition: This is acute inflammation of the meibomian glands due to *Staphylococcus aureus* organisms.

Clinical features and pathology: These are almost similar to external hordeolum.

RETINITIS PIGMENTOSA

Retinitis pigmentosa is retinal dystrophy affecting mainly rods than cones. This occurs as inherited (AD or AR or X-linked) or sporadic disorder.

Clinical features: Night blindness due to degeneration of rods and dark adaptation is not affected until late in the disease process.

MEIBOMIAN GLAND CARCINOMA/SEBACEOUS GLAND CARCINOMA OF EYELID

Eyelid is the most common site for sebaceous/meibomian gland carcinoma.

RETINOBLASTOMA

Retinoblastoma is a common intraocular malignancy of childhood. The incidence decreases with age and diagnosed usually before 4 years of age. It develops from primitive embryonal retinal cells (retinoblasts) either photoreceptors or neuronal cells.

Retinoblastoma is either familial or sporadic. Familial are usually multifocal and bilateral. They may be unifocal and unilateral. Familial retinoblastomas are at increased risk of developing osteosarcoma and other soft tissue tumours. Sporadic, non-hereditary tumours are usually unifocal and unilateral. There is no sex predilection.

Pathogenesis of Retinoblastoma

RB gene is a cancer suppressor gene. In familial form (heritable or germline mutation), all somatic cells inherit one mutation of RB gene on long arm of chromosome locus 13q14 and the second mutation is seen after birth. Mutations of RB gene on both the alleles lead to neoplastic proliferation (Knudson's two hit hypothesis).

In sporadic form (non-heritable or somatic mutation), both the mutations occur after birth.

Clinical Features

- Median age is 2 years; tumour may be present at birth.
- Presents with poor vision
- Strabismus (squint)
- Leukocoria or whitish hue of the pupil (cat's eye reflex)
- Painless proptosis having retrobulbar mass
- Nystagmus: Rarely with bilateral retinoblastoma

Pathology

Gross: The tumour arises from posterior part of retina, it is grey-white with nodular and friable areas. The mass may be endophytic or exophytic. In endophytic growth, the tumour mass is polypoidal protruding into the vitreous cavity. In exophytic growth, mass spreads outwards and separates the retina from choroid. Exophytic tumours have higher risk of choroid invasion while endophytic growth pattern has risk of vitreous seeding (Figs 44.1A and B).

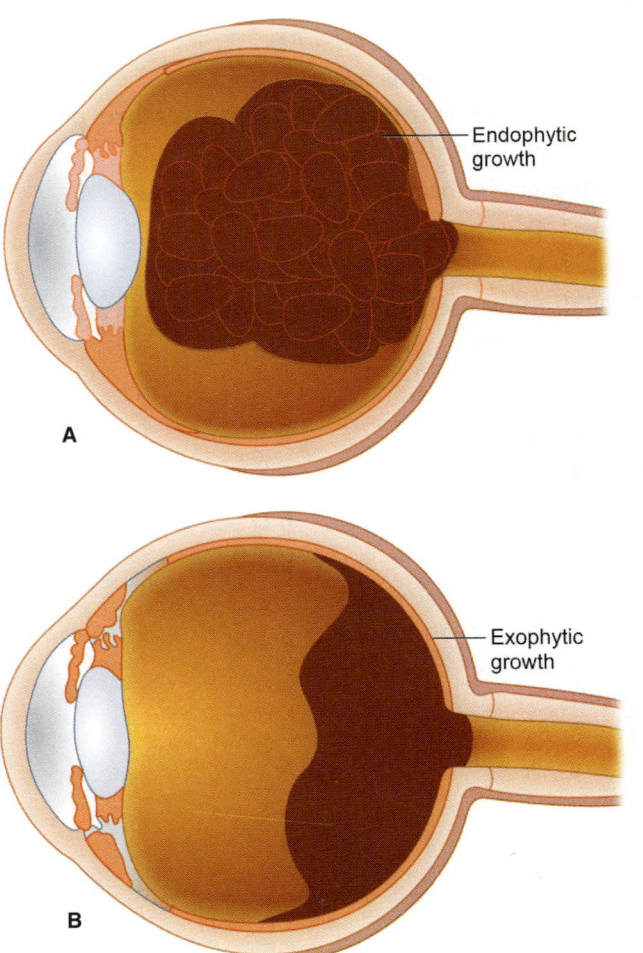

Fig. 44.1A and B: Gross appearance in retinoblastoma (schematic)

Microscopy Fig. 44.2): The tumour cells are small and round cells with hyperchromatic nuclei and scanty cytoplasm (undifferentiated cells). **Flexner-Wintersteiner rosettes** are present which are collection of cuboidal to low columnar cells around a central lumen. The nuclei are displayed away from the limiting membrane. Necrosis with or without calcification is a prominent feature.

The tumour cells may disseminate beyond the eye directly through optic nerve and subarachnoid spaces. Distant metastasis is seen in CNS, skull and other bones and lymph nodes.

Management includes chemotherapy and radiotherapy. Untreated tumours are fatal. Prognosis is good with early treatment with enucleation, chemotherapy and radiotherapy. Some tumours may regress on their own.

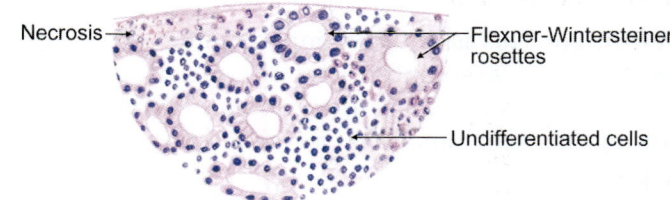

Fig. 44.2: Microscopy in retinoblastoma (schematic)

MALIGNANT MELANOMA OF EYE

Malignant melanoma can commonly arise from choroid, ciliary body and iris. It can also arise from eyelids and conjunctiva. The gross and histopathological features will be similar to melanomas occurring in othe areas.

SELF-ASSESSMENT EXERCISE

1. **Which of the following is false about retinoblastoma?**
   A. It is the most common malignant eye tumour of childhood
   B. Cause for cat's eye reflex
   C. Sporadic forms are multifocal
   D. Flexner-Wintersteiner rosettes are present histologically

2. **RB gene is located on following gene:**
   A. 13p   B. 13q
   C. 16p   D. 16q

3. **Malignant melanoma of eye can occur in all *except*:**
   A. Choroid
   B. Iris
   C. Ciliary body
   D. Lacrimal duct

4. **Chalazion is a chronic inflammatory granulomatous lesion of the following:**
   A. Meibomian gland
   B. Sweat gland
   C. Gland of Zeis
   D. All of the above

5. **All are true about trachoma *except*:**
   A. Causes blindness
   B. High socioeconomic group
   C. Intracytoplasmic inclusions
   D. Corneal opacities

Answers

1. C   2. B   3. D   4. A   5. B

Addendum

Following competencies which are not covered in the text are listed and described below.
1. Disseminated intravascular coagulation (DIC)
2. Blood components and their clinical use
3. Role of a pathologist in diagnosis and management of disease
4. Cellular aging
5. Obesity and its consequences
6. HLA system and immune principles in transplant and transplant rejection.
7. Tumour-like lesions, benign and malignant diseases of infancy and childhood.
8. Causes of splenomegaly.
9. Lung abscess.
10. CSF findings in meningitis.

DISSEMINATED INTRAVASCULAR COAGULATION (DIC)

The syndrome of DIC (synonyms: consumption coagulopathy, defibrination syndrome) is an acquired condition due to activation of coagulation system (intrinsic/extrinsic) leading to reduced coagulation factors and platelets resulting in bleeding. DIC can be acute or chronic. Acute DIC develops with sudden exposure of blood procoagulants and chronic DIC has compensated state. Causes include the following.

Acute DIC

1. Obstetric complications: Abruptio placentae, amniotic fluid embolism, abortion, intrauterine death and retained products
2. Malignancies: Acute promyelocytic leukaemia (AML-M3), metastatic mucus-secreting adenocarcinoma
3. Gram-negative septicaemia
4. Miscellaneous causes: Surgery (lung/heart), massive trauma, snake bite, severe burns, fat embolism and heat stroke

Chronic DIC

1. Disseminated or localized carcinoma
2. Septicaemia
3. Obstetric causes
4. Miscellaneous causes

Mechanism

The mechanism that activates intrinsic and extrinsic pathways of coagulation is complex. Endothelial injury, heat stroke, endotoxins, etc. activate intrinsic pathway.

Massive trauma, tissue injury, burns, obstetric complications, AML-M3, etc. release tissue thromboplastin activating extrinsic pathway. This leads to intravascular coagulation, leading to reduced platelets and coagulation factors resulting in profuse bleeding. There is release of plasmin with fibrin degradation products (FDPs) and D-dimer. Plasmin has inhibitory action on coagulation factors promoting further bleeding.

Clinical Manifestation of Acute DIC

1. Bleeding from venipuncture site
2. Bleeding from various sites: Gum bleeding, pulmonary haemorrhage, intracranial haemorrhage, etc.
3. Microangiopathic haemolytic anaemia
4. Acute renal failure
5. State of shock

Laboratory Diagnosis

- Platelets: Reduced
- PT: Increased
- APTT: Increased
- TT: Increased
- FDPs: Present
- D-dimer: Present
- Peripheral smear: Shows fragmented RBCs

Management

1. Primary cause to be treated
2. Transfuse platelets, fresh frozen plasma (FFP), and coagulation factors
3. Heparin therapy.

BLOOD COMPONENTS AND THEIR CLINICAL USE

The blood components are necessary for the following reasons.
1. From whole blood, various components can be prepared. Whole blood storage conditions are not optimal for all functional components of blood. For example, after 24 hours of storage at 1 to 6°C, whole blood has few viable platelets and granulocytes. Stable coagulation factors are well maintained during storage, but heat labile factors like factors V and VIII decrease with time and may not be adequate to correct specific deficiencies in patients. The separation of various components, allow storage of each component at the temperature and storage conditions required for *in vitro* survival.

2. Component preparation allows transfusion of specific portion of blood product that the patient requires.

3. Transfusion of required components avoids use of unnecessary whole blood transfusion which could be contraindicated in some conditions. For example, risk of hypervolemia in an elderly anaemic patient with congestive cardiac failure may not tolerate the transfusion of two units of whole blood.

4. Also, whole blood exposes to unnecessary antibodies. It also has white blood cells and platelets which can carry HLA antigens and can stimulate the patient's immune system.

Indications for Different Components

Red Cells Transfusion

1. Patients with symptomatic anaemia
2. Newborn exchange transfusion.
3. Major surgeries
4. Haemorrhage
5. Leukaemia
6. Intrapartum haemorrhage
7. Thalassaemia cases

Transfusion of Platelets

1. In prophylaxis of haemorrhage: Platelet count of <10 × 10^9/l, coagulation disorders, petechiae, ecchymosis

2. Prior to surgical or invasive procedures, with platelet count of <50 × 10^9/l

3. In case of microvascular bleeding without thrombocytopenia, when impairment of platelet function is confirmed by laboratory tests. Platelets are transfused, if this impairment cannot be treated by other ways (e.g. in case of congenital platelet disorders).

4. Performing epidural anaesthesia or analgesia, with platelet count of <100 × 10^9/l.

5. In case of normal vaginal delivery, thrombocytopenia of <50 × 10^9/l is safe without need for prophylactic platelet transfusion.

Transfusion of Fresh Frozen Plasma (FFP)

1. Coagulopathy and bleeding of different origin
2. Bleeding in case of disseminated intravascular coagulation (DIC)
3. Thrombotic thrombocytopenic purpura
4. Congenital or acquired deficiency of different coagulation factors, when there is no possibility to get a certain factor concentrates (e.g. V or XI)
5. Deficiency of specific plasma proteins (e.g. antithrombin III)
6. Bleeding due to warfarin therapy.

Transfusion of Cryoprecipitate

1. Factor VIII deficiency
2. Haemorrhage due to hypofibrinogenaemia or dysfibrinogenaemia
3. DIC syndrome
4. Von Willebrand's disease
5. Haemorrhage due to factor XIII deficiency

ROLE OF A PATHOLOGIST IN DIAGNOSIS AND MANAGEMENT OF DISEASE

Pathologists are medical specialists, who have considerable skills which enable them to contribute significantly to high quality of efficient and effective health care. The skills they develop because of training first as a medical practitioner and then as a specialist allow them to understand clinical disease processes, diagnostic methods and give them the specialised ability to report diagnostic tests.

A pathologist plays a crucial role in medical care. Sometimes he or she is the one who first gives the diagnosis and thus, helps the treating physician. The management of patients with disease inflammatory or neoplastic (either benign or malignant) is becoming ever more dependent on a knowledge of the pathology. The pathologist is well versed in diagnosing diseases on histopathology (tissues), haematology (blood), cytology (cells from tissues and fluids) and clinical pathology (urine, etc.), thus helps the clinician in treatment/management. The pathologist is also helpful in identifying the disease at an early stage of cancer by using Pap smears (e.g. carcinoma cervix), fine needle aspiration cytology (palpable and deep seat masses) and using tumour markers.

CELLULAR AGING

Cellular aging depends upon the biological changes taking place in the cells and tissue as we grow old. The changes of aging are due to following:
1. Functional and structural changes
2. Telomerase activity
3. Genetic factors
4. Increased oxidative stress

Functional and Structural Changes

There will be decline in muscle strength, cardiac reserve, nerve conduction, pulmonary function, kidney function, vascular elasticity and hair become grey. The muscle mass reduces and lipofuscin wear and tear pigment accumulates in cells and tissues. The size of the organ is smaller and appear brownish due to lipofuscin deposition. The changes are seen especially heart and brain.

Telomerase Activity

The ends of the chromosomes get shortened during mitosis and telomerase can replace these lost portions. Telomerase activity is reduced as cells age. Telomere shortening and chromosome instability are associated with premature aging syndromes and age-related diseases.

Genetic Factors

Progeria has genetic changes with changes occurring at early age and includes group of syndromes. Werner syndrome is an autosomal recessive disease with defects in WRN gene and these have hair loss, early cataract, atrophy of skin, osteoporosis and atherosclerosis. Hutchinson-Gilford syndrome has mutation of LMNA gene which produces abnormal protein Lamin A, that accumulates in the cells, produce early onset of baldness, cataract and coronary heart disease. Fanconi anaemia and Bloom's syndrome are also associated with progeria.

Increased Oxidative Stress

Increased oxidative stress with imbalance in reactive oxygen free radicals (ROS) production and removal mechanisms also contribute to aging. Increased ROS can cause damage to DNA, lipid peroxidation, and reduced protein synthesis.

OBESITY AND ITS CONSEQUENCES

Obesity is abnormal or excessive accumulation of body fat that threatens health and results with interaction of environment/lifestyle and genetic susceptibility factors.

Body Mass Index (BMI) Criteria

1. BMI of less than 25 kg/m^2 is normal.
2. 25 to 30 kg/m^2: Overweight
3. 30–35 kg/m^2: Moderate obesity
4. 35–40 kg/m^2: Severe obesity
5. More than 40 kg/m^2: Extremely high

Causes

1. Heredity
2. Sedentary lifestyle
3. Psychological problems
4. Fat and sugar rich diet

Pathogenesis

Obesity develops from imbalance in energy production and expenditure in the body. Mutation of leptin, disorders of adiponectin and ghrelin play role in pathogenesis of obesity. Leptin is a hormone produced from adipose tissue which acts on hypothalamus and suppresses food intake. Mutation of leptin cannot do this function. Adiponectin is another hormone produced from adipocytes which has anti-inflammatory, antidiabetic, antiatherogenic and cardioprotective properties. The secretion of adiponectin is reduced in obesity. Ghrelin is produced by stomach which increases appetite and stimulates release of growth hormones. Increased amounts of ghrelin can be observed in obesity.

Consequences of Obesity

1. Diabetes mellitus type 2
2. Atherosclerosis
3. Cardiovascular and lung diseases with premature death
4. Gallbladder diseases
5. Arthritis
6. Some cancers: Breast, colon, endometrial, esophageal, hepatocellular, renal, prostate, etc.

HLA SYSTEM AND IMMUNE PRINCIPLES IN TRANSPLANT AND TRANSPLANT REJECTION

Major histocompatibility complex (MHC) is a tightly linked cluster of genes, the products of which play a role in recognition and discrimination between self and non-self cells. These express proteins on the cell surface. They are of class I, II and III. These are located on chromosome 6p21.31 and also designated as human leucocyte antigen (HLA). These antigens are inherited in a dominant manner.

Class I MHC molecule is encoded by closely linked loci HLA-A, B and C. These are present on all nucleated cells. The antigen has polymorphic transmembrane α heavy chain (α1, α2 and α3) and non-polymorphic β2 microglobulin. Centre of α2 and α3 has a cleft to identify foreign peptides and present to CD8+ T cells for elimination.

Class II also has transmembrane molecules coded by genes in HLA-D region. These are: DP, DQ and DR. These are expressed on antigen presenting cells (APC), macrophages, dendritic cells and B cells. Class II molecules have two transmembrane chains α (α1, α2) and β (β1, β2). The centre of α2 and β2 has a cleft to identify non-self particles and present to T cells which in turn activate B cells for production of antibodies. Class III has genes for complement and cytokines. These are located in between class I and class II regions. Some of the diseases associated with MHC are:

1. Allergic disorders: HLA-A3
2. Ankylosing spondylitis: HLA-B27
3. Celiac disease: DR3, B8

4. Graves' disease: DR3, B8
5. Hashimoto thyroiditis: DR5
6. Type II diabetes mellitus: DR3, DR4, B8
7. Rheumatoid arthritis: DR4

Role of HLA in Transplant

Purpose of transplant: Damaged or non-functional tissues or organs require transplant. In allotransplant (one person to other), the transplanted tissue antigens are identified by the recipient's immune system unless donor and recipient are identical twins. If the recipient possesses all the antigens of the tissue to be transplanted, there will be no immune response or rejection. The patient is put on immunosuppression and HLA matching is done to prevent the rejection.

HLA molecules expressed on donor cells induce an antigenic stimulus by recipient's immune system which triggers immune rejection of transplanted tissue/organ/graft. Following are the types of rejections:

- **Hyperacute rejection** is caused within minutes to hours after transplant as vascularization is rapidly destroyed. This is because, recipient has pre-existing antibodies which are induced by prior blood transfusions, multiple pregnancies, or transplant. Antibodies bind to donor endothelial cells. Complement system is activated leading to thrombosis of the vessels which prevents vascularization. The transplanted organ becomes cyanotic, mottled and flaccid instead of becoming pink and turgid.

- **Acute rejection** begins as early as one week after transplant. The risk is highest in first 3 months. Recipient's CD8+ cells will recognize Class I MHC molecules on donor's nucleated cells and recipient CD4 T cells will recognize directly or indirectly MHC II molecules of the donor on APCs and destroy them. The cellular and humoral mechanisms play role. CD4 and CD8 cells are present in the interstitium along with oedema and mild haemorrhage. There can be deposition of antibody, complement and fibrin in the vessel wall causing vasculitis and thrombosis.

- **Chronic rejection,** there is indirect recognition of donor antigens processed and presented by recipient's MHC. There is activation of T cells with release of IL-2 and other cytokines which induce graft rejection. There is hyperplasia of the smooth muscle tissue of blood vessels with ischaemia, inflammation and fibrosis leading to loss of function of the transplant. This takes months to years after transplant.

    In renal transplant, above three major rejections are observed.

- **Graft versus host reaction** sometimes occurs wherein donor T cells attack host tissue leading to rejection.

TUMOUR-LIKE LESIONS, BENIGN AND MALIGNANT DISEASES OF INFANCY AND CHILDHOOD

The commonest tumour-like lesions, benign and malignant disorders of infancy and childhood are:

1. Hemangioma
2. Lymphangioma
3. Teratoma
4. Acute leukaemias
5. Retinoblastoma
6. Neuroblastoma
7. Hepatoblastoma
8. Paediatric CNS tumours (especially pilocytic astrocytoma)
9. Ewing's sarcoma
10. Osteosarcoma
11. Malignant lymphoma/Hodgkin disease

These are dealt in respective chapters.

CAUSES OF SPLENOMEGALY

1. Myeloproliferative diseases: Chronic myeloid leukaemia, myelofibrosis, polycythemia vera, essential thrombocythemia
2. Autoimmune haemolytic anaemia
3. Lymphoma/leukaemia
4. Metastasis
5. Storage diseases: Niemann-Pick, Gaucher
6. Cysts
7. Congestive: Cirrhosis, cardiac failure, etc.
8. Bacterial: Endocarditis, brucellosis, tuberculosis
9. Viral: Hepatitis, CMV, etc.
10. Protozoal: Malaria, etc.
11. Fungal

LUNG ABSCESS

Lung abscess has necrosis and cavitation.

Etiology: *Strept. pneumoniae, Staph. aureus, Strept. pyogenes, H. influenzae,* anaerobes.

Symptoms: Productive/copious foul smelling sputum, pleural pain present.

Clinical features: High fever, sputum production which is copious and fetid smelling, clubbing, fatigue, pleural rub, weight loss.

Diagnosis: Chest X-ray, CT, CT-FNA.

Complications: Bronchiectasis, recurrence of abscess, empyema.

CSF FINDINGS IN MENINGITIS

Pyogenic Meningitis

The following are the features.

i. CSF pressure increases to more than 180 mm H_2O

ii. Proteins increase with fibrinous coagulum to 100–500 mg/dl

iii. Sugar reduced to less than 40 mg/dl

iv. In centrifuged deposit, bacteria are present in 60–80% of the cases.

v. Cell count is very high, polymorphs range between 1000 to 10000 cells/cmm.

vi. Chlorides are reduced and may fall below 110 mmol/l.

Tuberculous Meningitis

The following are the features.

i. Pleocytosis with lymphocytes: 100 to 600 cells/cmm.

ii. Proteins elevated to 100–500 mg/dl, may exceed 2 g/l as the disease progresses.

iii. Glucose lowered to 30–45 mg/dl .

iv. Bacteria are present, but extremely difficult to demonstrate.

v. ZN staining and auramine staining can be applied.

vi. Pressure is increased.

vii. Opaque and on standing forms cobweb.

viii. Chlorides fall progressively, may be below 100 mmol/l.

Viral Meningitis

The following are the features.

i. Normal to moderate increase in CSF pressure.

ii. Cell count 5–300 cells/cmm and sometimes more than 1000 cells and lymphocytes predominate.

iii. Proteins: 30–100 mg/dl.

iv. Glucose: Normal/reduced.

Similes

1. **Ant hill:** External appearance in actinomycosis or fungal infections.

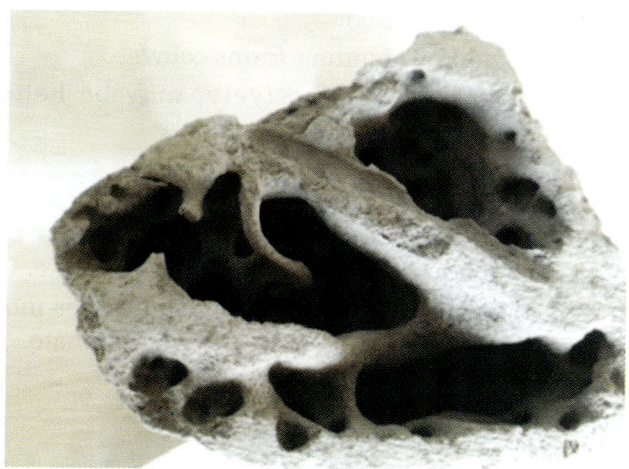

Ant hill: Actinomycosis or fungal infections

2. **Anchovy sauce:** Appearance of exudate/pus in Amoebic liver abscess.
3. **Antler horn pattern:** Cytology in fibroadenoma.
4. **Butterfly pattern of rash:** Malar rash in SLE (systemic lupus erythematosus).
5. **Bread and butter appearance:** Fibrinous pericarditis in rheumatic heart disease.
6. **Bite cells:** RBCs in G6PD haemolytic anaemia.
7. **Banana-shaped heart:** Shape of heart in hypertrophic cardiomyopathy.
8. **Banana-shaped gametocytes:** *P. falciparum* gamatocytes in RBCs.
9. **Button hole appearance:** Valves in rheumatic heart disease.

10. **Chicken wire collagen:** Perivenular collagen in alcoholic cirrhosis.
11. **Chicken wire appearance:** Anastomosing capillaries in oligodendroma and chondrosarcoma and liposarcoma.
12. **Crab:** For cancer.
13. **Cigar-shaped bundles:** Arrangement of *M. leprae* organisms in lepromatous leprosy.

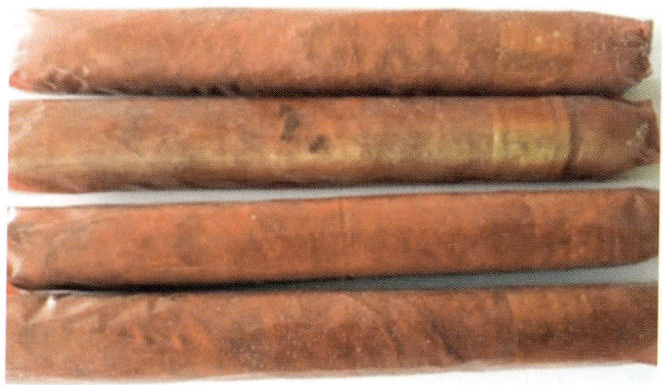

Cigar bundle: Lepra bacilli

14. **Cartwheel-shaped nuclei:** Chromatin arrangement in nuclei of plasma cells.
15. **Cobble stone appearance:** Mucosa of intestine in Crohn's disease.
16. **Cheese-like material:** Necrotic material in tuberculosis.
17. **Caterpillar appearance:** Wavy nuclei of Anitschkow cells in rheumatic heart disease.
18. **Coraline thrombus:** Propagating thrombus.

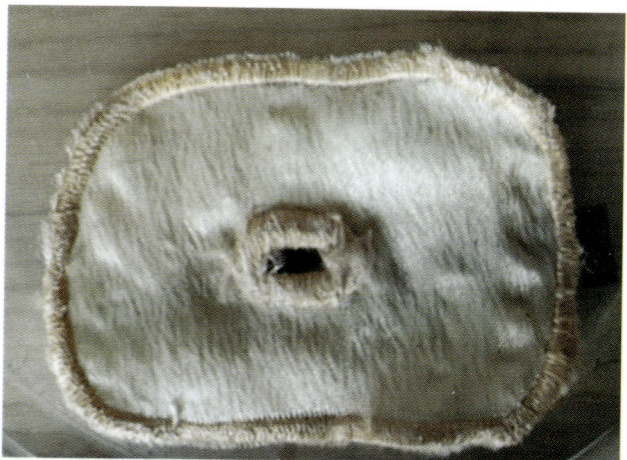

Button hole: Valves in rheumatic heart disease

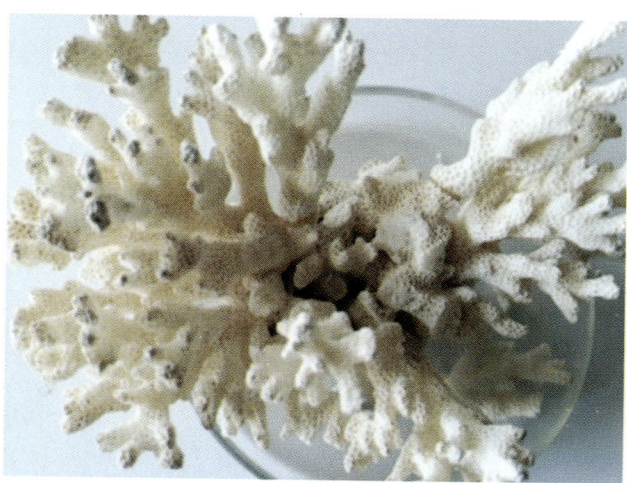

Corals (Coralline thrombus)

19. **Current jelly:** Postmortem clot due to stagnant blood, no time for separation of cells and plasma, red coloured giving jelly-like appearance.

20. **Chicken fat:** Postmortem clot due to stagnant blood slowly formed (blood separates into layers, lower red coloured due to RBCs, upper plasma layer) which is yellow or pale coloured.

21. **Coffee bean:** Nuclei with grooves, seen in cells of granulosa cell tumour and Brenner tumour.

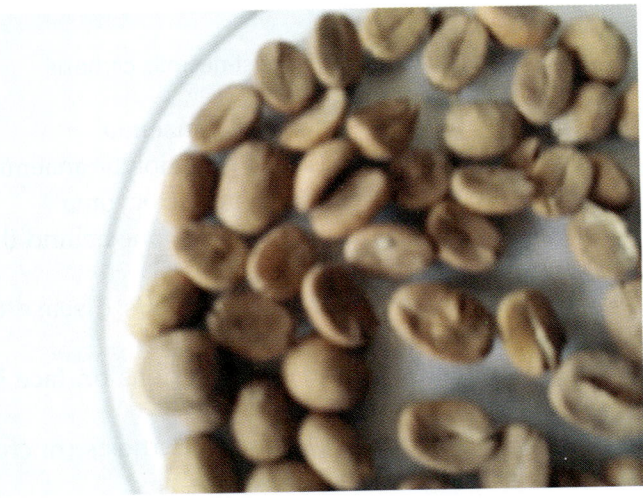

Coffee bean: Nuclei with grooves, cells of granulosa cell tumour and Brenner tumour of ovary

22. **Cartwheel appearance:** Cell arrangement in MFH, nucleus of plasma cell.

23. **Comedo appearance:** Necrotic material in DCIS (comedo carcinoma).

24. **Cambium layer:** Tumour cell arrangement in embryonal carcinoma.

25. **Carrot-shaped nuclei:** Nuclei of tumour cells in medulloblastoma.

26. **Crumple tissue paper appearance:** Cytoplasm of Gaucher cells.

27. **Cribriform pattern:** Adenoid cystic carcinoma, cribriform DCIS, prostatic carcinoma.

28. **Cob web:** Appearance of CSF due to increased proteins in tuberculous meningitis.

29. **Chinese letter:** Curvilinear bony trabaculae (woven bone) in fibrous dysplasia of bone.

30. **Club-shaped deformity:** Gross appearance of involved bone in osteoclastoma, one end bulged.

31. **Cannon ball appearance:** X-ray appearance of metastatic lesions in lung.

32. **Dumbell shaped:** Asbestos bodies.

33. **Dilapidated brick wall appearance:** Acantholytic cells in Hailey-Hailey disease (familial benign chronic pemphigus).

34. **Envelope-shaped crystals:** Oxalate crystals in urine.

35. **Egg shell crackling:** Thinned cortex of involved bone in osteoclastoma, with pressure gives egg shell crackling.

36. **Exodus ball:** Endometrial cells 6 to 10 days of menstrual cycle.

37. **Elephantiasis:** Filariasis obstructing lymphatics.

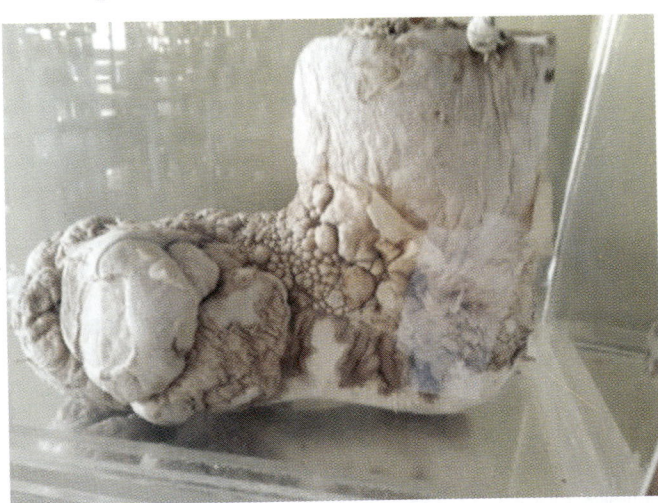

Elephantiasis foot (filariasis)

38. **Fern-like pattern:** Cervical mucin due to oestrogen activity.

39. **Fish mouth appearance:** Valves in rheumatic heart disease.

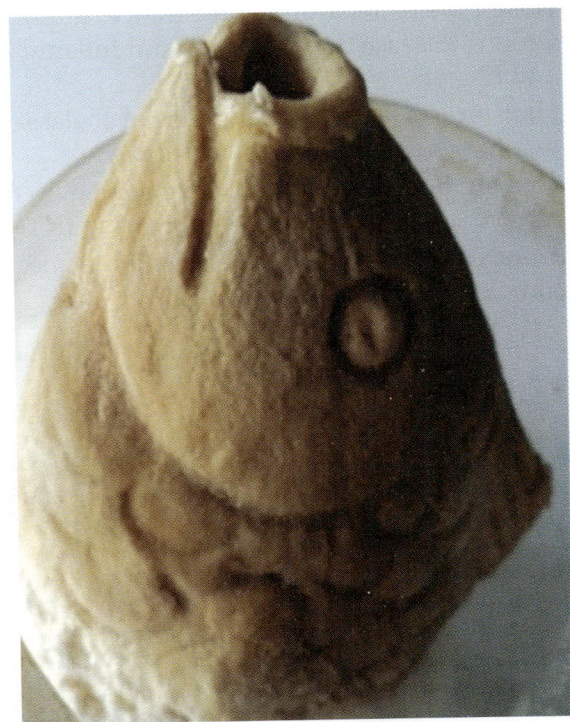

Fish mouth: Valves in rheumatic heart disease

40. **Fishnet pattern:** Immunofluorescence in pemphigus vulgaris.

41. **Fried egg appearance:** Cells of oligodendroglioma.
42. **Flea bitten kidney:** Kidney in RPGN and malignant HT.
43. **Grape-like structures:** Vesicular mole, gross appearance.

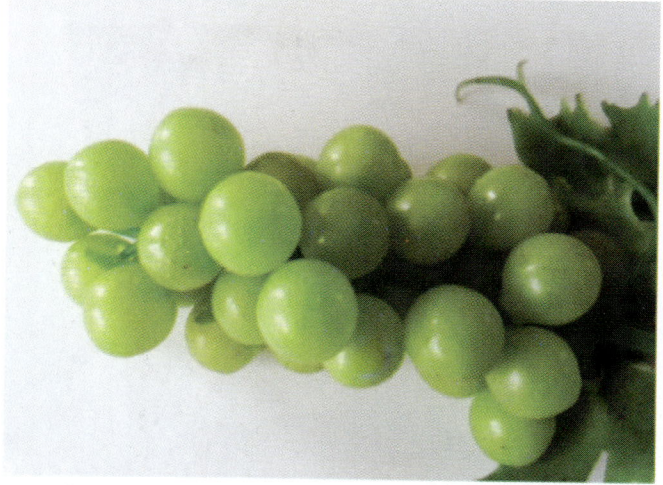

Grape-like structures: Vesicular mole, gross appearance

44. **Gritty sensation:** Dystrophic calcification of necrosis in carcinoma breast.
45. **Hair with flag sign:** Hair of PEM patients.
46. **Horseshoe kidney:** Both kidneys joined at the lower pole.
47. **Hose pipe or lead pipe appearance:** Intestine in Crohn's disease due to transmural inflammation and fibrosis.
48. **Hair on end appearance:** Bones in thalassaemia due to widening of medullary cavity.
49. **Herring bone pattern:** Cell arrangement in fibrosarcoma, similar to skeleton of herring fish.
50. **Honeycomb:** Gross appearance in bronchiectasis, lung in Hamman-Rich syndrome.

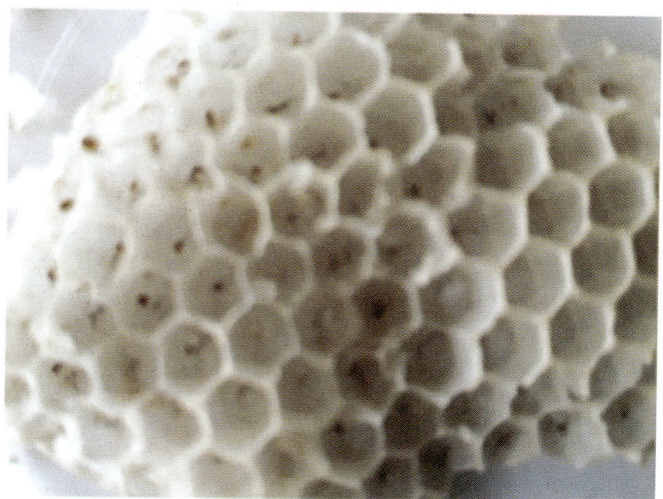

Honeycomb: Gross appearance in bronchiectasis

51. **Hobnail:** Macronodules in post-necrotic cirrhosis.

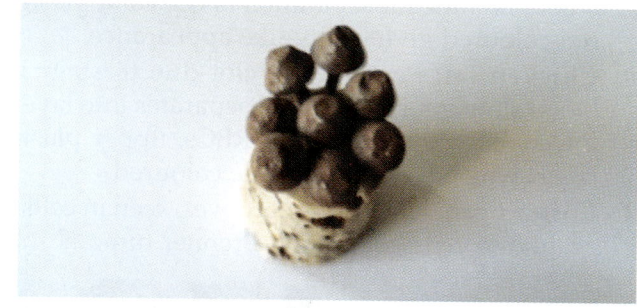

Hobnail: Macronodules in post-necrotic cirrhosis

52. **Holly leaf:** RBCs in sickle cell anaemia.
53. **Helmet cells:** Broken RBCs in haemolytic anaemia.
54. **Hair-like structures:** Pilocytic astrocyoma.
55. **Indian file:** Arrangement of cells, one behind the other in lobular carcinoma breast.
56. **Jigsaw puzzle appearance:** Paget's disease of bone, cylindroma.
57. **Leonine facies:** Nodular skin lesions on face in lepromatous leprosy.
58. **Laennec's cirrhosis:** Alcoholic cirrhosis (micronodules).
59. **Lines of Zahn:** Gross appearance of surface of thrombus (elevated areas of platelets and depressed areas of red cells, WBCs and fibrin).
60. **Leaf-like:** Stromal overgrowth, ductal epithelium stretched over it giving leaf appearance in phyllodes tumour of breast.
61. **Lardaceous spleen:** Amyloidosis involving sinusoids of spleen.
62. **Schiller dual body:** In yolk sac tumour.
63. **Needle-shaped crystals:** Gout (monosodium urate crystals).
64. **Rhomboid-shaped crystals:** Triple phosphate crystals.
65. **Millet seeds:** Lesions in miliary tuberculosis.

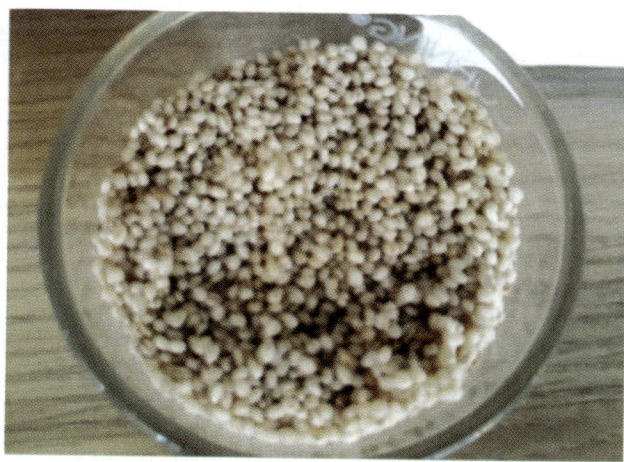

Millet seeds: Tiny lesions in miliary tuberculosis

66. Sago: Lesions of spleen in amyloidosis involving lymphoid follicles and terminal arteriole.

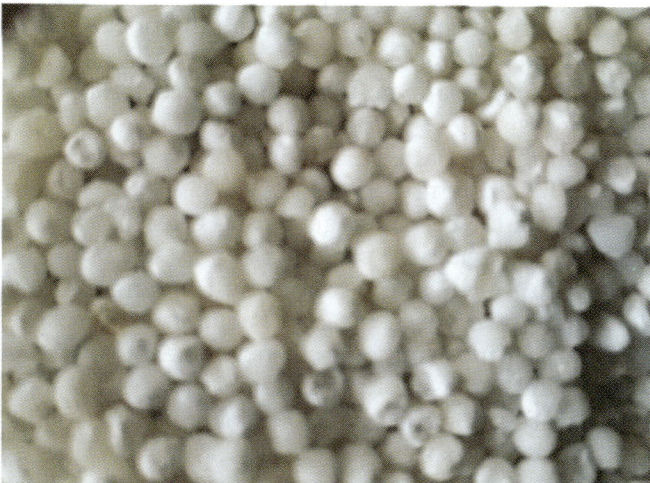

Sago: Spleen in amyloidosis

67. Tapioca appearance: Lesions of spleen in amyloidosis involving lymphoid follicles and terminal arteriole.

68. Nut meg: CVC liver, gross appearance.

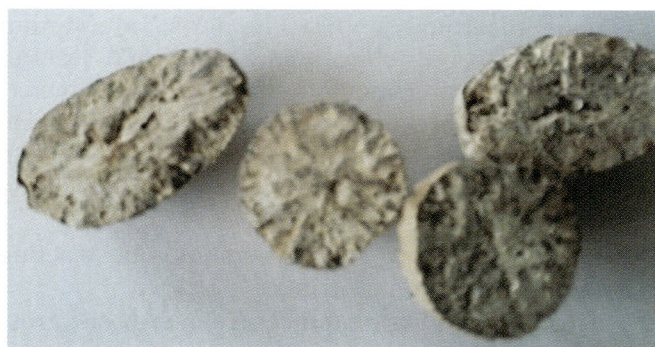

Nutmeg: CVC liver, gross appearance

69. Maple syrup odour: Smell of urine in enzyme deficiency involving metabolism of branched chain amino acids.

70. Ochronosis: Ocher-like (yellowish) discoloration due to accumulation of homogentisic acid in connective tissues.

71. Psammoma body: Dystrophic calcification in whorled appearance observed in papillary carcinoma thyroid, serous papillary carcinoma ovary, psammomatous meningioma.

72. Onion peal/skin appearance: X-ray appearance of periosteal reaction with new bone in Ewing's sarcoma, arrangement of keratined atypical cells in squamous cell carcinoma.

73. Sirenomalia (mermaid appearance): Anomalies of lower spine and lower limbs, partial or complete fusion of lower limbs.

74. Rice water: Stools in cholera.

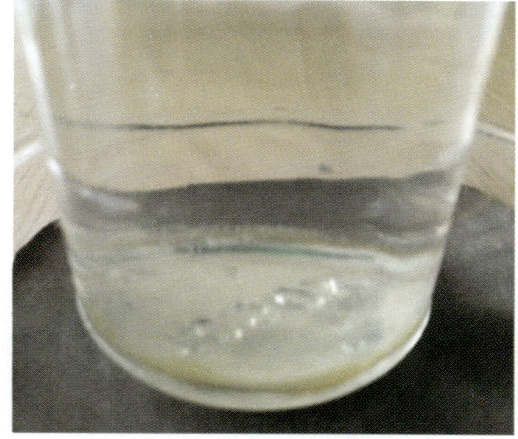

Rice water: Stools in cholera

75. Sickle-shaped of RBCs: RBCs in sickle cell HA.

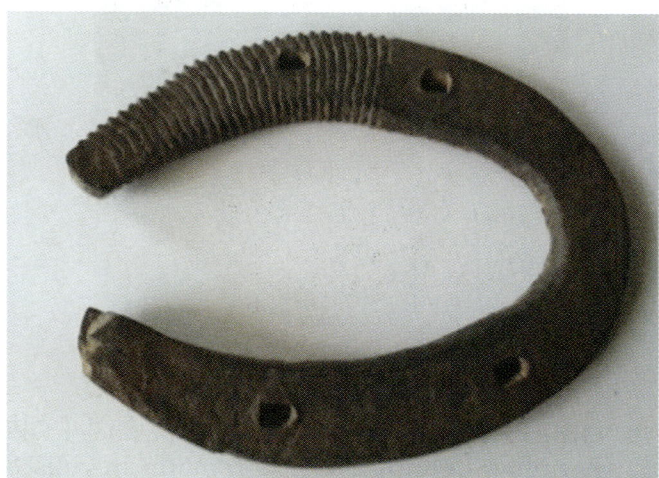

Sickle: Shape of RBCs in sickle cell HA

76. Potato tumour: Gross appearance of carotid body tumour.

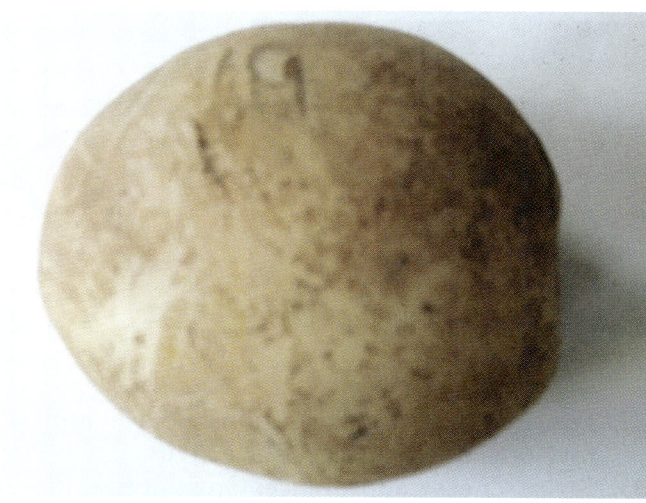

Potato tumour: Gross appearance of carotid body tumour

77. **Signet ring cells:** Malignant cells in mucinous carcinoma.

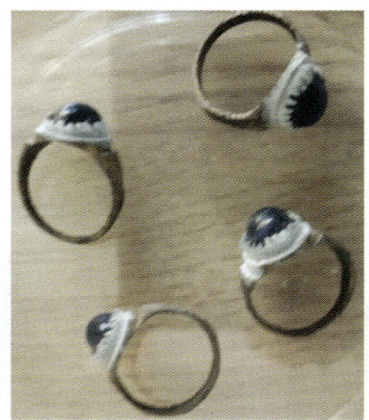

Signet ring: Malignant cells in mucinous carcinoma

78. **Portwine colour:** Colour of urine in porphyria.

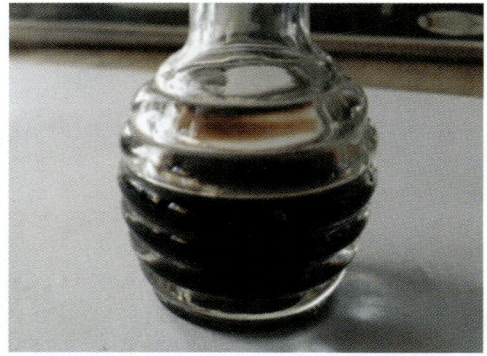

Portwine colour: Urine in porphyria

79. **Orphan Annie eye:** Appearance of nuclei with peripheral clumping of chromatin in cells of papillary carcinoma thyroid.

80. **Rubbery feel:** Hodgkin's disease, feel of the lymph nodes.

81. **Owl eye appearance:** RS cells in Hodgkin disease, mirror image nuclei.

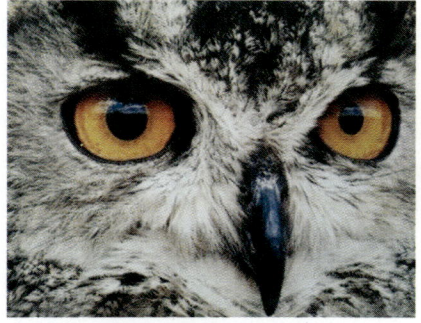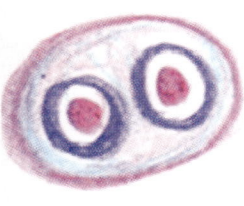

Owl eye: Mirror image nuclei of RS cells

82. **Punched out osteolytic lesions:** Bone in multiple myeloma due to osteoclastic activity.

83. **Swiss Cheese appearance:** Gross appearance in cystoglandular hyperplasia.

84. **Tadpole cells:** Cells in syringoma and individual cells with tapered cytoplasm in squamous cell carcinoma.

85. **Staghorn calculi:** Renal stones in pelvis, composed of struvite (magnesium ammonium phosphate) or calcium carbonate apatite.

86. **Moth eaten appearance:** Vacuolated cytoplasm in necrosis.

87. **Starry sky pattern:** Tingible body macrophages in Burkitt lymphoma.

88. **Navicular cells:** Progesterone effect of cervical cells especially in pregnancy.

89. **Onion skin appearance:** Cell arrangement in touch receptor also called Pacinian corpuscle.

90. **Pallisading arrangement:** Peripheral arrangement of cells in basal cell carcinoma.

91. **Safety pin appearance:** Donovanosis *C. granulomatis* organisms.

92. **Storiform pattern:** Arrangement of cells in fibrosarcoma and fibroma.

93. **Spider-like cells:** Lipoblasts in liposarcoma.

94. **Zebra bodies:** EM picture of lamellated inclusions in neuronal lysozymes in mucopolysaccharidosis/gangliosidosis.

95. **Rosettes and florets:** Homer Wright rosettes (cell arrangement around neuropil) in medulloblastoma/neuroblastoma/PNET, Flexner-Wintersteiner rosettes in retinoblastoma, ependymal rosettes with cell arrangement around a tubular lumen.

96. **Mutton or chicken leg appearance:** Gross appearance of osteosarcoma.

97. **Soap bubble appearance:** Osteoclastoma X-ray appearance.

98. **Saddle embolus:** Thromboembolus obstructing the main pulmonary trunk.

99. **Turkish towel appearance:** Adenomyosis, gross appearance.

100. **Tree bark appearance :** Syphilitic aortitis classically seen in ascending aorta and arch of aorta, intima showing scars and furrows due to endarteritis of vasavasorum, inflammation with predominantly plasma cells and other chronic inflammatory cells and destruction of media which is replaced by fibrosis.

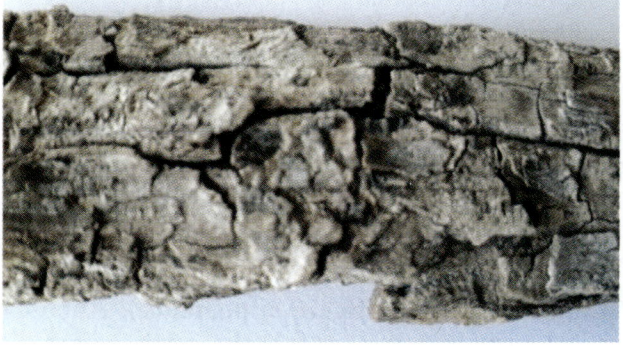

Tree bark: Syphilitic aortitis

101. **Tigered heart appearance:** Fatty heart in chronic ischaemia showing alternate dark-coloured normal muscle and pale-coloured muscle with fat accumulation.

102. **Thrush breast heart:** Fatty heart with normal dark-coloured muscle alternating with light-coloured muscle in fatty change heart appearing like patches on chest of bird called thrush.

103. **Portwine-stained skin areas:** This is due to hemangiomas or anomalies of blood vessels. It may be component of Sturge-Weber syndrome.

104. **Peau d'orange:** Over lying skin in carcinoma breast, appears like skin of orange due to obstructed lymphatics.

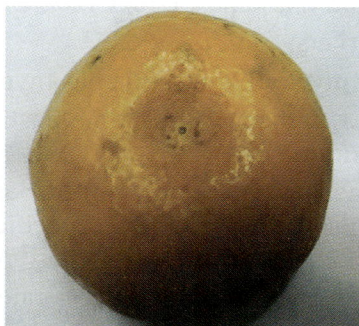

Peau d'orange: Skin in breast carcinoma

105. **Targetoid appearance:** Arrangement of tumour cells in concentric manner around normal ducts in lobular carcinoma breast.

106. **Turban tumour:** Numerous dome-shaped nodules on scalp in cylindromas.

107. **Tomb stone appearance:** Cells in coagulative necrosis.

108. **Spider naevi/angioma:** Due to excess oestrogen or cirrhosis and portal hypertension, there is failure of sphincteric muscle surrounding the cutaneous arteriole, central portion has dilated arteriole.

109. **Splinter haemorrhage:** Haemorrhages below nail in bacterial endocarditis.

110. **Salt and pepper appearance:** Nuclei of cells in carcinoid tumour.

111. **Strawberry like uterine cervix:** Erythematous punctate and papilliform appearance of cervix in *Trichomonas* infection.

112. **Zellballen:** Cell arrangement in paraganglioma or pheochromocytoma.

Pearls to Know

Anaemias

1. Red cells normally survive for 120 days.
2. Anticoagulants of choice in haematology laboratory are: EDTA, double oxalate, 3.2% or 3.8% trisodium citrate and heparin.
3. Warm antibodies in HA are: IgG antibodies.
4. A person with haemoglobin of 15 mg% will have PCV of 45%.
5. Low MCV and high RDW: Iron deficiency anaemia.
6. A unit of packed red cells will increase Hb by 3%.
7. Fanconi anaemia: AR disease with bone marrow failure. 90% of these cases have aplastic anaemia.
8. Paroxysmal nocturnal haemoglobinuria (PNH): Absence of GPI linked proteins with reduced anchorage of decay accelerating factors are unusually sensitive to complement-mediated lysis.
9. G6PD is required to generate NADPH.
10. NADPH protects RBCs from oxidative stress.
11. In sickle cell anaemia, there is substitution of valine for glutamic acid in 6th position of beta chains.
12. At less pH and low oxygen tension, Hb-S cells begin to sickle.
13. Cryohemolysis more than 20% is seen in HS.
14. In HS, there is spectrin deficiency.
15. DDs for normocytic normochromic anaemia
    i. Acute blood loss
    ii. Haemolytic anaemia
    iii. Chronic renal failure (erythropoietin deficiency)
    iv. Anaemia of chronic disorders: Infections
    v. Microangiopathic HA
    vi. Autoimmune HA
    vii. Transfusion reactions
    viii. Burns
16. DDs for microcytic anaemia (mnemonics—TICS)
    i. Iron deficiency anaemia
    ii. Thalassaemia
    iii. Anaemia of chronic diseases
    iv. Sideroblastic anaemia
17. DDs for macrocytic anaemia
    i. Vitamin B_{12} deficiency
    ii. Folic acid deficiency
    iii. MDS
    iv. Alcohol
    v. Chronic liver disease (cirrhosis)
    vi. Congenital BM failure (Shwachman-Diamond syndrome—BM dysregulation, sketetal abnormalities and exocrine pancreatic insufficiency)
    vii. Hypothyroidism
    viii. Reticulocytosis

Leukaemias

1. B lymphoid markers: CD10, CD19, CD20, CD79.
2. T cell markers: CD2, CD3, CD7.
3. M6 acute myeloid leukaemia has myelofibrosis.
4. T cell ALL can manifest as mediastinal mass of thymic origin.
5. CML: Massive spleen, increased basophils and eosinophils, immature WBCs specifically myelocytes, t(9:22) Philadelphia chromosome.
6. CML phases: Chronic phase, accelerated phase and blast crisis.
7. Chronic phase: Less than 10% myeloblasts in bone marrow.
8. Accelerated phase: Myeloblasts in bone marrow are between 11 to 19%.
9. Blast crisis: Blasts in bone marrow more than 20%.

Multiple Myeloma and Plasma Cell Disorders

1. Plasma cell neoplasms: There is clonal proliferation of plasma cells.
2. Plasmacytoma is multiple myeloma (MM) occurring in soft tissue.
3. Punched out lesions of multiple myeloma are due to: IL-6.
4. POEMS syndrome: Polyneuropathy, organomegaly, endocrinopathy, monoclonal gammopathy and skin changes.
5. CRAB features for multiple myeloma: Calcium elevated, renal insufficiency, anaemia and bony osteolytic lesions.
6. Bence Jones (BJ) proteins in urine: These are light chain gamma globulins excreted in plasma cell dyscrasias.
7. Increased ESR more than 100 mm at the end of first hour is characteristic in multiple myeloma and other plasma cell dyscrasias.
8. Waldenstrom macroglobulinaemia (WM): IgM producing malignant plasma cell disease presents with anaemia and hyperviscocity features.

9. M band on serum electrophoresis is diagnostic in multiple myeloma and Waldenstrom macroglobulinaemia.
10. Monoclonal gammopathy of undetermined significance (MUGS): Clonal plasma cells <10%.

Myeloproliferative Disorders

1. Primary myelofibrosis: Prefibrotic and fibrotic phases. Prefibrotic phase can have leukoerythroblastic blood picture, tear drop cells and splenomegaly.
2. JAK2 mutations positive disorders are: Polycythemia vera (PV). Essential thrombocythemia (ET), primary myelofibrosis (PMF).
3. Polycythemia vera (PV): Hb more than 16.5 gm% for males and 16 gm% for females, panmyelosis, JAK2 positive.
4. Essential thrombocythemia (ET): Platelet counts more than 4.5 lakh cells/cmm, increased megakaryocytes in bone marrow and JAK2 positive.

Myelodysplastic Syndrome (MDS)

1. MDS is a stem cell malignancy.
2. The cells in MDS are dysplastic.
3. MDS presents with ineffective blood cell production.
4. MDS can occur in old age with 5q deletion.
5. Monosomy 7, 5q deletion and other chromosomal abnormalities are known in MDS.
6. Abnormal localization of immature precursors (ALIP) is observed in MDS.
7. Neutrophils with hypogranularity, hypolobulation or hyposegmentation can be present in MDS.
8. Micromegakaryocytes are observed in MDS.

Haemorrhagic Disorders

1. Idiopathic thrombocytopenic purpura (ITP) is an acquired disorder with thrombocytopenia due to antibody formation. Megakaryocytes increased which are often in clusters. Often hypogranular and hypolobulation present. Cytoplasm is basophilic.
2. The monoclonal antibody specific immobilisation of platelet antigen (MAIPA): Positive (50–65%) in ITP.
3. Hermansky-Pudlak syndrome: Albinism and platelet dysfunction.
4. PGI2 and NO produced by endothelial cells have antiplatelet effect.
5. Glanzmann thrombasthenia: AR, GP IIb/IIIa receptor deficient or dysfunctional. These genes present on chromosome 17. With dysfunction or deficiency, there is defective aggregation of platelets.

6. Factors II, VII, IX, X and protein C and S are Vitamin K dependent factors.
7. Von Willebrand disease: AD with spontaneous bleeding from mucous membranes, platelet count is normal.
8. A newborn with bleeding from umbilical cord is: Factors X and XII deficiency.
9. A female with hemarthrosis is: Probably due to factor VIII inhibitors.
10. DIC has: FDPs, prolonged PT, APTT and reduced platelet count.
11. vWF produced from endothelium.
12. Factor VIII is always in combination with vWF.
13. Protein C, thrombomodulin, and thrombin produce activated protein C. This along with protein S inactivates FVa and FVIIIa.
14. Protein C cannot cleave factor Leiden Va.
15. Heparin-like molecules from endothelium activate antithrombin-III. This binds thrombin and inactivates vitamin K dependent activated factors.
16. Antiphospholipid antibody syndrome: Presence of antibodies against phospholipid binding plasma proteins. The syndrome presents with recurrent abortions.
17. Prothrombin time (PT): Assesses coagulation mechanism by extrinsic pathway and deficiency of common pathway (Factors VII, X, V , II and I).
18. Activated partial thromboplastin time (APTT): Assesses coagulation mechanism by intrinsic pathway and deficiency of common pathway. (Factors XII, XI, IX, VIII, X, V, II and I).
19. PT Normal and APTT prolonged in FVIII, IX, prekallikrein, HMWK deficiency and with presence of inhibitors.
20. PT increased in defects of FV, VII, X and fibrinogen deficiency.

Blood Grouping and Transfusion Medicine

I. Important points regarding blood groups

1. Antigens are present on the wall of RBCs.
2. ABO and Rh are important blood groups.
3. IgM antibodies are present in ABO system. These IgM antibodies can also be present in other rare blood groups (MNSs, P).
4. IgG antibodies may be produced in O blood group patients.
5. IgG antibodies can be produced in Rh system with immunological sensitization.
6. IgG antibodies can be also produced with immunological sensitization in other blood group systems such as Kell, Duffy, Kidd, MNSs and Lutheran.

7. IgG antibodies produce HDN and haemolytic transfusion reactions.

8. Compatible blood needs to be given to save the life.

II. Donation of blood and blood components

1. 8 ml per kg body weight blood can be given.

2. The plasma volume and platelets are replaced within 48 hours, granulocytes and other elements of plasma (proteins, etc.) within 7 days, red blood cells in 56 days and iron lost is replaced in 8 weeks.

3. Plasmapheresis can be done at an interval of 48 hours.

4. Platelet apheresis at an interval 48 hours.

5. Red blood cells/whole blood used within 35 days with CPDA1.

6. Platelets are used within 5 days.

7. Plasma and cryoprecipitate can be used up to one year.

III. Blood and blood components

1. One unit of whole blood will increase Hb by 1 g/dl and PCV by 3%.

2. 1 unit of packed red cells has 250 mg of iron.

3. Iron that can be removed by the body is 1 mg/day.

4. One unit of single donor platelets (SDP) will increase platelet count by 30,000–60000 platelets/cmm.

5. One unit of random donor platelets (RDP) will increase the platelet count by 4,000–6000 platelets/cmm.

6. Preserve the platelets at 22–24°C in agitator.

7. Transfuse platelets if less than 10,000. With antibodies to platelets, platelet transfusion may not be of use.

8. Platelet increase is observed after 1 hour and again at 20–24 hours of platelet transfusion.

9. Preserve the whole blood/PRBCs at 1–6°C.

10. FFP once collected from the blood bank can be preserved at 1–6°C and used within 6 hrs.

11. Do not transfuse red cells unless clear indication is present. Some of the indications are given below.
   - Chronic anaemias with Hb less than 6 g/dl.
   - Less than **7 g/dl** when patient is symptomatic and undergoing surgery.
   - Less than **8 g** with **CVS problems**.
   - With 6–10 g/dl only when severe bleeding or complications of inadequate hypoxia are expected.
   - **Blood loss of 30–40%** of circulating blood volume.
   - In **anaemia/severe heart or pulmonary disease/ when bleeding continues with 15–30% blood loss**.

- In **obstetrics, patients** Hb less than 7 g/dl, not amenable to timely therapies antenataly.
- In **concealed haemorrhage** with **abruptio placentae**, to replenish the concealed blood loss **irrespective of symptoms**.

IV. Important points to keep in mind regarding neonatal transfusion

- In neonates, 10–20 ml/kg body weight blood can be given.
- Blood less than 7 days is preferred for neonatal transfusion.
- In neonates, only antigen grouping is done.
- Blood given to neonate should be compatible with mother's serum.
- If mother's and baby's group are the same, use Rh negative blood of baby/mother's ABO group. If not the same use 'O' Rh negative blood.
- In neonates, rate of transfusion should be less than 10 ml/kg/hour.

V. The most common cause of transfusion of ABO incompatible blood and this can be due to:

- Errors in blood request form.
- Taking wrong sample into prelabelled sample tube.
- Incorrect labelling of the sample tube sent to the blood bank.
- Inadequate checks of the blood against the identity of the patient while starting a transfusion.

VI. Prevention of errors

1. Correctly label the blood samples and request forms. Place the patient's blood sample in the sample tube.

2. Always check the blood against the identity of the patient at the bedside before transfusion.

3. Proper identification of the patient from sample collection through to blood administration, proper labelling of samples and products is essential. Prevention of non-immune haemolysis requires adherence to proper handling, storage and administration of blood products.

VII. Different types of donors

- Voluntary donors
- Replacement donors
- Autologous donors

Voluntary donor is one who donates blood for storage at a blood blank for transfusion to an unknown recipient.

- A greater percentage of better quality of blood comes from voluntary donors.

- These donors are very important because the incidence of blood-transmitted infections is much less in blood drawn from these volunteers.

Replacement donor is a person, often a family member, donates blood for transfusion to a specific individual.
- The donor is selected by the recipient.
- Since there is pressure to donate, they may give blood even if there is risk behaviour.

Autologous donor is a person who donates blood to be stored and transfused back to the donor later usually during and/or after surgery.

VIII. Criteria for donor selection
- **Age:** 18–65 years.
- **Minimum body weight:** 45 kg.
- **A person can donate 8 ml/kg** body weight (up to 450 ml every three months).
- **Haemoglobin (Hb):** 12.5 gm% or above or Hct equal to more than 38%.
- **Donor screening:** Involves registration, consent of the donor, demographic information, medical history, limited physical examination and simple laboratory tests.
- **Demographic information:** It should be complete and correct so that the donor can be informed of any laboratory testing abnormality.
  1. Donor's full name
  2. Father's/Husband's name
  3. Age
  4. Gender
  5. Phone number
  6. Residential address
- **Medical history:**
  1. History of any long-term illness.
  2. Any medication, if patient is taking.
  3. Allergy to any substance/medication, etc.
- **Physical examination:** A qualified practitioner of medicine or blood bank officer will examine for the following:
  - General appearance: A donor should be healthy.
  - Pulse: 60–100 beats/minute.
  - Temperature: 37°C.
  - Blood pressure:
    - Systolic pressure: 100–140 mm Hg
    - Diastolic pressure: 60–90 mm Hg
  - Respiratory, cardiovascular, gastrointestinal, etc. systems should be normal and no problems should be detected by a rapid physical examination.
- **Informed consent:** If the donor has successfully passed the history and physical examination, informed consent is required prior to donation.

IX. Laboratory tests
Following are the tests done on a unit of blood donated.
1. Haemoglobin estimation
2. Blood grouping and crossmatching
4. Screening for unwanted antibodies
5. Screening for transfusion transmissible infections: Indian Govt. regulatory authorities for blood bank recommends following 5 tests to be mandatory. These are mentioned below.
   - HIV 1 and 2
   - Hepatitis B
   - Hepatitis C
   - Syphilis
   - Malaria

Tests must be performed at each donation regardless of number of earlier donations.

There are temporary deferrals or permanent deferrals for blood transfusion.

Introduction and History of Pathology
1. Hippocrates: Father of medicine. He established the basic principles of medicine.
2. Aulus Cornelius Celsus described the four cardinal signs of inflammation (rubor, calor, tumor and dolor).
3. William Harvey established circulation of blood.
4. Giovanni B. Morgagni conducted 700 postmortems with clinicopathological correlations and described morbid anatomy.
5. Huntarian museum at the Royal College of Physicians and Surgeons is named after John Hunter and William Hunter.
6. Thomas Hodgkin described the reasons for enlargement of lymph nodes, spleen and liver.
7. Carl Von Rokitansky conducted 30,000 autopsies.
8. Migration of Leukocytes in Inflammation is described by Julium Cohnheim.
9. Karl Landsteiner discovered A, B and O blood groups. AB blood group was discovered by A. Decastello and A. Sturli.
10. Pap smear is named after George Papanicolaou.
11. Monoclonal antibodies production credit goes to **George Kohler**.
12. **Albert Coons** is known for discoveries of fluorescein-labelled antibodies.
13. Combination of methylene blue and eosin is named after Romanowsky.
14. Gregor Johann Mendel discovered the fundamental laws of inheritance
15. Barry Marshall and Robin Warren discovered *Helicobacter pylori*.

Cell Injury

1. Moth eaten appearance is due to: Enzymatic digestion of cell organelles.
2. In Fenton reaction, ROS develop when ferrous iron is converted to ferric ion.
3. Superoxide dismutase takes off superoxide which in combination with hydrogen molecule gets converted to H_2O_2 and oxygen.
4. Antioxidants are: Endogenous and exogenous anti-oxidants (vitamin A, E, C and beta-carotenes) block the formation of free radicals.
5. Superoxide dismutase protects brain from injury by ROS.
6. Ionising radiation produces cell injury by release of free radicals especially OH ions.
7. During lactation, breast hyperplasia is seen.
8. Breast lesions during puberty and pregnancy are examples of hyperplasia.
9. Skeletal muscle of limbs in athletes is an example of hypertrophy due to increased muscle activity.
10. Myocardial fibres undergo only hypertrophy. No hyperplasia is seen as they are permanent cells.
11. Wear and tear pigment is lipofuscin which is yellow brown coloured.
12. Brown colour in brown atrophy of heart is due to deposition of wear and tear pigment, i.e. lipofuscin.
13. Undigested material from lipid peroxidation is: Lipofuscin.
14. Metaplasia can be epithelial or mesenchymal, reversible, occurs at stem cell level.
15. Commonest metaplasia in respiratory tract is: Ciliated pseudostratified columnar epithelium changes to stratified squamous epithelium.
16. Ducts of salivary glands with glandular epithelium may undergo metaplasia to stratified squamous epithelium due to chronic irritation by stones.
17. In Barrett's esophagus, squamous epithelium changes to columnar epithelium.
18. Osseous and mesenchymal metaplasia can be seen in leiomyomas and fibromas.
19. In cloudy degeneration, the parenchymal cells affected are rich in mitochondria.
20. Chaperones are responsible for proper protein folding.
21. Dutcher bodies are: Cytoplasmic inclusions found in the nucleus (intranuclear inclusions) of plasma cells.
22. Mott cells: Plasma cell with multiple Russell bodies.
23. Plasma cell with eosinophilic cytoplasmic inclusion is Russell body.
24. Neurofibrillary tangles are seen in: Amyloidosis brain.
25. Amyloid gives green birefringence with polarizing microscope.
26. Fatty heart is encountered in diphtheria and chronic ischaemia.
27. Mallory hyaline refers to: Damaged intermediate filaments.
28. Programmed cell death refers to: Apoptosis, observed in embryogenesis, deletion of auto-reactive T cells and virus infected cells.
29. Characteristic of apoptosis is chromatin condensation.
30. Anti-apoptotic molecules are: Bcl2 and Bcl-XL. These are present on the outer mitochondrial and ER membranes. These prevent leakage of cytochrome C into cytosol.
31. BAX and BAK are pro-apoptotic.
32. Cytochrome C binds to APAF1 and activates caspase 9.
33. With failure of calcium pump, influx of calcium activates many enzymes.
34. In cell injury, there is ATP depletion, ribosomes detach from rough endoplasmic reticulum with reduction in protein synthesis.
35. Death receptors are: TNFR and FAS-1.
36. Initiator caspase in intrinsic pathway of apoptosis is: Caspase 9.
37. Initiator caspase in extrinsic pathway of apoptosis is: Caspase 8.
38. Fat saponification is seen in: Chronic pancreatitis and traumatic injury to fat.
39. Wet gangrene is combination of coagulative and liquefactive nacrosis.
40. Coagulative necrosis: Organ is mummified, blackish colored and microscopy shows tomb stone appearance.
41. Fragmentation of nucleus: Karyorrhexis.
42. Fading with basophila of nucleus is referred to as: Karyolysis.
43. Pyknosis: Shrinkage of nucleus.
44. Autophagy: Self-destruction. Cell eats its own contents.
45. Hyperplasia is increase in number of cells in organ or tissue. This type of adaptation occurs in tissues which can undergo division.
46. Physiological causes of hyperplasia
   i. Hormonal stimulus can cause proliferation of the glands and stromal tissue:
      a. Breast during puberty and pregnancy
      b. Uterus in pregnancy
      c. Prostate enlargement called benign prostatic hyperplasia (BPH) or nodular prostatic hyperplasia (NPH)

ii. Compensatory hyperplasia which occurs after portion of tissue is resected or diseased as in liver, lung and kidney.

47. The pathological causes of hyperplasia:
    i. Endometrial hyperplasia due to excess estrogen hormone
    ii. Skin epithelium with HPV infection which causes hyperplasia of stratified squamous epithelial cells causing papilloma (viral wart).
    iii. Skin epithelium in psoriasis.
    iv. Pancreatic islet cell hyperplasia in infants of diabetic mothers.

48. Hypertrophy is an increase in the size of the cells resulting in increased size of the organs. In hypertrophy, there are no new cells.

49. Physiological causes of hypertrophy
    i. Uterus during pregnancy: Estrogen stimulates smooth muscle cells to undergo hypertrophy and hyperplasia.
    ii. Skeletal muscles of limbs in athletes: Skeletal muscles undergo hypertrophy due to increased muscle activity.

50. Pathological causes of hypertrophy: Hypertrophy of heart due to increase in demand as in hypertension or aortic valve incompetence/stenosis.

51. Atrophy is shrinkage in size of the cell, due to loss of cell substances.

52. Physiological causes of atrophy:
    i. Involution of branchial cleft, thyroglossal duct, and notochord.
    ii. Involution of Wolffian duct and Mullerian duct in females and males, respectively.
    iii. Atrophy of ovary, endometrium after menopause and atrophy of other tissues in old age.
    iv. Old age (senile atrophy).

53. Pathological causes of atrophy:
    i. Disuse atrophy of limb: Decreased workload (immobilisation of limb in plaster cast in fracture of limb bones)
    ii. Loss of innervation
    iii. Loss of blood supply
    iv. Pressure atrophy
    v. Lack of nutrients
    vi. Reduced hormones
    vii. Loss of endocrine stimulation

54. Metaplasia is a reversible change in which one adult cell type (epithelial or mesenchymal) is replaced by another adult cell type.

55. Epithelial metaplasia
    i. Respiratory epithelium (ciliated pseudostratified columnar epithelium) changes to stratified squamous epithelium in habitual cigarette smokers and vitamin A deficiency.
    ii. Endocervical epithelium may be change to stratified squamous epithelium.
    iii. Ducts of salivary glands with glandular epithelium may undergo metaplasia to stratified squamous epithelium due to chronic irritation by stones.
    iv. Ducts of pancreatic glands may change to stratified squamous epithelium due to stones.
    v. Transitional epithelium of bladder and pelvis of kidney may change to stiatified squamous epithelium due to irritation by renal stones.
    vi. Endometrial metaplasia may show different types of epithelia.
    vii. The lower end of esophagus which is usually lined by stratified squamous epithelium may change to columnar epithelium due to reflux esophagitis (Barrett's esophagus).

56. Mesenchymal metaplasia: The undifferentiated cells transform into other adult mesenchymal cells. Cartilagenous metaplasia or osseous metaplasias are more common.
    i. In old scars, necrotic areas, myositis ossificans foci of bone may develop.
    ii. Foci of bone may develop in the walls of diseased arteries destroyed by injury or inflammation.
    iii. In laryngeal and bronchial cartilage of old people, cartilage may undergo ossification.
    iv. Fibromas may show osseous metaplasia.
    v. Uterine leiomyoma may undergo osseous and mesenchymal metaplasia.

57. Though the metaplastic epithelium has survival advantages, the important protective mechanisms are lost, such as:
    i. Mucous secretion
    ii. Ciliary clearance of particulate matter as in respiratory tract.

58. The metaplastic epithelium may predispose to malignant transformation, if it is not reversed back or the causative agent is not removed.

59. Degenerations are retrogressive changes in the cells due to direct action of the injurious agents.

60. Hyaline degeneration is glassy, amorphous and homogenous material which stains pink/eosinophilic with H and E stain.

61. Physiological conditions with hyaline degeneration are:
    i. Arteries of atrophic uterus
    ii. Colloid in multinodular goiter
    iii. Corpora amylacea in prostate
    iv. Corpora albicans in ovary

62. Extracellular hyaline:
    i. Collagen in:
       a. Old scar tissue
       b. Keloid
       c. Thickened capillaries and vessels
    ii. Fibroma
    iii. Vessel wall in
       a. Diabetes mellitus
       b. Hypertension
    iv. KW lesions of kidney in diabetes mellitus
    v. Hyalinzation of islets of Langerhans in diabetes mellitus
63. Intracellular hyaline
    i. Mallory hyaline: Damaged prekeratin intermediate filaments. Commonly seen in fatty change, hepatitis or cirrhosis due to alcohol, Wilson's disease, Indian childhood cirrhosis, primary biliary cirrhosis, non-alcoholic steatohepatitis (NASH), hepatocellular carcinoma, etc.
    ii. Councilman bodies: Seen in yellow fever.
    iii. Russell bodies: These represent immunoglobulins in plasma cells.
    iv. Epithelial hyaline: These are commonly seen in epithelium of the proximal tubules due to excess absorption of plasma proteins.
    v. Zenker's degeneration: Striated muscles of diaphragm, abdomen and thigh show hyaline change in typhoid fever.
64. Abnormal accumulation of triglycerides within the parenchymal cells is referred to as fatty change.
65. Stains for demonstration of fat
    i. Oil red 'O'—fat stains red
    ii. Sudan III/IV—fat stains orange to red
    iii. Osmium tetroxide—with alpha naphthylamine reaction phospholipids are stained orange red; cholesterol and triglycerides are stained black.
    iv. Neutral fat is stained black with 1% osmic acid in saturated bichlorides or mercury.
66. Fatty change heart: Prolonged moderate hypoxia as seen in severe anaemia results in focal intracellular fat deposits, grossly, this gives yellowish appearance to the affected myocardial fibres and the normal fibres remain darker and red brown ('tigered' or 'thrush breast' effect). The myocardial fibers are uniformly and diffusely affected due to some toxins, e.g. diphtheria. The anaemia is more severe and profound.
67. Amyloid is an abnormal proteinaceous substance deposited extracellularly in various organs.
68. Special stains for amyloid
    i. H and E stain: Amyloid stains homogenous and pale pink

    ii. PAS stain: Amyloid stains magenta pink
    iii. Van Gieson: Amyloid stains yellow to yellow brown
    iv. Iodine (Gram's or Lugol's): Amyloid stains Mahogany brown turning to blue or violet with application of dilute sulphuric acid
    v. Metachromatic stains (e.g. 1% methyl violet, 1% toluidine blue): Amyloid stains pink, other tissues stain violet
    vi. Congo red: Amyloid stains orange
    vii. Congo red with polarisation: Apple green birefringence
    viii. X-ray diffraction: Cross beta pleated structure
    ix. Fluorescence with thioflavin T and S
69. Apoptosis is a process that helps to eliminate unwanted cells, by an internally programmed series of events, the process is tightly regulated and the cells are destined to die.
70. Necrosis has a spectrum of morphological changes that follow cell death in a living tissue, largely resulting from progressive degradative action of enzymes on lethally injured cells. The damage caused is irreversible.

Inflammation

1. Acute inflammation has vasodilatation, edema, and inflammatory response.
2. Chronic inflammation has inflammation and repair occurring at the same time.
3. ICAM1 and VCAM1 responsible for adhesion of neutrophils.
4. Proinflammatory cytokines are: IL-1, TNF and chemokines.
5. Pain is caused by: PGE_2, bradykinin, histamine, serotonin and neuropeptide.
6. Fever: IL-1, IL-8, TNF and PGE_2.
7. Cytokines: Signaling molecules produced by many cells.
8. Chemotaxis: C5a, LTB4, IL-8, PAF, 5-HETE.
9. Chemokines are chemoattractants for leucocytes.
10. CXC, CC, XC and CX3C are important chemokines. These mediate G protein coupled receptors.
11. IL-8 is a CXC chemokine.
12. CC chemokine is: Monocyte attractant protein (MCP1), eotaxin, macrophage inflammatory protein 1 alpha.
13. Platelet aggregation is by TXA2 and PAF.
14. Vasoconstriction is by TXA2, LTB4, LTC4, LTD4 and C5a.
15. Vasodilatation: Histamine, serotonin, bradykinin and C3a.

16. Increased vascular permeability: Histamine, serotonin, C3a, C5a, LTC4, D4 and E4.

17. C3a, C5a and C4a act as: Anaphylatoxins.

18. Inflammation is reaction of a living tissue to an injurious agent. Inflammation tries to eliminate, dilute or neutralize the harmful agents.

19. Vascular changes of inflammation are:
    i. The changes in vascular flow and caliber
    ii. Increased vascular permeability

20. The cellular events in inflammation
    i. Margination, rolling, pavementation, adhesion and transmigration
    ii. Chemotaxis
    iii. Recognition and attachment
    iv. Phagocytosis/engulfment
    v. Killing and degradation

21. The chemical mediators of inflammation are:
    Cell derived:
    i. Vasoactive amines: Histamine, serotonin
    ii. Lysosomal component
    iii. Platelet-activating factor
    iv. Cytokines
    v. NO and O_2 metabolites
    vi. Arachidonic acid metabolites
    Plasma derived:
    i. The kinin system
    ii. The clotting system
    iii. The fibrinolytic system
    iv. The complement system

22. Leucocytes express many types of toll-like receptors which identify toll proteins present on the microbes.

23. TLRs are present on neutrophils, macrophages, natural killer cells, epithelial cells and endothelial cells. Most important amongst these TLRs is TLR-4 which can bind LPS binding proteins on microbes and activate potent cytokines like IL-1 and TNF.

24. Granulomatous inflammation is a chronic inflammation characterised by focal collection of epithelioid cells (modified macrophages), giant cells and mantle of lymphocytes.

25. Morphological patterns of inflammation
    i. Serous inflammation
    ii. Fibrinous inflammation
    iii. Suppurative or purulent inflammation
    iv. Abscess
    v. Gangrene
    vi. Ulcer

Cell Cycle and Wound Healing

1. Labile cells: Epithelial cells lining different tracts, endometrium, bone marrow cells.

2. Continuously dividing cells are labile cells.

3. Liver, kidney and pancreatic cells are stable cells.

4. Neuronal and cardiac muscle cells are permanent cells.

5. If regeneration cannot occur, the injured cells are replaced by connective tissue.

6. Regeneration of liver is triggered by cytokines and growth factors. Surviving cells or progenitor cells proliferate.

7. VEGF drives angiogenesis.

8. Important growth factors for connective tissue are: PDGF, TGF-β, FGF$_2$.

9. TGF-β is important growth factor for formation of connective tissue.

10. Myofibroblasts are fibroblasts which have features of smooth muscle cells, including presence of actin filaments.

11. Myofibroblasts are involved in wound contraction.

12. Scar is remodeled by matrix metalloproteases which are dependent on zinc.

13. The granulation tissue is oedematous, reddish, velvety and formed in 3 days.

14. In wound healing initial collagen formed is type III, which is later replaced by type I.

15. An excessive amount of granulation tissue is called as 'Proud flesh'.

16. Excess production of ECM is encountered in hypertrophic scar and keloid which are abnormalities of tissue repair.

17. The cell cycle phases:
    i. Gap 1 (G_1) phase: This is pre-DNA synthetic phase, lasts for 6–12 hrs.
    ii. DNA synthesis phase (S phase): DNA synthetic phase lasts for 6–8 hrs.
    iii. Gap 2 (G_2) phase: This is pre-mitosis phase, lasts for 2–4 hrs.
    iv. Mitosis (M) phase: This is mitosis phase, and lasts for a short time (usually 1 hour).

18. Steps of wound healing by first intention:
    i. Haematoma formation and above this scab forms.
    ii. Within 24 hrs, neutrophils appear at the incision margin. The neutrophils migrate towards the fibrin clot. There is hyperaemia. The inflammatory cells remove clot and debris, if any.
    iii. The epithelial cells (basal cells) at the cut edge, show increased mitotic activity within 24–48 hrs.
    iv. By 3rd day, neutrophils are replaced by macrophages and granulation tissue is formed.
    v. By day 5, epidermis recovers normal thickness.

vi. By the 2nd week, there is continued collagen accumulation, deposition and regression of vascular channels. The leucocyte infiltration, oedema, and vascularity are reduced.

vii. By the end of first month, the tensile strength of the wound increases. The connective tissue is devoid of inflammatory cells and surface is covered by normal epidermis.

19. Wound healing by second intention:
   i. The tissue destruction is more and edges are ragged.
   ii. The edges cannot be approximated due to extensive loss of tissue.
   iii. As bleeding is heavy, large clot or haematoma formation is present.
   iv. Inflammation is more intense, necrotic debris and exudate formed is more.
   v. Epithelial cells migrate to replace the dead cells within a few days.
   vi. Larger amount of granulation tissue is formed to fill the large defect.
   vii. A large amount of collagen is laid down.
   viii. In 4–6 weeks, there is wound contraction, large skin defects are reduced to 5–10% of their original size by wound contraction.

20. Factors influencing wound healing:
   I. Local factors
   i. Location of wound on joints and bones.
   ii. Intervening tissue or foreign body have necrotic debris
   iii. Type of tissue
   iv. Mechanical variables local pressure, movement.
   v. Wound dehiscence
   vi. Infection
   vii. Growth factors
   II. General factors (systemic factors)
   i. Age: Older the age delay in healing
   ii. Nutrition status: Vitamin C deficiency, lack of zinc and protein energy malnutrition cases have delayed wound healing.
   iii. Blood supply: Atherosclerosed blood vessels and tissues with less blood supply have delayed wound healing.
   iv. Exogenous corticosteroids/increased glucocorticosteroids retards wound healing
   v. Diabetes and some haematological disorders: Diabetes has decreased phagocytic and chemotactic activity of inflammatory cells. Agranulocytosis leads to susceptibility of infection.
   vi. Radiation energy: Ultraviolet rays, X-rays in small doses stimulate wound healing whereas large doses delay healing.

vii. Smoking delays healing.
viii. Environmental temperature: Wound healing is slow in cold weather.

21. Steps of healing of fracture bone (simple fracture)
   i. Haematoma formation
   ii. Inflammatory reaction
   iii. Granulation tissue formation
   iv. Provisional callus formation (procallus/soft tissue callus/callus composed of cartilage and woven bone)
   v. Callus formation
   vi. Remodelling.

Thrombosis

1. Transudate is protein poor while exudate is protein rich.
2. Platelet GPIb binds to subendothelial collagen via vWF.
3. Platelet IIb/IIIa binds fibrinogen.
4. Normal endothelium releases factors which inhibit platelet aggregation. These are: Prostacyclin (PGI_2), NO and ADPase.
5. Normal endothelium has anticoagulant properties.
6. Thrombomodulin binds thrombin and activates protein C which is a inhibitor of Va and VIIIa.
7. Heparin-like molecules activate antithrombin III which binds thrombin and inactivate activated coagulation factors.
8. Protein C is a tissue factor pathway inhibitor.
9. Protein C requires protein S as co-factor.
10. Activated endothelial cells downregulate thrombomodulin, thus increased thrombin activity.
11. Stasis and turbulence are produced in aneurysms and atherosclerotic plaques.
12. Deep vein thrombosis (DVT) is associated with hypercoagulable state with bed rest and immobilization.
13. Most pulmonary emboli are silent as they are small.
14. Factor V Leiden is resistant to cleavage and inactivation by protein C. These have increased risk of thrombosis.

Infectious Diseases

1. Defects in complements are commonly prone for pneumococcal and Neisseria infections.
2. Defects of Toll-like receptors are prone for: Pyogenic infections.
3. Mutations of receptors: IL-12, TNF-γ and transcription factor STAT-1 impair generation of Th1 cells and are associated with atypical mycobacterial infections.

4. Gp of HIV 120 binds CD4 and CCR4 on T cells and CCR5 chemoreceptor on macrophages.

5. Koplik spots are pathognomonic of: Measles.

6. West Nile virus is an arthropod-borne virus, proliferates in skin dendritic cells and lymph nodes, can cross blood–brain barrier and can infect neurons too.

7. Cytomegalovirus (CMV) shows cytoplasmic and nuclear basophilic inclusions.

8. Shingles occurs in VZV; virus has latent infection in dorsal root ganglia and spreads to sensory nerves.

9. Dengue fever is arbovirus infection spread by *Aedes aegypti* mosquitoes. Dengue haemorrhagic fever has increased vascular permeability with plasma leakage and shock.

10. Ghon focus: 1 to 1.5 cm, subpleurally present in lower portion of the upper lobe or upper portion of the lower or middle lobe.

11. Apical tuberculosis on X-ray is called Simon's focus.

12. Rhinoscleroma: Chronic inflammatory cells, vacuolated histiocytes containg organisms (Mikulicz cells), plasma cells with Russell bodies and lymphocytes.

13. Fernandez and Mitsuda reactions are examples of delayed HS reaction in tuberculoid leprosy.

14. Destruction of vomer bone causes collapse of nasal bridge.

15. Syphilitic osteochondritis and periostitis affect all bones.

16. Eighth nerve deafness in syphilis is due to meningovascular syphilis.

17. Cryptococcus is yeast and has gelatinous capsule.

18. Aspergillus: Acute angle branching, septate, 5 to 10 µ in thickness.

19. Mucormycosis: Non-septate broad hyphae, often right angle branching, variable width (6 to 50 µ)

20. Leishmania donovani: Promastigote forms in sand fly, amastigote in macrophages of host cells.

Calcification

1. Metastatic calcification occurs in normal tissues with increased calcium levels.

2. Dystrophic calcification occurs in dead and dying tissues.

3. Increased bone catabolism occurring in multiple myeloma is an example of metastatic calcification.

4. Metastatic pulmonary calcification is a common complication of MM.

5. Intracellular deposits of calcium initially start in damaged mitochondria.

6. Intracerebral calcification (dystrophic calcification) occurs in toxoplasmosis.

7. Fibrosiderotic nodules with calcification are Gandy-Gamna bodies.

8. Phlebolith in pelvis can be confused with stones in the ureters. Psammoma bodies can be seen in papillary carcinoma thyroid, serous carcinoma ovary, psammomatous meningioma, etc.

Pigment Disorders

1. Lipofuscin is a wear and tear pigment. It is brownish granular and intracellular pigment. It is seen in brown atrophy.

2. Ochronosis is AR disease with absence of homogentisic acid oxidase, homogentisic acid is deposited in tissues as yellow to brown or black pigment.

3. Hemosiderin is stained by Perl's or Prussian blue stain.

4. Haemozoin is a haemoglobin-derived pigment from malarial parasites stained with Romanowsky stains (Giemsa, Wright, etc.) and methylene blue stain.

Hypersensitivity (HS) Reactions

1. Type I HS: Anaphylaxis, allergies and asthma.

2. Type II HS: Autoimmune haemolytic anaemia (AIHA), Goodpasture syndrome, haemolytic disease of newborn (HDN), drug reactions and graft rejection.

3. Antibody-mediated destruction and phagocytosis (Type II HS) occur in: Transfusion reactions, HDN, AIHA, drug reactions.

4. Type III HS: Kidney in systemic lupus erythematosus (SLE), acute glomerulonephritis (AGN), serum sickness, Arthus reaction.

5. Arthus reaction: Localised tissue reaction with vasculitis due to exposure of an antigen in a case with previously formed antibodies.

6. T cell-mediated (Type IV) HS reaction: Tuberulosis, sarcoidosis, etc.

7. Asthma is type I HS reaction.

8. Type I is IgE antibody mediated.

9. Type II HS is antibody dependent cell-mediated cytotoxicity (ADCC).

Autoimmune (AI) Disorders

1. MHC molecule (HLA): Class I expressed on all nucleated cells and platelets. Peptides derived from virus or tumour antigens are displayed on the surface and recognized by CD8 T lymphocytes.

2. Class II HLA display peptides derived from microbes or soluble proteins recognized by CD4 T cells.

3. Anergy: T cells have CD28 and APC has B7. APC without B7 is rendered anergic. No immune reaction occurs.

4. Regulatory T cells: Prevent immune reactions against self-reactive T cells.

5. Self-tolerance: Central and peripheral, breakdown leads to AI.

6. T cells recognizing self-antigens undergo apoptosis.

7. Polymorphisms of NOD2 are associated with Crohn's disease.

8. Diagnostic of SLE: Anti-DNA (double stranded) antibodies and anti-Smith antibodies

9. Systemic lupus erythematosus: Low levels of complement, DNA–anti-DNA complexes, antibodies to RBCs, white cells, platelets, antiphospholipid antibody (APLA) positive.

10. Libman-Sacks endocarditis is seen in SLE.

11. Sjögren's syndrome: Inflammation of lacrimal gland and salivary gland.

12. Salivary gland in Sjögren's disease has lymphocytic and plasma cell infiltrate and ductal cell hyperplasia.

13. Sjögren's syndrome has high incidence of B cell lymphoma.

Genetic Disorders

1. Fragile X syndrome patient is inactive, mental retardation, macro-orchidism, FMR1 gene mutations, CGG repeats are hypermethylated.

2. Gaucher's disease: Splenomegaly, hepatomegaly, failure to thrive, may have CNS manifestations.

3. DiGeorge syndrome: T cell markers are absent.

4. Child with failure to thrive, splenomegaly and diarrhoea suggest galactosaemia.

5. Niemann-Pick (NP) disease is due to: Deficiency of enzyme sphingomyelinase.

6. NP is a lipid storage disorder.

7. In NP disease, bone marrow, liver, and spleen have foamy RE cells or macrophages.

8. NP is AR disease.

9. Type Ia (Von Gierke's disease) is the most common type of glycogen storage disease.

10. Maple syrup urine disease: There is defect in metabolism of branched chain amino acids (valine, leucine and isoleucine). Urine smells of maple syrup, sweetish odour.

11. Cystic fibrosis: There is CFTR gene mutation with disruption of chloride channels, glands have thick and sticky mucus and allows growth of organisms.

12. If both the parents have CFTR gene, there will be 25% chance to get the disease, 25% normal and 50% chance to be carriers.

Neoplasia

1. Common malignant tumours in Indian males: Oral cancer and lung cancer.

2. Common malignant tumour in Indian females: Breast and cervical cancers.

3. Common malignancies in whites—carcinoma colon and malignant melanoma.

4. Common malignancy in USA: Lung cancer, carcinoma colon and malignant melanoma.

5. Common malignancy in Japan: Gastric cancer.

6. Schistosomiasis is common in: Africa and Middle East countries.

7. C-kit mutations are seen in: GIST.

8. Microsatellite instability seen in: HNPCC.

9. Choristoma is: Normal cells in abnormal location.

10. Hamartoma is: Normal cells in excessive number in normal location.

11. VHL tumour suppressor gene is mutated in: Angiomatosis and hemangioblastoma. VHL gene is on chromosome 3 and AD.

12. RET proto-oncogene is associated with: MEN type 2.

13. Mutation of PAX7 seen in rhabdomyosarcoma.

14. CA 15.3 is a breast cancer marker.

15. CA19.9 is a marker for pancreatic cancer.

16. CEA is a tumour marker for colonic cancer.

17. AFP is tumour marker for yolk sac tumour.

18. HTLV causes T cell lymphoma and leukaemia.

19. DNA viruses causing cancer are: HPV, HBV, EBV, human herpes virus 8

20. Oncogenic RNA viruses: HCV and HTLV-1.

21. Only action of promoter carcinogens cannot initiate malignancy.

22. Action of initiator carcinogens causes mutations.

23. Aflatoxin 1 from *Aspergillus flavus* causes HCC.

24. Asbestosis produces mesothelioma and lung cancer.

25. RB and P53 are tumour suppressor genes.

26. Telomerase is responsible for limitless replicative activity in cancers.

27. The most common oncogenic DNA viruses causing cancer are:

  i. Human papilloma virus (HPV): HPV commonly produces warts, and squamous cell carcinoma of cervix and skin.

  ii. Epstein-Barr virus (EBV): EBV is implicated in Burkitt's lymphoma, patients of organ transplantation, Hodgkin's lymphoma, nasopharyngeal carcinoma.

  iii. Hepatitis B virus (HBV): Hepatocellular carcinoma.

  iv. Kaposi's sarcoma herpes virus (KSHV, human herpes virus 8).

28. The oncogenic RNA viruses are:
    i. HTLV-1 (human T cell leukaemia virus): It causes T cell leukaemia and lymphoma in Japan and the Caribbean region.
    ii. HCV: Hepatocellular carcinoma.
29. Application of initiator in chemical carcinogenesis may cause mutation of genes such as RAS. Subsequent application of promoter leads to clonal expansion of initiated cell. These are: Pharbol esters, hormones, phenols and benzopyrines, azo dyes and aflatoxins.
30. Application of promoters alone does not cause mutations. However, act on a mutated cell.
31. Asbestos produces malignant mesothelioma and lung carcinoma. Crocidotile fibres have greater risk than shorter and thicker Amosite and flexible chrysolite fibres for mesothelioma and lung cancer.
32. Aflatoxin B1, a natural product of fungus *Aspergillus flavus*, is known to produce hepatocellular carcinoma.
33. Preneoplastic conditions include disorders that are associated with a significantly increased risk of cancer.
    i. Chronic atrophic gastritis of pernicious anaemia
    ii. Solar keratosis
    iii. Oral lichen planus
    iv. Oral submucous fibrosis
    v. Endometrial hyperplasia
    vi. Chronic gastritis
    vii. Ulcerative colitis
    viii. Adenomatous polyps of colon
    ix. Xeroderma pigmentosum
    x. Epidermolysis bullosa hereditaria
34. Mucin-secreting adenocarcinomas of pancreas, lung and GIT can have:
    a. Non-bacterial thrombotic endocarditis (marantic endocarditis)
    b. Hypercoagulability leading to venous thrombosis
    c. Trousseau's syndrome (migratory thrombosis in superficial veins and uncommon site).
35. Syndromes which can occur in lung carcinoma are:
    a. Hypercalcaemia (non-small cell carcinoma/sqamous cell carcinoma)
    b. SIADH (non-small cell carcinoma/sqamous cell carcinoma)
    c. Carcinoid (small cell carcinoma)
    d. Venous thrombosis (Trousseau phenomenon)
    e. Hypertrophic osteoarthropathy and clubbing of the fingers
    f. Dermatomyositis
    g. Myasthenia gravis
    h. Acanthosis nigricans
    i. Hypoglycaemia
36. Paraneoplastic syndromes which can occur in breast carcinoma are:
    a. Hypercalcaemia
    b. CNS and nerve disorders
37. Paraneoplastic syndromes which can occur in renal cell carcinoma are:
    a. Polycythaemia
    b. Hypercalcaemia

Lymph Nodes

1. Nodular lymphocyte predominant Hodgkin disease (HD): Express Pan B markers: CD19, CD20, PAX5, LCA , MUM1, CD15 and 30 negative.
2. RS cells are CD15 and CD30 positive.
3. Lacunar RS cells are present in nodular sclerosis HD.
4. Prognosis in nodular sclerosis HD: Good
5. Prognosis in mixed cellularity HD: Intermediate
6. EBV causes HD and nasopharyngeal carcinoma.
7. Favourable prognosis is seen in: NLPHD and NSHD.
8. Worst prognosis is seen in LDHD.
9. SLL may present as lymphocytosis, monoclonal gammopathy, or hypogammaglobulinaemia.
10. Richter syndrome: Transformation of SLL to large cell lymphoma which is aggressive type of lymphoma.
11. PAX5 postive in RS cells and B cell lymphomas.
12. In follicular lymphoma, t(14:18)(q32:q21) places Bcl2 close to IgH, thus overexpression of Bcl2.
13. t(2:5)(p23:q35) involves ALK (tyrosine kinase gene) close to nucleophosmin (NPM) with increased activity of tyrosine kinase.
14. t(8:14) in Burkitt's lymphoma, c-myc proto-onogene of chromosome 8 moves to chromosome 14 close IgH region.
15. t(11;14) Cyclin D1 overexpressed in mantle cell lymphoma and Cyclin D1 on chromosome 11 are placed near IgH on chromosome 14.
16. Mantle cell lymphoma is CD5 positive and CD23 negative.
17. SLL cells are: CD20 +, CD5+ and CD23+.
18. Follicular NHL cells are: Pan B cell markers +, CD10 + (CALLA+), Bcl2+, Bcl6 + in high grade follicular lymphoma.
19. DLBCL CD20+, CD30+, Ki-67+, Bcl2 overexpressed, Bcl6 +.
20. Myc overexpressed in Burkitt lymphoma. Express B cell markers, CD10 and Bcl6.

21. Germinal centre cell markers are: CD10 and Bcl6.
22. Lymphoblastic lymphoma: Common in children and adults, aggressive, T cell markers present in 85% of the cases. They are TDT +, CD1+, CD2+ and CD7+.
23. T cell rich DLBCL: B cells are less than 10%.
24. Peripheral T cell and NK cell lymphomas are highly aggressive with poor prognosis. Cells express CD2+, CD3+, CD45 RO+, CD5+ and CD7+.
25. Anaplastic large cell lymphoma: CD30+, Ki-1+.
26. Mantle zone lymphoma: CD5+, Cyclin D1+ due to t(11:14).

Respiratory Diseases

1. Nasopharyngeal carcinoma is associated with EBV.
2. Type II pneumocytes synthesize surfactant.
3. Type I pneumocytes are flat and occupy 95% of the alveolar surface.
4. Type II cells are involved in repair mechanisms.
5. *Histoplasma capsulatum* produced granulomas can undergo necrosis and cavitation. Disseminated histoplasmosis occurs in immunocompromised hosts.
6. *Pneumocystis carinii* pneumonia usually occurs when CD4 T cell count is below 200 cells/cmm.
7. Simon's focus: Apical tuberculosis on X-ray.
8. Infraclavicular lesion in tuberculosis is known as Assmann focus.
9. Schaumann bodies and asteroid bodies are seen in sarcoidosis.
10. Non-caseating granulomas are seen in sarcoidosis.
11. Most common cause of nosocomial pneumonia is *Staphylococcus aureus*.
12. Commonest cause of lung abscess is aspiration.
13. Bronchial artery is the source of haemoptysis in TB.
14. Hyaline membrane is made of fibrin and necrotic cells.
15. Deep vein thrombosis (DVT) is the commonest cause of pulmonary thromboembolism.
16. Creola bodies are seen in bronchial asthma.
17. Crushmann spirals are mucus plugs. Also present are eosinophils and Charcot-Leyden crystals.
18. Asthma has increased sensitivity to variety of stimuli with episodic bronchoconstriction.
19. Atopic asthma is IgE mediated.
20. Non-atopic asthma is respiratory infection (viral) and inhaled pollutants are common triggers. Family history in non-atopic asthma is not available. Th2 cells are activated to normal harmless antigens of the environment which produce cytokines which promote B cells and inflammation.

21. LTC4, D4, E4 and acetylcholine cause broncho-constriction. Histamine, prostaglandin D2 and PAF also induce bronchoconstriction.
22. Eosinophils are the cells found in asthma.
23. Reid index is increased in chronic bronchitis. Normal Reid index is 0.4 whereas its value increases in chronic bronchitis. Reid index is ratio of the thickness of the submucous glands to the thickness between the epithelium and the cartilage.
24. Bronchiectasis affects vertical air passages of lower lobes bilaterally with involvement of left side more frequent than right.
25. Chronic bronchitis: Persistent cough for 3 consecutive months for at least two years.
26. Chronic bronchitis has hyperplasia of mucous glands, goblet cell hyperplasia, chronic inflammation and bronchiolar wall fibrosis.
27. Smoking, pollutants and genetic predisposition plays role in emphysema.
28. Patients with antiprotease alpha-1 antitrypsin deficiency have tendency for emphysema. Severe alpha-1 antitrypsin deficiency (PiZZ) is autosomal co-dominantly inherited disorder. Normal individuals are PiMM and PiMZ state is associated with moderate deficiency of alpha-1 antitrypsin deficiency.
29. Alpha-1 antitrypsin is produced by liver and by neutrophils during inflammation.
30. Smoking and pollutants are cause of inflammation and release of elastases.
31. With loss of elastic recoil of the lung parenchyma, there is functional obstruction during expiration (functional outflow obstruction).
32. Panacinar emphysema is common with alpha-1-antitrypsin deficiency.
33. Both emphysematous and normal acini are present in centriacinar emphysema. Heavy smokers and chronic bronchitis patients have centriacinar emphysema.
34. Bronchiectasis: Causes include bronchial obstruction, infection and ciliary dyskinesia (Kartagener's syndrome). The airways are dialated.
35. Restrictive lung diseases are characterised by inflammation and fibrosis.
36. Goodpasture's syndrome is: Antibodies to non-collagenous domain of alpha-3 chain of collagen IV. There is necrotizing haemorrhagic interstitial pneumonitis.
37. Nuclear moulding, necrosis and high mitotic count are present in small cell carcinoma lung.
38. Azzopardi effect is present in small cell carcinoma. Dark blue DNA material from necrotic tumour cells encrusts the inner surface of the vessel.

39. Cancer suppressor gene deletions are: 3p, 9p and 17p.
40. TTF1 is positive in thyroid neoplasms and lung carcinomas.
41. Adenocarcinoma lung expresses TTF1 and CK7 and squamous cell carcinoma expresses P63 and CK5/6.
42. EGFR mutations are associated with adenocarcinomas in non-smokers.
43. Lung carcinomas with paraneoplastic syndromes: ADH inducing hyponatraemia, ACTH producing Cushing syndrome, paratharmone-related peptide inducing hypercalcaemia, calcitonin producing hypocalcaemia, gonadotropins inducing gynaecomastia and serotonin and bradykinin causing carcinoid syndrome.
44. Simple coal worker pneumoconiosis has macules and nodules. Progressive lesions have scars.
45. Amphiboles (chrysolite, amosite, crocidolite) are dangerous and act as initiators and promoters of cancer.
46. Asbestos bodies: Golden brown fusiform rods are asbestos fibres surrounded by iron containing proteinaceous material.
47. The most dangerous particle size for causation of pneumoconiosis is 1–5 µ.
48. Caplan syndrome is co-existence of pneumoconiosis with cavitating rheumatoid nodules.
49. Most common lesion in asbestosis is benign pleural plaques.
50. Bronchogenic carcinoma is the commonest asbestos-related cancer.
51. Heart failure cells are the hemosiderin laden macrophages.
52. Malignant mesothelioma is not associated with smoking.
53. Byssinosis: Occupational lung diseases due to textile fibres like: Cotton, hemp or linen fibres, etc.
54. Bagassosis: Occupational lung disease causing hypersensitivity pneumonitis due to inhalation of sugarcane dust.
55. Caplan syndrome is co-existence of pneumoconiosis with cavitating rheumatoid nodules.

Vascular Diseases

1. Hyaline arteriosclerosis is characteristic of benign nephrosclerosis.
2. Hyperplastic arteriosclerosis: Seen in malignant hypertension, onion skin concentric and laminated thickening of vessel wall are common features, can also have necrotizing arteriolitis.
3. Mycotic aneurysms are due to infective etiology (bacterial, fungal, etc.)

4. Ischaemia because of endarteritis to media and loss of elastic fibres with scarring is characteristic of syphilitic aneurysm.
5. Marfan syndrome is due to mutation of fibrillin which is required for elastic tissue synthesis.
6. Older individuals with large vessel involvement is characteristic of giant cell arteritis
7. Vasculitis of small vessels of lung tissue is seen in Wegener's syndrome.
8. Pulseless disease occurring below 50 years is: Takayasu arteritis.
9. Immune complex deposits in vessel wall with inflammation are seen in: PAN.
10. Young male smokers commonly have TAO or Buerger's disease.

Gastrointestinal Disease: Esophagus

1. Etiology of gastroesophageal reflux disease (GERD): Smoking, decreased physical activity, increased abdominal pressure, delayed gastric emptying, estrogen therapy.
2. GERD has: Basal cell hyperplasia, elongated papillae, intraepithelial eosinophils and venular dilatation, bile crystals may be present.
3. CMV can affect esophagus and rest of GIT. Multiple, superficial serpeginous or oval ulcers are present.
4. CMV has intranuclear eosinophilic and sometimes basophilic intracytoplasmic inclusions.
5. Barrett esophagus: There is metaplasia of squamous epithelium of lower esophagus which is replaced by columnar epithelium.
6. Bile acids act as tumour promoter in Barrett esophagus.
7. Barrett esophagus is associated with adenocarcinoma.
8. Plummer-Vinson syndrome is associated with iron deficiency anaemia.
9. Carcinoma esophagus is more common in: Upper and middle portion of esophagus.
10. Risk factors for esophageal carcinoma: Alcohol, tobacco, HPV infection, Barrett esophagus, nitrate and nitroso compounds, radiation exposure, etc.

Gastrointestinal Disease: Stomach and Intestinal Lesions

1. Peptic ulcer is most commonly located in first part of duodenum (anterior wall more often affected) and stomach (more commonly on lesser curvature) usually at antral and corpus junction. Majority are solitary. These are usually less than 2 cm. They may penetrate the muscle tissue. Round to oval,

sharply punched out, with straight walls, margins are usually levelled or slightly elevated. Base is smooth and clean, converging mucosal folds are present. The blood vessels at the margins may be thrombosed.

2. Cushing's ulcer: Seen in burns and acute erosive gastritis. Ischaemia and breakdown of protective mucosal barrier play role.

3. Vitamin B_{12} is absorbed from distal ileum.

4. Syndromes associated with polyposis of intestine: Turcot's syndrome, Gardner syndrome, PJ syndrome, adenomatous polyposis, HNPCC, Lynch syndrome, and Cowden syndrome.

5. Increased levels of 5-hydroxyindoleacetic acid and its excretion in urine is seen in carcinoid syndrome. Presents with flushing, diarrhoea and intermittent abdominal cramps.

6. Leukoplakia and erythroplakia can undergo malignant transformation.

7. CEA is tumour marker for adenocarcinoma colon, lung, ovary, pancreas and breast.

8. Carcinoid is most commonly arises from: Midgut.

9. Intestinal biopsy is diagnostic in: Celiac disease and fatty diarrhoea.

10. Sites of gastric ulcer: Lesser curvature and antrum (common), anterior and posterior wall and greater curvature (less common).

11. Ulcerative colitis predisposes to colonic carcinoma.

Lesions of Liver

1. Hepatitis C: Spreads by blood and blood products.
2. Hepatitis B: Spreads by blood and blood products.
3. Fibrolamellar variant of hepatocellular carcinoma (HCC) has good prognosis.
4. Adenomas of liver enlarge and cause symptoms and have malignant potential.
5. Right lobe of liver is prone for abscess due to the streaming effect of superior mesenteric artery.
6. *E. multilocularis* is endemic in US and likely to be fatal.
7. *E. granulosus* is common in certain parts of Europe and resectable without peritoneal soilage.

Lesions of Breast

1. Ductal epithelium has two layers.
2. Milk line runs from axilla to inguinal region. Ectopic breast tissue can be present in this line.
3. Fat necrosis of breast can mimic carcinoma breast and presents as painless mass.
4. Fibrocystic disease is associated with: Epithelial hyperplasia, cystic change, fibrosis, adenosis, chronic inflammation, apocrine metaplasia and fibroadenomatoid change.

5. Phyllodes tumour has proliferating stroma more than the epithelial component having leaf-like appearance.

6. Mondor disease is thrmbophlebitis of breast and contiguous tissue.

7. Fibroadenoma is estrogen responsive benign capsulated tumour which occurs in reproductive life.

8. Low grade phyllodes is similar to fibroadenoma, but more cellular and mitotically active.

9. High grade phyllodes has high cellularity, high mitotic rate, nuclear pleomorphism stromal overgrowth and infiltrative borders.

10. Bilaterality and multicentricity is more common with lobular carcinoma.

11. A breast carcinoma patient has five times more risk of developing carcinoma in contralateral breast.

12. Ductal carcinoma *in situ* (DCIS) is limited to ducts and lobular carcinoma *in situ* (LCIS) to lobules.

13. DCIS can be detected by mammography.

14. Atypical ductal and lobular hyperplasia has increased risk of malignancy.

15. Estrogen hormone therapy: Increases risk of carcinoma breast.

16. Radiation exposure increases risk of breast malignancy.

17. With longer duration of breastfeeding, there is reduced risk of carcinoma breast.

18. Mutations of BRCA1 and BRCA2 are seen in familial breast cancers.

19. BRCA1 is located on chromosome 17q21 and BRCA2 on 13q12.3.

20. Mucinous, medullary, colloid, tubular, apocrine, and secretory carcinomas of breast have good prognosis.

21. Medullary carcinoma breast has pushing borders, tumour cells grow in syncytial pattern and surrounding stroma is infiltrated with lymphocytes.

22. Metaplastic carcinoma: Pain present.

23. Sentinel lymph node (LN): First LN to receive tumour cells.

24. ER positive and HER2 negative cancers are most common and occur in elderly age.

25. HER2 positive and ER, PR negative breast carcinoma is common in younger females.

26. Triple negative breast carcinoma (basal-like) occurs in young females, as well as in African females.

27. Breast carcinoma—Luminal A: ER and PR positive and has good prognosis.

28. Breast carcinoma—Luminal B: ER and PR positive HER2 variable, higher histological grade than luminal A tumours.

29. Breast carcinoma—Basal-like: Poor prognosis, triple negative.

30. Medullary carcinoma breast: BRCA1 positive, ER and PR negative, HER 2 negative. However, has good prognosis.

Female Genital System: Cervix

1. Carcinoma cervix ranks the third most common cancer in women in the world.
2. According to latest data, the estimated new cases of cervical cancer are: 5,00,000.
3. With estrogen, spinnbarkeit test is positive. Mucous can withstand stretching up to 10 cm.
4. Presence of fern test positive after 21 days of menstrual cycle suggests: Anovulatory cycle.
5. Abnormal Pap smears followed by biopsy after abnormal colposcopic biopsy can detect cervical cancer in early stages.
6. Persistent infection with high risk HPV is the important causative factor in carcinoma cervix.
7. HPV-16 is the most common type of HPV causing carcinoma cervix and HSIL.
8. HPV infects immature basal cells of the stratified squamous epithelium or immature metaplastic epithelial cells. Viral replication occurs in mature cells.
9. Damage to the epithelium is necessary for HPV to gain entry into the cells.
10. Viral oncoproteins E6 and E7 interfere with the activity of the tumour suppressor genes.
11. E7 binds to active RB gene and degrades it.
12. E7 also inhibits p21 and p27 cyclin dependent kinase inhibitors. This enhances cell cycle progression and impairs DNA repair ability.
13. E6 protein binds to P53 and degrades it.
14. E6 upregulates telomerase, with immortalization.
15. E6 and E7 prevent cell cycle arrest.
16. Ki-67 activity normally limited to the basal layer. In high-risk HPV infection, Ki-67 expression extends to upper portion of stratified squamous epithelium.
17. P16 and Ki-67 suggest high risk HPV infection.
18. Koilocytes: Squamous epithelial cells with peri-nuclear halo, peripheral condensation of cytoplasm, and hyperchromatic moderately enlarged nucleus. These are superficial or intermediate squamous cells.
19. HSIL are caused by high-risk HPV.
20. Features of dyskeratosis are: Increased cell size, clumping of chromatin, irregular nuclear borders, hyperchromatic nucleus.
21. Recombinant HPV vaccine prepared from highly purified virus like particles is available for HPV types 6, 11, 16, 18, 31, 33, 45, 52 and 58.
22. Patients of CIN1 are followed up for 6 and 12 months and if negative both times, there after every three years Pap smear is repeated.
23. In carcinoma *in situ*, atypia is limited to the epithelium and basement membrane is intact.
24. Squamous cell carcinoma is the most common histological type followed by adenocarcinoma.
25. Microinvasion of squamous cell carcinoma cervix (Stage Ia1): Invasion is not deeper than 3 mm and width less than 7 mm.
26. Stage Ia2 squamous cell carcinoma cervix: Depth 3–5 mm and width less than 7 mm.
27. Women with normal cervical cytology and high risk HPV-DNA positive, cervical Pap smears repeated after 6 to 12 months.
28. For abnormal Pap smears colposcopy done, biopsied from acetowhite area.
29. LSIL is followed up and for HSIL conisation is done.
30. Cytoplasmic glycogen is absent in cancerous squamous cells of ectocervix (Lugol or Schiller test positive).
31. Lymph node metastasis seen in carcinoma cervix.
32. Pap smears in squamous cell carcinoma show: Necrosis, tadpole cells, atypical tumour cells.
33. Sarcoma botryoides (embryonal rhabdomyo-sarcoma) of cervix/vagina is a highly malignant tumour occurring in children. Microscopy has undifferentiated cells seen below the epithelium (similar to cambium layer of plants) and has poor outcome.

Female Genital System: Uterus and Placenta

1. Metaplasia in endometrium: Papillary, squamous, tubal (ciliated tall columnar epithelium), mucinous, granular cell, etc.
2. Endometriosis: Endometrial tissue in abnormal location. Encountered in ovaries, tubes and outer surface of uterus and intestine, uterine ligaments, urinary bladder and ureters, scar tissue after uterine surgery.
3. Infertility can be because of fallopian tube tuberculosis.
4. Leiomyoma: Common benign smooth muscle tumour. Can undergo mucoid/myxoid degeneration, red degeneration, etc. Other histological variants: Cellular leiomyoma, bizarre leiomyoma, epithelioid leiomyoma, angioleiomyoma, leiomyolipoma, intravascular leiomyoma.
5. Leiomyoma is estrogen-sensitive tumour. Can cause infertility, bleeding, rarely polycythaemia, pain, etc.
6. PEComa: Uncommon mesenchymal tumour, perivascular epithelioid cell neoplasm (PEComa).

7. Simple hyperplasia has 1% chance while complex hyperplasia with atypia has about 28% chance of going for endometrial carcinoma.

8. Endometrial cancer is common in: Nulliparous, elderly age, common in Jews, predisposing factors: HT, obesity, DM.

9. Patient of endometrial carcinoma is an eldely lady with history of abnormal bleeding.

10. Risk factors for endometrial carcinoma are: Estrogen excess as with anovulatory cycles, polycystic ovaries, use of estrogen agonists, HRT treatment, obesity, DM, etc.

11. Type I endometrial (endometrioid) carcinoma has microsatellite instability and PTEN and beta catenin genes mutations.

12. Type I endometrial carcinomas are estrogen dependent and endometrioid type.

13. Type II endometrial carcinomas are non-estrogen dependent, non-endometrioid, aggressive and have poor prognosis. Alterations of P53, human epidermal growth factor -2/neu, P16 and E-cadherin. Serous and clear cell histological types are most common.

Female Genital System: Ovary

1. Turner's syndrome: 45XO, short statured female, web neck, cubitus valgus, shield-like chest, renal abnormalities, streak gonads, etc.

2. Stein-Leventhal syndrome: It is polycystic ovarian syndrome with anovulatory cycles, high levels of LH, estrogen, androgens, insulin resistance and hyperinsulinaemia. They can have increased BMI, facial hair and acne.

3. Risk factors for ovarian carcinoma: Age 40–60 years, family history, BRCA1 and 2 mutations, nulliparity, streak ovaries, obesity, etc.

4. Screening test for detection of epithelial ovarian cancer: Serum CA-125.

5. CA125 also helps in detection of recurrence and monitoring with treatmentin epithelial ovarian cancer.

6. Lynch syndrome: AD, with HNPCC associated with other cancers (endometrium, ovary, etc.).

7. Yolk sac tumour has Schiller-Duval bodies.

8. Call-Exner bodies are present in granulosa cell tumour.

9. Patients of sex-cord tumours can have: Precocious puberty, AUB, and postmenopausal bleeding. They also can have hyper-estrogenic effects and sometimes with androgen effects.

10. Arrhenoblastoma is: Sex cord stromal tumour.

11. Granulosa cell tumours can have: Precocious puberty, endometrial hyperplasia and endometrial carcinoma.

12. Granulosa cell tumour produces estrogen and can produce endometrial hyperplasia, endometrial carcinoma and breast carcinomas.

13. Inhibin is a marker for stromal tumours of ovary.

14. Feminisation or masculinisation are encountered in sex cord stromal tumours.

15. Germ cell tumours occur in children and young females. Teratoma is common germ cell tumour followed by dysgerminoma.

16. AFP is raised in yolk sac tumour.

17. Krukenburg tumour is secondaries in ovaries from malignant tumour of breast, GIT, pancreas, spread occurs through transcoelomic spread or retrograde lymphatics. Microscopy has signet ring cells which are PAS positive.

Male Genital System

1. Anaplastic seminoma has worse prognosis.

2. Spermatocytic seminoma has good prognosis.

3. Verrucous carcinoma: Broad fonts, well differentiated squamous cell carcinoma and rare metastasis.

4. Schiller-Duval bodies are seen in endodermal sinus tumour.

5. AFP is raised in endodermal sinus tumour.

6. LDH and gamma-glutamyl transpeptidase (GGT) in testicular tumours are markers for bulk disease.

7. Raised LDH in testicular tumours has poor prognosis.

8. AFP is elevated in yolk sac tumour, HCC and hepatoblastoma.

Endocrinology

1. MEN I: AD, parathyroid tumours, pancreatic islet cell tumours and anterior pituitary hyperplasia or adenoma.

2. MEN 2A: AD, medullary carcinoma thyroid, thyroid hyperplasia, pheochromocytoma, Hirschsprung disease, lichen amyloidosis.

3. MEN 2B: Medullary carcinoma thyroid, pheochromocytoma, mucosal or GI neuromas, and Marfanoid body features.

Renal System

1. Kidneys remove waste and excess water, maintain electrolyte balance hormone produced by the kidneys helps to regulate blood pressure, help in RBC production, and keep our bones strong.

2. Microalbuminuria is excretion of 30–300 mg/day of albumin in urine.

3. Polycythemia and hypertension are the most common paraneoplastic features in renal cell carcinoma.

4. Major cause of papillary necrosis is analgesic nephropathy.

5. Michaelis-Gutmann bodies are seen in malakoplakia.

6. Tamm-Horsfall protein secreted by the thick ascending loop of Henle which forms the matrix of all casts.

7. Subepithelial deposits are seen in: PSGN (humps), MGN, RPGN, Heymann nephritis

8. Subendothelial deposits are seen in: Lupus nephritis, MPGNI.

9. Membranous deposits are seen in: MPGN II.

10. Mesangial deposits are seen in: IgA nephropathy.

11. Kidney in RPGN is enlarged, pale, often have petechial haemorrhages (flea-bitten kidney).

12. Primary causes of nephrotic syndrome: MGN, MCD, FSGS, MPGN, IgA nephropathy.

13. Secondary causes of nephrotic syndrome: DM, amyloidosis, drugs, infections, malignant diseases, hereditary nephritis.

14. The normal urine albumin creatinine ratio (ACR) in young adults is <10 mg/g (<1 mg/mmol).

15. Alport syndrome has deafness, corneal dystrophy and haematuria.

16. Most common cause of nephrotic syndrome in children is MCD.

17. Most common cause of nephritic syndrome in adults is FSGS.

18. Serum antibodies to alpha 3NC1 domain of collagen IV are seen in Goodpasture syndrome.

19. LM features of MPGN are: Glomeruli large, hypercellular, GBM is double contoured, tram track appearance or shows duplication.

20. Adult polycystic disease PKD1 is on chromosome 16 and ADPKD2 on chromosome 4.

Lesions of Bone

1. Multiple enchondroma: Ollier's disease.

2. Ollier's disease: Non-hereditary, childhood disease with enchondromatosis has risk of visceral and bone cancers.

3. Multiple enchondromas with hemangioma (spindle cell): Muffucci's disease.

4. Muffucci's disease has IDH1 mutation.

5. Gardner syndrome is: GI polyps (FAP), multiple osteomas, epidermoid cysts, desmoid tumours, and other benign tumours.

6. Aneurysmal bone cyst (ABC): 10 to 20 years of age, eccentric expansion, metaphysis involved, blood-filled spaces with thin shell of reactive bone. Plump fibroblasts, reactive woven bone and multinucleated osteoclastic giant cells are present. Pain and swelling are common symptoms. Rearrangements of 17p13 with NFkB increased activity.

7. Metaphysial fibrous defect: Painful, fibrous tissue with irregularly scattered osteoclasts.

8. Fibrous dysplasia: Bone is thinned out, expanded, curved fish hook bony trabaculae or resembling C and Y Chinese characters (woven bone).

9. Rice bodies: Causes include tuberculous bursitis or arthritis, rheumatoid athritis, tenosynovitis, inflammatory athritis.

10. Gout: Aspirated material preserve in alcohol to appreciate needle-shaped urate monohydrate sodium crystals. These are refractile crystals.

11. Pseudogout: Deposition of calcium pyrophosphate dihydrate crystals in joint cavities.

12. Paget disease: Also called osteitis deformans, three phases: Initial lytic phase, osteoclastic and osteoblastic phase and osteosclerotic phase. Mutations of RANK and inactivating mutations of OPG are known.

13. Osteoid osteoma: Cortex, less than 2 cm, nocturnal pain, relieved by aspirin, reactive bone present around nidus.

14. Osteoblastoma: Osteoblastoma similar to osteoid osteoma, however, larger than 2 cm. Pain is not relieved by aspirin.

15. Osteosarcoma (OS): Bimodal age occurs below 20 years of age and above 60 years of age.

16. Variants of osteosarcoma: Depending on location: Periosteal OS, parosteal OS, intramedullary OS, intracortical OS or surface OS.

17. Histological variants OS: Conventional OS (about 90%), telangiectatic OS, small cell OS, fibroblastic OS, chondroblastic OS, giant cell rich OS.

18. Osteosarcoma risk factors: Familial Paget's disease, NF type 1, P53/RB gene mutations, INK4a inactivation.

19. Osteosarcoma: X-ray characteristic with sunburst appearance and Codman's triangle.

20. Chondrosarcoma has osteolytic lesion with splotchy calcification or arcs and ring form of calcification.

21. Variants of chondrosarcoma (CS): Clear cell CS, myxoid CS, dedifferentiated CS, mesenchymal CS.

22. Giant cell tumour: Epiphysis involved, 20–40 yrs age group.

23. Giant cell tumour (GCT): RANKL (receptor activator of nuclear factor) over expressed, epiphysial tumour, RANKL inhibitor denosumab is the adjuvant therapy used in recent years. Rarely metastasize and a locally malignant tumour.
24. Ewing's sarcoma: Childhood bone tumour, aggressive tumour, CD99 positive.
25. Ewing's sarcoma: t(11;22) (q24:q12) with this translocation EWS-FLI1 fusion gene formed.
26. Metastasis to bone: Most common primaries are from breast, lung, thyroid and kidney.
27. Giant cell lesions of bone
    i. Gaint cell tumour of bone
    ii. Chondroblastoma
    iii. Osteosarcoma
    iv. Simple bone cyst
    v. Aneurysmal bone cyst
    vi. Osteoid osteoma
    vii. Osteoblastoma
    viii. Non-ossifying fibroma
    ix. Giant cell reparative granuloma
    x. Brown tumour of hyperparathyroidism.
28. Cystic bone lesions
    i. Solitary (simple, unicameral) bone cyst (SBC)
    ii. Aneurysmal bone cysts (ABC)
    iii. Giant cell tumour of bone
    iv. Adamantinoma
    v. Intraosseous ganglion cyst
    vi. Epidermal cyst in bone
    vii. Hydatid cyst of bone
29. Painful tumours
    i. Osteoid osteoma
    ii. Osteoblastoma
    iii. Chondroblastoma
    iv. Reparative granuloma
    v. Glomus tumour

    vi. Aneurysmal bone cysts (ABC)
    vii. Metaphysial fibrous defect

Lesions of Central Nervous System

1. Co-deletion of chromosome 1p and 19q is seen in oligodendroglioma.
2. *Isocitrate dehydrogenase 1 and 2 (IDH1 and IDH2)* are found in infiltrating astrocytomas and oligodendrogliomas.
3. Isocitrate dehydrogenase (IDH) mutation in diffuse gliomas has favourable prognosis, compared with IDH wild-type tumours.
4. Medulloblastoma with alterations in the WNT pathways is associated with a significantly indolent prognosis.
5. *RELA* fusion-positive are seen in ependymoma.
6. The *NF1* gene is located on chromosome 17q11.2, which encodes for a protein known as neurofibromin.
7. Microglia are derived from monocyte lineage, also called gitter cells or Hortega cells.

Skin Lesions

1. Precancerous conditions of skin: Xeroderma pigmentosum, Bowen's disease, bowenoid papulosis.
2. Pautrier abscess is seen in: Mycosis fungoides.
3. "Row of tomb stone" is seen in: Pemphigus vulgaris.
4. Fishnet pattern is seen in: Pemphigus vulgaris.
5. Acantholytic cells in pemphigus are derived from: Stratum spinosum.
6. Café au lait spots are seen in: NF1 or von Recklinghausen disease.
7. Lepra cells are macrophages seen in lepromatous leprosy.
8. Turbon tumour: Dermal cylindroma of scalp.
9. Langerhans' cell histiocytosis expresses CD1a and langerin.

Know Your Scientists

1. **Hippocrates (**460–377 BC): He was a Greek physician. He is called the **father of medicine**. He established the basic principles of medicine.
2. **Aulus Cornelius Celsus** (25 BC–50 AD): He was a Roman physician, first described the four cardinal signs of inflammation (rubor, calor, tumour and dolor).
3. **William Harvey** (1578–1657): Established circulation of blood.
4. **Giovanni B Morgagni** (1682–1771): He conducted 700 postmortems with clinicopathological correlations and described morbid anatomy.
5. **John Hunter and William Hunter**: Described inflammation, defense mechanism and repair mechanism. Also wrote a book on venereal diseases.
6. **Mathew Baillie:** Described morbid anatomy.
7. **Thomas Hodgkin** (1798–1866): Described the reasons for enlargement of lymph nodes, spleen and liver.
8. **Carl Von Rokitansky** (1804–1878): Conducted 30,000 autopsies, described endocarditis, lobar pneumonia, bronchopneumonia, anomalies like Rokitansky-Aschoff sinuses and septal defects of heart.
9. **Rudolf Virchow** (1821–1902): Virchow is known as father of cellular pathology or modern pathology. On his name are Virchow's method of autopsy, Virchow cell and Virchow triad which are described by him.
10. **Paul Ehrlich (**1854–1915): He was a German scientist, first identified mast cells and his prodigious laboratory talent led to the use of aniline dyes as metachromatic stains.
11. **Friedrich von Recklinghausen** (1833–1910): He is remembered for 'multiple neurofibromatosis'. Neurofibromatosis type I which is due to mutation of NF1 gene located on chromosome 17q11.2 is named after him.
12. **Sternberg and Reed:** These two scientists described the RS cells and histopathological changes in Hodgkin disease.
13. **Ludwig Aschoff (**1866–1942): Developed the concept of the reticuloendothelial system and described Aschoff cells, Aschoff sinus and Aschoff rule.
14. **Nikolai Anitschkov** (1885–1964): Described the histopathology of the heart in rheumatic fever.
15. **Paul Klemperer** (1884–1964): Introduced the concept of "collagen disease"and described the LE cell phenomenon.
16. **Albert Coons** (1912–1978): He is known for revolutionary discoveries of **fluorescein-labelled antibodies.**
17. **George Kohler** (1946–1995): George Kohler was awarded Nobel Prize in Physiology in 1984 along with other two scientists for the work on immune system and production **of monoclonal antibodies.**
18. **Dr James Holmer Wright:** He demonstrated that multiple myeloma is a tumour of plasma cells, that platelets arise from megakaryocytes, spirochetes can be identified in syphilis and neuroblastoma is of nerve cell lineage and contains "Homer Wright" rosettes.
19. **George Papanicolaou** (1883–1962): He was pioneer in cytopathology and early cancer detection, and inventor of the "Pap smear".
20. **Watson and Crick:** Described the structure of DNA and revolutionised genetic study.
21. **Karl Landsteiner** (1868–1943): In 1900, Karl Landsteiner (Austrian physician) discovered A, B and O blood groups. AB blood group was discovered in the year 1902 by A. Decastello and A. Sturli.
22. **James Paget** (1814–1899): He was a surgical pathologist, prepared catalogue of pathology museum of the Royal College of Surgeons in 1882.
23. **Julius Cohnheim** (1839–1884): He was a pathologist from Germany, described migration of leucocytes in inflammation.
24. **Richard Bright** (1789–1858): He was a physician from England, described Bright disease.
25. **Gregor Johann Mendel** (1822–1884): Experimented on green peas and discovered the fundamental laws of inheritance.
26. **DL Romanowsky** (1861–1921): Developed stain to stain blood cells. He used two basic stains methylene blue and eosin.
27. **Barry Marshall and Robin Warren:** In 2005, Barry Marshall and Robin Warren were awarded the Nobel Prize in Physiology for their pioneering work on *Helicobacter pylori.*
28. **JB Chatterjee:** Indian scientist worked on macrocytic anaemia.

29. **James Paget:** Described Paget's disease of breast and bone.
30. **VB Khanolkar:** Worked on leprosy, demonstrated bacilli in nerves and worked on cancer research
31. **Thomas Addison:** Described Addisonian anaemia (pernicious anaemia) and Addison's disease (adrenal insufficiency)
32. **Richard Bright:** Described Bright disease (nephritis).
33. **Rene Laennec:** Described alcoholic cirrhosis and invented stethoscope.
34. **Jean Baptiste Bouillaud:** Worked on rheumatic fever.
35. **Percivol Pott:** Pott's puffy tumour, Pott's fracture, Pott's spine and scrotal cancer in Chimney sweepers.
36. **BK Aikat:** Worked on tropical splenomegaly.
37. **Antonie van Leeuwenhoek:** Used microscope to observe bacteria.
38. **Robert Koch:** Physician and founder of modern microbiology. Discovered tuberculous bacilli in the year 1882 and described Koch's postulates. Causative agent for Anthrax was discovered.
39. **Dr Bhende and colleagues:** Indian scientists invented Bombay blood group in Bombay.
40. **Dr Dharmendra:** Indian scientist worked on leprosy. Published book on leprosy.

Normal Values

Haematology

Haematology		Normal range
Hb	Men	13.5–15.5 gm%
	Women	12.5–13.5 gm%
	Newborn	16–18 gm%
	10 to 12 yrs of age	12–13 gm%
MCV		80–98 fl
MCH		26–34 pg
MCHC		31–37 g/dl
RDW		11.5–14.5%
Platelet count		1.5–4 lakh cells /cmm
RBC count	Males	4.5–5.5 million cells/cmm
	Females	3.8–4.8 million cells/cmm
Reticulocyte count		0.5–2.0%
Total leucocyte count		4000–11000 cells/cmm
Adults		4000–11000 cells/cmm
At birth		10000–25000 cells/cmm
1–3 years		6000–18000 cells/cmm
4–7 years		6000–18000 cells/cmm
8–12 years		4500–13500 cells/cmm
Absolute eosinophil count		40–440 cells/cmm

Differential count	Adults	Children
Neutrophils	60–70%	20–30%
Lymphocytes	20–40%	60–70%
Monocytes	02–08%	02–08%
Eosinophils	01–08%	01–08%
Basophils	00–01%	00–01
PCV	Males	47 ±7 (40–54%)
	Females	42 ±5 (37–47%)
ESR (Westergren's method)	Males	5–15 mm/1st hour
	Females	5–20 mm/1st hour
Bleeding time		2–7 minutes
Clotting time		4–9 minutes
Hess/Tourniquet test	Less than 10 petechiae	Negative/normal

Biochemistry

Biochemistry		
Urea		16–45 mg/dl
Serum creatinine		0.6–1.2 mg/dl
RBS		60–160 mg/dl
FBS		90–110 mg/dl
PPBS		90–140 mg/dl
Uric acid		2–7 mg/dl
SGOT (AST)		5–45 IU/L
SGPT (ALT)		5–40 IU/L
GGT		9–48 U/L
Alkaline phosphatase		20–80 IU/L (adults)
Total bilirubin		0.1–1.3 mg/d
Direct bilirubin		0.1–0.4 mg/dl
Indirect bilirubin		0.2–0.8 mg/dl
Calcium, serum		9–11 mg/dl
Cholesterol		150–250 mg/dl
HDL cholesterol		30–60 mg/dl
LDL cholesterol		80–150 mg/dl
Triglycerides		75–160mg/dl
Creatine kinase	Male	25–90 U/L
	Female	10–70 U/L
Total proteins		6–8 g/dl
Albumin		3.5–5.0 g/dl
Globulin		1.8–3.6 g/dl
Thyroxine (T_4)		5.1–14.1 µg/dl
Triiodothyronine (T_3)		85–202 µg/dL
TSH		0.3 and 4 mIU/L
Haemoglobin A1c		4–6.5%
Serum iron	Male	27–138 µg/dL,
	Female	33–102 µg/d
Serum ferritin	Male	29–248 µg/L
	Female	10–150 µg/L
TIBC	Male	174–351 µg/dL
	Female	194–372 µg/dL
Plasma transferrin	Male	194–348 µg/dL
	Female	181–416 µg/dL
Free erythrocyte Protoporphyrin		17–27 µg/dL

References

1. Gale E, Torrance J, Bothwell T. Quantitative Estimation of Total Iron Stores in Human Bone Marrow. J Clin Invest 1963 Jul; 42:1076–82.

2. Arber DA, et al. The 2016 revision of the WHO classification of myeloid neoplasms and acute leukemia. Blood 2016; 127:2391–2405.

3. WHO 2008 classification of MDS/MPD.

4. International myeloma working group 2011, Criteria for myeloma diagnosis.

5. International myeloma working group updated criteria for the diagnosis of multiple myeloma. The Lancet Oncology 2014; 12: e538–e548.

6. Palumbo, et al Revised International Staging System for Multiple Myeloma: A report from International Myeloma Working Group. J of Clinical Oncology, 2015:33 No. 26:2863–2869.

7. Vincent RS. Risk stratification of MM multiple myeloma: 2016 update on diagnosis, risk stratification and management. Am J Haemology 2016; 91:719–734.

8. Tefler A, Vardiman JW. Classification and Diagnosis of myeloproliferative neoplasms: The 2008 WHO criteria and point of care diagnostic algorithms. Epub 2007. 2008; Jan 22:14–22.

9. The 2016 WHO classification MPN and MDS/MPN, WHO classification of tumors of hemopoietic and lymphoid tissues.

10. The IPSS-revised for MDS. Greenberg P, Tuechler H, Schanz, et al. Revised International prognostic scoring system for myelodysplastic syndromes. Blood 2012; 120:2454–2465.

11. Bernadt MC and Andrews RK. Haematologica 2011; 96: 355–359.

12. Zumla A, Geraint James D. Granulomatous Infections: Etiology and Classification. In: Clinical Infectious Diseases 1996; 23:146–58.

13. Dey NC, Grueber HLE and Dey TK. Medical Mycology, Ist Central edition, 2006, New Central Book Agency(P) Ltd. Kolkata, India.

14. Tan EM, et al. Arthritis Rheum 1982;25:1271 and Hochberg MC. Arthritis Rheum. 1997; 40:1725

15. Weening JJ, et al (2004). International Society of Nephrology/ Renal Pathology Society (ISN/RPS) classification.

16. Petri M, et al. Arthritis and Rheumatology.2012 SLICC SLE criteria.

17. Survillance, epidemiology and end results (SEER), Cancer statistical branch 2011.www.seer.cancer.gov

18. 2016 WHO Classification of mature lymphoid, histiocytic and dendritc neoplasms, From WHO classification of tumours of haemopoietic and Lymphoid tissues, Lyon, IARC, 2016.

19. Swerdlow SH, Campo E, Harris NL. WHO classification hemopoietic and lymphoid tissues. 4th edition IARC; Lyon 2008.

20. Travis WD, et al. The WHO classification of tumours of Lung, Pleura, Thymus and heart. 5th ed. Lyon, France, IARC press, 2015.

21. Modified from Stary HC, Chandler AB, Dinsmore RE, et al. A definition of advanced types of atherosclerotic lesions and a histological classification of atherosclerosis: a report from the Committee on Vascular Lesions of the Council on Arteriosclerosis, American Heart Association. Circulation 1995; 92:1355–1374.

22. Classification of salivary gland neoplasms, 4th Ed. Of the WHO classification of Head and Neck tumours. 2017.

23. Shafer's Textbook of Oral Pathology (6th edition), Oral and Maxillofacial Pathology (3rd edition)–Neville, Damm, Allen, Bouquot, Cawson's Essentials of Oral Pathology and Oral Medicine (7th edition), Oral Pathology Clinical and Pathological Correlations by Regezi 4th edition.

24. Playford RJ. Gut 2006; 55:442.

25. Wang KK, Sampliner RE. Updated guidelines 2008 for diagnosis Barrett esophagus. Am J GE 2008;103:788.

26. Liang, et al. Peptic ulcer disease risk in CKD.PLOS one. 2014; 9(2):e87952

27. Lauren's classification. Acta Pathol Microbiol Scand 1965; 64:31–49.

28. Lauwers GY, et al. Classification of tumours of the digestive system 4th Ed, Lyon: IARC; 2010.

29. Odze RD, Goldblum JR. Surgical pathology of the GI tract, liver, biliary tract and Pancreas 2nd Ed. 2009, Saunders Elsevier, Philadelphia.

30. Dasgupta A, Singh N, Bhatia A. Abdominal Tuberculosis: A Histopathological Study with Special Reference to Intestinal Perforation and Mesenteric Vasculopathy, 2009.

31. Boland CR, Goel A. Microsatellite instability in colorectal cancer Gastroenterology 2010; 138:2073–87

32. WHO classification of tumors of the liver and intrahepatic bile ducts.

33. Lakhani S, et al. WHO classification of Histological Typing of tumours of the Breast, 4th Ed, Lyon: IARC; 2012.

34. Cervical cancer vaccine: National Cancer Institute information on vaccine against HPV.

35. Kurman RJ, et al. The WHO classification of tumours of female reproductive organs. Lyon: IARC; 2014.

36. Carcinoma of the cervix: FIGO staging (FIGO, revised 2009). J Gynaecol Obstet 2009; 105:103–104.

37. New classification system of endometrial hyperplasia WHO 2014. Geburtsh Frauenheilk. 2015; 75:135–136.

38. Lacey JV Jr., et al. Endometrial hyperplasia, J Clin Oncol. 2010; 28:788–792.

39. FIGO surgical staging of endometrial carcinoma.

40. 2014 FIGO staging of ovarian cancer.

41. Classification of Testicular tumours: From The 2016 WHO Classification of tumours of the urinary system and male genital organs, 4th edition, IARC.

42. Moore RA. Benign Hypertrophy of prostate: A morphological study. J Urol 1943; 50:680–710.
43. 2014 WHO/ISUP grading for prostatic cancer.
44. Kin YJ. Korean Soc Pediatr Nephrol 2013; 17: Kidney Int. 2012; 82:465–473
45. WHO 2016 classification of Kidney tumors.
46. WHO/International society for urological pathology grading system for renal cell carcinoma and other prognostic parameters. Am J Surg Pathol 2013; 37:1490–504.
47. Contemp Clin Dent 2017; 8:175–78.
48. Bone Mineral 1992; 19:159–74.
49. WHO 2013 classification of bone tumors.
50. Desai SS, Nirmala A Jambhekar. Pathology of Ewing's sarcoma/PNET: Current opinion and emerging concepts Indian J Orthop. 2010 Oct-Dec; 44(4):363–368.
51. Louis DN, et al. The 2016 WHO classification of tumours of the CNS: A summary. Acta Neuropathol Springer Verlag Berlin Heidelberg 2016.
52. Cohen A, Holmen S, Colman H. Curr Neurol Neurosci Rep 2013; 13:345–354; Chen JR, Yao Y, Xu HZ, et al. Medicine (Baltimore) 2016:95;e2583.
53. Tateishi K, et al. Neurosurgery 2017; 64:134–138.
54. Faulker C, et al. J Neuropath Exp. Neurol. 2015; 74:867–872.
55. Fleming ID, Cooper JS, Henson DE, Hutter RVP, Kennedy BJ, Murphy GP, et al., (editors). American Joint Committee on Cancer staging manual. 5th edition. Philadelphia: JB Lippincott, 1997.
56. Friedman RJ, et al. Volume of malignant melanoma is superior to thickness as a prognostic indicator. Preliminary observation. Dermatologic clinics. 1991; 9:643–8.

BOOK REFERENCES

Haematology

1. Brown BA, Hematology principles and procedures. Lea and Febriger, 1993.
2. Dacie JV, Lewis SM. Practical Haematology. 8 edn. Edinburg: Churchill Livingstone, 1994.
3. Firkin F, Chesterman C, Penington D, Rush B.de Gruchy's climical Hematology in Medical practice. 6thadapted edn. 2013, Wiley. India Pvt. Ltd.
4. Hillyer CD, Silberstein LE, Ness PM, Anderson KC, (eds). Blood Banking and Tranfusion medicine–Basic principles and practice, Philadelphia: Churchill Livingstone, 2003.
5. Mollison PL, Engelfriet CP, Contreras M. Blood transfusion in clinical Medicine. 10th edn. Blackwell Science, 1997.
6. Rodak BF. Diagnostic Hematology. Philadelphia: WB Saunders Company, 1995.
7. Rudmann SV. Textbook of blood banking and transfusion medicine. Philadelphia: WB Saunders Company, 1995.
8. Wintrobe's Clinical Hematology 13th Ed. 2014 Wolter Kluwer Health/Lippincott Williams and Wilkins.

General Pathology and Systemic Pathology

1. Damjanov J, Linder J. Anderson's Pathology. 10th edn. St. Louis: Mosby, 1996.
2. Cotran RS, Kumar V, Collins T. Robins and Cotran Pathologic Basis of Disease. 8th Ed. Saunders Elsevier. 2010.
3. Fuster V, Alexander WR, O Rourke RA. Hurst's The Heart, 10th edn. (International edn.), The McGraw Hill Companies Inc. 2001.
4. Rubin R, Stayer DS (editors). Rubin's Pathology. (Clinico-pathologyic Foundation of Medicine) 5th edn. Wolter Kluwer Health/Lippincott Williams And Wilkins, 2008.
5. Rosai J. Rosai and Ackerman's Surgical Pathology. 10th edn. St. Louis: Mosby, 2011.
6. Sternberg's diagnostic surgical pathology 6th edn. 2015.
7. Underwood JCE, Cross SS (editors). General and Systemic Pathology, 5th edn. Churchill Livingstone Elsevier, 2009.

Cytology

1. Bibbo M. Comprehensive Cytopathology. 2nd edn. Philadelphia: WB Saunders company, 1997.
2. Gray Winifred, McKee GT. Diagnostic Cytopathology. 2nd edn. Churchill Livingstone, 2003.
3. Kini SR. Colour Atlas of Differential Diagnosis in Exfoliative and Aspiration Cytopathology. Baltimore: William and Wilkins, 1999.
4. Koss LG. Diagnostic cytology and its histopathological basis. 4rd edn. Philadelphia: JB Lippincott, 1992.
5. Naib Z. Cytopatholgy. 4th ed. Boston: Little, Brown and Company, 1996.
6. Orell SR, Sterrett GF , Whitaker D. Fine Needle Aspiration Cytology. 4th edn. Australia: Churchill Livingstone, 2005.
7. Young JA. Fine Needle Aspiration Cytopathology. 1st ed. London: Blackwell Scientific Publication, 1993.

Clinical Pathology

1. Frankel S, Reitman S, Sonnenwirth AC, (eds). Gradwohl's Clinical Laboratory Methods and diagnosis. 7th ed. St.Louis: The CV Mosby Company, 1970.
2. Godkar PB, Godkar DP. Textbook of Medical Laboratory Technology. 2nd ed. India: Bhalani Publishing House, 2003.
3. Henry JB. Clinical diagnosis and management by laboratory methods. 20th ed. Philadelphia: WB Saunders, 2001.
4. Fine LG, Salehmoghaddam S.Chapter Proteinuria In:Clinical Methods Walker KH, Hall DW, and Hurst WJ(Editors), 3rd edn, Emory University School of Medicine, Atlanta, Georgia, Boston: Butterworths; 1990.
5. Satyanarayana U. Biochemistry. 2nd ed. India: Books and Allied (P) Ltd, 2004.

Index